OCULAR TRAUMA
Principles and Practice

Edited by

Ferenc Kuhn, M.D., Ph.D.

Director of Clinical Research
Helen Keller Foundation for Research
and Education

Vice President
United States Eye Injury Registry

Associate Professor of Clinical Ophthalmology
University of Alabama at Birmingham
Birmingham, Alabama

Visiting Professor
Department of Ophthalmology
University of Pécs
Pécs, Hungary

Dante J. Pieramici, M.D.

Co-Director
California Retina Research Foundation

Co-Director
California Eye Trauma Registry
Santa Barbara, California

Secretary/Treasurer
United States Eye Injury Registry
Birmingham, Alabama

Visiting Assistant Professor Ophthalmology
Wilmer Eye Institute, Johns Hopkins University
Baltimore, Maryland

Thieme
New York • Stuttgart

Thieme New York
333 Seventh Avenue
New York, NY 10001

The unique logo shows an injury that involves the adnexa as well as the anterior and posterior segments; the eyeball is turned an impossible 90 degrees in the orbit, symbolizing the confusion severe ocular trauma might cause.

Consulting Medical Editor: Esther Gumpert
Editorial Assistant: Owen Zurhellen
Director of Production and Manufacturing: Anne Vinnicombe
Production Editor: Vani T. Kurup
Marketing Director: Phyllis Gold
Sales Manager: Ross Lumpkin
Chief Financial Officer: Peter van Woerden
President: Brian D. Scanlan
Illustrators: Juan Garcia and Karen Kimble
Compositor: Preparé Inc. / Emilcomp SRL
Printer: Sfera International

Library of Congress Cataloging-in-Publication Data on file with publisher

Important note: Medical knowledge is ever-changing. As new research and clinical experience broaden our knowledge, changes in treatment and drug therapy may be required. The authors and the editors of the material herein have consulted sources believed to be reliable in their efforts to provide information that is complete and in accord with the standards accepted at the time of publication. However, in view of the possibility of human error by the authors, editors, or publisher of the work herein, or changes in medical knowledge, neither the authors, editors, publisher, or any other party who has been involved in the preparation of this work, warrants that the information contained herein is in every respect accurate or complete, and they are not responsible for any errors or omissions or for the results obtained from use of such information. For example, readers are advised to check the product information sheet included in the package of each drug they plan to administer to be certain that the information contained in this publication is accurate and that changes have not been made in the recommended dose or in the contraindications for administration. This recommendation is of particular importance in connection with new or infrequently used drugs.

Some of the product names, patents, and registered designs referred to in this book are in fact registered trademarks or proprietary names even though specific reference to this fact is not always made in the text. Therefore, the appearance of a name without designation as proprietary is not to be construed as a representation by the publisher that it is in the public domain.

Printed in Italy

5 4 3 2 1

TNY ISBN 1-58890-075-4
GTV ISBN 3-13-125771-7

CONTENTS

Section I: General Considerations

Section VI: Appendices

FOREWORD

It was with great pleasure and humility that I accepted the invitation to write an introduction to this unique, definitive, yet innovative volume on ocular trauma.

The field of eye injuries and their management has appeared over the last quarter of a century to be a conflict between two opposing forces. On the one hand, we see the countless new ways that eye injuries occur, such as by lasers, bungee cords, paintball games, terrorist bombings, and many others. On the other hand, we are witnessing a quantum leap effect in efforts to prevent, catalog, and treat eye injuries. These include efforts to prevent eye injuries through legislative and labor-law practices; the use of protective eyewear on the job, at home, and in sports; and the massive epidemiological studies of eye trauma (e.g., the United States Eye Injury Registry). This time period has also seen revolutionary advances in the surgical management of ocular trauma: vitrectomy surgery; endolaser and endoscopy; use of the intraocular gases, heavy liquids, and silicone oil; keratoprosthesis and advanced implant surgery; rare earth magnets and increasingly sophisticated micro-instrumentation; powerful antibiotics and anti-inflammatory agents; and many others.

This wealth of new information, techniques, and data challenges us and calls for a reassessment of ocular trauma and its treatment. The editors and this new volume boldly take on the challenge to give us a state-of-the-art update on ocular traumatology.

The concept, organization, and presentation of this book are challenging, engaging, and unconventional.

The challenging feature of this text comes through in its approach to eye trauma, with several chapters that are unique among similar texts on this subject.

The chapters on the patient's perspective on eye trauma, the terminology and classification of eye trauma, and a rigorously scientific prognostication on final visual outcome are timely and pertinent. The editors have the advantage of intensive involvement in the development of concepts such as the BETT (the terminology of eye trauma) and the OTS (Ocular Trauma Score), and this is positively reflected in the book. The United States Eye Injury Registry Data Bank has served as a wellspring of valuable information on the epidemiology of eye trauma, and this knowledge also inspires a large section of this text. Chapters on patient and family counseling, visual rehabilitation, and medical/legal issues are mandatory reading in the context of medical and surgical practice today.

The engaging aspects of this book are due to the organized yet free-style approach that draws on the expertise of eye surgeons and traumatologists from across the world. The "outline" and "talking points" approach appears deceptively simple but manages to convey a huge amount of rigorous and vital scientific data concisely. The chapters on trauma to specific eye tissues are refreshing little gems and highlight the authors' mastery of their subject. The color photographs, the appendix, and particularly the sections on management, "pearls," "pitfalls," and "special considerations" have a very immediate and practical appeal. The critical editing of the text contributes to a reassuringly complete, polished, final product despite the huge amount of germane data it encompasses and the multiplicity of its authors.

Finally, the unconventional style of this volume breaks with previous writing traditions and, as a result, the editors' have accomplished their goal of content that is "easy to find" and "easy to use." The authors also assume a "myth-buster" approach to their subject with a chapter specifically on "myths and truths" about eye injuries. The open yet business-like tone of presentation, which reads at times almost like an e-mail from a good friend, contributes to this new and refreshing approach. It is interesting that the editors invite constructive criticism of the text via e-mail, suggesting that this may not be the final word that we have heard from them on the subject of ocular trauma.

Z. Nicholas Zakov, M.D., F.A.C.S.
President, United States Eye Injury Registry
Retina Associates of Cleveland
Assistant Clinical Professor of Ophthalmology
Case Western Reserve University School of Medicine
Cleveland, Ohio

PREFACE

Joseph Murray, a 1990 Nobel laureate once said that a scientist possesses curiosity, imagination, and persistence. Emil Fischer, a 1902 Nobel laureate thought that scientific progress was usually not made by brilliant personal achievement but by collaboration of teams of researchers. How true both of these statements are of those who treat patients with eye injuries!

Ocular trauma is a field where there are no controls; where retrospective reviews substitute for prospective studies and subjective observations are more common than rigorous science; where randomization is nearly impossible but the potential for selection bias is great.

Yet, this is the very beauty of this multidisciplinary specialty, a wall into which all of us can place our own brick, if we just keep an open mind, learn from personal experience, and make these observations available for others.

This is what *Ocular Trauma: Principles and Practice* is, a group of experts sharing their knowledge with colleagues throughout the world. As such, this book is simply an updated version of the many wonderful books previously published. However, we also wanted to make *Ocular Trauma* "user-friendly" in its format, and we very much hope that this attempt was successful. We encourage all readers to first read the section on *About This Book* and *Serious Eye Injury: The Patient's Perspective.* We can learn so much from those unique trauma experts, our patients.

In the last 50 years, there have been many quiet victories in the understanding and management of eye injuries. Unlike more high-profile ocular disease entities, these victories have typically occurred without multi-million dollar sponsorships or the allure of heightened clinical revenue. Credit for these advances goes to the large number of researchers and clinicians who have decided to study ocular injuries just like any other eye disease process, and who, with limited resources, have made priceless discoveries.

This book is dedicated to the Father of modern trauma management in the vitrectomy era, *Dr. Klaus Heimann*, who unfortunately did not live to see the day when so many of the people he helped fall in love with eye injury treatment joined together to write about the current approaches in this field.

The last decade saw the birth of organizations such as the *International Society of Ocular Trauma*, an idea of *Dr. Giora Treister*; and, more recently, the founding of the *World Eye Injury Registry*, following the path of the *United States Eye Injury Registry.* Through Internet reporting, these organizations indeed make this a small world.

The editors would like to thank the international group of experts for their tireless efforts in contributing their expertise to this book. We think their efforts will be obvious to the readers for years to come. To the reader we present this book with the hope that it will offer surprise, comfort, and challenge. *Surprise* in the magnitude of new and useful information about eye injuries. *Comfort* in the quality of care that can be offered today to our patients who present with potentially blinding and disfiguring injuries. *Challenge* by identifying the shortcomings of our current treatment options so that others will improve on them.

We would like to thank the many individuals who throughout our professional life and during the completion of this book have helped, supported, inspired, challenged, and encouraged us: *Bálint Kovács, LoRetta Mann, Viktória Mester, Robert Morris, Brandy Palmerino*, and the people at Thieme, *Esther Gumpert, J. Owen Zuerhellen*, and, most of all, *Vani T. Kurup*. Finally, we thank our families for their support, and ask for their forgiveness for the countless hours we spent elsewhere.

Ferenc Kuhn
Dante J. Pieramici

CONTRIBUTORS

PATIENTS

Ellen M. Bomer
4710 Rutledge Dr., NW
Huntsville, Alabama, USA
ebomer@bellsouth.net

Emily and Jeff Lyons
267 W. Valley Ave., #365
Homewood, Alabama, USA
www.emilylyons.com
emily@emilylyons.com

SPECIALISTS

D. Virgil Alfaro, III, M.D.
Associate Clinical Professor
Medical University of South Carolina
Retina Consultants
Charleston, South Carolina, USA
dralfaro@bellsouth.net

**Kah-Guan Au Eong, M.Med.(Ophth),
F.R.C.S.(Edin), F.R.C.S.(Glasg),
D.R.C.Ophth.(Lond), F.A.M.S.(Ophth)**
Consultant Ophthalmologist and Head, Research
Department of Ophthalmology
Tan Tock Seng Hospital
Singapore, Singapore
Kah_Guan_Au_Eong@ttsh.com.sg

Yaniv Barkana, M.D.
Department of Ophthalmology
Assaf Harofe Medical Center
Zerifin, Israel
idityaniv@yahoo.com

Michael Belkin, M.A., M.D.
Director
Ophthalmic Technologies Laboratory
Goldschleger Eye Research Institute
Tel Aviv University, Sheba Medical Center
Israel
belkin@netvision.net.il

Wesley D. Blakeslee, J.D.
Associate General Counsel
Johns Hopkins University
Baltimore, Maryland, USA
blakesleew@jhu.edu

Claude Boscher, M.D.
Retinal Consultant, American Hospital of Paris
Département d'Ophtalmologie
Neuilly, France
cboscher@wanadoo.fr

Michael A. Callahan, M.D., F.A.C.S.
Professor of Ophthalmology
Director of Ophthalmic Plastic and
    Reconstructive Surgery
University of Alabama at Birmingham
Birmingham, Alabama, USA
isurgeons@aol.com

Nauman A. Chaudhry, M.D.
New England Retina Associates
New London, Connecticut, USA
naumanchaudhry@aol.com

August Colenbrander, M.D.
Emeritus Director, Low Vision Rehabilitation Service
California Pacific Medical Center
Affiliated Senior Scientist

Smith-Kettlewell Eye Research Institute
San Francisco, California, USA
gus@ski.org

Nathan Congdon, M.D., M.P.H.
Assistant Professor of Ophthalmology
Wilmer Eye Institute
Johns Hopkins University
Baltimore, Maryland, USA
ncongdon@jhmi.edu

José Dalma-Weiszhausz, M.D.
Attending Physician, Retina Service
Association for the Prevention of Blindness
Coordinator, Ophthalmology Service
Hospital Angeles de las Lomas
    Mexico City, Mexico
Secretary and founding member, Pan-American
    Association of Ocular Trauma
Former President, Mexican Retina Association
    Mexico
jdalma@data.net.mx

Ronald P. Danis, M.D.
Professor of Ophthalmology
Indiana University School of Medicine
Indianapolis, Indiana, USA
rdanis@iupui.edu

Nicholas E. Engelbrecht, M.D.
Vitreoretinal Fellow
Emory University Eye Center
Atlanta, Georgia, USA
neengel@emory.edu

Donald C. Fletcher, M.D.
Associate Professor, Department of Ophthalmology
University of Alabama at Birmingham
Helen Keller Foundation Chair for Research in Low
    Vision Rehabilitation
Birmingham, Alabama, USA
floridafletch@msn.com

Harry W. Flynn, Jr., M.D.
Professor of Ophthalmology
Bascom Palmer Eye Institute
University of Miami School of Medicine
Miami, Florida, USA
Hflynn@med.miami.edu

Christopher A. Girkin, M.D.
Assistant Professor
Director, Glaucoma Service
Department of Ophthalmology
University of Alabama at Birmingham
Birmingham, Alabama, USA
cgirkin@uabmc.edu

M. Bowes Hamill, M.D.
Associate Professor
Baylor College of Medicine
Texas Medical Center
Houston, Texas, USA
mhamill@bcm.tmc.edu

J.B. Harlan, Jr., M.D.
Assistant Professor of Ophthalmology, School of
    Medicine
Director of Ocular Trauma
Wilmer Eye Institute, Johns Hopkins University
Baltimore, Maryland, USA
jharlan@jhmi.edu

Martin L. Heredia-Elizondo, M.D.
Retina and Vitreous Investigator
Medical University of South Carolina
South Carolina, USA
herediamartin@hotmail.com

Joel H. Herring, M.D.
Vitreoretinal Surgeon
Mississippi Retina Associates
Jackson, Mississippi
Research Fellow
Helen Keller Foundation for Research
    and Education
Birmingham, Alabama, USA
jherring00@aol.com

David Kent, F.R.C.Ophth.
Clinical Fellow in Diseases of the Vitreous & Retina
Wilmer Eye Institute, Johns Hopkins University
Baltimore, Maryland, USA
dakent@jhmi.edu

Kenneth R. Kenyon, M.D.
Associate Clinical Professor, Harvard Medical
    School
Senior Surgeon, Massachusetts Eye &
    Ear Infirmary
Senior Clinical Scientist, Schepens Eye
    Research Institute
Boston, Massachussetts, USA
Consultant, Augenklinik Ludwig Maximilians
    Universitaet
Muenchen, Germany
kkenyon@compuserve.com

Bernd Kirchhof, M.D.
Professor
University of Cologne
Department of Ophthalmology
Augenklinik der RWTH, Germany
Bernd.Kirchhof@post.rwth-aachen.de

Lanning B. Kline, M.D.
Professor and Chairman
Department of Ophthalmology
University of Alabama at Birmingham
Birmingham, Alabama, USA
lkline@uabmc.edu

Derek Kuhl, M.D., Ph.D.
Clinical Instructor
Department of Ophthalmology
Baylor College of Medicine
Houston, Texas, USA
dkuhl@bcm.tmc.edu

Ferenc Kuhn, M.D., Ph.D.
Director of Clinical Research
Helen Keller Foundation for Research
    and Education
Vice President, United States Eye Injury Registry
Associate Professor of Clinical Ophthalmology
University of Alabama at Birmingham
Birmingham, Alabama
Visiting Professor, Department of Ophthalmology
University of Pécs
Pécs, Hungary
fkuhn@mindspring.com

Jennifer L. Lindsey, M.D., B.S.
Medical Resident
Department of Ophthalmology
Baylor College of Medicine
Houston, Texas, USA
jluiz@bcm.tmc.edu

John A. Long, M.D., F.A.C.S.
Assistant Professor of Ophthalmology
Chief, Oculoplastic and Reconstructive Surgery
University of Alabama at Birmingham
Birmingham, Alabama, USA
eyeliddoc@mindspring.com

Tamer A. Macky, M.D.
Assistant Lecturer
Department of Ophthalmology
Cairo University, Cairo, Egypt
macky@www.com

Richard Maisiak, Ph.D., M.S.P.H.
Professor
School of Medicine
University of Alabama at Birmingham
Birmingham, Alabama, USA
rmaisiak@uabmc.edu

LoRetta Mann, C.O.T.
Technical Director
United States Eye Injury Registry

Birmingham, Alabama, USA
loretta@useironline.org

Kristin Hammersmith Matelis, M.D.
Resident
Wilmer Eye Institute, Johns Hopkins University
Baltimore, Maryland, USA
krmatelis@jhmi.edu

Viktória Mester, M.D.
Consultant Vitreoretinal Surgeon
Mafraq Hospital
Abu Dhabi, United Arab Emirates
Chairman, Hungarian Eye Injury Registry
viktoriamester@hotmail.com

William F. Mieler, M.D.
Professor of Ophthalmology
Baylor College of Medicine
Houston, Texas, USA
wmieler@bcm.tmc.edu

Robert A. Mittra, M.D.
VitreoRetinal Surgery P.A.
Clinical Assistant Professor
University of Minnesota
Attending Surgeon, Phillips Eye Institute
Minneapolis, Minnesota, USA
ramittra@aol.com

Robert Morris, M.D.
President, International Society of Ocular Trauma
Associate Professor of Ophthalmology
University of Alabama at Birmingham
President, Helen Keller Foundation for
    Research and Education
Birmingham, Alabama, USA
bobmorris@helenkellerfoundation.com

Daniel E. Neely, M.D.
Assistant Professor of Ophthalmology
Indiana University School of Medicine
Indianapolis, Indiana, USA
deneely@iupui.edu

Suzanne Nelson, R.N., B.S.N.
Director of Clinical Services
Retina Specialists of Alabama, LLC
Birmingham, Alabama, USA
snelson@retinanetwork.com

Eugene W.M. Ng, M.D.
Vitreoretinal Fellow
Wilmer Eye Institute, Johns Hopkins University
Baltimore, Maryland, USA
eng@jhmi.edu

Joel A. Pearlman, M.D., Ph.D.
Assistant Chief of Service,
Associate Director of the Ocular Trauma Service
Wilmer Eye Institute, Johns Hopkins Hospital
Baltimore, Maryland, USA
jpearlman@jhmi.edu

Robert L. Phillips, M.D., F.A.C.S.
Associate Professor
Cornea and External Disease
University of Alabama at Birmingham,
Birmingham, Alabama, USA
rphillips@uabmc.edu

Dante J. Pieramici, M.D.
Co-Director, California Retina Research Foundation
Co-Director, California Eye Trauma Registry
Santa Barbara, California
Secretary/Treasurer, United States Eye
    Injury Registry
Birmingham, Alabama, USA
Visiting Assistant Professor Ophthalmology
Wilmer Eye Institute, Johns Hopkins University
Baltimore, Maryland, USA
dpieramici@yahoo.com

David A. Plager, M.D.
Associate Professor of Ophthalmology
Director, Pediatric Ophthalmology and Adult
    Strabismus Service
Indiana University School of Medicine
Indianapolis, Indiana, USA
dplager@iupui.edu

Sharath C. Raja, M.D.
Vitreoretinal Surgeon
Retina & Vitreous Consultants of Wisconsin Ltd.
Milwaukee, Wisconsin, USA
scraja1@worldnet.att.net

Wolfgang F. Schrader, M.D.
Consultant
Head of the Section Posterior Segment Diseases
Universitätsaugenklinik
Würzburg, Germany
w.schrader@augenklinik.uni-wuerzburg.de

Stephen G. Schwartz, M.D.
Assistant Professor
Department of Ophthalmology
Medical College of Virginia

Virginia Commonwealth University
Richmond, Virginia, USA
sgschwartz@hotmail.com

D. Donald C. Stephens, M.D.
Instructor/Fellow
Department of Ophthalmology,
University of Alabama at Birmingham
Birmingham, Alabama, USA
dstephens@uabmc.edu

Paul Sternberg, Jr., M.D.
Thomas M. Aaberg Professor of Ophthalmology
Director, Vitreoretinal Service
Emory University Eye Center
Atlanta, Georgia, USA
ophtps@emory.edu

Thomas M. Tann, M.D.
Clinical Instructor of Ophthalmology
University of Alabama at Birmingham
Birmingham, Alabama, USA
tomtann@home.com

Paul F. Vinger, M.D.
Clinical Professor of Ophthalmology
Tufts University School of Medicine
Boston, Massachusetts, USA
vingven@tiac.net

Michael D. Wagoner, M.D.
Professor of Ophthalmology
University of Iowa Hospitals
Iowa City, Iowa, USA
wagonerm@horus.ophth.uiowa.edu

S. Robert Witherspoon, B.S.
St. Louis School of Medicine
St. Louis, Illinois, USA
withersr@slu.edu

C. Douglas Witherspoon, M.D.
Executive Vice President
United States Eye Injury Registry
Associate Professor of Clinical Ophthalmology
University of Alabama at Birmingham
Director of Clinical Research
Helen Keller Foundation for Research
    and Education
Birmingham, Alabama, USA
cdwitherspoon@retinanetwork.com

ABOUT THIS BOOK

This book has some notable differences when compared to previous works on ocular trauma. Using contributions by colleagues with special interest, expertise, and experience in ocular trauma, we wanted to provide the reader with:

- an up-to-date collection of information on the management of patients with eye injuries; presented in a format that is:
  - easy-to-find; and
  - easy-to-use.

For this reason, we encouraged all contributors to follow certain guidelines regarding both substance and format so that the book:

- provides material that is clinically relevant for daily practice;
- assists the reader who treats patients with eye injuries in making decisions not only about
  - "what to do",
  - "how to do it", and
  - "*why* to do it", but also
  - "what *not* to do";
- is easy to use because the text is in the form of bulleted (•) lists, rather than lengthy paragraphs,
  - forcing *structured thinking* on the authors[a] and
  - saving the reader from having to "read between the lines" to find the information);
- *highlights* information that is especially useful, via the use of "Pearls", "Pitfalls", and "Special Considerations."

We edited the book as best as we could to:

- *eliminate duplicate materials*; and
- *resolve conflicting information* to provide the reader with a coherent approach.

In addition, we:

- included *topics that are never or only occasionally discussed* (e.g., the patient's perspective; the terminology and classification of ocular trauma; predicting the outcome of severe eye injuries; counseling; rehabilitation; designing the management strategy[b]);
- presented a systematic approach to management on a *tissue-by-tissue basis*, instead of the traditional method, which suggests that the injured eye can be divided into an anterior segment and a posterior segment;[c]
- frequently used *footnotes*, which provide useful additional information but whose inclusion in the body of the text would interrupt the logic/flow of the chapter;
- drew extensively on the largest data collection of epidemiological/clinical information on serious eye injuries, the *United States Eye Injury Registry* and one of its affiliates, the *Hungarian Eye Injury Registry;*[d]

---

[b] We highly recommend a thorough reading of Chapter 8 as it contains elements necessary for the clinician to develop a comprehensive yet individualized thought process

[c] This is done in recognition of the fact that life (i.e., trauma) does not accept excuses on the attending surgeon's part such as "well, I know nothing about fixing a retinal break"

[d] This allowed us to communicate information that is relevant although not necessarily published yet

---

[a] Also assuming a similar approach on the reader's part

- compiled a list of *abbreviations*; since these all are grouped together, it is not necessary for the reader to look for explanations hidden somewhere in the book;
- used *color*, rather than black and white, photographs—the latter have very little value in the context of eye trauma;
- provided an *international* flavor, not restricting the list of authors or specific management issues to what is the standard in a single country (which may have a rather unique medicolegal environment).

We hope that these measures indeed help the reader, who *is* the ultimate judge. We therefore invite you to send your comments directly to us via email.

Ferenc Kuhn
Dante J. Pieramici

SERIOUS EYE INJURY: THE PATIENT'S PERSPECTIVE

Editors' note

There are ocular diseases that can be prevented, and there are those that can be treated. For those illnesses that can be neither prevented nor cured, solace is usually found in the fact that they progress slowly, allowing time for patient and family to adapt. A blinding injury, however, occurs instantaneously. The physician must possess all attributes of empathy (see Chapter 5) to truly understand what it means to lose one's eyesight. During their constant daily flow of activities, it is rare that ophthalmologists take a break and consciously put themselves in their patient's place. The best way to open our own eyes is to read what our patients can teach us.

ELLEN

On August 7, 1998, the American Embassy in Nairobi, Kenya, became front-page news.

As a child of God and a person possessing strong faith, I was blessed and did not have to join my deceased eldest son in Heaven. I heard very little (my eardrums ruptured); my head, face, and arms were severely burned and lacerated: the window in our office blasted spears into my body with such force that after two years I continue to have small glass pieces expelled from my face and chest. I was alive – only to realize that I could not see. The bomb did not kill me, but it left me blind. I began to bargain with God for one eye. Please let me have at least one eye. That would be all right.

I was evacuated to an army medical center in Germany where surgery was performed to close the hole in the sclera of my right eye. My left eye was lost. I was then transported back to a United States hospital for further treatment. For many days I was unaware of my surroundings, suspended in time with intermittent pain that consumed my energy.

It seemed like hundreds of doctors were pulling, stretching, directing me to open my eyes, advising me that they were cautiously optimistic that I would eventually have useable vision. We learned much later that, considering the amount of damage I had sustained, they were amazed that I even had light and hand motion perception. Only a few years earlier the ophthalmologists would only have been able to replace my eyes with a prosthesis.

As time passed, I began to lose hope that I would ever regain useable vision. I was an independent, educated and confident person before the bombing, and the thought of giving up and accepting blindness was horrible. I was determined to live and continue my life as close as possible to what it was before the bomb. We started looking for rehabilitation centers so I could regain some of my lost independence. A member of the NFB threw us a life preserver that started me back on that long road.

I eventually enrolled in an NFB residential school, the most difficult thing I have ever done: I was screaming inwardly while accepting eternal blindness. For the first time in my 52 years, I felt totally alone. I did not want to be in this place, but I had nowhere to hide or run. The staff was very caring and professional, teaching me the difference between a "blind person" and a "person who happens to be blind".

After 5 months I graduated, and, with my new-found confidence, began looking for doctors to give me the miracle of sight that was ripped from me. After another set of surgeries[a] and 2 years following the bombing, I am slowly regaining usable vision.

I always knew that God would not have me remain blind. It is amazing to me the relationships bonded between patients and eye doctors. I guess one's trust in the dedication of these specialists forges a strong sense of personal esteem and hope that they can give you back a quality of life that was lost.

I firmly believe that each individual has an inner strength to preserve and achieve wondrous things. It is unfortunate that it took such a crisis in my life for me to realign my priorities. I was given another chance and now I know that personal relationships are more important than material worth. People are good and, given the opportunity to shine, they will.

EMILY

It should have been like any other day: wake up, take a shower, go to work. But as I woke up, it quickly became obvious that something was horribly wrong. I wasn't sure where I was, but certainly not in my bed at home. I felt indescribable pain throughout my body. I couldn't open my eyes.

Through the darkness I heard the voices of two nurses, trying to gently force my swollen eyelids open. One nurse said that I was to receive five different drops each hour in the right eye. There was no worry about the left eye since it was gone.

Somewhere in the mental fog, I recalled that my husband had told me that I was in the hospital because of some injuries. What a weird dream I must be having. However, the pain told me that this was reality. It slowly sank in that I might be blind for the rest of my life.

Being afraid of the dark took on a whole new meaning. Fear of the dark had been part of the motivation for Thomas Edison to invent the light bulb. They say he died many years later with the lights on. I was afraid that I would not be so fortunate. Having the lights on would make no difference to me.

An ophthalmic surgeon came in and told me that my left eye had an injury that was beyond repair and that my husband had to give permission to "clean up the remaining tissues." No matter how it is said, the

way it comes across is someone taking a knife and cutting your eye out. My husband said that his mind went numb and his body physically ached when he signed the enucleation papers.

The surgeon went on to say that he didn't know about the right eye. A piece of metal was lodged in the eye, injuring internal tissues and causing it to be filled with blood. The eye had also developed cataract. The surgeon said that it was impossible to determine without exploratory surgery exactly how much damage the eye has sustained and how much hope for recovery remained.

My husband's first thought was that I would not see my daughters grow up, that I would always have an image of them as children. He said that he had prayed "If she can't see to drive, I will take her wherever she wants to go. If she can't read, I will read to her. But please, please let her see well enough to watch her children grow up." The surgeon described the upcoming operation as "opening a surprise package." If the ciliary body was intact, my eye would retain its normal size. If the optic nerve was undamaged, I should be able to at least detect light. If the macula was OK, there was hope for useful vision. Otherwise… I would have to go through life with a white cane.

While in the waiting room, my husband was comforted by a volunteer whose one eye was prosthetic. He showed my husband that the loss of one eye was something that a person could live with. The "emotional medicine" we have received has been so important to us. The big question was, what would happen to my remaining eye?

The exploratory surgery revealed an eye with potential for function and the surgeon went on to reconstruct it. When I woke up, I saw again. The picture was not what it used to be, but I saw well enough to make me the happiest person alive.

Five weeks after the bombing, I had another eye examination. The surgeon held a strong lens in front of me. I said that he must be married because I could make out his ring. My husband, who was with me in the examination room, told me that he would not trade being with me that day for the world.

For months afterwards, I had Coke-bottle glasses. They allowed me to see that there were blobs of food on my plate, even if I couldn't tell what the food was. I was told of a 5% risk of postoperative macular swelling, and indeed I found myself in that 5%. I cannot describe the horror and shear panic of waking up from an afternoon nap with another drastic vision loss. The macular swelling eventually subsided and I have not developed severe retinal scarring.

Months later, a second ophthalmologist performed an operation on the front of my eye, completing the

___
[a] The surgeons mentioned are *Robert Morris, Robert Phillips,* and *C. Douglas Witherspoon; all from Birmingham, Alabama.*

miracle. I now have an IOL, but my injured cornea suffers from astigmatism of six diopters and I have to wear a special bitoric contact lens. Reading still requires a great deal of effort. I must look through my lens implant, my contact lens, strong reading glasses, and a magnifying glass. When I give a speech, it is printed in

48

-point text – but everything is relative. I can drive a few blocks to the store. And I will see my children grow. I thank all ophthalmologists who were part of my miracles.

During my time in the darkness, I learned what some people experience their entire lives. My other senses became more important to me. People were recognized by the sound of their footsteps, their perfume, their voice, and how their face felt. I had to remember things because I could not write them down. Even though I had a college degree, I was suddenly illiterate: I had to have my medical instructions read by someone else. I was dependent on someone else to tell me which door was the Lady's room. I learned what it was like to be a prisoner, and no metal bars were needed to keep this blind person in her room. I dared not venture outside of my tiny world.

As we grow older, it seems only natural to wish we were young again. Children have to have someone hold their hand when they cross the street, be taken to the restroom, cooked for, dressed, bathed, read to, and be constantly watched over; children are afraid of the dark. Being a 42-year-old child is not what you are supposed to be.

When I went to physical rehabilitation, I recognized each piece of equipment by touch and the type of pain it caused, not by appearance. I longed for the day when I would be able to put a face with each hospital staff member that I had become so dependent on.

I became aware of how many phrases in the English language are related to vision. *"I see." "Watch out." "See you later." "Look out." "Watch where you're going." "What's the matter with you, are you blind?" "When will I see you again?" "Her guardian angel is watching over her." "The lights are on, but nobody is home." "He has been kept in the dark." "It came to me in a flash." "You look great." "Good to see you." "Blind as a bat."* And I was blinder than a bat, if there is such a word as blinder.

Of all phrases, my favorite now comes from the Bible in John, Chapter 9, also used in *Amazing Grace*. "I once was blind, but now I see." It is such a simple sentence, but I cannot think of any words that have more meaning and give more joy.

We live in such a sight-oriented society. Without sight, there is no beauty. After all, "beauty is in the eye of the beholder." Other than the change in temperature, a sunset is pointless. Television and movies are just not the same when all you can do is listen, and how do you tell about a rainbow to someone who has always been blind? I had a new answer for the age-old question of "Why is the sky blue?" My new answer was "it isn't," just as the grass and trees are not green, and a fire truck is not red. Clouds no longer exist during the day; moon and stars no longer exist at night. In fact, the sky no longer has a "day." It is always dark as night. There is no longer a debate over the ocean being green or blue, murky or clear, it is just foul-tasting water. Childhood love poems have no meaning because roses are not red and violets are not blue.

People who are blind are still people. They are not deaf or stupid, they just don't see like we do. You don't have to speak louder or more slowly. Sometimes I think that many blind persons are aware of things that sighted people miss.

Sometimes at night, when I'm in bed and there is little light in my room, it appears that I have both of my eyes again. It is my little vacation from vision loss. But I know that my left eye will still be gone when daylight returns. There is no real vacation from vision loss; it will be with me every day of the rest of my life.

Emily's Husband

Working as a lab and x-ray technician, I soon fell into the habit of thinking of diseases and injuries instead of people. A heart attack meant I would be doing cardiac enzymes; an arm in a sling meant I would be taking an x-ray. Nameless faces, that's what they were.

My wife went to work that day like on any other day, but this time a bomb containing dynamite and 1.5 inch nails detonated. My wife spent 10 hours in surgery with many surgeons fighting for her life. She survived, but her life of physical ability was gone.

That first day an ophthalmologist told me that there was no hope for her left eye. For what seemed like several minutes, my mouth started to open to ask a question. "Are you sure?" "Can we get a second opinion?" "Please, isn't there anything you can do?" None of the questions made it out, because I already knew the answers. They wouldn't be standing in front of me if there were another option. All I could do was slowly nod my head to indicate that I understood. After the doctors broke the news with the phrase "we need your approval to clean up the remaining tissues," I had to sign the consent form for them to cut my wife's eye out.

The emotion I felt while signing the consent form cannot be described. Sadly, the devastation was not over. I was told that the right eye was also badly damaged, although there was some hope. My first thought was that if there was "hope," then there was also a chance that she would be totally blind. Suddenly, a white cane became the most terrifying object I could imagine.

I am grateful beyond words for the miracle of sight that has been restored to my wife. Vision is so much more than light perception and optics. It is the world. What impressed me most throughout our ordeal was the way that the medical staff was able to deal with our emotions, how they treated us as human beings, never as nameless faces.

Ellen M. Bomer
Emily Lyons
Jeff Lyons

ABBREVIATIONS

A	Appendix		**ERG**	Electroretinogram
AC	Anterior chamber		**ETDRS**	Early Treatment Diabetic Retinopathy Study
AIDS	Acquired immunodeficiency syndrome		**EVS**	Endophthalmitis Vitrectomy Study
ALK	Automated lamellar keratoplasty		**FA**	Fluorescein angiography
ALT	Argon laser trabeculoplasty		**FDA**	Food and Drug Administration
APD	Afferent pupillary defect		**GFLI**	Gas-forced liquid infusion
ASTM	American Society for Testing and Materials		**GRIN**	Gradient index
BB	0.18 inch-diameter pellet (for air gun or shotgun)		**HECC**	Hockey Equipment Certification Council
BETT	Birmingham Eye Trauma Terminology		**HEIR**	Hungarian Eye Injury Registry
BSS	Balanced salt solution		**IBO**	Indirect binocular ophthalmoscope/y/ic
C₃F₈	Perfluoropropane gas		**ICCE**	Intracapsular cataract extraction
CAI	Carbonic anhydrase inhibitor		**ICD**	International Classification of Diseases
CCD	Charge-coupled device (i.e. video camera)		**ICIDH**	International Classification of Impairments, Disabilities and Handicaps
CDC	Centers for Disease Control and Prevention		**ICG**	Indocyanine green angiography
CME	Cystoid macular edema		**ICR**	Intrastromal corneal ring
CNS	Central nervous system		**ILM**	Internal limiting membrane
CNV	Choroidal neovascularization		**im**	Intramuscular
CT	Computed tomography		**IR**	Infrared
ECCE	Extracapsular cataract extraction		**IOFB**	Intraocular foreign body
ECH	Expulsive choroidal hemorrhage (see the first footnote in Chapter 22)		**IOL**	Intraocular lens
			IOM	Internal (permanent) magnet
EEM	External (electro-) magnet		**IOP**	Intraocular pressure
EIRA	Eye Injury Registry of Alabama		**iv**	Intravenous
EMP	Epimacular proliferation (macular pucker)		**J**	Joule
			LASIK	Excimer laser—assisted in situ keratomileusis
ER	Emergency room		**LMA**	Laryngeal mask airway

MMP	Matrix metalloproteinase	**PVR**	Proliferative vitreoretinopathy
mph	Miles per hour	**RPE**	Retinal pigment epithelium
MVC	Motor vehicle crash	**PRK**	Photorefractive keratectomy
MVR	Microvitrectomy (e.g., blade)	**RBC**	Red blood cells
MRI	Magnetic resonance imaging	**RK**	Radial keratotomy
NA	Not applicable	**RR**	Relative risk
NCAA	National Collegiate Athletic Association	**SCH**	Suprachoroidal hemorrhage (see the first footnote in Chapter 22)
NEI	National Eye Institute (U.S.)		
NEISS	National Electronic Injury Surveillance System	SF_6	Sulfur hexafluoride gas
		SGMA	Sporting Goods Manufacturer's Association
NETS	National Eye Trauma System		
NFB	National Federation of the Blind	**SO**	Sympathetic ophthalmia
NLP	No light perception (vision)	**sp.**	Species
NPO	Nothing per os (nothing by mouth)	**TKP**	Temporary keratoprosthesis
OTS	Ocular Trauma Score	**TON**	Traumatic optic neuropathy
PECC	Protective Eyewear Certification Council	**TPA**	Tissue plasminogen activator
PC	Posterior chamber	**U**	Unit
PFCL	Perfluorocarbon liquid	**USEIR**	United States Eye Injury Registry
PK	Penetrating keratoplasty	**UV**	Ultraviolet
PMMA	Polymethyl methacrylate	**VEP**	Visually evoked potential/response
p. os	Oral/ly	**VKH**	Vogt-Koyanagi-Harada syndrome
PRK	Photorefractive keratectomy	**WEIR**	World Eye Injury Registry
psi	pound per square inch	**WHO**	World Health Organization
PTK	Phototherapeutic keratectomy	**vs.**	versus

SECTION I

GENERAL CONSIDERATIONS

Chapter 1

BETT: The Terminology of Ocular Trauma

Ferenc Kuhn, Robert Morris, and C. Douglas Witherspoon

CURRENT PROBLEMS

 Trauma can result in a wide spectrum of tissue lesions of the globe, optic nerve, and adnexa, ranging from the relatively superficial to vision threatening. Our understanding of the pathophysiology and management of these disorders has advanced tremendously over the last 30 years, and it is critical that a standardized classification system of terminology and assessment be used by both ophthalmologists and non-ophthalmologists when describing and communicating clinical findings. A uniform classification system enables this accurate transmission of clinical data, facilitating the delivery of optimal patient care as well as further analysis of the efficacy of medical and surgical interventions.

Without a standardized terminology of eye injury types, it is impossible to design projects such as the development of the OTS, to plan clinical trials in the field of ocular trauma, and to communicate unambiguously between ophthalmologists. Multiple examples from the literature demonstrate the lack of definitions, with obvious implications.

Blunt injury
- If the *consequences* are blunt, it is a *contusion* (closed globe injury).[1]
- If the inflicting *object* is blunt, it is either a contusion or a *rupture* (open globe injury).[2] To add to the confusion, the two terms have even been thrown together as *contusion rupture*.[3] Because the word "blunt" is ambiguous and contusion and rupture

have vastly different implications, it is best to eliminate "blunt" from the eye injury vocabulary.

Blunt nonpenetrating globe injury[3]
- Do *sharp* nonpenetrating injuries also occur?

Blunt penetrating trauma[4]
- Aren't *all* penetrating injuries sharp?

Sharp laceration[5]
- Is there a laceration that is *blunt*?

Blunt rupture[6]
- Is there a rupture that is *sharp*?

An unambiguous system in ocular traumatology must satisfy the following three criteria.

1. *Each term has a unique definition.* Currently, it is exceptional that definitions in publications are provided at all or that their use is enforced.[7]
2. *No term can be applied for two different injuries.* Unfortunately, numerous examples show that the same term is used to describe two distinctly different clinical entities. For example, *perforating* can mean an injury with an entrance wound only[8] or one with *both* an entrance and an exit wound.[9]
3. *No injury is described by different terms.* Unfortunately, numerous examples show just the opposite. For example, an injury with both entrance and exit wounds is referred to as *double penetrating*,[10] *double perforating*,[11] and *perforating*,[12] or the same injury is alternatively referred to either as *penetrating* or as *perforating* even within the same article.[13]

Birmingham Eye Trauma Terminology[a]

BETT satisfies all criteria for unambiguous standard terminology by:

- providing a clear definition for all injury types (Table 1–1); and
- placing each injury type within the framework of a comprehensive system (Fig. 1–1).

The key to BETT's logic is to understand that all terms relate to the whole eyeball as the tissue of reference.[b] In BETT, a *penetrating corneal injury* is unambiguously an *open globe* injury with a corneal wound; the same term had two potential meanings before:

1. An injury penetrating into the cornea (i.e., a partial-thickness corneal wound: a *closed globe* injury) or

2. An injury penetrating into the globe (i.e., a full-thickness corneal wound: an *open globe* injury).

BETT[15] has been endorsed by several organizations including the American Academy of Ophthalmology, International Society of Ocular Trauma, Retina Society, United States Eye Injury Registry and its 25 international affiliates, Vitreous Society, and the World Eye Injury Registry. It is mandated by several journals such as *Graefe's Archives*, *Journal of Eye Trauma*, *Klinische Monatsblätter*, and *Ophthalmology*.

Therefore, it is desirable that BETT becomes the language of everyday clinical practice.

---

[a]Standardizing injury types also has far-reaching prognostic implications (see Chapter 3). For instance, many variables characterize an object (e.g., aerodynamics, kinetic energy).[14] The most important, kinetic energy (E), is determined by the mass (m) and the velocity (v); $E = 1/2mv^2$. Blunt objects need higher kinetic energy to enter the eye (rupture) and are thus capable of inflicting more damage than sharp objects (laceration). Even when the blunt object causes a closed globe injury (contusion), the visual consequences can be more devastating (e.g., choroidal rupture at the fovea) than in eyes with an open globe trauma (e.g., retinal tear).

[b]When the tissue of reference changes, the terminology must reflect that; for example, in the sentence in Chapter 24: "The IOFB must possess certain energy to *perforate* the eye's protective wall", the tissue of reference is obviously the sclera/cornea. If the object *penetrates* either of these tissues, it does not become intraocular but remains intrascleral/corneal (see reference 72). Perforation means that the object entered the tissue on one side and left it on the other side, thus becoming an IOFB.

Table 1–1 Terms and Definitions in BETT*

Term	Definition and Explanation
Eyewall	Sclera and cornea *Although technically the eyewall has three coats posterior to the limbus, for clinical and practical purposes, violation of only the most external structure is taken into consideration*
Closed globe injury	No full-thickness wound of eyewall
Open globe injury	Full-thickness wound of the eyewall
Contusion	There is no (full-thickness) wound *The injury is due to either direct energy delivery by the object (e.g., choroidal rupture) or the changes in the shape of the globe (e.g., angle recession)*
Lamellar laceration	Partial-thickness wound of the eyewall
Rupture	Full-thickness wound of the eyewall, caused by a blunt object *Because the eye is filled with incompressible liquid, the impact results in momentary increase in IOP. The eyewall yields at its weakest point (at the impact site or elsewhere; e.g., an old cataract wound dehisces even though the impact occurred elsewhere); the actual wound is produced by an inside-out mechanism*
Laceration	Full-thickness wound of the eyewall, caused by a sharp object *The wound occurs at the impact site by an outside-in mechanism*
Penetrating injury	Entrance wound *If more than one wound is present, each must have been caused by a different agent* Retained foreign object(s) *Technically a penetrating injury, but grouped separately because of different clinical implications*
Perforating injury	Entrance *and* exit wounds *Both wounds caused by the same agent*

*Some injuries remain difficult to classify. For instance, an intravitreal BB pellet is technically an IOFB injury. However, because this is a blunt object that requires a huge impact force if it enters, not just contuses, the eye, there is an element of rupture involved. In such situations, the ophthalmologist should either describe the injury as "mixed" (i.e., rupture with an IOFB) or select the most serious type of the mechanisms involved (see Chapter 3).

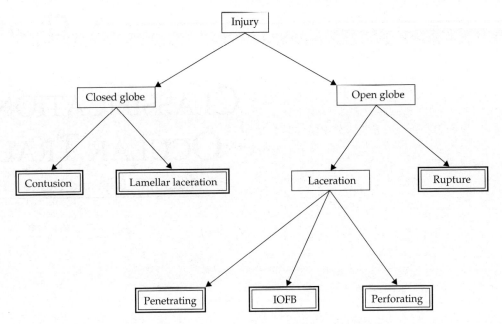

Figure 1-1   BETT. The double-framed boxes show the diagnoses that are used in clinical practice.

REFERENCES

1. Joseph E, Zak R, Smith S, Best W, Gamelli R, Dries D. Predictors of blinding or serious eye injury in blunt trauma. *J Eye Trauma*. 1992;33:19–24.

2. Russell S, Olsen K, Folk J. Predictors of scleral rupture and the role of vitrectomy in severe blunt ocular trauma. *Am J Ophthalmol*. 1988;105:253–257.

3. Liggett PE, Gauderman WJ, Moreira CM, Barlow W, Green RL, Ryan SJ. Pars plana vitrectomy for acute retinal detachment in penetrating ocular injuries. *Arch Ophthalmol*. 1990;108:1724–1728.

4. Meredith TA, Gordon PA. Pars plana vitrectomy for severe penetrating injury with posterior segment involvement. *Am J Ophthalmol*. 1987;103:549–554.

5. De Juan E, Sternberg P Jr, Michels RG. Penetrating ocular injuries. *Ophthalmology*. 1983;90:1318–1322.

6. Klystra JA, Lamkin JC, Runyan DK. Clinical predictors of scleral rupture after blunt ocular trauma. *Am J Ophthalmol*. 1993;115:530–535.

7. Alfaro V, Liggett P. *Vitreoretinal Surgery of the Injured Eye* Philadelphia: Lippincott Raven; 1998.

8. Punnonen E, Laatikainen L. Prognosis of perforating eye injuries with intraocular foreign bodies. *Acta Ophthalmol*. 1989;66:483–491.

9. Ramsay RC, Knobloch WH. Ocular perforation following retrobulbar anesthesia for retinal detachment surgery. *Am J Ophthalmol*. 1978;86:61–64.

10. Ramsay RC, Cantrill HL, Knobloch WH. Vitrectomy for double penetrating ocular injuries. *Am J Ophthalmol*. 1985;100:586–589.

11. Topping TM, Abrams GW, Machemer R. Experimental double-perforating injury of the posterior segment in rabbit eyes. *Arch Ophthalmol*. 1979;97:735–742.

12. Hutton WL, Fuller DG. Factors influencing final visual results in severely injured eyes. *Am J Ophthalmol*. 1984;97:715–722.

13. Hassett P, Kelleher C. The epidemiology of occupational penetrating eye injuries in Ireland. *Occup Med*. 1994;44:209–211.

14. Dziemian A, Mendelson J, Lindsey D. Comparison of the wounding characteristics of some commonly encountered bullets. *J Trauma*. 1961;1:341–353.

15. Kuhn F, Morris R, Witherspoon CD, Heimann K, Jeffers J, Treister G. A standardized classification of ocular trauma terminology. *Ophthalmology*. 1996;103: 240–243.

Chapter 2

CLASSIFICATION OF OCULAR TRAUMA

Sharath C. Raja and Dante J. Pieramici

 The Ocular Trauma Classification Group has developed a classification system[1] based on BETT[2] (see Chapter 1) and features of globe injury at initial examination. Mechanical[a] trauma to the eye is subdivided into open and closed globe injuries because these have different pathophysiological and therapeutic ramifications (Tables 2–1 and 2–2). The system categorizes trauma by four parameters:

1. *Type*, based on the mechanism of injury.[3–9] The *type* of the injury should be determined based on the history as reported by the patient or witnesses regarding the circumstances of the incident. If a patient is unconscious or unreliable (see Chapters 8, 9, and 30), typing may be based on clinical examination. If media opacity or other clinical factors preclude adequate examination, ultrasonography, x-ray, or CT scanning may assist.

2. *Grade*, as defined by visual acuity measurement at the initial examination.[3,4,7–16,b] Testing may be done with a Snellen acuity chart or a Rosenbaum near card and should be performed with the patient's corrective lenses if possible. A pinhole vision may be used if necessary.

3. *Presence/absence of a relative APD*.[3,17] The *presence of an APD*, as measured by the swinging flashlight test (see Chapter 9), is a gross indicator of aberrant optic nerve and/or retinal function. If the affected eye is nonreactive for mechanical or pharmacologic reasons, observing the consensual response in the fellow eye (i.e., looking for a "reverse" APD) is advised.

4. *Extent (i.e., zone) of the injury*: wound location in open globe injuries or the most posterior extent of damage in closed globe injuries.[3–5,7,8,10,14–16] The *zone of injury* depends on whether the injury is open or closed globe.

> **PEARL...** Precise determination of the zone of injury is frequently possible only after surgical exploration of the wound.

For *open globe injuries*, zone I injuries are confined to the cornea and limbus. Zone II injuries involve the anterior 5 mm of the sclera (i.e., not extending into the retina). Zone III injuries involve full-thickness defects whose most anterior aspect is at least 5 mm posterior to the limbus. In cases involving perforating injury, the most posterior defect, usually the exit site, is used to judge the zone of involvement.

---

[a] Injuries due to chemical, electrical, or thermal agents are not included in this protocol.

[b] Visual acuity at initial examination has been demonstrated to be the most reliable predictor of final visual outcome in open globe injuries (see Chapter 3).[10]

TABLE 2–1 OPEN GLOBE INJURY CLASSIFICATION

Type

    A. Rupture
    B. Penetrating
    C. IOFB
    D. Perforating
    E. Mixed

Grade (Visual acuity)

    A. ≥20/40
    B. 20/50 to 20/100
    C. 19/100 to 5/200
    D. 4/200 to light perception
    E. NLP

Pupil

    A. Positive, relative APD in injured eye
    B. Negative, relative APD in injured eye

Zone (see Fig. 2–1)

    I. Cornea and limbus
    II. Limbus to 5 mm posterior into sclera
    III. Posterior to 5 mm from the limbus

TABLE 2–2 CLOSED GLOBE INJURY CLASSIFICATION

Type

    A. Contusion
    B. Lamellar laceration
    C. Superficial foreign body
    D. Mixed

Grade (Visual acuity)

    A. ≥20/40
    B. 20/50 to 20/100
    C. 19/100 to 5/200
    D. 4/200 to light perception
    E. NLP

Pupil

    A. Positive, relative APD in injured eye
    B. Negative, relative APD in injured eye

Zone (see Fig. 2–2)

    I. External (limited to bulbar conjunctiva, sclera, cornea)
    II. Anterior segment (includes structures of the anterior segment and the pars plicata)
    III. Posterior segment (all internal structures posterior to the posterior lens capsule)

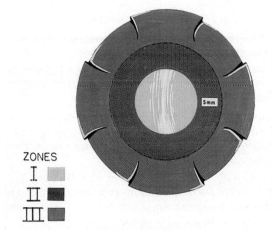

FIGURE 2–1 Zones for open globe injury. Zone I, wound involves only cornea. Zone II, wound extends into anterior 5 mm of sclera. Zone III, wound involves sclera extending more than 5 mm from the limbus.

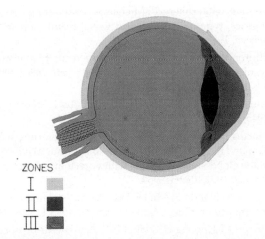

FIGURE 2–2 Zones for closed globe injury. Zone I, injury involves only conjuntivae, sclera, or cornea. Zone II, injury to structures in the anterior chamber including the lens and zonules. Zone III, injury to posterior structures including the vitreous, retina, optic nerve, choroid, and ciliary body.

Closed globe injuries are zoned according to the most posterior tissue displaying evidence of structural alteration. Zone I injuries include superficial injuries of the bulbar conjunctiva, sclera, or cornea. Zone II injuries encompass damage to the lens apparatus or structures of the anterior segment. Zone III injuries include damage to the retina, vitreous, posterior uvea (e.g., ciliary body, choroid), and optic nerve. When clinical circumstances preclude assessment of posterior structures, standardized B-scan ultrasonography may be necessary to delineate the extent of the damage.

---

c Exceptions include CT or echography when the presence of an intraocular foreign body cannot be ruled out during clinical examination.

PEARL... These four parameters (type, grade, presence/absence of a relative APD, extent of injury) are ideally evaluated after determining whether the injury is open or closed globe. The data can easily be collected by ophthalmologists at the time of initial examination and usually do not require specialized equipment or testing.*c* Primary care personnel are typically able to determine most of what is necessary for classifying the injury; however, forceful investigation (e.g., trying to open squeezed eyelids) must never be attempted (see **Chapters 8 and 9**).

References

1. Pieramici DJ, Sternberg P, Aaberg TM, et al. A system for classifying mechanical injuries of the eye (globe). *Am J Ophthalmol.* 1997;123:820–831.

2. Kuhn F, Morris R, Witherspoon D, et al. A standardized classification of ocular trauma. *Ophthalmology.* 1996;103:240–243.

3. de Juan E, Sternberg P, Michels R. Penetrating ocular injuries: types of injuries and visual results. *Ophthalmology.* 1983;90:1318–1322.

4. Hutton WL, Fuller DG. Factors influencing final visual results in severely injured eyes. *Am J Ophthalmol.* 1984; 97:715–722.

5. Snell AC. Perforating ocular injuries. *Am J Ophthalmol.* 1945;28:263–281.

6. Martin DF, Meredith TA, Topping TM, Sternberg P, Kaplan HJ. Perforating (through-and-through) injuries of the globe: surgical results with vitrectomy. *Arch Ophthalmol.* 1991;109:951–956.

7. Grossl S, Nanda S, Mieler WF. Assault-related penetrating ocular injury. *Am J Ophthalmol.* 1993;116:26–33.

8. Gilbert CM, Soong HK, Hirst LW. A two-year prospective study of penetrating ocular traumata the Wilmer Ophthalmological Institute. *Ann Ophthalmol.* 1987;19: 104–106.

9. Esmali B, Elner SG, Schork A, Elner VM. Visual outcome and ocular survival after penetrating trauma. *Ophthalmology.* 1995;102:393–400.

10. Sternberg P, de Juan E, Michels RG, Auer C. Multivariate analysis of prognostic factors in penetrating ocular injuries. *Am J Ophthalmol.* 1984;98:467–482.

11. Barr CC. Prognostic factors in corneoscleral lacerations. *Arch Ophthalmol.* 1983;101:919–924.

12. Moncreiff WF, Scheribel KH. Penetrating injuries of the eye: a statistical survey. *Am J Ophthalmol.* 1945;28: 1212–1220.

13. Williams DF, Mieler WF, Abrams GW, Lewis H. Results and prognostic factors in penetrating ocular injuries with retained intraocular foreign bodies. *Ophthalmology.* 1988;95:911–916.

14. Brinton GS, Aaberg TM, Reeser FH, Topping TM, Abrams GW. Surgical results in ocular trauma involving the posterior segment. *Am J Ophthalmol.* 1982;93:271–278.

15. Eagling EM. Perforating injuries of the eye. *Br J Ophthalmol.* 1976;60:732–736.

16. Kearns P. Traumatic hyphema: a retrospective study of 314 cases. *Br J Ophthalmol.* 1991;75:137–141.

17. Joseph E, Zak R, Smith S, et al. Predictors of blinding or serious eye injury in blunt trauma. *J Trauma.* 1992;33:19–24.

Chapter 3

THE OTS: PREDICTING THE FINAL VISION IN THE INJURED EYE

Ferenc Kuhn, Richard Maisiak, LoRetta Mann,
Robert Morris, and C. Douglas Witherspoon

 In cases of serious eye trauma, it is invaluable for both patient and ophthalmologist to obtain, as early as possible, reliable information regarding the expected outcome of the injury. Unfortunately, no comprehensive method is available to calculate objectively the eye's functional prognosis.

- Several variables have been found to have predictive value in certain published reports, only to be described in other studies as not having any impact on the outcome (Table 3–1).

TABLE 3–1 PROGNOSTIC VALUE OF SELECTED VARIABLES: CONTROVERSIAL LITERATURE DATA

Variable	Prognostic Value (references)	No Prognostic Value (references)
Age	1–3	4
Cause of injury	5–7	8
Endophthalmitis	9	10
Extent of wound	5, 7, 9, 11–15	16
Facial fracture	8	17
Hyphema	4, 18	1
Initial visual acuity	1–4, 9, 10, 12, 14, 15, 19–22	11, 23, 24
Injury type	2, 12, 13, 19–21, 25–27	4, 11, 23
IOFB	16, 23, 26	12, 14
IOFB location	22, 23	1
Laterality of eye injured	8	17
Lens injury	3, 4, 11, 12, 18, 21	1, 16
Lens: absence	9	
Lens: presence	28	
NLP initial vision	6, 29	30, 31
Perforating injury	12	23
Retinal detachment	1, 14, 16, 19, 24, 32	33
Sex	34	2, 4
Tissue prolapse	4, 9, 19, 22	1
VEP, ERG	14, 35	30, 31
Vitreous hemorrhage	4, 6, 12, 16, 19, 21, 27	1
Wound location	3, 6, 9, 11, 12, 19–21, 27, 32	1, 10, 14

- In addition, even among studies finding a factor to have prognostic significance, the cutoff values are controversial (Tables 3–2 and 3–3).

- Finally, individual factors such as the type of surgery should also be taken into consideration (Table 3–4).

TABLE 3–2   WOUND LENGTHS SIGNIFYING PROGNOSTIC IMPORTANCE

Length (mm)	References
2	21
3	11
4	10
5	36
6	7, 16
9	9, 17
10	2, 5, 12, 13, 21, 24
11	15
12	4, 14
15	19

TABLE 3–3   WOUND LOCATIONS SIGNIFYING PROGNOSTIC IMPORTANCE

The Boundary Is Between	References
Anterior versus posterior	2, 13, 26, 32
Sclera versus limbus	6, 12
Limbus versus cornea	12
Limbus versus cornea or sclera	5
Corneal versus scleral, anterior to muscle insertion	3
Scleral, anterior to muscle insertion versus scleral, posterior to muscle insertion	3
Equator	20
Scleral versus limbus or cornea	21, 27
Scleral, posterior versus scleral, anterior	19

TABLE 3–4   SURGICAL INTERVENTIONS WITH AND WITHOUT PREDICTIVE VALUE

Intervention	Prognostic Value (references)	No Prognostic Value (references)
Number of operations	10, 19	21
Prophylactic cryopexy	21	37
Prophylactic scleral buckling	14, 16	24, 38
Vitrectomy	39	2
Timing of vitrectomy*	16, 40	11, 12, 14, 23–25
Prophylactic antibiotics[†]	41	42
PPV versus tap for endophthalmitis[‡]	43	44
Silicone oil versus gas[§] for PVR	45	46
PPV versus external magnet for IOFB	47	10, 40, 48
IOL implantation: primary versus secondary	49	43, 47, 50

*Also depends on how early is defined: 3 days in one study[40], 14 days in another[16].

[†]Also depends on the type of drug used.

[‡]Original study involved postoperative, not post-traumatic, infections.

[§]Also depends on the type of gas used.

On the basis of BETT (which already implied prognostic significance; see Chapter 1) and a support grant[a] from the National Center for Injury Prevention at the CDC, we used information from the USEIR and the HEIR to develop a simple system, the OTS (see Table 3–5), to prognosticate the outcome of the injury.

The OTS is easy to calculate and has major significance for the patient, ophthalmologist, and other public health professionals (Table 3–6). It is recommended that the OTS be at hand (e.g., in the form of a wall chart) wherever patients with eye injuries are treated.

[a] Grant R49-CCR 411716-02.

PEARL...   The OTS uses a *limited number of variables* (readily determined at the time of the initial evaluation or surgery) and *basic mathematics* to give the ophthalmologist a 77% chance to predict the final functional outcome within ± one visual category shortly after the eye injury. Having access to early prognostic information allows appropriate counseling of the patient (see Chapter 5) and contributes to making the correct triage and management decisions.

TABLE 3–5   CALCULATING THE OTS

Step 1: The Variables and the Raw Points	Variables Used	Raw Points
	Initial vision	
	NLP	60
	LP/HM	70
	1/200–19/200	80
	20/200–20/50	90
	≥20/40	100
	Rupture	−23
	Endophthalmitis	−17
	Perforating injury	−14
	Retinal detachment	−11
	APD	−10

Step 2: Calculating the sum of the raw points: A + B + C + D + E + F

Step 3: Conversion of raw points into the OTS and calculating the likelihood of the final visual categories

Sum of the Raw Points	OTS	NLP	LP/HM	1/200–19/200	20/200–20/50	≥20/40
0–44	1	74%	15%	7%	3%	1%
45–65	2	27%	26%	18%	15%	15%
66–80	3	2%	11%	15%	31%	41%
81–91	4	1%	2%	3%	22%	73%
92–100	5	0%	1%	1%	5%	94%

TABLE 3–6   THE SIGNIFICANCE OF THE OTS

For the patient	Anxiety relief Quality of life issues Economical decisions
For the ophthalmologist	Counseling Triaging Management Rehabilitation Research (standardized reporting; internationally valid comparisons)
For public health officials	Determining the national/regional "injury scene" Planning of intervention strategies Evaluation of interventions

References

1. Chiquet C, Zech JC, Gain P, Adeleine P, Trepsat C. Visual outcome and prognostic factors after magnetic extraction of posterior segment foreign bodies in 40 cases. *Br J Ophthalmol.* 1998;82:801–806.

2. Esmaeli B, Elner SG, Schork A, Elner VM. Visual outcome and ocular survival after penetrating trauma. *Ophthalmology.* 1995;102:393–400.

3. Sternberg PJ, de Juan EJ, Michels RG, Auer C. Multivariate analysis of prognostic factors in penetrating ocular injuries. *Am J Ophthalmol.* 1984;98:467–472.

4. Barr CC. Prognostic factors in corneoscleral lacerations. *Arch Ophthalmol.* 1983;101:919–924.

5. Bastiaensen L. The visual prognosis of a perforation of the eyeball: a retrospective study. *Doc Ophthalmol.* 1981;50:213–231.

6. Cinotti A, Maltzman B. Prognosis and treatment of perforating ocular injuries. *Ophthalmic Surg.* 1975;6:54–61.

7. Rudd JC, Jaeger EA, Freitag SK, Jeffers JB. Traumatically ruptured globes in children. *J Pediatr Ophthalmol Strabismus.* 1994;31:307–311.

8. Joseph E, Zak R, Smith S, Best WR, Gamelli RL, Dries DJ. Predictors of blinding or serious eye injury in blunt trauma. *J Trauma.* 1992;33:19–24.

9. Edmund J. The prognosis of perforating eye injuries. *Acta Ophthalmol.* 1968;46:1165–1174.

10. Williams DF, Mieler WF, Abrams GW, Lewis H. Results and prognostic factors in penetrating ocular injuries with retained intraocular foreign bodies. *Ophthalmology.* 1988;95:911–916.

11. Baxter RJ, Hodgkins PR, Calder I, Morrell AJ, Vardy S, Elkington AR. Visual outcome of childhood anterior perforating eye injuries. *Eye.* 1994;8:349–352.

12. De Juan E, Sternberg PJ, Michels R. Penetrating ocular injuries. *Ophthalmology.* 1983;90:1318–1322.

13. Gilbert CM, Soong HK, Hirst LW. A two-year prospective study of penetrating ocular trauma at the Wilmer Ophthalmological Institute. *Ann Ophthalmol.* 1987;19:104–106.

14. Hutton WL, Fuller DG. Factors influencing final visual results in severely injured eyes. *Am J Ophthalmol.* 1984;97:715–722.

15. Russell SR, Olsen KR, Folk JC. Predictors of scleral rupture and the role of vitrectomy in severe blunt ocular trauma. *Am J Ophthalmol.* 1988;105:253–257.

16. Brinton G, Aaberg T, Reeser F, Topping T, Abrams G. Surgical results in ocular trauma involving the posterior segment. *Am J Ophthalmol.* 1982;93:271–278.

17. Cherry P. Factors influencing prognosis in indirect traumatic rupture of the globe. *Ann Ophthalmol.* 1979;11:275–279.

18. Lath NK, Patel MM. Visual prognosis in blunt eye trauma. *Cent Afr J Med.* 1986;32:268–271.

19. Groessl S, Nanda SK, Mieler WF. Assault-related penetrating ocular injury. *Am J Ophthalmol.* 1993;116:26–33.

20. Matthews GP, Das A, Brown S. Visual outcome and ocular survival in patients with retinal detachments secondary to open- or closed-globe injuries. *Ophthalmic Surg Lasers.* 1998;29:48–54.

21. Pieramici DJ, MacCumber MW, Humayun MU, Marsh MJ, de Juan EJ. Open-globe injury. Update on types of injuries and visual results. *Ophthalmology.* 1996;103:1798–1803.

22. Punnonen E, Laatikainen L. Prognosis of perforating eye injuries with intraocular foreign bodies. *Acta Ophthalmol.* 1989;66:483–491.

23. Ahmadieh H, Soheilian M, Sajjadi H, Azarmina M, Abrishami M. Vitrectomy in ocular trauma. Factors influencing final visual outcome. *Retina.* 1993;13:107–113.

24. Martin DF, Meredith TA, Topping TM, Sternberg PJ, Kaplan HJ. Perforating (through-and-through) injuries of the globe. *Arch Ophthalmol.* 1991;109:951–956.

25. Dalma-Weiszhausz J, Quiroz-Mercado H, Morales-Canton V, Oliver-Fernandez K, De Anda-Turati M. Vitrectomy for ocular trauma: a question of timing? *Eur J Ophthalmol.* 1996;6:460–463.

26. Miyake Y, Ando F. Surgical results of vitrectomy in ocular trauma. *Retina.* 1983;3:265–268.

27. Sternberg PJ, de Juan EJ, Michels RG. Penetrating ocular injuries in young patients. *Retina.* 1984;4:5–8.

28. Liggett PE, Gauderman WJ, Moreira CM, Barlow W, Green RL, Ryan SJ. Pars plana vitrectomy for acute retinal detachment in penetrating ocular injuries. *Arch Ophthalmol.* 1990;108:1724–1728.

29. Adhikary H, Taylor P, Fitzmaurice D. Prognosis of perforating eye injury. *Br J Ophthalmol.* 1976;60:737–739.

30. Morris R, Kuhn F, Witherspoon CD. Management of the recently injured eye with no light perception vision. In: Alfaro V, Liggett P, eds. *Vitrectomy in the Management of the Injured Globe.* Philadelphia: Lippincott Raven; 1998:113–125.

31. Witherspoon CD, Kuhn F, Morris R, Collins P, Phillips R. Anterior and posterior segment trauma. In: Roy FH, ed. *Master Techniques in Ophthalmic Surgery.* Baltimore: Williams & Wilkins; 1995:538–547.

32. Rubsamen PE, Cousins SW, Winward KE, Byrne SF. Diagnostic ultrasound and pars plana vitrectomy in penetrating ocular trauma. *Ophthalmology.* 1994;101:809–814.

33. Johnston P. Traumatic retinal detachment. *Br J Ophthalmol.* 1991;75:18–21.

34. Cardillo JA, Stout JT, LaBree L, et al. Post-traumatic proliferative vitreoretinopathy. The epidemiologic profile, onset, risk factors, and visual outcome. *Ophthalmology.* 1997;104:1166–1173.

35. Jayle G, Tassy A. Prognostic value of the electroretinogram in severe recent ocular trauma. *Br J Ophthalmol.* 1970;54:51–58.

36. Schmidseder E, Mino de Kaspar H, Klauss V, Kampik A. Post-traumatic endophthalmitis after penetrating eye injuries. Risk factors, microbiological diagnosis and functional outcome. *Ophthalmologe.* 1998;95:153–157.

37. Jaccoma E, Conway B, Campochiaro P. Cryotherapy causes extensive breakdown of the blood-retinal barrier. A comparison with argon laser photocoagulation. *Arch Ophthalmol.* 1985;103:1728–1730.

38. Hermsen V. Vitrectomy in severe ocular trauma. *Ophthalmologica.* 1984;189:86–92.

39. Liggett P, Pince K, Barlow W, Ragen M, Ryan S. Ocular trauma in an urban population. *Ophthalmology.* 1990;97: 581–584.

40. Coleman D. Early vitrectomy in the management of the severely traumatized eye. *Am J Ophthalmol.* 1982;93: 543–551.

41. Baum J, Peyman G, Barza M. Intravitreal administration of antibiotic in the treatment of bacterial endophthalmitis. III. Consensus. *Surv Ophthalmol.* 1982;26:204–206.

42. Donahue S, Kowalski R, Eller A, et al. Empiric treatment of endophthalmitis. Are aminoglycosides necessary? *Arch Ophthalmol.* 1994;112:45–47.

43. Mittra R, Mieler W. Controversies in the management of open-globe injuries involving the posterior segment. *Surv Ophthalmol.* 1999;44:215–225.

44. Group, E V S. Results of the Endophthalmitis Vitrectomy Study. *Arch Ophthalmol.* 1995;113:1479–1496.

45. Group TSS. The Silicone Study Group: vitrectomy with silicone oil or perfluorocarbon gas in eyes with severe PVR: results of a randomized clinical trial. *Arch Ophthalmol.* 1992;110:780–792.

46. Abrams G, Azen S, McCuen B, Flynn H, Lai M, Ryan S. Vitrectomy with silicone oil or perfluorocarbon gas in eyes with severe PVR. Results of additional and long-term follow-up. *Arch Ophthalmol.* 1997;115: 335–344.

47. Mester V, Kuhn F. Ferrous intraocular foreign bodies retained in the posterior segment: Management options and results. *Int Ophthalmol.* 2000;22:355–362.

48. Pavlovic S, Schmidt KG, Tomic Z, Dzinic M. Management of intra-ocular foreign bodies impacting or embedded in the retina. *Aust N Z J Ophthalmol.* 1998; 26:241–246.

49. Rubsamen P, Irwin W, McCuen B, et al. Primary IOL implantation in the setting of penetrating ocular trauma. *Ophthalmology.* 1995;102:101–107.

50. Mietz H, Konen W, Heimann K. Visual outcome after trauma or complicated retinal detachment surgery. *Retina.* 1994;14:212–218.

Chapter 4

EYE INJURY EPIDEMIOLOGY AND PREVENTION OF OPHTHALMIC INJURIES

Ferenc Kuhn, Viktória Mester, LoRetta Mann,
C. Douglas Witherspoon, Robert Morris, and Richard Maisiak

 Epidemiology involves systematic observation (*data collection*) leading to the development and execution of a strategy (*planning and implementing an intervention*). Subsequent observation (*testing the efficacy of the intervention*) determines whether the recommended strategy (*preventive measure*) has been successful.

SPECIAL CONSIDERATION

Epidemiology was born during the fight against infectious disease, one of the two major causes of early death throughout recorded human history. Trauma, the other major cause of early death, has long been considered a result of random, unrelated, and unpreventable factors rather than a *disease* and, as such, has received far less attention.

Through the development of scientific and public health models, injuries are now *defined* and *measured*; and interventions are *designed*, *tested* for effectiveness, and *implemented* if their efficacy is proved.

PEARL... Injuries are no longer perceived as unavoidable events.

Although the eyes represent only 0.1% of the total body surface and only 0.27% of the anterior body surface, their significance to individuals and society is disproportionally higher: most of the information reaches humans through vision. Consequently, the socioeconomic impact of ocular trauma can hardly be overestimated. Those affected often have to face:

- loss of career opportunities;
- major lifestyle changes; and, occasionally,
- permanent physical disfigurement.

In addition to the physical and psychological[1] costs of eye injuries to the individual, the direct and indirect financial costs to society are enormous (Table 4–1). The cost-effectiveness of well-planned preventive measures based on sound epidemiologic data has repeatedly been demonstrated.[2–4]

In industrialized nations, trauma has become the most common reason for extended hospitalization of ophthalmologic patients. In the United States alone[5] there are almost 2.5 million incident cases of eye injuries each year; the number of people with trauma-related visual impairment was close to 1 million in 1977 with 40,000–60,000 incident cases of trauma-related visual impairment annually.

THE UNITED STATES EYE INJURY REGISTRY

The prerequisite for the scientific study of injury is acquisition of data[6] to design appropriate preventive and therapeutic interventions; the same surveillance system is used to monitor the effectiveness of preventive, acute care, and rehabilitative interventions.

TABLE 4–1 COST ESTIMATES OF EYE INJURIES

Publication Year, Reference	Finding	Remark
1990[12]	Hospital charges for ocular injuries: $200 million each year	Excluding those admitted to the Veterans Administration system, physicians' fees, outpatient follow-up charges, medication expenses, and indirect costs
1988[9]	Those with open globe injuries lose an average 70 days of work	This generates additional indirect costs
1988[9]	40% of those with work-related open globe injuries pursue legal action	This generates additional indirect costs
2001*	Total cost in 1995 of the 140,000 disabling eye injuries at the workplace: $3,920,000,000; of this, the total direct cost of workers compensation claims was $924,840,000	When the cost of nondisabling eye injuries is included, the total easily exceeds $4 billion

*Prevent Blindness America Statement on the Scope of the Eye Injury Problem, Schamburg, IL.

> **PEARL...** Prevention requires developing and maintaining a comprehensive and standardized eye trauma surveillance system in a defined population[7] to identify risk factors.

Established in 1988,[8] the USEIR satisfies the following criteria:

- collects information at hospitals and emergency rooms as well as at physicians' offices;
- uses single-page initial and 6 months follow-up reporting forms (Figs. 4–1 and 4–2);
- surveys all types of eye injuries—open globe, closed globe, and adnexal; but
- limits data collection to *injuries resulting in permanent and significant structural or functional change to the eye.*[a]

In the USEIR, the reporting forms as well as the data collecting and handling processes are standardized (see Chapter 1) and, regardless of whether the information is sent in paper or electronic format (floppy or zip disc or via the Internet), the data undergo multiple quality checks before becoming available for research.

Although an eye injury is a sudden and usually unanticipated event to the person involved, general trends can be identified if the surveillance is on a sufficiently large scale, such as in the USEIR. Its affiliates currently operate in 25 countries,[b] allowing comparison of findings from different geographic locations or across national borders and making it easier to highlight areas amenable to prevention.[c]

OCULAR TRAUMA EPIDEMIOLOGY: GENERAL FINDINGS

Annual Incidence Rate[d] of Hospitalization for Eye Injuries

The annual incidence rate of hospitalization for eye injuries is 8.1 in Scotland[13]; 12.6 in Singapore[7]; 13.2 in the United States[14]; and 15.2 in Sweden[15].

Cumulative Lifetime Prevalence[e]

The cumulative lifetime prevalence of eye injuries is 860[16] to 14,400[17]; see Table 4–2 for additional information.

Who is at Risk

- Approximately 80% of those injured are males;[17–22] male/female ratio in the USEIR is 4.6:1 and in the HEIR is 4.3:1.

[a] The vast majority of injuries are minor ones[9] that do not result in visual or other impairment.

[b] The HEIR is the affiliate with the longest existence and has compiled the largest pool of information.

[c] Such studies with conclusions based on differences in national eye trauma scenes and consequent suggestions for prevention have already been published by the USEIR and the HEIR; others are in progress.[10,11]

[d] Per 100,000 population/years; the findings are also determined by local customs, that is, which injuries result in admission and which are treated on an outpatient basis. It appears that worldwide, 5 to 16% of the patients are admitted.[12]

[e] Per 100,000 population.

U.S. EYE INJURY REGISTRY
INITIAL REPORT

1) Check appropriate responses 2) Fill out comments 3) File bilateral injury reports seperately
4) Submit Data via USEIRONLINE.org 5) Write Down Record ID _____

IDENTIFICATION:

Patient's Initials: _____

Patient's Home ZIP: _____

Medical Rec. # _____

Age: _____ Sex: ☐ M ☐ F

Injury Date: _____/_____/_____

Eye: ☐ Right ☐ Left

Race: _____

Initial Rx MD: _____

Initially Treated At: _____

Reporting MD: _____

Exam Date for Report:

_____/_____/_____

Report Filer's Name: _____

_____

Contact for 6 mo F/U: _____

_____

BILATERAL INJURY: ☐ Yes ☐ No
EYE PROTECTION:
☐ Yes ☐ No ☐ Unknown
☐ Regular ☐ Safety ☐ Sun
Glass Shattered? ☐ Yes ☐ No
☐ Unknown
PATIENT A BYSTANDER:
☐ Yes ☐ No ☐ Unknown
WORK-RELATED:
☐ Yes ▸ *List Occupation below*
☐ No ☐ Unknown
Occupation: _____
PLACE:
☐ 01 Industrial Premises
☐ 05 Farm
☐ 10 Home
☐ 20 School
☐ 30 Place for Recreation & Sport*
☐ 40 Street and Highway*
☐ 60 Public Building*
☐ 98 Unknown
☐ 99 Other*
*Specify: _____
INJURY'S ZIP: _____
INTENT: ☐ 52 Unintentional
☐ 50 Assault ☐ 98 Unknown
☐ 51 Self-inflicted (intentional)
DRUG USE: ☐ Y ☐ N ☐ Unknown
Describe: _____
ALCOHOL USE: ☐ Yes ☐ No
☐ Unknown

Ⓘ SOURCE:
☐ 00 Hammer on Metal
☐ 10 Sharp Object*
☐ 11 Nail
☐ 25 Fall
☐ 20 Blunt Object*
☐ 30 Gunshot
☐ 31 BB/Pellet Gun
☐ 40 Motor Vehicle Crash
☐ 50 Fireworks*
☐ 60 Burn
☐ 70 Explosion
☐ 90 Lawn Equipment*
☐ 98 Unknown
☐ 99 Other*
*Description of Source: _____
_____

Ⓙ TISSUES INVOLVED:
☐ 00 Lids
☐ 09 Lacrimal System
☐ 10 Cornea
☐ 19 Sclera
☐ 20 Iris
☐ 22 Anterior Chamber
☐ 30 Lens
☐ 40 Vitreous
☐ 50 Retina
☐ 55 Macula
☐ 58 Choroid
☐ 60 Extraocular Muscle
☐ 70 Orbit
☐ 80 Optic Nerve
☐ 99 Other*
*Describe: _____
_____

Ⓚ VISION (OF BOTH EYES):
DATE: _____/_____/_____
RE   LE
☐ 00- - - - - NLP - - - -☐ 00
☐ 10 - - - - - - LP - - - - - -☐ 10
☐ 20 - - - - - - HM - - - - - -☐ 20
☐ 30 1/200 to 4/200 (CF) ☐ 30
☐ 40- - 5/200 to 19/200 - -☐ 40
____ If > 19/200 Specify Accuity ____
☐ 91 - - - Not Tested - - -☐ 91
☐ 98 - - - - Unknown - - - -☐ 98
☐ 99 - - - - - Other - - - - -☐ 99
ⓀⓀ EYE NORMAL PRIOR TO INJURY?
☐ Yes ☐ Unknown
☐ No *(Explain)* _____
_____

Ⓛ COMMENTS: *(Please describe the injury as much as possible):*

Ⓜ INITIAL DIAGNOSES:
OPEN GLOBE INJURY: ☐ Yes ▸ ☐18.5 Postequatorial Extension ☐ No
LACERATION: ☐ 00.0 Perioc. ☐ 02.0 Lacrim. ☐ 08.1 Contusion
PARTIAL THICKNESS WOUND: ☐ 09.1 Corneal ☐ 09.2 Scleral
CORNEAL BURN: ☐ 12.0 Thermal ☐ 12.1 Alkal. ☐ 12.2 Acid
RUPTURE: ☐ 10.3 Corneal _____ mm ☐ 18.3 Scleral _____ mm
☐ 13.3 Corneoscleral _____ mm
PENETRATING INJURY:
☐ 10.4 Corneal _____mm ☐ 18.4 Scleral _____mm ☐ 13.4 Corneoscleral _____mm
IOFB: ☐ 90.0 Magnetic ☐ 90.1 Ant. Segment ☐ 90.2 Post. Segment
☐ 91.0 Nonmagnetic ☐ 91.1 Ant. Segment ☐ 91.2 Post. Segment
PERFORATING INJURY: ☐ 18.2 Perforating Injury ☐ 18.21 Corneoscleral
☐ 18.22 Scleroscleral
UVEA IN WOUND: ☐ 18.1 Scleral ☐ 10.1 Cornea ☐11.1 In Visual Axis
WOUND DEHISCENCE: ☐ 19.0   HYPHEMA: ☐ 20.0 _____%
IRIS PUPIL: ☐ 22.0 Iris Laceration/Dialysis ☐ 22.3 Afferent Pupil Defect
IOP: ☐ 24.0 Angle Recession ☐ 26.0 Glaucoma, Secondary ☐ 28.0 Hypotony
LENS: ☐ 30.0 Cataract (Traumatic) ☐ 32.0 Subluxed Lens ☐ 32.1 Dislocated Lens
VITREOUS: ☐ 40.0 Hemorrhage ☐ 42.0 Penetration
RETINA: ☐ 50.0 Retinal Hemorrhage ☐ 55.5 Macular Hemorrhage
☐ 51.0 Retinal Edema ☐ 55.2 Macular Edema ☐ 52.0 Retinal Defect
☐ 52.1 Tear ☐ 52.2 Giant Tear ☐ 52.3 Laceration ☐ 52.4 Dialysis
☐ 53.0 Retinal Detachment ▸ *Number of Quadrants?* ☐ 1 ☐ 2 ☐ 3 ☐ 4
RD TYPE: ☐ 53.1 Hemorrhagic ☐ 53.2 Tract. ☐ 53.3 Rhegm. ☐ 53.5 Macular
CHOROID: ☐ 58.0 Hemorrhage ☐ 58.1 Rupture
OPTIC NERVE INJURY: ☐ 82.0 Optic Nerve
ORBITAL: ☐ 70.0 Fracture ☐ 71.0 Foreign Body ☐ 73.0 Hemorrhage
INFLAMMATION: ☐ 95.0 Uveitis ☐ 92.0 Endophthalmitis ▸ *Organism:* _____
☐ 99.0 Other or comments: _____
_____

Ⓝ INITIAL OPERATION: Date: _____/_____/_____
REPAIR EYELID WOUND: ☐ 00.0 Full-thickness ☐ 00.1 Partial-thickness
REPAIR LACRIMAL: ☐ 02.0 GLOBE: ☐ 18.0 Exploration of Globe
REPAIR CORNEAL: ☐ 10.4 Laceration ☐ 10.3 Rupture
REPAIR SCLERAL: ☐ 18.4 Laceration ☐ 18.3 Rupture
REPAIR CORNEOSCLERAL: ☐ 13.4 Laceration ☐ 13.3 Rupture
IOFB: ☐ 90.1 IOFB Removal by Magnet from Anterior Segment
☐ 90.2 IOFB Removal by Magnet from Posterior Segment
☐ 91.1 IOFB Removal by Forceps from Anterior Segment
☐ 91.2 IOFB Removal by Forceps from Posterior Segment
CORNEA: ☐ 19.2 Corneal Transplant ☐ 19.3 Temporary Keratoprosthesis (TKP)
REPAIR WOUND DEHIS: ☐ 19.0 Dehiscence HYPHEMA: ☐ 20.0 Removal
IRIS: ☐ 22.0 Iridectomy ☐ 22.1 Iridoplasty ☐ 22.2 Iridotomy
LENS: ☐ 30.0 ECCE ☐ 30.2 Phaco ☐ 30.3 Pars Plana Lensectomy
IOL: ☐ 36.1 AC ☐ 36.2 PC
VITRECTOMY MECHANICAL: ☐ 44.0 Anterior ☐ 44.1 Posterior
VITRECTOMY OPEN-SKY: ☐ 44.2
ANTIBIOTICS: ☐ 45.0 Intravitreal ☐ 45.1 Intracameral
RD PROPHYLAXIS: ☐ 53.0 Cryopexy ☐ 53.1 Laser ☐ 53.2 Buckle
RD REPAIR: ☐ 53.01 Cryopexy ☐ 53.11 Laser ☐ 53.5 Buckle ☐ 53.3 Vitrectomy
☐ 53.7 Air ☐ 53.4 Gas ☐ 53.6 Silicone Oil ☐ 53.8 Pneumatic Retinopexy
REPAIR EXTRAOCULAR MUSCLE: ☐ 60.0
ORBIT: ☐ 70.0 Fract. Repair ☐ 71.0 FB Removal ☐ 75.0 Decomp.
☐ 93.0 Evisceration ☐ 94.0 Enucleation ☐ 97.0 None ☐ 98.0 Unknown
OTHER: ☐ 99.0 Other or Comments: _____

FIGURE 4-1 The revised initial reporting form of the USEIR.

U.S. EYE INJURY REGISTRY
6 MONTH FOLLOW-UP REPORT

1) Check appropriate responses 2) Fill out comments 3) File bilateral injury reports seperately
4) Submit Data via WEIRONLINE.org 5) Write Down Record ID _____

IDENTIFICATION:

Patient's Initials: _____

Patient's Home ZIP: _____

Medical Rec. # _____

Age: _____   Sex: ☐ M ☐ F

Injury Date: ____/____/____

Eye: ☐ Right ☐ Left

Race: _____

Reporting MD: _____

Exam Date for Report:

____/____/____

Report Filer's Name: _____

_____

CORRECTED VISION:

DATE: ____/____/____

☐ 00 NLP
☐ 10 LP
☐ 20 HM
☐ 30 1/200 to 4/200 (CF)
☐ 40 5/200 to 19/200
Specify VA _____
☐ 91 Not Tested
☐ 98 Unknown
☐ 99 Other _____
Description of follow up vision test:

_____

LENS STATUS:

☐ 10 Phakic - Clear
☐ 20 Phakic - Cataract
☐ 30 Phakic - Unknown
☐ 40 Aphakic - Clear
☐ 50 Aphakic - Membrane
☐ 60 Aphakic - Unknown
☐ 71 Pseudophakic - AC
☐ 80 Pseudophakic - PC

HOSPITALIZATION DUE TO INJURY?

☐ Yes ☐ No ☐ Unknown

VISUAL FIELD:

☐ 10 100%
☐ 20 75%
☐ 30 50%
☐ 40 25%
☐ 50 < 25%
☐ 60 0%
☐ 98 Unknown

VISUAL LOSS CONTR. FACTORS:

☐ 01 Eyelid
☐ 10 Cornea
☐ 21 Glaucoma
☐ 22 Pupillary Opacity
☐ 30 Cataract
☐ 40 Vitreous Opacity
☐ 50 Retina
☐ 55 Macula
☐ 58 Choroid
☐ 70 Orbit
☐ 80 Optic Nerve
☐ 97 None
☐ 98 Unknown
   99 Other _____

Ⓡ VISUAL FUNCTION:

☐ 10 Stable
☐ 20 Improving
☐ 30 Decreasing
☐ 98 Unknown

ⓇⓇ POTENTIALLY IMPROVABLE WITH ADDITIONAL TREATMENT?

☐ Yes ☐ No ☐ Unknown

Ⓣ REHAB. STATUS:

☐ 10 Former Job _____
☐ 20 Limited Job _____
☐ 30 Unemployed
☐ 40 Retraining
☐ 50 Student
☐ 51 Child
☐ 98 Unknown
☐ 99 Other _____

Ⓥ COMMENTS: _____

_____
_____
_____
_____

Ⓦ LATE DIAGNOSES:

LID: ☐ 01.0 Eyelid Deformity
☐ 03.0 Lacrimal Obstruction
☐ 04.0 Conjunctival Scarring
CORNEA: ☐ 10.5 Corneal Scar
▸ In Visual Axis? ☐ 14.1 Y ☐ 14.2 N
☐ 10.6 Corneal Edema
▸ In Visual Axis? ☐ 14.1 Y ☐ 14.2 N
IRIS: ☐ 22.1 Iris Deformity
☐ 22.2 Pupillary Membrane
☐ 24.0 Angle Recession
☐ 26.0 Glaucoma, Secondary
▸ Controlled? ☐ 26.1 Yes ☐ 26.2 No
LENS: ☐ 28.0 Hypotony
☐ 28.1 Phthisis
☐ 30.0 Cataract, Traumatic
☐ 32.0 Subluxed
▸ ☐ 32.1 Dislocated Lens
☐ 34.0 Aphakia
☐ 36.0 Pseudophakia
▸ ☐ 36.1 AC IOL ☐ 36.2 PC IOL
HEMORRHAGE: ☐ 40.0 Vitreous
☐ 50.0 Retinal ☐ 55.5 Macular
EDEMA: ☐ 51.0 Retinal Traumatic
☐ 55.2 Macular
DEFECT: ☐ 52.0 Retinal ☐ 52.1 Tear
☐ 52.2 Giant Tear ☐ 52.3 Laceration
☐ 52.4 Dialysis ☐ 52.5 Hole
☐ 53.0 Retinal Detachment
▸ Number of Quadrants?
☐ 1 ☐ 2 ☐ 3 ☐ 4
☐ 53.1 Hemorrhagic ☐ 53 .2 Tractional
☐ 53.3 Rhegmatogenous
☐ 53.5 Macular
☐ 57.0 Proliferative Vitreoretinopathy
▸ PVR Stage ☐ A ☐ B ☐ C ☐ D
☐ 1 ☐ 2 ☐ 3
☐ 55.0 Macular Degeneration/Scarring
☐ 55.1 Epimacular Membrane
☐ 55.3 Macular Hole
CONTUSION: ☐ 55.4 Maculopathy
   54.0 Retinopathy

Ⓦ LATE DIAGNOSES (CONT.):

CHOROIDAL: ☐ 58.0 Hemorrhage ☐ 58.1 Rupture
☐ 64.0 Strabismus
OPTIC NERVE: ☐ 88.0 Atrophy ☐ 82.0 Injury
☐ 92.0 Endophthalmitis Organism _____
☐ 95.0 Uveitis ☐ 93.0 Sympathetic ophthalmia
☐ 96.0 Enophthalmos ☐ 97.0 Proptosis
☐ 98.0 Unknown
☐ 99.0 Other or Comments (use space below)

_____
_____
_____
_____

Ⓧ ADDITIONAL OPERATIONS:

	DATE #2	DATE #3	DATE #4				
	____/____/____	____/____/____	____/____/____				
				#2	#3	#4	
REPAIR EYELID WOUND				☐	☐	☐	00.3 Oculoplastic Surgery, Eyelids
LACRIMAL				☐	☐	☐	02.0 Repair Lacrimal System
				☐	☐	☐	18.0 Exploration of Globe
IOFB EXTR., MAGNET				☐	☐	☐	90.1 Anterior Segment
				☐	☐	☐	90.2 Posterior Segment
IOFB EXTR., FORCEPS				☐	☐	☐	91.1 Anterior Segment
				☐	☐	☐	91.2 Posterior Segment
LENS				☐	☐	☐	30.0 ECCE
				☐	☐	☐	30.2 Phaco
				☐	☐	☐	30.3 P.P. Lensectomy
IOL				☐	☐	☐	36.1 AC IOL
				☐	☐	☐	36.2 PC IOL
VITRECTOMY				☐	☐	☐	44.0 Vitrectomy, Open Sky
				☐	☐	☐	44.1 Vitrectomy, Total Pars Plana
WOUND DEHIS				☐	☐	☐	19.0 Repair
CORNEA				☐	☐	☐	19.2 Transplant
				☐	☐	☐	19.3 Temporary Keratoprosthesis (TKP)
IRIS				☐	☐	☐	22.0 Iridectomy
				☐	☐	☐	22.2 Iridotomy
				☐	☐	☐	22.1 Iridoplasty
IOP				☐	☐	☐	26.0 Glaucoma Procedure
ANTIBIOTICS				☐	☐	☐	45.0 Vitreous
				☐	☐	☐	45.1 AC
RD PROPHYLAXIS				☐	☐	☐	53.0 Cryopexy
				☐	☐	☐	53.1 Laser
				☐	☐	☐	53.2 Buckle
RD REPAIR				☐	☐	☐	53.01 Cryopexy
				☐	☐	☐	53.11 Laser
				☐	☐	☐	53.5 Buckle
				☐	☐	☐	53.3 Vitrectomy
				☐	☐	☐	53.4 Gas
				☐	☐	☐	53.7 Air
				☐	☐	☐	53.6 Silicone Oil
				☐	☐	☐	53.8 Pneumatic Retinopexy
EXTRAOCULAR MUSCLE				☐	☐	☐	60.0 Repair
ORBIT				☐	☐	☐	70.0 Fracture Repair
				☐	☐	☐	71.0 F.B. Removal
ENVIS/ENUC				☐	☐	☐	93.0 Evisceration
				☐	☐	☐	94.0 Enucleation
ENOPHTHALMOS REPAIR				☐	☐	☐	96.0 Enopthalmos Repair
MISC.				☐	☐	☐	97.0 None
				☐	☐	☐	98.0 Unknown
				☐	☐	☐	99.0 Other or Comments (use space below)

_____
_____
_____
_____

FIGURE 4–2   The revised 6-month follow-up reporting form of the USEIR.

Table 4–2   Incidence and Prevalence Estimates of Eye Injuries

Publication Year, Reference	Finding*	Country and Remark
1988[43]	Prevalence of trauma-related bilateral blindness: 200/100,000	Nepal; interview-based study
1990[44]	Of all monocular blindness cases, 40% caused by trauma	United States; population-based
1986[20]	Incidence rate of acute, hospital-treated eye injuries: 423/100,000 population/years	United States; based on emergency room and hospital records; all ages studied
1989[22]	Incidence rate of hospitalized cases of eye injuries: 13.2/100,000 population/years	United States; based on hospital discharges; all ages studied
1988[19]	Incidence of eye injuries requiring medical treatment: 975/100,000	United States; interview-based
1995[45]	Incidence of "penetrating eye injuries": 3.6/100,000	Australia; hospital-based study
1995[45]	Incidence of eye injuries requiring hospitalization: 15.2/100,000	Australia; hospital-based study
1966[13]	One-year cumulative incidence of blinding outcome from serious ocular trauma: 0.41/100,000 population/years	Scotland; hospital-based study
1994[46]	Annual incidence of "perforating eye injuries": 3.3/100,000	Sweden; hospital-based study

*The great variability is due in part to differences in study design.

- Most of those injured are young with an average age around 30 years.[9,18,21,22] The average age in the USEIR is 33 years and in the HEIR is 29 years. Patients younger than 30 years in the USEIR: 57% and in the HEIR: 42%. The age range in the USEIR is 0–101 years and in the HEIR is 0–85 years. The estimated risk of sustaining ocular trauma when two persons are compared is 80% higher for the individual who is 10 years younger.[19]

- Less educated and less wealthy persons are more prone to partake in risk-taking activities and thus to be injured.[18,19]

- Nonwhites have a 40 to 60% higher risk.[22] Black or Hispanic races in the United States are more at risk between ages 25 through 65 years.

- The combined effect of race and sex cannot be ignored: in one survey, 23% of black men, 20% of white men, 12% of black women, and 8% of white women reported at least one injury in their lifetime.[17]

- Other risk factors include self-reported dangerous behaviors (e.g., traffic violations, marijuana use)[19]; and alcohol and drug use, unemployment, and unsettled social environments[12].

The Site

- The workplace has traditionally been the most common site of ocular trauma. Although occupational injuries are still the most frequent in certain settings,[9,19] their significance is decreasing.[8,18,20,23,24] In 1996, the estimated annual incidence of severe work-related ocular injury was 2.98 per 100,000 employed persons, resulting in an estimated 3745 acute hospitalizations. The annual incidence was higher among men, Hispanics, and those 20 to 24 years of age (5.02,

3.72, and 4.64 per 100,000 employed, respectively).[25] Males injured at the workplace in the USEIR and in the HEIR: 96%. Eye injury in industrial premises in the USEIR and the HEIR: 13%. In the USEIR, most of these injuries are sustained by those working as laborers and in construction; in the HEIR, as mechanics and unskilled workers.

- The proportion of domestic injuries has been increasing[26,27] (USEIR and the HEIR: 39%).

- Streets and highways in industrialized nations are common sites of ocular trauma (USEIR: 11%; HEIR: 17%).[25]

The Source

- Blunt objects are the most common cause for ocular trauma[28] (USEIR: 31%; HEIR: 45%). The typical objects in the United States are rocks, fists, baseballs, and lumber, as opposed to fists, wood branches, rocks, and champagne corks in Hungary. Champagne corks are responsible for 0.06% of all injuries in the USEIR and for 1.4% in Hungary. The statistically different rates ($P = 0.000001$) may be due to the presence of highly visible warning labels on the bottles in the United States (Fig. 4–3) ; such labels are absent in Hungary.

- Work-related injuries are an important source (USEIR, 21%; in the HEIR, 27%).

- MVC is an important source of ocular trauma in industrialized nations,[18,22,29,30] responsible for up to 12% of all reported eye injuries in an urban setting.[18] Glass splinters from heat-toughened windshields are a common cause of eye injury; laminated windshields offer more protection by preventing the glass splinters from dislodging.[30] In a similar crash, a per-

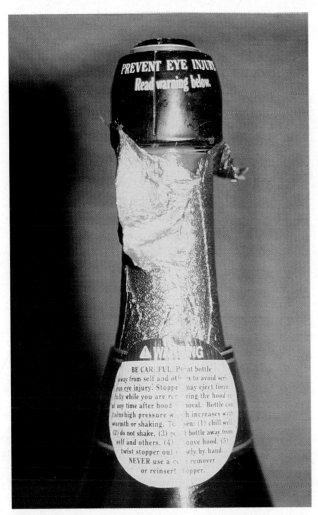

FIGURE 4–3 This champagne bottle is difficult to open without noticing the conspicuous warning icon on the cap and its reference to the label below.

son unprotected by an air bag has a 2.5 times higher risk of sustaining an eye injury than a person in a car in which the air bag has deployed;[31] air bag deployment offers measurable protection[f].

• Sports and recreational activities appear to be gaining significance as sources of ocular trauma in industrialized nations; basketball and baseball are most frequently implicated in the United States.[9,20,23] In the USEIR, 12% of all cases are sport related; in the HEIR, 9%.

• Firearms and BB guns are responsible for a very high percentage of serious ocular trauma in countries where they are legal. In the USEIR they repre-

sent 12%; in the HEIR (where they are illegal), the rate is less than 1%.

• Hammering on metal and nails is a common and easily preventable cause of eye injury (see Chapter 24); its proportion among all serious eye injuries is 5% in the USEIR and 9% in the HEIR.

• Fireworks are a major source wherever they are legal: 4.4% in the EIRA. In Hungary (where private fireworks use is forbidden by law), the rate is 0.1% ($P = 0.000001$).[10]

Intention

• Violence is usually responsible for 15% or less of ocular trauma cases[9,20,21,23] (USEIR: 16%), but in urban environments the figure can reach 43%.[18] Such injuries are usually severe: up to 34% of those assaulted may present with NLP initial vision.[33]

• Race is a risk factor in becoming a victim of assault, with double the rate among nonwhites.[22] Black men have a 2.3 times higher chance than white men of having visual impairment as a result of trauma.[17]

PREVENTION

The goal of data collection is to identify trends on the basis of which primary, secondary, and tertiary prevention is developed.[g] Among the many examples showing the benefits of systematic data collection and implementation of prophylactic measures are the effects of seat belt laws, which have reduced the incidence of eye injuries by 47% to 65%.[34–36]

> **PEARL...** Campaigns organized toward educating the public should have two major goals: pinpointing activities or environments associated with an increased risk of eye injury (e.g., hammering) and providing the necessary information regarding prevention (use of safety eyewear, its type and availability, and instructions for use).

---

[f]Most reports claiming that a certain eye injury was caused by an air bag fail to prove unequivocally a cause-effect relationship: the injury sustained during the MVC may simply be coincidental.[32] Furthermore, even if an eye injury was caused by the air bag, its deployment may have saved the person's life.

[g]The purpose is to prevent tragedies such as one witnessed by one the authors (F.K.): a 17-year-old male presenting with his left eye virtually cut in half by a butcher's knife he was using as a student at a meat processing factory. The workers were provided with metal gloves but no eye protection. The eye had to be removed. When the father visited his son, he was noticed to wear a prosthesis in his left orbit; 23 years earlier he sustained an identical injury at the same plant.

There are efficient and convenient protective devices available for the public,[37] offering adequate (front plus side) protection without interfering with the peripheral visual field and without fogging up during use. The efficacy of such polycarbonate shields is well proved by combat experience.[38] Even though war-related eye injuries, as a percentage of all war injuries, showed a steady increase from the mid-19th century (1.76% in the Crimean War [1854–1856], 6.8% in the Lebanon War [1982]), not a single eye was injured in the Israeli Defense Forces among soldiers wearing proper goggles.[38] The experience is similar in sports such as ice hockey, racquetball, and squash.[2–4] A more current example of data collection resulting in effective proposals to reduce eye injury incidence in sports is paint ball trauma and war games.[39]

The general belief is that conventional glasses offer little protection and may even contribute to the injury by shattering.[40] Recent data from the USEIR suggest that in certain circumstances the opposite may be true; further studies are needed to answer this important question.[11] It remains to be seen, for instance, whether wearing standard prescription glasses should be discouraged in the front seat of air bag-equipped cars because the fracture of the glass may be responsible[41] for eye injury.

The USEIR has estimated that in the United States alone, 500,000 years of eyesight are lost annually due to injury. Nevertheless, "injury is probably the most under-recognized major health problem facing the nation. The study of injury presents unparalleled opportunities for reducing morbidity and for realizing savings in both financial and human terms."[47]

PEARL... Reporting to the USEIR is now possible over the Internet (USEIRonline.org), and the WEIR is operational. All ophthalmologists, regardless of the physical location of their practice, have the opportunity to contribute to ocular trauma control by reporting their experience in a standardized fashion over the Internet (WEIRonline.org).

Summary

Systemic collection of standardized data on the occurrence of eye injuries can help the ophthalmologist play a key role in successfully preventing ocular trauma. The USEIR model, whether reporting over the Internet or on paper, has proved to be an efficient epidemiological tool. Use of this model in other countries has allowed research involving valid comparisons between regions and even countries. Such comparisons have highlighted injury patterns that may be different in different geographical areas, pinpointing areas where prophylaxis (e.g., legislation, public campaigns) was effective.

References

1. Steiner G, Peterson L. Severe emotional response to eye trauma in a child: awareness and intervention. *Arch Ophthalmol.* 1992;110:753.

2. Easterbrook M. Eye protection in racquet sports. *Curr Ther Sports Med.* 1990;2:356–362.

3. Pashby T, Pashby R, Chisholm L, Crawford J. Eye injuries in Canadian hockey. *Can Med Assoc J.* 1975; 113:663.

4. Pashby T. Eye injuries in Canadian hockey. Phase II. *Can Med Assoc J.* 1977;117:671.

5. National Society to Prevent Blindness. *Vision Problems in the U.S.: Data Analysis.* New York: National Society to Prevent Blindness; 1980:25–26.

6. Committee on Trauma Research, National Research Council. *Injury in America: A Continuing Public Health Problem.* Washington, DC: National Academy Press; 1985.

7. Wong T, Tielsch J. A population-based study on the incidence of severe ocular trauma in Singapore. *Am J Ophthalmol.* 1999;128:345–351.

8. Morris R, Witherspoon C, Helms H, et al. Serious eye trauma in Alabama. *Ala Med.* 1988;58:36–40.

9. Schein OD, Hibberd PL, Shingleton BJ, et al. The spectrum and burden of ocular injury. *Ophthalmology.* 1988;95:300–305.

10. Kuhn F, Morris R, Witherspoon CD, et al. Serious fireworks-related eye injuries. *Ophthalmic Epidemiol.* 2000; 7:139–148.

11. May D, Kuhn F, Morris R, et al. The epidemiology of serious eye injuries from the United States Eye Injury Registry. *Graefes Arch Clin Exp Ophthalmol.* 2000;238:153–157.

12. Negrel A, Thylefors B. The global impact of eye injuries. *Ophthalmic Epidemiol.* 1998;5:143–169.

13. Desai P, MacEwen C, Baines P, Minassian D. Incidence of cases of ocular trauma admitted to hospital and incidence of blinding outcome. *Br J Ophthalmol.* 1966;80: 592–596.

14. Klopfer J, Tielsch J, Vitale S, et al. Ocular trauma in the United states, eye injuries resulting in hospitalization, 1984–1987. *Arch Ophthalmol.* 1992;110:838–842.

15. Blomdahl S, Norell S. Perforating eye injury in the Stockholm population: an epidemiological study. *Acta Ophthalmol.* 1984;62:378–390.

16. Brillant G, ed. *Trauma in the Epidemiology of Blindness in Nepal. Report of the 1981 Nepal Blindness Survey.* San Rafael, Calif: The SEVA Foundation; 1988.

17. Katz J, Tielsch J. Lifetime prevalence of ocular injuries from the Baltimore Eye Survey. *Arch Ophthalmol.* 1993;111:1564–1568.

18. Liggett P, Pince K, Barlow W, Ragen M, Ryan S. Ocular trauma in an urban population. *Ophthalmology.* 1990;97:581–584.

19. Glynn R, Seddon J, Berlin B. The incidence of eye injuries in New England adults. *Arch Ophthalmol.* 1988;106:785–789.

20. Karlson T, Klein B. The incidence of acute hospital-treated eye injuries. *Arch Ophthalmol.* 1986;104:1473–1476.

21. Maltzman B, Pruzon H, Mund M. A survey of ocular trauma. *Surv Ophthalmol.* 1976;21:285–290.

22. Tielsch J, Parver L, Shankar B. Time trends in the incidence of hospitalized ocular trauma. *Arch Ophthalmol.* 1989;107:519–523.

23. White M, Morris R, Feist R, Witherspoon C, Helms H, John G. Eye injury: prevalence and prognosis by setting. *South Med J.* 1989;82:151–158.

24. Dannenberg A, Parver L, Brechner R, Khoo L. Penetrating eye injuries in the workplace; the National Eye Trauma System Registry. *Arch Ophthalmol.* 1992;110:843–848.

25. Kuhn F, Mester V, Witherspoon CD, Morris R, Maisiak R. Epidemiology and socioeconomic impact of eye injuries. In: *Vitrectomy in the Management of the Injured Globe.* Philadelphia: Lippincott Raven; 1998:17–24.

26. Chapman-Smith JS. Eye injuries: a 12-month survey. *N Z Med J.* 1979;90:47–49.

27. Johnston SS. Symposium on ocular trauma. *Trans Ophthalmol Soc UK.* 1975;95:305–310.

28. MacEwan C, Naines P, Desai P. Eye injuries in children: the current picture. *Br J Ophthalmol.* 1999;83:933–936.

29. Strahlman E, Elman M, Daub E, Baker S. Causes of pediatric injuries. *Arch Ophthalmol.* 1990;108:603–606.

30. Kuhn F, Collins P, Morris R. Epidemiology of motor vehicle crash–related serious eye injuries. *Accid Anal Prev.* 1994;26:385–390.

31. Kuhn F, Morris R, Witherspoon C. Eye injury and the air bag. *Curr Opin Ophthalmol.* 1995;6(3):38–44.

32. Kuhn F, Morris R, Witherspoon C, Byrne J, Brown S. Air bag: friend or foe? *Arch Ophthalmol.* 1993;111:1333–1334.

33. Dannenberg A, Parver L, Fowler C. Penetrating eye injuries related to assault. The National Eye Trauma System Registry. *Arch Ophthalmol.* 1992;110:829–852.

34. Cole MD, Clearkin L, Dabbs T, Smerdon D. The seat belt law and after. *Br J Ophthalmol.* 1987;71:436–440.

35. Chapman-Smith JS. Eye injuries produced by vehicle safety glass. *N Z Med J.* 1978;88:239.

36. Briner A. Penetrating eye injuries associated with motor vehicle accidents. *Med J Aust.* 1976;1:912–914.

37. John G, Witherspoon C, Morris R, White M, Feist R. Field evaluation of polycarbonate versus conventional safety glasses. *South Med J.* 1988;81:1534–1536.

38. Belkin M, Treister G, Dotan S. Eye injuries and ocular protection in the Lebanon War, 1982. *Isr J Med Sci.* 1984;20:333–338.

39. Vinger P, Sparks J, Mussack K, Dondero J, Jeffers J. A program to prevent eye injuries in paintball. *Sports Vision* 1997;3:33–40.

40. Keeney A, Fintelmann E, Renaldo D. Clinical mechanisms in non-industrial trauma. *Am J Ophthalmol.* 1972;74:662.

41. Gault J, Vichnin M, Jaeger E, Jeffers J. Ocular injuries associated with eyeglass wear and airbag inflation. *J Trauma.* 1995;38:494–497.

42. Tielsch J, Parver L. Determinants of hospital charges and length of stay for ocular trauma. *Ophthalmology.* 1990;97:231–237.

43. Brilliant GE. *The Epidemiology of Blindness in Nepal. Report of the 1981 Nepal Blindness Survey.* San Rafael, Calif: The SEVA Foundation; 1988.

44. Dana M, Tielsch J, Enger C, et al. Visual impairment in a rural Appalachian community. *JAMA.* 1990;264:2400–2405.

45. Fong L. Eye injuries in Victoria, Australia. *Med J Aust.* 1995;162:64–68.

46. Byhr E. Perforating eye injuries in a western part of Sweden. *Acta Ophthalmol.* 1994;72:91–97.

47. Foege W. *Injury Control. A Review of the Status and Progress of the Injury Control Program at the Centers for Disease Control.* Washington, DC: National Academy Press; 1988.

COUNSELING THE PATIENT AND THE FAMILY

Robert Morris, Ferenc Kuhn,
C. Douglas Witherspoon, and D. Donald C. Stephens

Although any injury is stressful, eye trauma, among non life-threatening injuries, is especially so.[1] Blindness has regularly been found the most feared of all disabilities in Gallup polls, and any threat to vision is emotionally wrenching.

Of all causes of sight loss, injury is the most sudden and dramatic because it is instantaneous (Fig. 5–1). Humans rely heavily on vision to avoid bodily trauma, and therefore it is particularly shocking if the eye itself is injured. This makes counseling of eye trauma patients and their families uniquely important. Adequate and skilled counseling is especially critical in cases of serious injuries that require surgical intervention.

COUNSELING GOALS

Counseling must be
- comforting;
- informative;
- truthful;
- accurate;
- compassionate;
- patient;
- dynamic; and
- continuing at least until the conclusion of treatment.

Comforting the Patient

Because the first contact occurs in the emergency setting, the physician–patient relationship does not enjoy the usual benefits of an orderly, planned encounter. In view of the stress associated with an unexpected injury, it is especially important for the ophthalmologist to communicate calmness and seriousness of purpose. Careless words or gestures may quickly handicap this delicate and growing relationship.

The counselor is preferably the treating physician, instilling confidence and hope to the extent that hope is justified by increasingly detailed knowledge of the prognosis.

PEARL... Although it is true that the final visual outcome often remains in doubt for weeks or even months, the physician should encourage the patient not to give up hope unless the eye has permanently (see Chapter 8) lost all potential for vision.

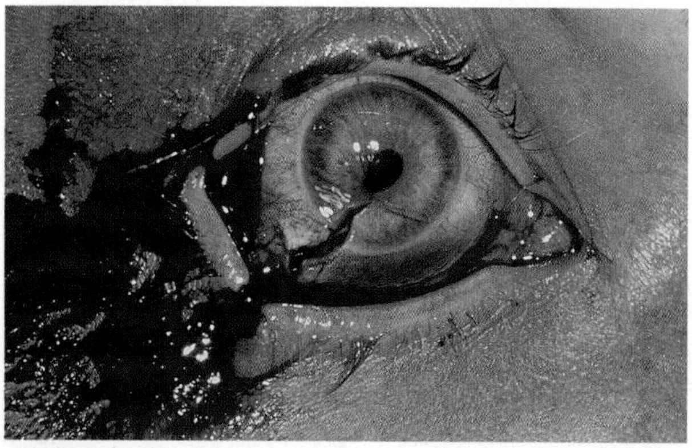

Modern techniques of globe reconstruction enable visual recovery in eyes that would have been considered lost even as recently as a few years ago. The external

FIGURE 5–1 Corneoscleral laceration at presentation.

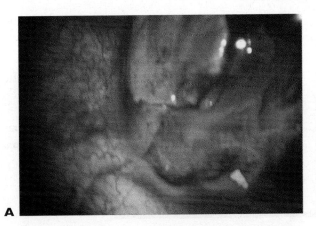
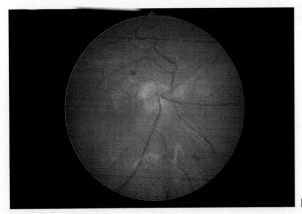

FIGURE 5–2   **(A)** Preoperative photograph of retinal prolapse through a severe corneoscleral laceration, an injury unsalvageable only years ago. **(B)** Reattached retina under silicone oil.

appearance of the injury's severity and the loss of light perception must not by themselves guide management (see Fig. 5–2 and Chapter 8). It is the vitreous surgeon's responsibility to distinguish reasonable hope from futility in the search for vision.

SPECIAL CONSIDERATION

Hope for visual improvement may increase or decrease throughout the course of therapy; counseling therefore has to continue through the entirety of the patient–physician relationship. The patient's occasional inappropriately optimistic or pessimistic attitude must be recognized by the physician, who, even if it is extremely time consuming, must respond to it.

The physician who is not effectively communicating with the patient and family[a] may engender false hope or unnecessary anxiety. Without a reasonable measure of compassion and empathy, the physician will fail to observe these reactions, which may lead to:

• sudden depression when a poor prognosis is belatedly understood; or
• unnecessary suffering when the outcome is clearly better than the patient has come to expect.

No matter what the treatment outcome, it will be more acceptable to, and appreciated by, the patient at the conclusion of the treatment if the physician has maintained effective communication throughout their encounters.

Informing the Patient

Providing comfort to the patient and family is inseparable from the goal of providing information to obtain the patient's participation and informed consent because realistic decisions cannot be based on inaccurate information. Major recent milestones in the ophthalmologist's ability to provide an injury-specific prognosis include the BETT,[2] the classification of injuries,[3] and the OTS (see Chapters 1, 2, and 3).

After the initial assessment, the counseling physician should keep the patient and family regularly apprised of the eye's response to the applied treatment and of additional treatment options. The latter is especially important for gaining both acceptance of the recurrent surgical intervention commonly needed after injury and patience to allow full recovery without avoidable frustration or depression.

The constant flow of information from the ophthalmologist is also important to facilitate the patient's cooperation (e.g., positioning after the application of certain vitreous substitutes; see the Appendix). The patient must plan life adjustments and will deeply appreciate the accurate and timely information that enables such planning.

As required, vocational and psychological counseling must also be offered, as well as low-vision rehabilitation (see Chapter 6).

PEARL...   The emotions associated with eye injury and its treatment run the gamut from depression to exhilaration. Compassion, competence, and commitment on the part of the treating physician *and* support staff are appreciated by the patient.

---

[a] Providing guidance while also listening to the patient.

Specific Counseling Issues

No list of specific counseling issues can be totally comprehensive, given:

- the variability of eye injuries and the response of the eyes to treatment;
- the different patient-family personalities; and
- the physicians' treatment philosophies.

Issues to be addressed specifically at appropriate points during the treatment are listed in Table 5–1. Additional comments include the following:

- The ophthalmologist must be able to adjust the counseling strategy according to each patient's situation.
- Outcomes and risks should be described quantitatively to the extent possible. Otherwise, estimates

Table 5–1 Steps in Specific Counseling

At initial presentation	Physician introduction
	Estimate of severity
	Eye anatomy
	Description of injury
	Treatment goals (vision, cosmesis, comfort)
	Treatment philosophy and options; risks and benefits
	Prognosis
	Statement of physician's commitment and concern
	Patient's responsibilities
	If indicated, permission for primary enucleation
	Informed consent to treatment plan
After primary surgery	Results of surgery and need for further diagnostic tests
	Prognosis change
	Potential complications (especially infection)
	Patient instructions (pain, monocular vision checkup, positioning, medical treatment, activity)
	Monocular status, fellow eye health and stability assurance
Prior to secondary surgery/enucleation	Revision of goals, treatment plan, prognosis
	Discussion of SO
	Informed consent for further surgery/enucleation
	Informed consent for certain vitreous substitutes (e.g., silicone oil)
After each reconstructive surgery	Results
	Further prognosis refinement
	Potential complications (infection; hemorrhage; retinal detachment; glaucoma/hypotony/phthisis; cataract; corneal decompensation/distortion; traumatic mydriasis/diplopia/metamorphopsia; PVR; loss of the eye; SO)
	Anesthesia risk
	Patient instructions
	Consent for further treatment
At treatment conclusion (or as appropriate during treatment)	Lifetime examination plan
	Safety precautions
	Rehabilitation (personal, occupational)
	Further treatment options (e.g., secondary IOL, pupilloplasty, iris reconstruction/implant, penetrating keratoplasty, muscle surgery)
	Amblyopia prophylaxis/treatment
	Singular binocular vision versus reserve eye
	Prosthetic fitting if appropriate

such as "possible," "probable," "unlikely," and "remotely possible" should be considered.

- The presence of a family member or members during counseling is especially helpful to ensure effective communication. It provides a more familiar and supportive environment as well as more accurate interpretation and subsequent recollection of the conversation.

- The use of drawings or pictures is often helpful in communicating the nature of an injury and the subsequent surgical repair.

- The physician is usually a total stranger to the patient. The treating doctor's heartfelt commitment to trying everything possible to achieve the best outcome produces an atmosphere of trust.

- Early on, it often helps to reassure the patient specifically about the health of the fellow eye and to refute the understandable anxiety that the remaining eye might be strained from overuse if the injured eye does not recover (see the Appendix).

- An eye injury can be physically painful, and suffering patients are difficult to counsel. The physician should alleviate the pain immediately. The patient will not only be grateful but also be more willing to participate in critical decision making.

- Approximately 7% of eyes with open globe injury suffer endophthalmitis[4] (see Chapter 28), and almost one third of patients experience glaucoma after vitrectomy.[5] For timely recognition, the patient should be informed of the early symptoms of these conditions and urged to report them immediately.

- The possible need for multiple operations (Fig. 5–3) and the long-term threat of intraocular scarring, both of which may limit vision, should be mentioned in advance.

- If the injured eye is aphakic, has only ambulatory final vision, and optical correction is not elected (e.g., because of metamorphopsia), the patient should at least be acquainted with the concept that the potential for improved vision with adequate correction is available in the future.

- Injuries in children were found to have prognostic factors similar to those for adults.[6] When an injury is severe or traumatic cataract is present, a less favorable outcome may be caused by amblyopia.[7] The importance of amblyopia therapy and lifelong protection of the unaffected eye should be emphasized to the patient and family (see Chapter 30).

- After enucleation, the prosthetic socket has the potential to harbor pathogens. Therefore, the patient should be made aware that if surgery on the remaining eye is ever needed, cultures of *both* the prosthetic socket and the eye should first be done.[8]

- Approximately 3% eye injuries are bilateral, most commonly those resulting from MVC, shotgun incidents, or alkaline burns (USEIR data). Extensive psychological support is needed for the person who suffers sudden, irreversible blindness.

- An injured eye with an opaque cornea and posterior segment trauma is best explored and treated by timely use of a TKP to perform complete vitrectomy (see Chapter 25). The patient must understand that TKP vitrectomy is an exploratory procedure initially. Preoperative permission based on the patient's informed consent should be sought for *enucleation, functional reconstruction,* or *cosmetic reconstruction,* depending on the findings during direct inspection of the optic nerve and retina (see Chapter 8).

- Patients with severe injury must be told about the risk of SO (see Chapter 29), posing a serious, although rare, threat to the fellow eye after open globe injury.[9] The patient must be involved in selecting the treatment option.

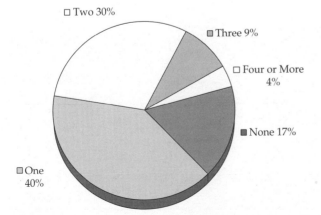

FIGURE 5–3 Graph illustrating the need for multiple operations for patients with serious eye injury (USEIR).

PEARL... Counseling represents the difference between treating solely the eye and treating the person. Counseling is an art. As Pericles stated 500 years ago, "The art of medicine cannot be learned from books, nor can it be inherited". The art of counseling the eye trauma victim is learned over a lifetime from other physicians during formal training and from one's personal counseling experiences. The effort to develop this art will be greatly appreciated and richly awarded with personal satisfaction.

Summary

Proper communication between the physician, patient, and family is a critical part in the management of severe ocular injuries. Thorough and honest discussions should begin preoperatively and continue throughout the postoperative period. Understanding the prognosis for severe ocular injuries will help the physician disseminate accurate information.

References

1. Hine RV. *Second Sight*. Thorndike, Me: Thorndike Publishers; 1993:213.
2. Kuhn F, Morris R, Witherspoon CD, Heimann K, Jeffers JB, Treister G. A standardized classification of ocular trauma. *Ophthalmology*. 1996;103:240–243.
3. Pieramici DJ, Sternberg P Jr, Aaberg TM Sr, et al. A system for classifying mechanical injuries of the eye (globe). The Ocular Trauma Classification Group. *Am J Ophthalmol*. 1997;123:820–831.
4. Brinton GS, Topping TM, Hyndiuk RA, et al. Posttraumatic endophthalmitis. *Arch Ophthalmol*. 1984;102:547–550.
5. Weinberg RS, Peyman GA, Haumonte FU. Elevation of intraocular pressure after pars plana vitrectomy. *Graefes Arch Clin Exp Ophthalmol*. 1976;200:157–162.
6. Rostomian K, Thach AB, Isfahani A, Pakkar A, Pakkar R, Borchert M. Open globe injuries in children. *JAAPOS*. 1998;2:234–238.
7. Alfaro DV, Chaudhry NA, Walonker AF, Runyan T, Saito Y, Liggett PE. Penetrating eye injuries in young children. *Retina*. 1994;14:201–205.
8. Morris RE, Camesasca FI, Byrne JB, et al. Postoperative endophthalmitis resulting from prosthesis contamination in a monocular patient. *Am J Ophthalmol*. 1993;116:346–349.
9. Albert DM, Diaz-Rohena R. A historical review of sympathetic ophthalmia and its epidemiology. *Surv Ophthalmol*. 1989;34:1–14.

Chapter 6

REHABILITATION OF PATIENTS WITH OCULAR TRAUMA

Donald C. Fletcher and August Colenbrander

 Because the visual system alone provides more input to the brain than all other senses combined, vision loss can have a devastating impact on people's lives.

PEARL... In our daily medical practice, we usually narrow our focus on acute care, to minimize the impact of a disease on an organ or system. Trauma, however, has a much greater impact; for example, eye injury affects the quality of life of the individual far beyond the globe.

Health care promotes *health: a condition of optimal physical, mental, and social well-being* (WHO definition).

With a focus different from that of acute care, *rehabilitation medicine*, irrespective of the organ system involved, tries to reduce the functional impact of the impairment so that the individual can maintain:

- independence;
- productive activity; and
- life satisfaction.

REHABILITATION GOALS

Rehabilitation is best approached (see Table 6–1) via the following four terms[1,a].

1. *Disorder* (describing aspects of the *organ's* condition, i.e., anatomic/structural changes).

[a]Used by the WHO for the ICD (ICD-9 and ICD-9-CM in the United States)[2,3] and the ICIDH.[4]

TABLE 6-1 ASPECTS OF VISION LOSS*

	The Organ		The Person	
Aspects	Structural change, anatomic change	Functional change at the organ level	Skills, abilities of the individual	Societal, economic consequences
Neutral terms	Health condition	Organ function	Skills, abilities	Social participation
Loss, limitation	Disorder, injury	Impairment	Disability	Handicap
ICIDH	Disorder	Impairment	Disability	Handicap
ICIDH	Structural change	Functional change, impairment	Activity + performance code	Participation + performance code
Application to vision	Eye diseases	"Visual functions" measured quantitatively (e.g., visual acuity)	"Functional vision" described qualitatively, (e.g., reading ability)	Vision-related quality of life

*Vision loss can be approached from different points of view. The different aspects are sometimes described by different names.

2. *Impairment* (describing aspects of the *organ's* condition, i.e., functional changes such as visual acuity field loss at the organ level).
3. *Disability* (describing aspects of the *person's* condition, i.e., generic skills and abilities).
4. *Handicap* (describing aspects of the *person's* condition, pointing to the social and economic consequences of a loss of abilities).

PEARL... In colloquial use, persons with severe vision loss are often called "blind." This term is inappropriate as most people have residual vision.

Improving participation is the ultimate goal of all medical and social interventions. There are obvious links between them: a disorder may cause an impairment, which may cause a loss of abilities, which may cause a lack of participation. Each of these links may be aggravating or compensating, and the very possibility of rehabilitation depends on this flexibility. For example:

- medical/surgical interventions can reduce disorder-related impairment;
- assistive devices may improve abilities in the presence of a given impairment;
- changes in the human and physical environment may increase participation regardless of reduced abilities.

The art of rehabilitation is to manipulate each of these links so that a given disorder results in the least possible loss of participation.

TEAMWORK

Figure 6–1 illustrates that different interventions, provided by different professionals, are needed at different points in the chain. Because ophthalmologists are early participants, it is their responsibility to call upon other team members appropriately.

RANGES OF VISION LOSS

The simplest scale, adopted by the WHO in 1974, has three ranges:

1. normal vision (normal and near-normal);
2. low vision (moderate, severe, profound); and
3. blindness (near blindness, total blindness).

Visual disorder	Visual impairment	Visual disability	Visual handicap
← the organ →		← the person →	
Anatomical changes	Functional changes	Skills and abilities	Social and economic consequences
← quality of the eye →		← quality of life →	
Medical and surgical intervention	Visual aids, adapted equipment	Social interventions, training counseling, education	

*An ophthalmologist is quite comfortable dealing with items listed on the left but probably less comfortable dealing with items on the right. Patients need attention to all aspects of their vision loss; ideally, teamwork develops between the different professionals working on the right side: occupational therapists; social workers; nurses (diabetic educators, psychiatric etc.); special education teachers; orientation and mobility specialists.

FIGURE 6–1 Modes of intervention. (From *International Classification of Impairments, Activities and Participation [ICIDH-2-Beta-2]*. Geneva: World Health Organization, under development. Available at www.who.ch/icidh.)

By acknowledging the "low-vision" range,[b] this scale has abandoned the old dichotomy between those who are considered "legally sighted" and those who are considered "legally blind."[c]

---

[b] Gerald Fonda, M.D., started the first Low Vision Service (1953) at the New York Lighthouse and has been credited with coining the term "low vision." The word *low* indicates that it is not normal vision; the word *vision* indicates that it is not blindness. The term has gradually replaced other terms such as "partially sighted," "partially blind," and "residual vision." The revision proposals for the Eye Section of ICD-9 were prepared by the Committee on Information of the International Council of Ophthalmology and the Committee on Terminology of the American Academy of Ophthalmology. They became official when accepted by the World Health Assembly (Geneva, 1976) and also became part of ICD-9-CM in the United States.

[c] For rehabilitation purposes, "blindness" is reserved for total vision loss.

PITFALL

Although labeling (or pronouncing) patients as legally blind may give them certain benefits, it is often counterproductive to efforts to convince them that their remaining vision is still useful. To call a person with severe vision loss "legally blind" is as preposterous as calling a person who is severely ill "legally dead."

For more detailed reporting, the three main ranges can be divided into seven subranges, each equivalent to four lines on a standardized acuity chart[d] (see Table 6–2).

---

[d] Official U.S. Health Care classification ICD-9-CM 3, category 369.

TABLE 6–2   LEVELS OF VISUAL PERFORMANCE AND CORRESPONDING READING AIDS

Classification of Visual Performance		Disability Estimates	Visual Devices for Reading
(Near) normal vision	Normal (20/12, 20/16, 20/20, 20/25)	Normal performance and normal reading distance. (The scale extends beyond 20/20 and "normal" [average] vision is >20/20)	Reading distance ≥33 cm. Regular bifocals (up to 3 D)
	Near normal (20/30, 20/40, 20/50, 20/60)	Individuals can function fairly normally but have no visual reserve. Normal performance using shorter reading distance	Reading distance 33–20 cm. Stronger bifocals (3–5 D). Low-power magnifier (5 D)
Low vision	Moderate low (20/70, 20/80, 20/100, 20/125, 20/160)	Educational assistance is often made available. (Near) normal performance with magnifiers and other devices	Reading distance 16–10 cm. Half eyeglasses (6–10 D) (with prisms for binocularity). Stronger magnifiers (>8 D). Video-magnifier
	Severe low (20/200, 20/250, 20/300, 20/400)	This corresponds to what was previously called "legal blindness" in the United States. Slower than normal with visual devices	Reading distance 8–5 cm (cannot be binocular). High-power reading lens (12–20 D). High-power magnifiers (>16 D). Videomagnifier
	Profound low (20/500, 20/600, 20/800, 20/1000)	This is the "legal blindness" level for many European countries and for the WHO. Reading more laborious with visual devices	Reading distance 4–2 cm (cannot be binocular). High-power reading lens (24–48 D). High-power magnifiers (>28 D). Videomagnifier. Talking books and vision substitution*
Blindness	Near (20/1250, 20/1600, 20/2000, 20/2500)	Vision is unreliable but can still be an adjunct to nonvisual skills	Videomagnifier. Talking books and vision substitution*
Blindness	Total (NLP)	The term "blindness" should be used only for eyes with NLP vision	Talking books and vision substitution*

*Vision substitution is any technique in which a sense other than vision is used to accomplish the task, for example, Braille or using a computer with voice synthesis.

REHABILITATION ISSUES

Ocular trauma most commonly results in monocular, not bilateral, vision loss. However, even minimal monocular impairment can lead to:

- a perceived loss of depth perception; and
- a vague awareness that vision is not what it used to be.

With a significant decrease, especially if the affected eye is the dominant eye, the patient's view of the world can drastically change.

These problems almost invariably improve with time. The visual system has remarkable plasticity even into the geriatric years. With experience, the brain finds innovative ways to interact with the environment. For example, people who previously used *binocular parallax* for stereopsis now use *movement parallax* by shifting their head to left and right to see an object from different viewpoints, or they may turn the object itself.

PEARL... The key to rehabilitation of almost all people with visual impairment, whether monocular or binocular, is not to let them give up. Patients should be strongly encouraged not to stop performing activities they have a reasonable chance of making adaptations for. The old adage "practice makes perfect" definitely applies to the visual system: there are eye surgeons and jewelers who are monocular and golfers who are bilaterally blind.

The effects of ocular trauma on the individual are far greater than just visual impairment (e.g., loss of work or school, restrictions on physical activity during recovery). These can have dramatic effects on the individual even if full visual recovery is eventually achieved. The physician must play an important role in minimizing the negative consequences of the trauma by stating emphatically and repeatedly that normal physical activity can and should be resumed.

REASSURANCE THERAPY

PEARL... Lack of confidence can multiply the functional impact of vision loss. Reassurance therapy should therefore be a part of every ophthalmologist's therapeutic armamentarium by providing a credible and acceptable prognosis (see **Chapters 3** and **5**).

- Be as specific as possible with respect to the patient's particular situation regarding what the patient can and cannot do.
- Seek out and stress all positive aspects.
- Do not volunteer negative and threatening facts unless the patient truly must know them (e.g., informed consent for surgery requires general knowledge that not every operation is successful).
- Be realistic (even somewhat pessimistic): avoid raising the patient's expectations so high that they exceed the physician's ability to deliver (see Chapters 7 and 8).
- Banish unwarranted fears—patients usually imagine that problems are worse than they actually are.
- Be aware of the power of the placebo effect[5] lest you grossly overvalue the effect of your medication or intervention and avoid the negative placebo: it is one of the most toxic and destructive elements in the practice of medicine.
- *Refer the patient to a practitioner who has experience with vision loss.*

PEARL... Having good vision, ophthalmologists probably exaggerate their own fears of vision loss, making it difficult to realize how well patients can cope with the loss. It is very helpful for the physician to visit a local agency for the "blind"; with such personal experience, your subsequent comments to your patients will be much more convincing.

SUMMARY

Traditional eye care treats the eye's anatomic abnormalities; low-vision rehabilitation addresses the consequences. For this, a team approach is needed in which the ophthalmologist is one of several professionals. Such a team must include the patient.

PEARL... In the *traditional* model, the physician is the source of the action while the patient is asked for compliance. In the *rehabilitation* model, the patient is the source of the action while the physician provides guidance.

Rehabilitation training teaches patients how best to use residual vision and offers practical adaptations for activities of daily living. It builds the confidence necessary for ongoing creative problem solving. Even when nothing can be done for the fovea or other eye structures, rehabilitation can do much to improve the individual's life.

PEARL... Ophthalmologists should render care to the *person*,[e] not just to the eyeballs. Every effort should be made to help patients achieve a positive attitude about their ability to use residual vision successfully and live a full and enjoyable life as a visually impaired person. As Victor Frankel said, "everything can be taken from a man but one thing, the last of the human freedoms—to choose one's attitude in any given set of circumstances, to choose one's own way."[6]

[e]Tables 6–3 through 6–5 show the relations between disability of the eye or eyes and disability of the person.

TABLE 6–3 VISUAL ACUITY AND THE CORRESPONDING PERCENTAGES OF CENTRAL VISION LOSS

Visual Acuity			Loss of Central Vision (%)
English	Metric 6	Metric 4	
20/15	6/5	4/3	0
20/20	6/6	4/4	0
20/25	6/7.5	4/5	5
20/30	6/10	4/6	10
20/40	6/12	4/8	15
20/50	6/15	4/10	25
20/60	6/20	4/12	35
20/70	6/22	4/14	40
20/80	6/24	4/16	45
20/100	6/30	4/20	50
20/125	6/38	4/25	60
20/150	6/50	4/30	70
20/200	6/60	4/40	80
20/300	6/90	4/60	85
20/400	6/120	4/80	90
20/800	6/240	4/160	95

TABLE 6–4 PERCENTAGES OF VISUAL SYSTEM IMPAIRMENT IN RELATION TO IMPAIRMENT OF THE WHOLE PERSON

Visual System	Whole Person	Visual System	Whole Person	Visual System	Whole Person	Visual System	Whole Person	Visual System	Whole Person	Visual System	Whole Person
0	0	15	15	30	28	45	42	60	57	75	71
1	1	16	15	31	29	46	43	61	58	76	72
2	2	17	16	32	30	47	44	62	59	77	73
3	3	18	17	33	31	48	45	63	59	78	74
4	4	19	18	34	32	49	46	64	60	79	75
5	5	20	19	35	33	50	47	65	61	80	76
6	6	21	20	36	34	51	48	66	62	81	76
7	7	22	21	37	35	52	49	67	63	82	77
8	8	23	22	38	36	53	50	68	64	83	78
9	8	24	23	39	37	54	51	69	65	84	79
10	9	25	24	40	38	55	52	70	66	85	80
11	10	26	25	41	39	56	53	71	67	86	81
12	11	27	25	42	40	57	54	72	68	87	82
13	12	28	26	43	41	58	55	73	69	88	83
14	13	29	27	44	42	59	56	74	70	89	84
										90–100	85

Table 6–5 Loss of Eye Versus Impairment Of The Visual System and Impairment Of The Whole Person

	Impairment of The Visual System (%)	Impairment of The Whole Person (%)
Total loss of vision, one eye	25	24
Total loss of vision, both eyes	100	85

References

1. Colenbrander A. Dimensions of visual performance, Low Vision Symposium, American Academy of Ophthalmology. *Trans Am Acad Ophthalmol Otolaryngol.* 1977;83:332–337.

2. *International Classification of Diseases, 9th Revision—Clinical Modification (ICD-9-CM).* 1st ed. Ann Arbor, Mich: Commission on Professional and Hospital Activities; 1978. Later editions by U.S. Public Health Service, 1980 and by Med-Index, 1991.

3. *International Classification of Diseases, 9th Revision (ICD-9).* Geneva: World Health Organization; 1977.

4. *International Classification of Impairments, Disabilities and Handicaps.* Geneva: World Health Organization; 1980.

5. Havener W. *Low Vision Rehabilitation—Caring for the Whole Person.* Chapter 8. American Academy of Ophthalmology. Monograph 12.

6. Frankel V. *Man's Search for Meaning.* 4th ed. Boston: Beacon Press; 1992.

Chapter 7

MEDICOLEGAL ISSUES

Wesley D. Blakeslee

 This chapter, based on the United States legal system, reviews ocular trauma surgery-related medicolegal issues from two perspectives: that of the physician as *defendant* and as *expert witness*. Both arise from the physician's obligation to provide quality and competent care. While the role as surgeon and healer is most important for the patient's well-being, the physician's significance as authority and expert witness must be neither overlooked nor minimized.

In many cases, liability or compensation remains irrelevant, but if compensation becomes an issue, the surgeon's role as witness often substantially affects the patient.

PROFESSIONAL LIABILITY

The legal definition of negligence is *the doing of an act (or an omission) that a reasonably prudent person under the same circumstances would not do (or fail to do).*

PITFALL

Medical negligence is the failure of the physician to act in accordance with ordinary medical care and skill.

The physician must act as any reasonably competent physician would act under the same circumstances, which will vary depending on factors such as specialization, the availability of facilities, and advances in the profession.

To maintain a successful claim of negligence, the plaintiff must show that:

- the physician failed to adhere to the standard of medical skill and care ordinarily exercised in similar circumstances[1,a]; and that
- the physicians' failure to observe the proper standard of care was a direct cause of the injuries of which the patient complains in the malpractice action.[2]

Although the law provides special rules in emergency situations, the physician must still provide care in accordance with the standard of medical skill and care ordinarily exercised in emergencies.[3]

Because medical negligence claims are based upon a failure to adhere to a medical standard of which the trier of fact (judge or jury) has no knowledge, the establishment of a claim virtually always requires the testimony of an expert witness on behalf of the plaintiff, with rebuttal by an expert witness of the defendant. Although treatises and textbooks may be introduced to describe the standard or rebut an expressed opinion, the standard of care and whether there has been a breach of that standard is dependent upon expert testimony.

---

[a]A specialist in a full-facility metropolitan medical center will generally be held to a higher degree of skill than a general surgeon called upon to perform emergency surgery in a rural hospital with minimal equipment. Some states in the United States use a locality rule that requires the proof of care and skill in the particular locality, but the majority rule is that a *global general standard of care* is applied.

Sources of Litigation in Ocular Trauma

Informed Consent

The physician owes the patient the duty to properly inform[b] or advise of the potential risks of any medical treatment and to obtain consent for any procedure contemplated.[c] The disclosure must include:

- the diagnosis made by the physician;
- the nature and purpose of any proposed treatment;
- the risks and consequence of the treatment (including other risks associated with the surgical procedure, such as those of anesthesia);
- feasible treatment alternatives; and
- the prognosis if the treatment is not undertaken.[5]

The typical informed consent claim arises when a known serious consequence occurs of which the patient claims not to have been informed. To prevail, the patient must satisfy the trier of fact that had he been forewarned of the consequence, he would not have undergone the procedure.

▼ PITFALL

Informed consent claims are not common in emergency surgeries where there is only one logical course to take (e.g., intraocular foreign body removal)[d]: the patient can hardly argue that surgery would have been refused had he been told of the potential complication. However, secondary reconstructive surgery often presents more than one choice. If the particular course taken results in a devastating complication of which the patient was not warned, malpractice action is likely.

Defective eyewear

Defective eyewear that fails to protect from a known hazardous condition may result in a claim against the medical practitioner who prescribed it (e.g., to prevent

sports-related injuries). The physician who supplies safety eyewear must be familiar with its types and the safety standards that apply.[e] If the product itself is defective, the manufacturer will likely be the primary target, but the medical practitioner may be brought in under a number of theories. Such claims may include:

- failure to prescribe appropriate lens material (i.e., polycarbonate);
- failure to warn not only concerning the material but also of the fact that injuries can still occur while wearing safety glasses; and
- failure to inspect the eyewear prescribed.[6–10]

Improper or Incomplete Localization or Removal of IOFBs

The sources of litigation include:

- failure to use proper available equipment resulting in failure to find the IOFB;
- incorrect location of the IOFB; and
- failure to remove *all* particles if multiple IOFBs are present.[10,11]

Equipment Usage and Failure

The physician should:

- always use the diagnostic tools reasonably necessary and which are available;
- have knowledge of the limitations and proper use of the equipment;
- be cognizant of the ability of the staff to operate specialized equipment; and
- train new residents and staff in the usage of the equipment.

PEARL... Equipment failure is not the fault of the physician. Always retain the failed part and follow up on the diagnosis of the failure: it may provide a defense in a resulting claim.[12]

Failure to Diagnose and Delay in Diagnosis

The nature of the emergency situation and the overwhelming demands upon the physician may lead to a *failure to diagnose*, especially because some complications may initially be obscured by others.

Delay in diagnosis is another frequent source of claims (e.g., the injury does not appear to be an emergency; the patient does not present immediately but contacts the physicians' office for an appointment).

---

[b]In some states, verbal and written consent is required prior to health care delivery via telemedicine; a sample document may be downloaded from www.omic.com

[c]"Every human being of adult years and sound mind has a right to determine what shall be done with his own body; and a surgeon who performs an operation without his patient's consent, commits an assault, for which he is liable in damages" (Justice Benjamin Cardozo, then on the Court of Appeals of New York).[4]

[d]See Chapter 24 on whether IOFB surgery is indeed an *emergency* in all cases.

[e]Such standards will likely be introduced in litigation and used to assess the suitability of the eyewear in question.

Failure to Warn of Future Complications

Many conditions (e.g., cataract, retinal detachment) may develop years following the trauma. Proper follow-up must be arranged by the initial treating physician (see Chapter 8) or the patient must be clearly warned and instructed to be reexamined for that particular possibility.[12]

Anesthesia

Significant eye injuries and claims have been reported in association with anesthesia. Patient movement during ophthalmic surgery represented 30% of the claims in one study, resulting in blindness in all cases with significant awards.[13] Although problems due to anesthesia may not directly involve the ophthalmologist, use of an anesthesiologist with a known history of problems may be considered as negligence in itself.[12]

Retrobulbar Injection

Penetration of the globe during retrobulbar injection is uncommon, but it often leads to malpractice claims. Use of a blunt needle and being aware of the possibility, particularly in high-risk cases, may reduce the incidence of this complication.[14]

PREVENTING CLAIMS[f]

Making an Assessment of the Injury and a Reasonable Prognosis

Injury often leads to significant loss of vision in eyes with good prior vision. Consequently, the patient's lifestyle is greatly altered and employment opportunities are also diminished (see Chapter 6). Particularly when the cause of the injury is not compensable, the patient may look to the eye surgeon to find fault and obtain compensation. It is therefore of extreme importance to (see Chapters 3 and 5 for additional details):

- advise the patient as soon as possible of the potential for permanent impairment;
- avoid giving false hope ("complete or near-complete recovery")[10];
- establish a good physician-patient relationship, which can often prevent a claim from being brought even when the visual outcome is poor;

[f]Bad medical results result in good malpractice cases.

- treat the patient with care, compassion, and respect; and
- provide thorough explanations of the eye's condition.

Medical Records

A complete, legible, and accurate medical record may be the best defense in a malpractice action.

PITFALL

A physician should *never* alter or rewrite a record, particularly following an adverse result or hint of a malpractice action. Nothing solidifies the belief of wrongdoing in the juror's mind better than showing that the physician tried to cover up the wrongdoing by changing the record.

If an addendum to the record is absolutely necessary, the physician should:
- clearly explain why the information (addendum) was not part of the original record;
- add it immediately after the event or when the physician is presented with the typewritten record and realizes that additional information is needed; and
- date and sign it.[15]

Videotaping

At present, there are no statistical analyses of the effect of surgical videotapes on malpractice claims. It appears, however, that videotaping of surgeries will not be beneficial to defendants in most malpractice litigation.

> **PEARL...** Malpractice cases are battles of experts, with the standard of care being expressed by the plaintiff's expert(s). However, as the plaintiff's experts were not present during the surgery and will be able to testify only from the record, a videotape provides a powerful weapon (i.e., more ammunition) for the plaintiff's experts to find fault with the technique and procedures as they are recorded. The experts can challenge the description of conditions encountered by the operating physician, as the videotape provides a picture to accompany the description.[g]

The Physician as an Expert

The majority of workplace injuries are subject to workers' compensation benefits. Many transportation[h] incidents involve issues of compensation. Many injuries involving failure of safety glasses result in claims for compensation either as product liability or as malpractice in the prescribing of the glasses.[7–9]

Expert Opinions of the Treating Physician

In compensable cases, medical expert opinion is generally needed to establish causation between, and the nature and extent of, permanent impairment and the injury. The manner in which the physician describes the injury may have a great impact on the patient's ability to obtain fair compensation.

---

[g] In one reported opinion, it was the plaintiff who wanted the videotape and the defense that fought to keep the tape from being produced, suggesting just such a result.[16] Although the court in that case held that a videotape of an operation was not a medical record (as defined by statute) that would have allowed the patient to get a copy of the record *prior to* litigation for the purpose of framing the issues in a malpractice suit, that result is not likely to be universal. That case specifically did not involve discovery *after* suit is filed, which is certain to be permitted in most jurisdictions.

[h] The NETS found that 21% of open globe injuries occur at the workplace and 8% involve transportation[17]; data from the USEIR are very similar: 18% at the workplace and 10% on streets and highway.

> **PEARL...** Causation between eye damage and the trauma is seldom in doubt, but subsequent complications (e.g., cataract, retinal detachment) may not be so obvious. Even when obvious, an expression of the causal connection is still necessary for the patient to receive compensation.

Physicians should be aware of the evidentiary requirements in their own jurisdiction regarding the manner in which opinions must be expressed. In most jurisdictions, an opinion must be expressed in reasonable medical certainty or a reasonable medical probability.[18–21] In some jurisdictions these have the same meaning, whereas in others the term *certainty* must be used. An opinion that something is *possibly* caused by, or *may be* caused by, is generally insufficient to establish the causal connection between the incident and the injury; use of such language can needlessly undermine the patient's claim.

If a complication may develop later, expressing this possibility as "a retinal detachment may occur in the future" is of little help to the patient.[6] Instead, the physician can state that the injury has placed the patient, with reasonable medical certainty, at greater risk of a future retina detachment. Alternatively, the physician can express with reasonable medical certainty which future complications are likely to occur and the treatment required. This provides an accurate assessment of the nature of the injury and the effect on the patient that can be evaluated and compensated.

> **PEARL...** In most workers' compensation claims, disability is awarded when disability occurs; additional award can be made in the future when and if an additional disability arises. However, in a liability claim, the patient has only one opportunity to either settle or litigate the case, and all damages must be concluded in that litigation or settlement.

Nature and Extent of Permanent Impairment

The nature and extent of permanent impairment are typically measured in cases of loss of visual acuity and impairment of visual field.

However, a patient can suffer additional complications such as:

- diplopia;
- reduction in reading speed;
- increased fatigue and/or headache; and
- cosmetic impairment.

In preparing reports of the patient's injuries caused by the trauma, the physician should not overlook these conditions but should make a fair and reasonable assessment of the nature and extent of the permanent impairment. It is also important to express the opinion in the required language (e.g., "with reasonable medical certainty") in situations in which the patient's condition may improve.

Workers' Compensation Issues

Physicians are typically well aware of the broad control of the physician-client relationship that is typical of workers' compensation statutes. There may be a prescribed fee schedule regulating what may be charged for services. Often specialized reports must be prepared and filed with the state, the employer, and the insurer. Although most physicians learn these rules out of business necessity, many fail to learn the manner in which the workers' compensation statute determines benefits.

In most states, eyes are referred to as "scheduled members," which have a specific measure of compensation based on the percentage of loss of visual acuity and visual field. Related effects may be compensated as part of the eye or as a separate impairment. Workers' compensation statutes often contain thresholds, the crossing of which substantially increases the payment to the injured worker (see Table 7–1).

TABLE 7–1 THE RELATIONSHIP BETWEEN PERCENTAGE OF VISION LOSS AND COMPENSATION*

Percentage of Loss of Vision	Permanent Disability Payment ($)
30	8,550
31	16,458
99	52,328
100	140,614

*From the State of Maryland; the employee makes $631 per week injured on or after January 1, 2000.

PITFALL

The preparing of reports and expressing opinions for patients is often viewed as an annoyance by busy physicians, and the task is commonly delegated to others in the office. The physician must understand that lack of diligence in preparing records or reports and in expressing opinions can have a serious impact on patients. It can also result in a successful malpractice claim against the physician who acts without proper regard for the patient.[12]

REFERENCES

1. *Malpractice-Care-non Local Testimony*, 37 ALR 3rd 420 (1971). Contrast *Dunham v Elder*, 18 Md App. 360, 306 A2d 568 (1973) with *Shilkret v Annapolis Emergency Hospital Association*, 276 Md 187, 349 A2d 245 (1975).
2. *Johns Hopkins Hospital v Genda*, 355 Md 616, 258 A2d 595 (1969).
3. Grove AS Jr. Legal aspects of ocular trauma. *Int Ophthalmol Clin*. 1974;14:193–203.
4. *Schloendorff v The Society of the New York Hospital*, 211 NY 125; 105 NE 92 (1914).
5. Rosoffs AJ. Informed consent in the electronic age, 25 *Am J Law Med*. 367, 1999.
6. Classe JG. Legal aspects of sports vision. *Optom Clin*. 1993;3:27–32.
7. Classe JG. Legal aspects of sports-related ocular injuries. *Int Ophthalmol Clin*. 1998;28:211–214.
8. Kaplan PJ. Ocular sports injuries. Legal aspects. I. Patients perspective. *Int Ophthalmol Clin*. 1981;21:203–207.
9. Hinson DB. Ocular sports injuries. Legal aspects. II. Lawyers perspective. *Int Ophthalmol Clin*. 1981;21;209–218.
10. Bettman JW. A review of 412 claims in ophthalmology. *Int Ophthalmol Clin*. 1980;20:131–142.
11. Bettman, JW. Seven hundred medicolegal cases in ophthalmology. *Ophthalmology*. 1990;97:1379–1384.
12. Bettman JW. How to reduce medicolegal involvement in cases of trauma. *Ophthalmology*. 1980;87:432–434.
13. Gild WM, Posner KL, Caplan RA, Cheney FW. Eye injuries associated with anesthesia. A closed claims analysis. *Anesthesiology*. 1992;76:204–208.
14. Boniuk V, Nockowitz R. Perforation of the globe during retrobulbar injection: medicolegal aspects of four cases. *Surv Ophthalmol*. 1994;39:141–145.
15. Jenkins PA, Gorney M. Accurate medical records your first line of defense. The Doctors Company Risk Management Handbook. 1999. Available at: http://www.the-doctors.com/Resources/Handbook/Handbook99/index_accurate.htm. Accessed September 6, 2000.
16. *Hill v Sprenger*, 132 Misc2d 1012, 506 NY S2d 255 (1986).
17. Parver LM, Dannenberg AL, Blacklow B, Fowler CJ, Brechner RJ, Tielsch JM. *Characteristics and Causes of Penetrating Eye Injuries Reported to the National Eye Trauma System Registry, 1985–91*. US Department of Health and Human Services; Public Health Reports; Sep-Oct 1993;108:625–632.
18. *Bentley v Carroll*, 355 Md 312; 734 A2d 697 (1999).
19. *Loretta Jones Murray, Executrix and Personal Representative of the Estate of Weston Murray, Deceased v United States of America*, 215 F3d 460 (4th Cir. 2000).
20. *Boyd v Baeppler*, 215 F3d 594 (6th Cir. 2000).
21. *Henderson v Sheahan*, 196 F3d 839 (7th Cir. 1999).

Chapter 8

DESIGNING THE MANAGEMENT STRATEGY

Ferenc Kuhn

 Treating a patient with eye injury requires specific knowledge of the anatomy, physiology, and pathophysiology of all tissues of the globe; surgical expertise or manual skills do not by themselves suffice. It is equally important, though rarely discussed in the literature, for the ophthalmologist to develop *strategic thinking* so that a systematic philosophy is utilized in every case, even if the injured eye presents unique difficulties for which no published recommendation is available.

> **PEARL...** Strategy is the general foundation based on which the specifics (tactics, plan) are developed.

This chapter provides an overview of the fundamentals in strategic thinking, based on which surgeons can develop their own, individualized approach.

> **PEARL...** The goal is more than optimal treatment of the injured eye; it is treatment of a *person* who has a traumatized organ. Ophthalmologists dealing with ocular trauma are not "tissue reconstruction specialists" but *physicians*.

When designing the strategy (plan) to treat the eye's specific injuries, the surgeon must understand that the relationship between the injured person and the ophthalmologist is one of *chance*, not of choice as with that of patients who present for elective surgery.

The ophthalmologist's (and the medical staff's) attitude, behavior, words, and metacommunication determine whether the patient develops sufficient confidence and trust in the treating physician—without which it is much more difficult to involve the patient as a *partner*.

The "partnership" is crucial because the patient is commonly:

- asked to follow instructions such as positioning after intravitreal gas injection;
- required to take *all* prescribed medications for *extended* periods of time *exactly* as directed; and, most importantly,
- involved in the decision-making process itself, helping to determine whether one procedure or another should be performed or whether the eye should be removed rather than reconstructed.

Proper communication with the patient requires the ophthalmologist to explain:

- the management options and their risks versus benefits and the short- and long-term implications, including a carefully pessimistic estimation of the final outcome;
- the potential for multiple surgeries;
- the potential for visual rehabilitation services;
- the advantages of safety eyewear; and
- the need for periodic follow-ups even if full vision has been restored (see Chapters 3, 5, and 6 for further details).

Such systematic thinking will result in the development of the best possible management plan (see Sections II through VI for the specifics of treating the individual tissue injuries).

HISTORY AND EVALUATION

Appropriate plans are impossible to design unless the ophthalmologist has a fairly accurate knowledge of:

- how the injury occurred; and
- what its consequences are (i.e., which tissues are involved and to what extent).

It is also mandatory to know whether the injured eye had prior surgery; for instance when struck by blunt force, eyes with ECCE or RK[1] wounds can rupture years after the procedure.[a]

The details of evaluating the injured patient and eye are presented in Chapters 9 and 10 with additional details in the appropriate chapters. Here we emphasize only a few fundamental rules:

- in conscious and cooperating patients, always assess the visual acuity in *both* eyes, one eye at a time;
- avoid inflicting iatrogenic damage (e.g., extrusion of intraocular tissues) to the eye (e.g., by forceful opening of the lids in children who *will not* or in adults who *cannot* obey instructions);

---

[a] This highlights the need for correct patient information when seeking consent for such elective surgeries (see Chapter 27).

[b] Accurate details (i.e., all the necessary information) will be obtained under microscopic examination of the anesthetized patient.

[c] Also keep in mind your country's legal environment; see Chapter 7 regarding documentation.

- once the diagnosis of an open globe injury requiring surgery is made, delay determining nonsignificant details until the patient is asleep[b];
- order only those diagnostic tests that are essential[c];
- document your oral communications with the patient and all details of the injury, especially if the incident occurred at the workplace using
  - drawings (e.g., show the location and extent of the eyewall's wound; Fig. 8–1);
  - pre- and postoperative photographs; and
  - intraoperative video or videos (see Chapter 7 for the potential drawback);
- try to have a witness present throughout your discussions with the patient; because of their understandable anxiety, patients frequently do not remember what they were told or remember inaccurately.

> **P**EARL... **Do not order tests whose results will not influence your subsequent treatment decisions. Conversely, the results of radiological tests should be checked by the ophthalmologist.**

Proper documentation is critical for treatment, research, and legal purposes and in case of referral. If you participate in a surveillance system such as the USEIR, it is wise to instruct your staff to attach the initial reporting form to every trauma chart. If you see many patients with eye injuries but are not part of a data collection system, you should consider joining or establishing one (see Chapters 4 and 9) or at least designing a special chart for trauma patients.

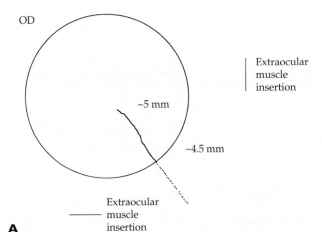

A

OD

~5 mm

~4.5 mm

Extraocular
muscle
insertion

Extraocular
muscle
insertion

The irregular wound starts somewhat nasally from the corneal epicenter in the right eye. It spreads toward and crosses the limbus at 5 o'clock. As the conjunctiva is dissected, a continuation of the wound onto the sclera is seen in almost a straight line. The wound's corneal length is approximately 5 mm, the scleral is approximately 4.5 mm, possibly extending over the anterior retina.

B

FIGURE 8–1   The power of a simple drawing **(A)** versus a lengthy description **(B)**.

Traditional versus Planned Approach to Eye Trauma

According to the *traditional* concept, surgeons operating on injured eyes should proceed in a sequential fashion, reacting to the actual situation (as determined by the trauma as well as by the body's reaction to the injury and to the applied therapeutic measures; see Fig. 8–2A). This approach requires:

- assessing the injury's consequences;
- performing certain manipulations as appropriate;
- reassessing the eye's condition;
- performing additional manipulations as appropriate; and
- repeating the process as many times as needed.

Example: eye with penetrating injury caused by a wire at the home; mild traumatic cataract with a large anterior capsule rupture; significant vitreous hemorrhage. This eye would undergo (1) primary wound closure, (2) secondary surgery with cataract removal (possibly with IOL implantation), (3) simultaneous or delayed vitreous hemorrhage removal if no sign of spontaneous resorption of the blood is seen after a few months, (4) treatment of retinal pathology if necessary, and (5) restoration of the lost refractive power if IOL implantation has not been performed earlier.

This traditional thinking is best characterized by the analogy of a person climbing a tree and making decisions "on the go" regarding which branch to step onto next. This traditional approach is not entirely wrong—but it forces the surgeon to view the restoration process as a series of individual surgical tasks as they emerge with time: the surgeon remains *passive*.

An alternative, *strategically planned* approach involves thinking "backwards from the desired endpoint" (see Fig. 8–2B) based on the following order of goals:

- full restoration of the eye's visual functions;
- partial restoration of the eye's visual functions if the former is impossible; or
- full restoration of the eye's normal anatomy (even if no visual function is achievable), depending on
  - comfort;
  - cosmesis; and
  - the patient's desire or decision when all factors, including SO (see Chapter 29), have been taken into consideration.

In the preceding example, the eye would undergo wound closure with cataract and vitreous hemorrhage removal to allow examination of the retina and treatment of any pathologic condition that requires intervention. IOL implanta-

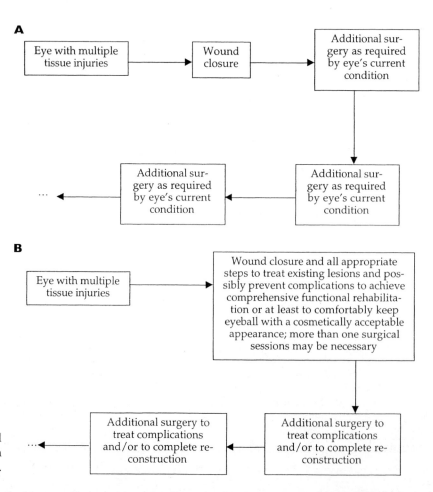

FIGURE 8–2 The traditional **(A)** and the suggested **(B)** way of thinking in approaching the eye with an eye injury.

tion would be performed if further vitreoretinal intervention appears unlikely (see Chapter 21) *and the IOL power can reasonably be determined.* (Alternatively, all steps beyond wound toilette and closure may be performed a few days later—see below.)

A person with this conceptual thinking, when trying to climb a tree, would inspect the tree and design a plan, selecting from the ground a route that appears to offer the safest way to reach the highest possible altitude. Obviously, during the actual climb, the original plan may have to be modified, just as the surgeon must remain flexible to alter the initial strategy should the eye's actual condition warrant it.

At first, there may not appear to be a tangible difference between these two approaches. However, the second concept requires that the ophthalmologist play an *active* role, appreciating the eye's condition in a comprehensive way.

> **P**EARL... An injured globe should be considered as a polytraumatized organ: a certain tissue injury may affect the condition of other tissues.

In the example, the ophthalmologist whose approach is based on strategic thinking would review the following: the lens injury makes it likely that the cataract will not remain stationary, the presence of vitreous hemorrhage in case of a penetrating injury significantly increases the chance of tractional retinal detachment,[2] and there is a measurable risk of direct retinal injury. It is therefore advisable to remove all media opacity early to allow direct inspection of the retina by the surgeon to determine whether and what kind of intervention is necessary to keep the retina attached and achieve early and maximal visual rehabilitation.

This planned approach also requires immediate steps for low-vision rehabilitation (see Chapter 6) if the eye's condition leaves no hope for significant functional improvement (see Chapter 3), e.g., a macular impact site is found during surgery in the example above.

THE SURGEON: KNOW YOUR CAPABILITIES *AND* LIMITATIONS

Reconstruction of a traumatized globe can be a complex procedure; life does not recognize artificial boundaries such as "anterior" versus "posterior" segment. If an ophthalmologist cannot address all treatable lesions (see Table 8–1), it is usually preferable not to perform any surgery but to *refer* the patient. To decide in favor of intervention, the physician must have adequate *experience* and *expertise* as well as access to the required *equipment* and *personnel* and *facility*.

If any one of these is missing, deferral or referral is probably a better option for both ophthalmologist and

patient. Do not attempt, for instance, to remove traumatic cataracts if vitrectomy instrumentation is unavailable[d] or you have no experience in its use; do not try to close corneal/scleral wounds if a good microscope is not available. Violation of these basic rules can worsen the eye's condition. Before deciding to "go in", the ophthalmologist should do a brief (self) assessment.

> **P**EARL... The most fundamental rule in the treatment of an injured globe: *If you can't, don't.*

> **PITFALL**
>
> An error all too commonly seen is the "forced" use of the technique a surgeon is most familiar or comfortable with instead of using the technique most suitable to solve the particular problem (i.e., trying to adopt the eye to the intervention rather than selecting the technique with the highest success rate). *Typical examples: the application of phacoemulsification to remove a traumatic cataract despite the risk of vitreous prolapse (instead of using vitrectomy instrumentation); prophylactic blind cryopexy of a scleral wound[e] (instead of removing the vitreous hemorrhage to inspect the retina underneath the wound and applying laser if a retinal break is present).*

Conversely, an ophthalmologist is rightly called a "trauma expert" if possessing sufficient expertise in treating all globe injuries.

An institution is de facto an eye trauma center if the following are in place:

- appropriate on-call system with all specialists available;
- complete technical infrastructure;
- data collection system (tracking both epidemiological and clinical information);
- active pursuit (follow-up) of all accessible patients; and
- continual quality control process with periodical external reviews.

---

[d]Unless you are absolutely certain that the posterior lens capsule is intact and no vitreous prolapse is present (see Chapter 21).

[e]Blind application of cryopexy is especially harmful; in addition, the cryospot's size on the sclera is irrelevant in judging spot size on the retina because tissues have different moisture content and the blood-rich choroid also plays a role.

TABLE 8-1   SURGICAL OPTIONS IN THE TREATMENT OF INJURED EYES*

Procedure	Example
Reappose/reattach	Closure of corneal wound/retinal detachment
Reformat	Injection of BSS into the AC
Remove/excise	Traumatic cataract/prolapsed uvea
Reduce	SCH
Replace	Vitreous with air
Reposition	Prolapsed uvea/dislocated IOL
Seal	Retinal break
Reconstruct[†]	Anterior segment

*Breaking down the four basic elements in surgery (excisional; reconstructive; transplant; inductive).
[†]May be a combination of all of the above.

RECONSTRUCTION VERSUS ENUCLEATION:[f] THE SIGNIFICANCE OF NLP VISION

Enucleation is a point of no return. Ophthalmologists rarely review enucleated eyes with the pathologist, although such clinicopathologic correlations should be routinely performed and would reduce unindicated removals of eyes.[g]

Truly *medical* reasons to perform primary enucleation are very few:

- when the eye is destroyed or cannot be reconstructed anatomically (i.e., wound or wounds are too large and posterior) and/or
- most of the globe's contents, including a substantial portion of the retina, are lost, leaving no hope for any function.

> **PEARL...** Loss of light perception in the immediate postinjury period does *not* by itself justify enucleation. We have found that of NLP eyes reconstructed on the basis of the ophthalmologist's judgment (i.e., excluding eyes reconstructed solely because of the patient's request), 64% improved.[3] Even a preoperatively nonrecordable bright-flash ERG is compatible with visual recovery if appropriate and timely reconstruction is persued.[3]

Several reversible factors may be responsible for NLP initial vision:

- media opacity (corneal edema, hyphema,[4] cataract,[5] vitreous hemorrhage[h]);
- retinal edema (commotio retinae);
- retinal detachment/subretinal hemorrhage; and
- the patient's mental condition.

> **PEARL...** No eye in the first few weeks after an injury should be enucleated based solely on its inability to detect light or because "the globe appears so badly damaged." Patients can be offered exploration and direct inspection by the vitreoretinal surgeon as a decision point.

It must also be mentioned that even in cases of TON being responsible for NLP vision, treatment, rather than abandonment, is recommended (see Chapter 37).

Secondary enucleation may be performed if:

- the eye chronically and despite reconstruction efforts remains NLP; *and*
- the risk of SO is determined to be higher than usual (see Chapter 29).

Even if this is the case, the ophthalmologist must, however, discuss all options with the patient, and not simply "prescribe" eye removal. Most patients prefer

---

[f]See Chapter 31 for decision making as to whether enucleation or evisceration should be performed.

[g]In a review of pathological specimens of ruptured eyes enucleated because they were NLP, we found retinal or optic nerve injury incompatible with *visual* recovery in only 50% of the cases.[2]

[h]We have found experimentally that even small amounts of blood in the vitreous can block 97% of incoming light from reaching the macula.[2]

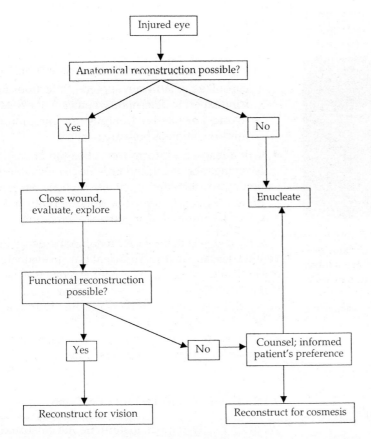

FIGURE 8–3 Decision making: enucleation or reconstruction? Note that NLP is not a decisive factor in designing the management strategy. Anatomical reconstruction is defined as a globe whose external integrity has been restored (i.e., wound or wounds closed with most of the intraocular contents preserved).

retaining the reconstructed eye to enucleation[i] (see Fig. 8–3), which has tremendous psychological implications (see "The Patient's Perspective").

Finally, the country's legal environment (see Chapter 7) must be kept in mind. This may tempt physicians to justify removal, instead of reconstruction, of the injured eye—even if no hard evidence from the literature supports this practice. The conceptual differences in management strategy are clearly reflected in the following enucleation rates[j]:

- 18%[6] among American servicemen in Desert Storm (1991), 21% in Vietnam,[7] as opposed to 10%[8] in the Six-Day Israeli-Arab war (1967; vitrectomy was not yet available)
- 5.5%[9] in Senegal and 6%[10] in Cameroon, as opposed to 14.2%[11] in Finland and 12.3%[12] in the United Kingdom;
- 12% in the USEIR, as opposed to <1% in the HEIR.

It is a general philosophy in both Hungary and Israel[13] not to remove blind eyes on the basis of a fear

of SO. It must also be mentioned that only two cases of SO were reported after the Second World War and none in the Korean, three Israeli-Arab (Six-Day, Yom Kippur, Lebanon), Vietnam, Iran-Iraq, and Desert Storm wars.[14]

OPEN VERSUS CLOSED GLOBE INJURY; INTERVENTION VERSUS REFERRAL

Open globe injuries usually require wound closure. Even when the wound is small and self-sealing,[k] closure may be required if there is a risk of late reopening (e.g., during vitrectomy).

Closure of corneal (and to a lesser extent scleral) wounds must be:

- nontraumatic;
- anatomic; and
- watertight (see Chapters 14 through 16 and the Appendix).

The attending ophthalmologist must decide whether to perform the operation and how urgently, or whether to refer the patient. Eyes with a protruding IOFB

---

[i]Assuming that the eye has a reasonable chance of comfort and acceptable cosmesis.

[j]The criteria for which cases were included in the study may also have been different.

[k]Try Seidel's test using a 2% sterile fluorescein strip to determine whether the wound leaks (see Chapter 9).

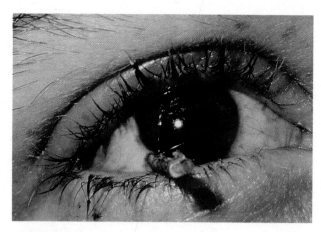

FIGURE 8-4   A nail has lodged in the eye. Removing it in an uncontrolled fashion (e.g., pulling it out without general anesthesia and a careful evaluation of the nail's internal position as well as the injuries it may have caused) may result in additional, iatrogenic trauma. It is best to refer the child to the closest facility where comprehensive management is available. The child must be immobilized while in transit.

(see Fig. 8-4) are usually better off without the attending ophthalmologist's removal attempt (see Chapter 24).

THE RULES OF TRANSPORTATION

If it is decided that the patient is best referred and transported to a facility where the chances of proper management are better, keep in mind the following.

- Shield[l] the eye appropriately (see Chapter 14); in children, sedation or securing of the hands may also be necessary (see Chapters 9 and 30).
- Use systemic (*never p. os*) medication as necessary against pain, nausea and coughing, high blood pressure, and extreme anxiety.
- It is usually *not* necessary to start antibiotic therapy.
- Tetanus prophylaxis[m] is appropriate, especially if the injury involves high risk. The type of injection depends on both the immunization history of the patient (the recommendations also vary by country) and the type of injury.[n] It is best to:

  - take the patient's vaccination history regarding past tetanus shots (i.e., whether active immunization has been completed and whether and when booster shots have been administered); and to
  - consult a pediatrician/surgeon/infectious medicine expert to determine whether active (tetanus toxoid) or passive (tetanus immunoglobulin) immunization or both are needed.

- Call ahead and inform the colleague or institute receiving the patient, and provide as much information as possible; document all you have observed/done and send along the documentation (e.g., CT scans, rather than just the test's reading).

Closed globe injuries rarely require emergency intervention. Usually there is sufficient time to evaluate the eye and seek consultation even if the retina is detached (functional recovery is not expected to be adversely affected if the retina will be reattached within a few days[15]) or the IOP is elevated and hyphema/lens swelling is present (no permanent damage occurs with timely intervention; see Chapters 17 and 20).

THE TIMING OF INTERVENTION

Wounds rarely require instantaneous closure. It is usually preferable to wait a few hours until appropriate expertise/equipment/personnel are available or to refer the patient to a facility where these requirements are met—especially because the initial intervention may involve much more than the introduction of stitches. Hastily and improperly closed wounds not only may need to be resutured[o] but can cause additional harm, for example, by increasing corneal decompensation. The risk of endophthalmitis does not significantly increase in the first 24[16] or even 36[17] hours, although special attention should be given to eyes that are at high risk. Table 8-2 provides a few guidelines.

ANESTHESIA[p]

When treating (occasionally, as mentioned earlier, evaluating) the patient with (suspected) eye injury, the patient must:

- feel no pain;
- be in stable condition; and

---

[l]Because it increases anxiety, bilateral shielding is not recommended unless serious bilateral open injuries are present.

[m]See also the Appendix.

[n]Lacerations are much more dangerous than ruptures; small (punctate) wounds are worse than large wounds; the risk also increases if there is contamination by soil, vegetable matter, or manure.

---

[o]In a consecutive series of eyes with ruptures, we found that resuturing was necessary in 18% (V. Mester and F. Kuhn, unpublished data from the HEIR).

[p]The author wishes to thank Ronald H. Vinik, MD (Birmingham, AL), for his invaluable contribution to this section.

TABLE 8-2 THE TIMING OF INTERVENTION IN TRAUMA INVOLVING THE GLOBE*

Timing	Condition	See Further Details in
Absolute emergencies	Chemical injury (alkali > acid)	Chapter 11
	ECH	Chapter 22
	Appearance of intraocular gas bubble†	Reference 23
	Orbital abscess	Chapter 12
	Vision loss due to expanding orbital hemorrhage	Chapters 12 and 36
Urgent	High-risk IOFB	Chapter 24
	Endophthalmitis	Chapter 28
≤24 hours	IOFB‡	Chapter 24
	Open wounds requiring surgical closure	Chapters 14 and 15; Appendix
Within a few days (24 to 72 hours preferred)	Medically uncontrollable IOP elevation in the presence of hyphema	Chapters 17 and 20
	Medically uncontrollable IOP elevation as a result of lens injury	Chapter 21
	Retinal detachment	Chapter 23
	Thick submacular hemorrhage	Chapter 23
Within 2 weeks	IOFB‡	Chapter 24
	Secondary reconstruction if retina is detached	Chapter 25
	Media opacity in the amblyopic age group	Chapters 21 and 30

*Commonly, although not universally, accepted suggestions; individual cases require individual decisions. Not all conditions are listed.

†We recently treated a 6-year-old boy who was injured when his father's knife slipped as he was dismembering a pig. We closed the wound and—because this is a high-risk injury—injected prophylactic intravitreal antibiotics. IBO was then performed and a small gas bubble was discovered, which had not been present preoperatively. Immediate consultation followed (the time was 3 AM) involving ophthalmologists, surgeons, traumatologists, microbiologists, and experts in infectious medicine. The conclusion was that to prevent a potentially lethal infection, enucleation should be performed. This was discussed with the parents, who gave consent. However, there was something odd about the case; we felt uneasy and repeatedly reviewed the surgical videotape. Finally, and to everybody's relief, we noticed that when injecting the antibiotics, a tiny air bubble was also injected into the vitreous cavity. The final vision in this eye was 20/20.

‡See Chapter 24 about the controversy regarding timing.

- be immobilized (or at least eye movements must be eliminated).

There are several methods to achieve this. *General anesthesia* is preferred because ideally it:

- does not require retro/peribulbar injection, which could elevate the IOP and possibly lead to (further) tissue extrusion;
- puts no time limit on the surgery;
- provides absolute immobility (including avoidance of coughing/bucking);
- satisfies a psychological goal by preventing claustrophobia, which may develop under the surgical drapes; and
- allows ventilatory assistance in a supine position.

Local anesthesia, usually supplemented by iv sedatives, has obvious drawbacks and may be in the form of:

- topical anesthesia*q*;
- local infiltration; or
- regional anesthesia (e.g., careful retro- or peribulbar[18] or sub-Tenon injection).

LMA anesthesia,[19] in which patients are unconscious without being paralyzed or intubated and breathe

---

*q*Wound closure under bupivacaine initially, followed by cocaine; placement of temporary sutures to close the open globe wound as appropriate; and administration of retro- or peribulbar anesthesia thereafter.

spontaneously. The patient may have concomitant anesthetic blocks to eliminate the nociceptive element and consequently reduce the amount of the hypnotic component administered. The hypnotic may be an inhalational or intravenous anesthetic delivered by an iv infusion.

The advantages of an LMA are the following.

- Simple to insert.
- Provides good unobtrusive airway.
- No need for intubation.
- No need for muscle relaxants (e.g., succinylcholine) to paralyze the patient or for reversal at the end of surgery.
- Minimal cardiovascular perturbation.
- Spontaneous ventilation.
- No need for retrobulbar injection.

LMA is unsuitable for patients with:

- residual stomach contents or the potential of blood contamination of the airway (LMA does *not* seal off the larynx as does a cuffed endotracheal tube); and
- gastric regurgitation or reflux disease.

It is a commonly held view that if the patient ate recently (usually perceived as 6 hours before the scheduled surgery), general anesthesia cannot be performed. If the ophthalmologist has strong reasons to require earlier intervention, however, there are several options available such as emptying the stomach or using rapid-sequence induction of general anesthesia with precurarization, which allows succinylcholine use.[20]

> **PEARL...** The important message for the anesthetist is not precurarization and succinylcholine use: the most potent stimulus for IOP elevation is *intubation*. Consequently, adequate depth of anesthesia is more important than the choice of muscle relaxant.[21]

PRIMARY SURGERY: WOUND CLOSURE VERSUS COMPREHENSIVE RECONSTRUCTION

Limiting the initial surgery to wound toilette[r] and closure has the following advantages:

- it is simple, requiring less skill and expertise than a comprehensive reconstruction;

---

[r]Excision/reposition of prolapsed tissues and cleaning of contaminated tissues.

- the risk of acute complications (e.g., ECH development) is reduced;
- a thorough evaluation of the eye's condition is possible postoperatively; and
- consultation is available with colleagues in person or via telephone or (mass) e-mail.

Truly comprehensive primary management (including vitreoretinal surgery), although increasingly popular, is performed only for certain indications such as IOFB removal (see Table 8–3). If the surgeon decides to perform comprehensive reconstruction, primary use of silicone oil in eyes with severe posterior segment injuries offers certain advantages[22] (see the Appendix for further details).

THE POSTOPERATIVE PERIOD AND SECONDARY RECONSTRUCTION

Mainly, there are the three "I"s to fight against:

- infection (see Chapter 28);
- inflammation (see Chapters 17, 20, and 23); and
- IOP elevation (see Chapter 20).

> **PEARL...** It is very important to explain to the patient why close follow-up and self-testing of the injured eye are necessary, even in cases of excellent visual recovery (e.g., late IOP elevation after a contusion; retinal detachment several years after injury).

Many eyes that underwent primary surgery (and many eyes that did not need surgery initially) require subsequent operation(s) (see Table 8–4 and the appropriate chapters in Sections III through V). These surgeries may be indicated to fight:

- against the original consequences of the trauma (e.g., PK for reduced corneal clarity following a severe corneal laceration);
- against the consequences of the initial repair (e.g., a retinal tear created at the vitreous base by inappropriate removal of a traumatic cataract);
- against the consequences of the body's wound healing attempt (e.g., PVR, glaucoma); and/or
- for improved cosmesis/comfort/convenience (e.g., IOL implantation to replace contact lens wear).

The risks and benefits of intervention should always be carefully balanced (e.g., PK for irregular astigmatism causing only limited distortion; extraction of minimal,

Table 8–3   The Advantages and Disadvantages of Comprehensive Initial Management of the Injured Eye

Advantages

Often better visibility through a central corneal wound than a few days after injury*

Immediate and continual visualization of the retina

Potentially avoiding the inconvenience and cost of additional surgery or surgeries

Potentially preventing endophthalmitis by removing the inoculated media such as the vitreous

Potentially preventing the development of retinal detachment by treating retinal breaks or traction-causing bands early

Potentially reducing postinjury inflammation and thus preventing scar formation (e.g., PVR)[24] and secondary IOP elevation

Earlier visual rehabilitation/prevention of amblyopia in the appropriate age group

Disadvantages

Less time to evaluate the eye's condition: increased chance of finding "surprise injuries" (e.g., breached posterior lens capsule, small peripheral retinal tear) and higher risk of inaccurately diagnosing certain conditions (e.g., lens injury)

Limited or no opportunity to consult experts who could provide valuable advice

Less likely that all elements of surgical success (expertise, experience, equipment, personnel, facility) are available

Increased risk of wound leakage occurring during vitrectomy

Higher risk of difficult-to-control intraocular hemorrhage

Increased difficulty in detaching and removing the posterior hyaloid face

Increased difficulty in assessing certain tissues or conditions and their change over time (e.g., ciliary body, macular hole, subretinal hemorrhage)

Difficulty in determining whether an IOL can be implanted safely and, if the decision to implant is made, determining the ideal IOL power

Temptation to implant silicone IOL if no (severe) posterior segment injury is present, making complete silicone oil removal impossible should silicone oil be needed subsequently

*Sufficient application of topical, even systemic, corticosteroids has an important role in maintaining/achieving corneal clarity.

Table 8–4   Selected Indications for Secondary Intervention on the Injured Eye*

Intervention	Indication/Comment
Exploration because of a persistent suspicion of an occult scleral wound	The IOP is not necessarily low even if an unsutured wound is present
Resuturing the corneal wound	Distortion, leakage; the sooner the better
Penetrating keratoplasty	Reduced transparency making posterior segment surgery impossible; irregular astigmatism
Hyphema removal	Impossible to visualize posterior segment; elevated IOP; blood staining of cornea may threaten
Iridoplasty	To compartmentalize globe; for cosmetic reasons; to reduce glare
Cataract removal	The eye's condition, not the surgeon's preference, should determine the method
IOL implantation	With the exception of children in the amblyopic age range, this should be performed only if the retina is stable
Ciliary body	Scar removal to prevent phthisis (endoscopy)
Vitreous removal	To remove hemorrhage, membranes, IOFB; to fight infection
Retina	To eliminate surface traction (cellophane, EMP, macular hole); to reattach (performing retinectomy if necessary); to remove IOFB
Subretinal space	To remove blood, membranes, IOFB
?RPE/choroid removal	It may have beneficial effect on PVR prevention in areas of retinectomy[†]; needs confirmation in future studies
Extraocular muscle surgery for globe deviation	For visual (double vision) or cosmetic reasons

*See individual chapters for details.   †The author's observation.

stationary cataract; removal of symptomless, old IOFBs). It is best, as emphasized earlier, to discuss all options and their implications with the patient and arrive at a decision with which both patient and ophthalmologist feel comfortable.

For functional eyes that are (becoming) phthisical, *complete*[s] silicone oil fill may be the only option to maintain globe integrity (see also Chapter 19 and the Appendix).

INSTRUMENTATION

Although instrumentation is beyond the scope of this chapter, it must be emphasized that using a wide-angle (panoramic) viewing system during vitreous surgery offers tremendous advantages by:

• allowing visualization of a much wider field than the area where the surgeon's intraocular instruments operate;

---

[s]In aphakic eyes not just the vitreous but also the AC must be completely filled to keep the eye pressurized and prevent aqueous access to the endothelium. It appears paradoxical, but this is what may prevent the development of (band) keratopathy. These eyes maintain corneal clarity as long as the silicone oil is in apposition to the entire endothelial surface. Once the oil is removed or emulsifies, the cornea inevitably becomes cloudy.

• bringing, with some manipulation, even the vitreous base into view;
• allowing adequate fundus visualization even in the presence of moderate corneal/lens opacity; and
• allowing adequate fundus visualization even if the pupil is small.

The disadvantages (e.g., learning curve; expense; increased risk of lens-touch in phakic eyes) are minimal compared with the advantages such viewing systems offer; once a surgeon becomes familiar with the system, it is difficult to "go back."

The Appendix contains additional information on the instruments required for eye trauma repair.

CONCLUDING THOUGHTS

There are a few additional points that may be useful to remember.

• Treating eyes with severe injuries is like navigating through uncharted territory. Knowledge of published information and sufficient personal experience are requisite, but there is no absolutely proven recipe ("cookbook approach") for each individual situation. Trauma management is significantly different from surgery for other diseases (see Table 8–5).
• There are usually several options to choose from, and it is impossible always to select the most opti-

TABLE 8–5 BASIC DIFFERENCES BETWEEN SURGERY FOR TRAUMA AND SURGERY FOR OTHER DISEASES

Variable	Tissue		Surgeon's Maneuvers		Example
	Significant Tissue Damage Present	Dislocation	Typically Focused on How Many Goals	How Often Different from Those Originally Planned	
Surgery on anterior segment	Typically no	Very rare	Few	Rarely is an individualized plan needed	Cataract removal and IOL implantation
Surgery on posterior segment	Yes	Common	Several	Commonly	Retinal detachment caused by horseshoe tear and complicated by mild vitreous hemorrhage
Surgery for trauma	Yes	Very common	Numerous	Very commonly; management plan frequently has to be redesigned	Corneal wound with iris prolapse, hyphema, lens injury, vitreous hemorrhage, retinal impactation

mal one. It is therefore inappropriate to blame one-self for a chosen option that was less than ideal—but the surgeon should learn from the experience and utilize the new information next time.

- There are many controversial issues; some will be resolved with time, while others may never find an answer.

- Trauma management does not tolerate dogmas; the surgeon must develop an individualized approach (management strategy) but has to remain flexible to change the thought process if it does not prove successful or new results emerge.

- There are no prospective, randomized, double-masked studies in the field of eye injuries. Personal experience and vigilance, an open mind, knowledge of the literature, and seeking out what others do in similar situations (e.g., through participation in trauma meetings) must substitute for the scientifically supported suggestions that are increasingly common in other fields ("evidence-based medicine").

- The Internet offers a great opportunity to seek rapid advice from a large group of practicing physicians and to search for existing information.

- The ophthalmologist must accept that the success rate in trauma management is rather low and recharge emotional batteries from cases in which the outcome was better than expected. The ophthalmologist should understand that for patients who face blindness, even partial sight is cherished. Because the trauma patient is likely to be grateful for even minimal vision, and later loss of the good eye through trauma or other disease is possible, do not give up on eyes easily.

- Do not choose the field of eye trauma if you don't like challenges; there are other opportunities within the profession that offer satisfaction with less stress and energy consumption. Conversely, the satisfaction felt in solving these greater challenges should compensate for the hardship.

- Keep a surgical diary to record your observations, thoughts, ideas, comments, techniques, whether they are general or relate to a specific situation. In the latter case, record the date and chart number as well. Such a compilation can be the key to lifelong learning.

PITFALL

We ophthalmologists should accept[t] that the eye we are about to treat belongs to the patient, not to us. Although trauma is obviously different from elective cases, on many occasions the patient not only *can* but *should* have a say in what is going to happen. In such instances (e.g., whether surgery is to be performed or deferred for a traumatic macular hole), the ophthalmologist's role is not the communication of a predetermined (and usually scientifically unsupported) statement (e.g., "I am not going to operate unless your vision is worse than 20/50"). The ophthalmologist should instead explain the options, point out the risks and benefits, provide actual prognostic figures, and make a decision together with, not instead of, the patient.

SUMMARY

Treating patients with serious eye injuries can be a difficult, even frustrating process. The ophthalmologist must remember that mastering the details of the management of individual tissue lesions allows "seeing the tree" only and does not provide *vision* of the entire forest. To develop a comprehensive understanding that leads to strategic thinking *before* making actual reconstruction efforts, the surgeon should follow a fairly rigorous thought process; Figure 8–5 provides the structure for this undertaking. Such an approach will reward both the patient and the treating physician.

---

[t] As should *all* physicians.

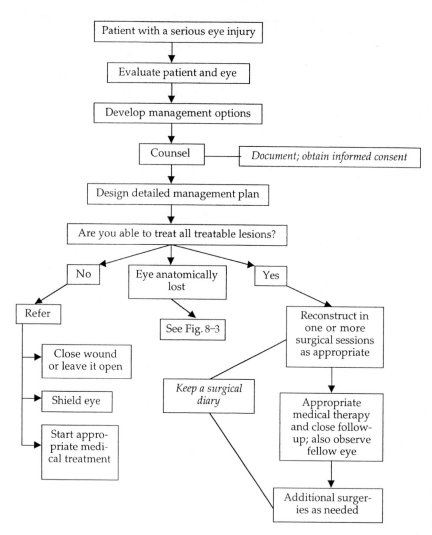

FIGURE 8-5 Designing the management strategy for patients with serious eye injury. See text for details.

References

1. Kuhn F, Johnston W, Mester V, Török M, Berta A. Informed consent and radial keratotomy. *Ann Ophthalmol*. 2000;32:331–332.

2. Cleary PE, Ryan SJ. Histology of wound, vitreous, and retina in experimental posterior penetrating eye injury in the rhesus monkey. *Am J Ophthalmol*. 1979;88:221–231.

3. Morris R, Kuhn F, Witherspoon C. Management of the recently injured eye with no light perception vision. In: Alfaro DV, Liggett PE, eds. *Vitrectomy in the Management of the Injured Globe*. Philadelphia: Lippincott Raven; 1998:113–124.

4. Striph G, Halperin L, Stevens J, Chu F. Afferent pupillary defect caused by hyphema. *Am J Ophthalmol*. 1988; 106;352–353.

5. Lam B, Thompson S. A unilateral cataract produces a relative afferent pupillary defect in the contralateral eye. *Ophthalmology*. 1990;97:334–338.

6. Mader T, Aragones JV, Chandler AC, et al. Ocular and ocular adnexal injuries by U.S. military ophthalmologists during Operations Desert Shield and Desert Storm. *Ophthalmology*. 1993;100:1462–1467.

7. Hoefle F. Initial treatment of eye injuries. *Arch Ophthalmol*. 1968;79:33–35.

8. Treister G. Ocular casualties in the Six-Day War. *Am J Ophthalmol*. 1969;68:669–675.

9. Negrel A, Carvalho D. Fréquence et gravité des traumatismes oculo-palpébraux en milieu african. *Med Afr Noire*. 1977;24:657–672.

10. Moukouri E, Moli M. Traumatismes oculaires en milieu camérounais a Yaounde. *Med Trop.* 1991;51:307–312.

11. Punnonen E. Epidemiological and social aspects of perforating eye injuries. *Acta Ophthalmol.* 1989;67:492 198.

12. Canavan YM, O'Flaherty MJ, Archer DB, Elwood JH. A 10-year survey of eye injuries in Northern Ireland, 1967–76. *Br J Ophthalmol.* 1980;64:618–625.

13. Belkin M. Ocular injuries in the Yom Kippur War. *J Ocular Ther Surg.* 1983;2:40–49.

14. Wong T, Seet B, Ang C. Eye injuries in 20th century warfare: a historical perspective. *Surv Ophthalmol.* 1997; 41:433–459.

15. Davies E. Factors affecting recovery of visual acuity following detachment of the retina. *Trans Ophthalmol Soc UK.* 1972;92:335–344.

16. Thompson W, Rubsamen P, Flynn H, Schiffman J, Cousins C. Endophthalmitis after penetrating trauma. *Ophthalmology.* 1995;102:1696–1701.

17. Barr C. Prognostic factors in corneoscleral lacerations. *Arch Ophthalmol.* 1983;101:919–924.

18. Lo M, Chalfin S. Retrobulbar anesthesia for repair of ruptured globe. *Am J Ophthalmol.* 1997;123:833–835.

19. Myles P, Venema H, Lindholm D. Trauma patient managed with the laryngeal mask airway. *Med J Aust.* 1994; 161:640.

20. Libonati MM, Leahy JJ, Ellison N. The use of succinylcholine in open eye surgery. *Anesthesiology.* 1985;62: 637–640.

21. Vinik H. Intraocular pressure changes during rapid sequence induction and intubation: a comparison of rocuronium, atracurium, and succinylcholine. *J Clin Anesth.* 1999;11:95–100.

22. Lemmen K, Heimann K. Fruh-Vitrektomie mit primarer Silikonolinjektion bei schwerstverletzten Augen. *Klin Monatsbl Augenheilkd.* 1988;193:594–601.

23. Bhargava S, Chopdar A. Gas gangrene panophthalmitis. *Br J Ophthalmol.* 1971;55:136–138.

24. Ryan S, Allen A. Pars plana vitrectomy in ocular trauma. *Am J Ophthalmol.* 1979;88:483–491.

Chapter 9

EVALUATION

J. B. Harlan, Jr., Eugene W. M. Ng, and Dante J. Pieramici

GENERAL EVALUATION

Prior to taking a history and performing an examination focused on the eye, the ophthalmologist must "take a step back" and assess the *whole patient*. In many cases with multiple injuries or polytrauma, an ER trauma team initiates the treatment, first focusing on any life-threatening injury (see Chapter 10). In this scenario, the ophthalmologist is usually called for consultation after the patient is stabilized and may have no immediate role in the triage process. Typically, however, the eye trauma patient presents directly to the ophthalmologist. In such cases, it is important to keep in mind that the patient may have sustained nonglobe injuries (e.g., occult stab/gunshot wound to the chest, fracture, closed head trauma) that may be life threatening and must be addressed first.

> **PEARL...** Always be suspicious of an undiagnosed injury to other organ systems.

Initial Systemic Triage

When accepting an ocular trauma patient directly or from another facility, the general status of the patient should be ascertained so that the appropriate triage pathway can be chosen (i.e., transfer to a general trauma ER or to an eye hospital).

- Record vital signs along with an assessment of the mental status.

- Quickly examine the patient for evidence of obvious bone or severe soft-tissue injury before concentrating on the eye examination.

- Transfer the ocular trauma patient immediately to a general ER or trauma facility if during the rapid primary assessment any of the following signs are present:
  - unstable vital signs;
  - impaired mental status; or
  - serious nonocular injuries.

Once it is determined that the patient is stable and the eye injury can be addressed, a more general medical/surgical history should be taken, documenting:

- all medical conditions;
- current medications;
- drug allergies;
- prior surgeries;
- history of any complications during anesthesia;
- tetanus immunization status (toxoid is recommended in all cases of open globe injury when immunization is not up to date or when an adequate vaccination history cannot be obtained; also see Chapter 8 and the Appendix); and
- the time when the patient last ate or drank (see Chapter 8).

Special Considerations for the Elderly Patient

Falls resulting in eye/orbital trauma may also cause fractures of the hip, long bones, and skull with or without subdural/intracerebral hemorrhage. Any underlying or associated conditions and the cause of the fall should be ascertained as:

- falls associated with loss of consciousness or syncope may indicate underlying cardiovascular disease (e.g., arrhythmia) or hypotension, requiring further investigation;
- significant, even potentially life-threatening, internal bleeding may occur despite mild trauma if the patient is receiving anticoagulation therapy;
- elderly patients may have underlying dementia, making it difficult to obtain a clear history of the events leading to the injury. In such cases, it can be helpful to interview family members and/or caregivers (see Chapter 10).

The examiner must always be alert to the possibility of abuse or neglect. Understanding the patient's home environment/living arrangement is critical for discharge planning in the aftermath of a serious eye injury. In many instances, family members and/or social services need to be engaged to effect a smooth transition from hospital to home/assisted living.

Special Considerations in Children (Also see Chapters 8 and 30)

Eliciting an accurate history can be difficult due to:

- unwillingness of the child to admit engaging in forbidden behavior (e.g., playing with a BB gun or fireworks);
- reluctance on the caregiver's part to volunteer basic information about the circumstances and mechanism of the injury. This should alert the ophthalmologist to the possibility of child abuse, poor supervision, neglect, or significant occult injury. A complete ophthalmic examination with meticulous documentation should be performed. If abuse is suspected, a social worker should be contacted so that the appropriate protective service agencies can be engaged.

> **P**EARL... **Inability to perform an adequate pediatric examination in the office should prompt the scheduling of a formal examination under sedation or general anesthesia.**

OPHTHALMOLOGIC EVALUATION[a]

History

Although a thorough ophthalmic examination usually reveals the nature of the ocular injury, a focused history may rapidly direct the examiner to the critical findings as well as provide important information for guiding initial management and assessing prognosis. A precise, well-documented history in the medical record is also useful for future legal proceedings (see Chapter 7).

It is best to allow the patient to tell his "story." It is important to resist the temptation to interrupt and interrogate the patient immediately in a busy ER setting, although periodic redirection is commonly necessary. The history should include the following.

The context and events leading up to the injury

- Location; and appropriate associated factors such as the use or misuse of safety glasses; seat belt use; air bag deployment and whether the injury has indeed been caused by it.[b]

A detailed description of the mechanism of the injury

- Blunt objects may cause rupture or contusion, as opposed to sharp objects that lead to laceration (see Chapter 1) with a usually more favorable prognosis[1] (see Chapter 3).
- It is a critical part of the Standardized Ocular Trauma Classification System[2,3] (see Chapter 2).

The exact time of the injury

- Knowing the time from injury to presentation is mandatory in planning the treatment strategy (see Chapter 8). Unlike fresh, open wounds, a quiet eye with a 1-week-old, self-sealing corneal laceration may be managed more conservatively.

The place of the injury

- Open globe injuries occurring in a rural setting have a much higher risk of infection than comparable injuries in nonrural settings.[4]

The composition of the IOFB (see Chapter 24) and the identity of any chemical agent (see Chapter 11)

Prior ocular history

- Ophthalmic surgery and/or trauma (risk factors for rupture, see Chapter 27).
- The preinjury vision and the visual potential of the fellow eye.
- Any ocular medications.

---

[a]The appropriate chapters contain additional information.

[b]Rather than a coincidental deployment of the air bag (see Chapter 4).

External Inspection

Key aspects of external inspection include the following.

- Inspect the head, scalp, face, periorbital tissues, and eyelids under bright illumination. Check for lacerations, ecchymoses, obvious protruding foreign bodies, lid and periorbital edema, ptosis, and the presence/absence of enophthalmos or exophthalmos by Hertel prism measurements.
- Inspect the globes without the aid of magnification for evidence of:
  - protruding foreign bodies (see Chapter 24);
  - gross prolapse of intraocular contents; and
  - occult open globe injury in case of appropriate history (e.g., fistfight; hammering; previous eye surgery/trauma), reduced vision, small lid wound, irregular (peaked) pupil, and hemorrhagic chemosis (Fig. 9–1);
  - pronounced unilateral exophthalmos (may suggest a traumatic carotid-cavernous fistula).
- Palpate the scalp, face and periorbital soft tissue for:
  - occult subcutaneous foreign bodies and signs that, even without Hertel measurement asymmetry, strongly suggest the presence of an orbital fracture:
  - crepitus;
  - step-off deformities; and
  - infraorbital hypesthesia.

PEARL... If lid edema is present, a speculum or retractor may be used to visualize the globe, but extreme care should be taken not to exert pressure on the globe, causing extrusion of ocular contents (see Fig. 9–2 and Chapter 8). In cases of very swollen lids or an uncooperative patient, it is better to forgo speculum/retractor use and proceed directly to an imaging study (see later in this Chapter).

Young children[c] may need to be restrained (see Chapters 8 and 30). If this is impossible or the child feels more secure when in direct contact with the parent, follow the steps given below.

1. An assistant and parent sit at the same level facing each other.
2. The child is positioned supine with legs straddling the parent's waist.
3. The child's head is placed on the assistant's lap.
4. The parent holds the child's hands and legs.
5. The assistant holds the child's head still while the physician performs the examination.

---

[c] Usually those younger than 5 years old.

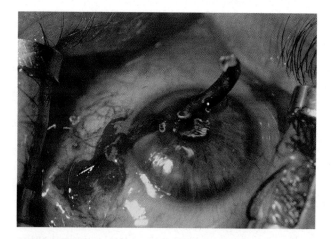

FIGURE 9–1 A penlight or flashlight can be used to assess the eye rapidly. Gentle traction with a lid speculum exposes the globe, revealing a full-thickness injury. The IOFB is not removed until the patient is in the operating room.

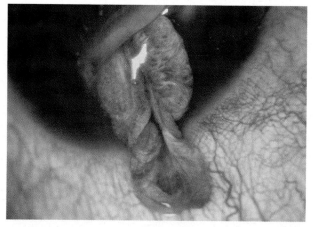

FIGURE 9–2 Shortly after slit-lamp examination, this patient developed a hemorrhagic choroidal detachment with extrusion of intraocular contents.

TABLE 9–1   METHODS TO REDUCE ANXIETY DURING EXAMINATION*

Explain procedures to the patient in advance, especially children.

Reassure the patient that you can help him/her.

Never patch both eyes unless both eyes are injured. Covering both eyes only heightens concern about impending blindness.

Place the patient in a calm, quiet setting and be mindful of the patient's privacy/modesty.

Be realistic but not overly pessimistic about potential outcomes. The patient should understand the severity of the eye injury, but this message should be delivered with compassion as well as candor. In all but the most hopeless of cases, the examiner should impart a sense of hope and optimism in discussions regarding prognosis.

*See also Chapters 5, 7, and 8.

If an adequate examination is not possible without the risk of extrusion of ocular contents, the examination should be carried out under sedation. A qualified anesthesiologist or critical care specialist should administer anesthesia in a monitored setting, with access to advanced life-support medication and equipment (see Chapter 8).

Anxiety is commonly present and should be addressed (see Table 9–1).

Visual Function Testing

Central Vision

The presenting visual acuity is a crucial prognostic indicator (see Chapter 3).

Visual acuity is measured in *each eye separately*, using an occluder or eye patch. Particularly in younger patients, care should be taken to ensure that the patient does not "cheat" or inadvertently use the fellow eye.

Whenever possible, a standardized chart (e.g., *Snellen, ETDRS*) should be used.

- Illiterate charts (e.g., *E, Landholt C*) should be used for patients unable to read.
- For preliterate children use *Allen cards*, *HOTV letters*, or the *E game*.
- In infants, fixation and smooth pursuit can be assessed by using *colorful targets, toys*, or a *hand light*.

If feasible, the patient's *best correction* should be used to record the visual acuity.

- Because it is rarely possible/practical to perform a formal refraction in an ER setting, the pinhole acuity can be used as a substitute.

For patients with severe ocular injuries or who are immobilized on a stretcher:

- a near card is utilized;
- if vision is too poor to be measured with standard charts, a gross assessment of the visual acuity should be obtained (e.g., counting fingers at a specific distance; hand motions; light perception with projection; light perception without projection; bare light perception; and NLP);
- light perception must be tested using a strong light source (e.g., IBO or slit lamp, *never* a candle).

Optic Nerve/Retinal Testing

- The presence/absence of an APD is a crucial indicator of gross visual function.[d] The test is performed utilizing a bright light source (e.g., the IBO at its highest setting). The light source is alternately directed at each eye in a swinging or back-and-forth fashion. The eye with the relative afferent deficit paradoxically *dilates* when exposed to the light source because the consensual pupillary response in one eye always mirrors the direct pupillary response in the fellow eye.

PEARL... The absence or presence of an APD can be assessed even if the iris is injured. Rather than examining the direct pupillary response in each eye with each swing, only the reactive, intact pupil is observed. If an APD is present, the pupil of the fellow eye dilates when the light is shone into the injured eye.

[d]May be absolute or relative.

The presence of an APD may indicate optic nerve damage or significant retinal damage and has prognostic significance (see Chapter 3).

> **PEARL...** APD caused by media opacity (e.g., hyphema, dense cataract) is very rare.

- The *patient's subjective perception of brightness* when confronted with a light source is used to estimate optic nerve function. The IBO or a hand-held transilluminator is directed at the normal eye and the patient is instructed that this level of brightness represents a value of 100%. The light is then redirected into the injured eye, and the patient is asked to compare the levels of brightness. If the level is reduced, the patient is asked to quantify the relative amount of brightness (e.g., 10%, 50%, 80%).
- Rapid assessment of the patient's *peripheral visual field* can provide additional information about the eye's overall visual function. Field abnormalities may indicate optic nerve damage or retinal injury.
  - Gross visual field testing can be performed quickly and effectively by finger confrontation.[e]
  - Formal kinetic/static perimetry is not performed in the acute ER setting, even though it is a sensitive means of following TON over time.
- *Color vision* testing may also detect optic nerve deficits. Color plates (e.g., *Hardy-Rand-Rittler, Ishihara*) can be used in cases in which the vision is 20/400 or better. If color plates are not available, a red object can be used to test for *red desaturation*: when optic nerve damage is present, the red object is perceived as grayish or "washed out" when compared with the color seen by the normal fellow eye.

Motility

- The assessment of ocular motility is most relevant in cases of known or suspected cranial nerve and/or orbital injury.
- Significant periorbital edema, hemorrhage, or lack of patient cooperation often prohibits formal motility testing.
- *Forced duction testing* may be useful to rule out muscle entrapment if orbital wall fracture is suspected (see Chapter 36). The test is contraindicated in case of (potential) open globe injury.

Slit Lamp

> **PEARL...** Although slit-lamp biomicroscopy and IBO are the preferred methods, a rapid assessment can often be made with the use of a simple pen- or flashlight.

Conjunctiva

Foreign bodies and/or chemical precipitates may be sequestered in redundant folds of chemotic conjunctiva or hidden in the fornices (see also Chapters 11 and 13).

- The fornix should be carefully probed and the lids everted using topical anesthetic (see Chapter 13).
- Hemorrhagic chemosis raises the possibility of orbital fracture and/or open globe trauma.
- Lacerations of the conjunctiva may not be obvious initially but can be detected with gentle manipulation of the conjunctiva using a cotton-tip swab. Once a conjunctival laceration is identified, attention should be focused on ruling out an underlying scleral wound or a subconjunctival foreign body.

Cornea

The examination begins on the surface, then proceeds more deeply (see also Chapter 14).

- *Epithelial defects* may require topical fluorescein staining.
- *Fresh wounds*[f] must be carefully evaluated to determine whether they are full thickness. A full-thickness wound leaks aqueous (although gentle pressure may have to be applied), which can be highlighted by using 2% fluorescein. Under blue light, egress of aqueous fluid dilutes the topical fluorescein dye, forming a green stream in the middle of a more stagnant pool of bright yellow dye ("Seidel positive"; see also Chapters 14 and 19).
- *Superficial foreign bodies.* If the foreign body spans the cornea into the AC, it is an open globe injury and the object is best removed in the operating room; see Fig. 9–3.
- *Abrasions*, *opacities*, and *ulcerations.* The examiner should always assume an open globe injury until proved otherwise.

Sclera

The conjunctiva may remain intact overlying a full-thickness wound or the two wounds may be distant from each other (see Chapter 13). Hemorrhage in or under the conjunctiva may also hide the scleral

---

[e]One eye is covered with a patch or an occluder while the tested eye fixates on the examiner's nose. The examiner's and patient's heads should be at the same level. Fingers from one or both hands are presented to the patient centrally and in each of the four quadrants. Simultaneous presentation of fingers in different quadrants is used to determine visual neglect or sensory inattention.

[f]They should be sketched in the chart, indicating their height, width, and estimated depth when possible (see Chapter 8).

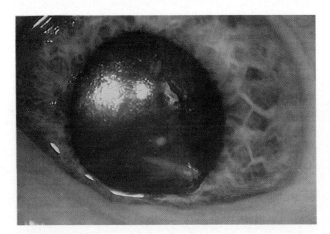

FIGURE 9–3   A transcorneal pricker extends into the AC. Although the external end could be grasped at the slit lamp, it was removed and the wound sutured in the operating room.

lesion. If the presence of a scleral wound cannot be ruled out under the slit lamp, exploratory surgery may have to performed.

Anterior Chamber

The AC should be examined for (see also Chapter 17):

- the presence of cells (inflammatory, pigmented, or RBCs), flare, fibrin, hypopyon, and IOFBs; and
- depth:
  - *deepening* can be seen with posterior dislocation or subluxation of the crystalline lens, iridodialysis, and scleral rupture;
  - *shallowing* can occur with anterior dislocation or subluxation of the crystalline lens, vitreous prolapse, a corneoscleral wound that leaks, SCH or serous choroidal detachment, aqueous misdirection, and angle closure.

Iris and Angle

The iris and angle are frequent sites of anatomic damage following both closed and open globe injury and require careful investigation (see also Chapters 17 and 20).

Using direct illumination and retroillumination techniques, the *iris* is examined for:

- sphincter tears;
- iridodialysis;
- full-thickness laceration (stromal defect); and
- iridodonesis lens subluxation.

The *angle* is examined using gonioscopy unless the injury is open globe[8] or hyphema is present. A careful examination in eyes with self-sealing wounds, however, can be useful in identifying an IOFB in the angle

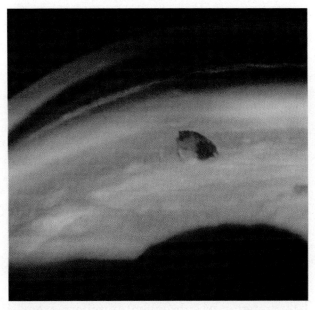

FIGURE 9–4   An occult IOFB in the AC foreign body is visualized with the aid of a goniolens.

or, with gentle pressure, an occult wound (Fig. 9–4). Use a four-mirror goniolens with contact lens solution.

Crystalline Lens

The crystalline lens should be examined for:

- phacodonesis;
- dislocation;
- defects in the anterior capsule with or without leakage of cortical material;
- posterior capsular defects or "feathering";
- sectoral cataract;
- intralenticular IOFB; and
- zonular rupture (as signaled by vitreous prolapse into the AC; see Chapter 21).

Intraocular Pressure

Knowledge of the IOP is important for all traumatized eyes, although actual measurement should be deferred in eyes with open globe injury. Following contusion, the IOP may rise acutely, particularly when blood/inflammatory cells are present.

- Abnormally low IOP may indicate occult penetration or rupture but may also be seen with ciliary body injury or retinal detachment.
- Elevated IOP usually occurs in the setting of outflow obstruction from:
  - inflammation and/or hemorrhage in the AC; or
  - mechanical angle closure in the setting of anatomic disruption: anterior movement of the lens–iris diaphragm with aqueous misdirection; anterior rotation of the ciliary body with SCH; pupillary block from a dislocated lens and/or inflammatory membrane.

---

[8]If a wound is open/leaking, gonioscopy should be deferred until after surgical closure in the operating room, at which time a Koeppe lens may be utilized under the microscope to visualize the angle.

> **PEARL...** Remember that abnormally high IOP does not rule out an (occult) open globe injury, even rupture.

Ophthalmoscopy[h]

The posterior segment should be examined in a timely fashion[i] before the view is compromised by media opacity (e.g., corneal decompensation, hyphema, traumatic cataract, vitreous hemorrhage) or by diminished patient cooperation. In most cases, mydriatics should be used.

> **PITFALL**
>
> Mydriatic use should be meticulously documented in the medical record to avoid misinterpretation of subsequent pupillary examinations performed by physicians of other specialties (e.g., neurology, neurosurgery, internal medicine).

All topical medications should be administered from fresh, unopened, sterile bottles to avoid iatrogenic intraocular infection or, in the case of antibiotics, drug toxicity.

In open globe injuries with iris prolapse, the dilated examination should be deferred until the wound is surgically closed. In such cases the posterior segment can be assessed initially with nondilated indirect examination, CT scan, or ultrasound.

In cases of severe ocular injury, IBO may be the best and only way to examine the posterior segment. When the media are clear in a closed globe injury, a more thorough examination of the posterior segment may include the use of a 90 diopter lens and/or contact lens biomicroscopy when it is not contraindicated.

Scleral depression may be necessary, although it is not recommended acutely if:

- a hyphema is present;
- an open globe injury is suspected[j]; or
- significant periocular injury (e.g., orbital fracture, major lid laceration) is present: in these cases, defer the examination until 4 to 6 weeks after injury.

Table 9–2 provides an overview of different ophthalmoscopic findings.

Imaging Studies

When the posterior segment cannot be visualized with IBO, an imaging study is recommended to rule out pathology that may require immediate intervention.

Ultrasonography

Echographic imaging can be employed to characterize accurately the internal ocular anatomy and to detect IOFBs.[5,6] In the hands of an experienced echographer,[k] ultrasound is reliable in detecting (Figs. 9–5 through 9–10):

---

[h]The slit lamp and a high-powered lens (e.g., 90 diopters) may also be used to examine the vitreous and retina.

[i]The initial examination may allow the only chance for days to weeks to view the posterior segment.

[j]Use of a wide-angle viewing system during vitrectomy usually allows meticulous examination of the retinal periphery.

[k]Preferably with clinical experience.

TABLE 9–2   POTENTIAL POSTERIOR SEGMENT FINDINGS FOLLOWING SEVERE OCULAR INJURY

Finding	Contusion	Laceration	Rupture
Vitreous hemorrhage	Yes	Yes	Yes
Vitreous pigment	Yes	Uncommon	Uncommon
Vitreous base dialysis	Yes	Uncommon	Yes
Retinal flap tear	Yes	Yes	Yes
Posterior vitreous separation	Yes	Uncommon	Yes
IOFB	No	Yes	Uncommon
Commotio retinae	Yes	Uncommon	Uncommon
Macular hole	Yes	Uncommon	Uncommon
Choroidal rupture	Yes	No	Uncommon
Sclopetaria	Yes	No	Yes
Subretinal hemorrhage	Yes	Yes	Yes
Optic nerve avulsion	Yes	Uncommon	Uncommon
Retinal detachment	Uncommon	Uncommon	Yes
Hypotony maculopathy	Yes	Yes	Yes
Lens dislocation	Yes	No	Yes
Endophthalmitis	No	Yes	Uncommon

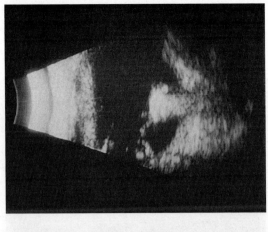

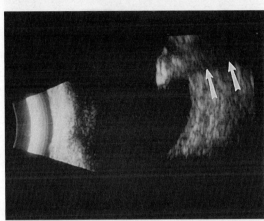

FIGURE 9–5   B-scan ultrasound of a patient with a large metallic IOFB. Transverse (top) and longitudinal (bottom) sections demonstrate anterior location of the large echodense object in the vitreous cavity with echolucent shadow (arrows).

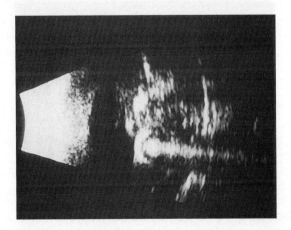

FIGURE 9–6   An intraocular pellet (BB) with typical ultrasonographic appearance.

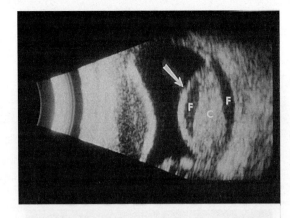

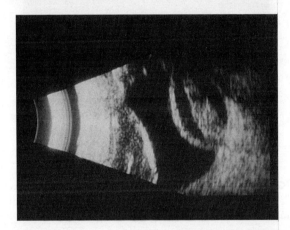

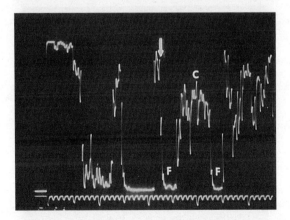

FIGURE 9–7   (Top) Transverse orientation showing bullous choroidal detachments (arrow) and subchoroidal hemorrhage, partially fluid (F), partially clotted (C). (Center) Longitudinal orientation showing choroidal detachments with fluid and clotted subchoroidal hemorrhage. (Bottom) Corresponding A-scan image showing the high choroidal spike (arrow) with areas of both high (C) and low (F) internal reflectivity from the clotted and fluid hemorrhage, respectively.

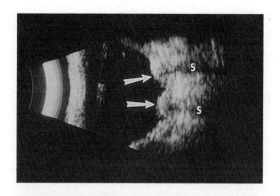

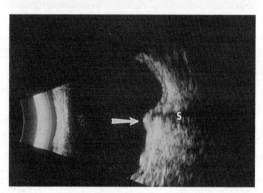

FIGURE 9–8 B-scan ultrasound of a ruptured globe showing multiple folds of the posterior sclera (arrows). The folds can produce a shadow (S) that may be confused with an IOFB.

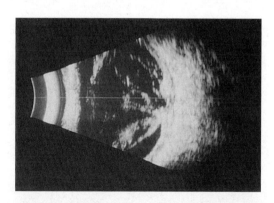

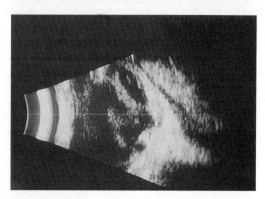

FIGURE 9–9 B-scan ultrasound: transverse section at decreased gain shows a large posterior scleral rupture with blood and vitreous to the wound.

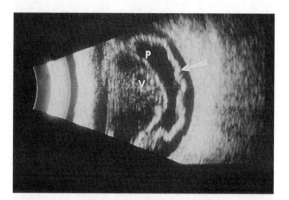

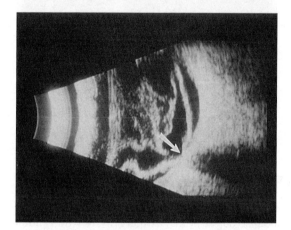

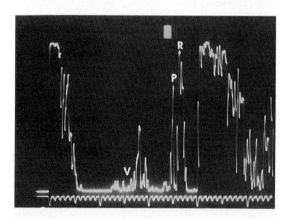

FIGURE 9–10 B-scan ultrasound. (Top) Transverse section showing dispersed vitreous hemorrhage (V), posterior vitreous detachment (P), and a dense, thick, folded retinal detachment (arrow). (Center) Longitudinal section showing the attachment of the retina to the disk (arrow). (Bottom) A-scan image showing low chain of spikes (vitreous hemorrhage, V), medium to high spike (posterior vitreous detachment, P), and maximally high spike (retinal detachment, R).

- retinal detachment;
- posterior vitreous separation;
- vitreous hemorrhage and opacities;
- choroidal detachment (can differentiate between serous and hemorrhagic);
- retinal tears and areas of vitreoretinal adhesion;
- choroidal and scleral ruptures;
- vitreous incarceration; and
- IOFBs, both radiolucent and radiopaque.[7,8]

Advantages:

- Unlike MRI and CT, ultrasound provides real-time images of the eye and orbit.
- The relatively high frequency of the sound waves (10 MHz) affords outstanding resolution (0.1 to 0.01 mm), an ideal choice to image intraocular structures.
- Multiple cross-sectional and radial cuts of the eye can be rapidly obtained at the bedside or in the operating room.
- Serial echography permits following the clinical course of various conditions (e.g., choroidal detachment resolution, membrane and retinal detachment development).
- Ultrasonography is less expensive than radiological studies.

Disadvantages:

- Because ultrasound requires direct contact with the eyelids and/or globe, it should not be used in eyes with a high risk of extrusion of intraocular contents (e.g., large wound, uncooperative patient). In these cases, echography can be performed in the operating room after the globe has been closed and the patient is under general anesthesia.
- Training and skill are required.
- It is not useful in diagnosing orbital fractures.

Radiological Imaging: CT

CT has replaced radiography as the most common and useful radiological imaging study in patients with severe peri/ocular trauma.

Advantages:

- Unlike ophthalmic ultrasound, CT is readily available in most hospitals.
- May be superior to ultrasound in determining the size and site of an IOFB.[7]
- No direct contact with eyelids or globe is required.
- Ideal imaging study to rule out orbital fractures.

- Faster and less expensive than MRI, with less motion artifact.
- Less likely to cause claustrophobia than MRI.

Disadvantages:

- Generally contraindicated for pregnant patients.
- May not be readily available if patient presents to private ophthalmic office.
- Intraocular structures not as well imaged as by ultrasound.
- Cannot be performed in the operating room.

Indications:

- No IBO view of the posterior segment.
- Suspected occult rupture/laceration.
- Suspected IOFB (see Chapter 24 for additional details).
- Suspected orbital/facial fractures.

The CT study ideally includes both axial and coronal sections. For coronal sections, the patient must either be in a prone position with the head resting on the chin or in a supine position with the head extended back on the vertex.[1] Direct coronal scans are particularly useful to evaluate the orbital roof, orbital floor, and inferior and superior rectus muscles; and to localize foreign bodies (Figs. 9–11 and 9–12).[9] Although not as sensitive as ultrasound,[7] CT is informative regarding intraocular anatomy (Figs. 9–13 through 9–17).[10]

PEARL... Generally, 1.5- to 2.0-mm-thick axial and 2.0- to 4.0-mm-thick coronal sections are used. In certain cases (see Chapter 24), the radiologist—who is usually responsible for setting the parameters—should be advised to use thinner cuts. Intravenous contrast enhancement, although useful for vascular lesions (e.g., orbital varix, arteriovenous malformation, carotid-cavernous fistula), is rarely necessary for ocular/orbital trauma.

---

[1]This may not be possible in an unconscious or uncooperative patient, in a patient who must be immobilized due to suspected neck injury, or in a child. In such instances, computer-reconstructed coronal views may be generated, but their quality is suboptimal compared with that of direct coronal sections.

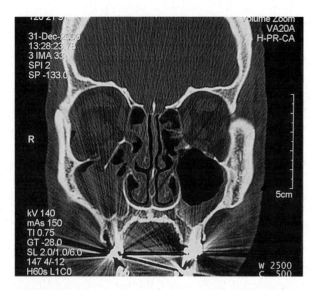

FIGURE 9–11   Coronal CT scan of a patient with right orbital floor and medial wall fractures. There is prolapse of the inferior rectus muscle into the maxillary sinus.

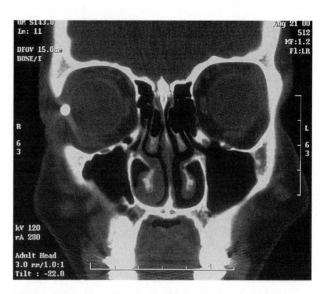

FIGURE 9–12   Coronal CT scan of a patient with an orbital BB lodged adjacent to the right eye.

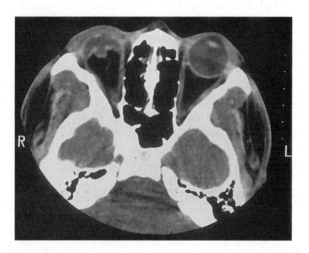

FIGURE 9–13   Axial CT scan of a severely deformed right eye. This is often referred as the "flat-tire" sign and suggests a poor visual prognosis in this open globe injury.

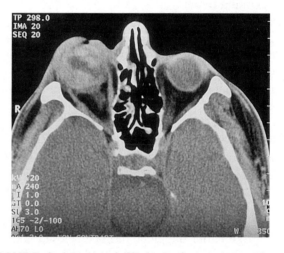

FIGURE 9–14   Axial CT scan of acute hemorrhagic choroidal detachments in an eye with corneal laceration; note the hyperdense uveal contours.

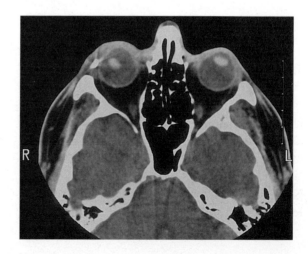

FIGURE 9–15   Axial CT scan of a patient struck with a piece of metal. The hyperdense foreign body adjacent to the globe did not penetrate the eye, as indicated by the uniform corneoscleral contour. The lens is dislocated into the vitreous.

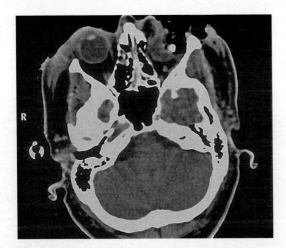

FIGURE 9-16 Axial CT scan of a patient who was ejected from a motor vehicle. A radiolucent wooden foreign body presses against the left globe temporally. Note the radiopaque metallic foreign body within the wooden foreign body.

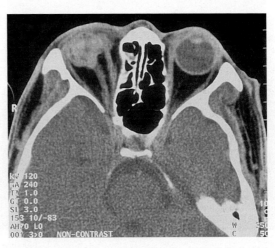

FIGURE 9-17 Axial CT scan of a patient struck in the right eye with a bungee cord. The rupture site was not apparent on clinical examination. The CT scan shows disruption of the normal corneoscleral contour and vitreous opacities (hemorrhage).

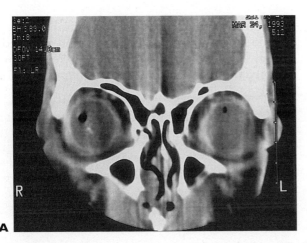

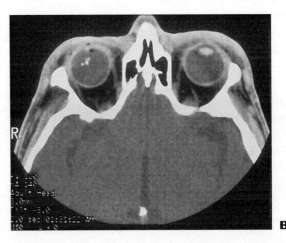

FIGURE 9-18 (A) Coronal CT scan reveals evidence of IOFB and intraocular air in the right eye following a blast injury. Air is also seen in the asymptotic left eye. (B) Axial view confirms the location of the IOFB in the right eye and confirms bilateral open globe injuries.

The sensitivity and specificity of CT in the detection of open globe injury are 73%[m] and 95%, respectively.[11] Common CT findings suggesting open globe injury include:

- eyewall deformity (Fig. 9–13);
- intraocular air (Figs. 9–18 and 9–19);
- IOFB;
- intraocular hemorrhage; and
- eyewall wound (Fig. 9–20).

[m]Too low to be used as an isolated screening tool.

PEARL... The CT findings may have prognostic significance: eyes with a poor visual outcome (<20/200) have significantly more pathology than eyes with a good visual outcome. Vitreous hemorrhage, absence of the lens, and severe distortion of the eyewall are among the CT findings most strongly associated with poor visual outcome.[11]

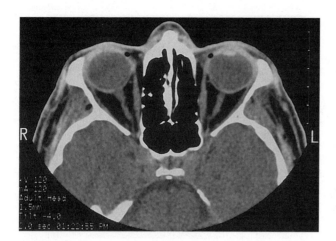

FIGURE 9–19   Intraocular air is generally seen only post-operatively or following open globe injury. Air exterior to the globe is a normal finding as in this case. The air is most often located in the upper lid.

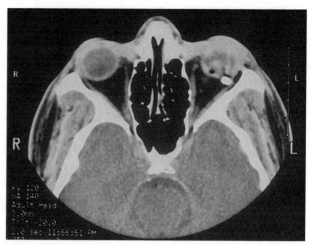

FIGURE 9–20   Following perforating ocular injury, a large posterior wound may be present on CT scan. The globe is usually disorganized and accompanied by intraocular air and hemorrhage. The foreign body often comes to rest in the orbit.

Radiological Imaging: MRI

Although MRI is an excellent tool for evaluating vascular lesions, its role in an acute ocular trauma setting has yet to be defined.

Advantages:

- MRI is able to generate axial, coronal, and sagittal views simultaneously, thus eliminating the need to reposition the patient.
- Superior image quality of soft tissues compared with CT.
- May be helpful in the evaluation of nonmagnetic IOFBs (e.g., wood, glass).[12–14]
- May be used for pregnant patients.

Disadvantages:

- Limited availability.
- Motion artifact.
- Cannot be used in cases of:
  ○ suspected magnetic IOFB[15];
  ○ pacemakers;
  ○ implanted magnetic hardware (e.g., cochlear implant); or
  ○ patients with advanced life support equipment.
- May cause claustrophobia.
- Less effective than CT for assessing orbital fractures.
- Longer image acquisition time.

Radiological Imaging: Plain Radiography

With the availability of CT, the use of conventional x-ray techniques in the evaluation of ocular trauma

has decreased significantly. If more advanced imaging modalities are unavailable, however, plain radiographs can still serve as a valuable screening tool for orbital fracture and intraocular/intraorbital foreign body.[16]

> **PEARL...**   It is critical for the ophthalmologist to review the images personally because most radiologists have limited experience with ocular injury.[n]

Electrophysiology

Electrophysiological testing can be useful to evaluate the visual potential of the injured eye in patients who are unable to communicate with the examiner (e.g., cognitive impairment, young age).

Although *standard-flash* ERG has been shown to have prognostic value in diabetic patients with vitreous hemorrhage,[17] even a nonrecordable *bright-flash* ERG in the presence of recent, massive traumatic vitreous hemorrhage does not necessarily indicate permanent visual loss (see Chapter 8).[18]

The ERG is used to assess the level of retinal degeneration in cases of chronic metallic IOFB (see Chapter 24).[19–21]

---

[n]A large study conducted at a teaching hospital demonstrated that, in the absence of any prior clinical information, ophthalmologists had a higher specificity and sensitivity in detecting open globe injury on CT than an experienced neuroradiologist.[11]

Surgical Exploration

Indications

The indications for surgical exploration are:

- the patient is uncooperative or too young to permit adequate clinical examination;
- the clinical findings and the results of the imaging tests are contradictory;

Procedure

- General anesthesia is preferred.
- An adequate conjunctival peritomy° is performed and the globe is scrutinized under the operating microscope for evidence of scleral rupture/laceration.
- The eyewall is thoroughly inspected (carefully use retractors or traction sutures if necessary), especially in the areas most prone to rupture:
  - ○ immediately posterior to the insertions of the rectus muscles;
  - ○ at the limbus;
  - ○ at the equator; and
  - ○ at sites of previous injury or surgery (see Chapter 27 and Fig. 9–21).
- The cornea and AC are inspected under high magnification.
- A Koeppe lens may be used to examine the angle for occult IOFBs.
- Coaxial illumination is used to detect subtle lenticular irregularities.

°360-degree if necessary.

- IBO or careful ultrasonography can also be performed.

The *endoscope* may serve both diagnostic and therapeutic purposes (see the Appendix).

Photodocumentation (see also Chapters 7 and 8)

Photodocumentation is useful because:

- photographs may be superior to chart sketches;
- photographs may serve as key forensic evidence in subsequent civil and/or criminal litigation stemming from the injury;
- serial photographs are an excellent means to document the injury's clinical course;
- archived clinical photos have great educational and research value.

PEARL... Proper photodocumentation should include external pictures taken with a 35-mm film or digital camera. Slit-lamp and fundus photos should also be obtained, although this can be difficult in the middle of the night in a general ER. Modern ultrasound machines can save the images digitally; Polaroid photographs can be taken with older machines. Surgical videotapes are also valuable (see Chapter 7 regarding its potential dangers), and conventional or digital "still" images at various phases of the operation may be captured too.

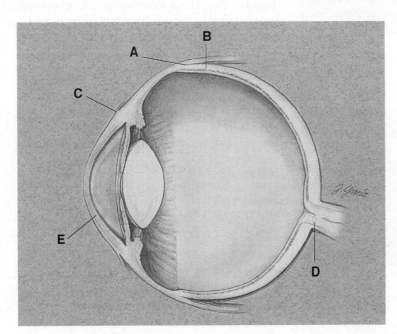

FIGURE 9–21 Diagram indicating the sites most likely to result in ocular rupture following severe blunt injury. **(A)** Just posterior to the rectus insertions where the sclera is thinnest. **(B)** At the equator. **(C)** At the corneoscleral limbus. **(D)** At the insertion of the optic nerve. **(E)** At the site of pervious intraocular surgery, particularly when the surgical incision was in the cornea.

Reporting of Ocular Injuries to the National Database

Growing awareness of the societal impact of ocular injury and rapid technological advances have aided the development of increasingly effective techniques for both prevention and treatment. The introduction of a standardized terminology[2,3] (see Chapters 1 and 2) and the creation in the United States of a national eye trauma database (USEIR; see Chapter 4) have provided a powerful foundation for the discovery of future management techniques through accurate and meaningful research. Any US ophthalmologist and/or institution[p] involved in the care of ocular trauma patients is strongly encouraged to contribute to the database of the USEIR, whether in paper or electronic format (USEIRonline.org).

Malingering and Hysteria

Definitions

The *malingering* patient is someone who deliberately feigns disease in order to achieve a specific desired end, such as personal injury compensation or disability benefits. In contrast, the *hysterical* patient truly experiences clinical symptoms independent of volition, yet there is no underlying organic disease. This phenomenon is more appropriately termed "psychogenic illness" and can occur in various forms.[22]

Body Dysmorphic Disorder   The patient focuses on a perceived physical defect that in reality is nonexistent or barely noticeable (e.g., perceived ptosis, anisocoria).

Somatization Disorder   The patient presents with multiple, recurrent, vague, somatic complaints. Anxiety and depression are usually present.

Hypochondriasis   The patient presents with many specific complaints involving multiple organ systems. Such patients typically practice excessive self-observation.

Conversion Disorder   The patient presents with sudden, dramatic loss or alteration of a particular single physical function (e.g., acute blindness, tunnel vision).

> **PEARL...** When the examiner suspects nonorganic disease, the first objective is to perform a thorough ophthalmic examination. Nonorganic disease must always be a diagnosis of exclusion; occult organic disease must always be ruled out before a diagnosis of nonphysiologic visual loss can be made.

---

[p] With the foundation of the World Eye Injury Registry, based on the USEIR model, reporting is now open for all ophthalmologists throughout the world (WEIRonline.org; see also Chapter 4).

Empathic reassurance is the most productive approach to patients with nonorganic visual disturbances. The clinician should always maintain a caring, professional demeanor and avoid direct confrontation.

> **PEARL...** A patient with psychogenic complaints who truly believes he is ill obviously does not have the capacity to understand or withstand a direct confrontation, and confronting the malingerer serves only to provoke a defensive posture, escalating the level of emotion and tension in the clinical encounter.

Once convinced that no underlying organic disease (injury) is present, the ophthalmologist's objective is to "trick" the patient into doing or seeing things that would be impossible in the presence of true disease. The examiner must project a sincere, empathic attitude and avoid direct confrontation.

Techniques for Patients Claiming Hand Motion to NLP Vision[22,23]

Finger Touch Test   Have the patient touch the tips of the index fingers together. An organically blind patient will be able to perform this maneuver because it is based on proprioception, not visual cues. A patient with nonorganic visual loss, especially a malingerer, will be unable to do this. Similarly, the patient with organic disease will have no difficulty signing his/her name, yet the malingerer may struggle.

Test for Pupillary Reactivity   A severe unilateral visual deficit in the presence of clear media cannot exist without an APD. True bilateral blindness is associated with nonreactive pupils except in cases of postgeniculate injury (cortical blindness, which can be detected using MRI).

Mirror Test   Have the patient look into a large mirror held in front of him. Tilt, twist, and rotate the mirror in various directions. If nystagmoid movements occur, vision has to be better than light perception.

Prism Test   Place a loose prism over the "blind" eye and have the patient fixate on a distant target. A report of double vision rules out monocular blindness.

Optokinetic Drum Test   Use a rotating optokinetic drum or horizontally moving striped tape to attempt to induce horizontal jerk nystagmus. If nystagmus is induced, vision must be at least 20/400.

Color Plate Test Ask the patient to read color plates, explaining that different nerves are used to see color. Correct reading of color plates in one or both eyes indicates at least 20/400 visual acuity.

Titmus Fly Test Test the patient with the Titmus Fly/Random Dot stereo plates. If the patient is able to perceive a three-dimensional effect, both eyes are being used.

Techniques for Patients Claiming 20/40 to Hand Motion Vision[22,23]

Visual Acuity Testing Begin visual acuity testing with the smallest line (usually 20/10). When the patient reports difficulty, appear amazed and show the patient the 20/15 line, stating that the letters are double the size of the previous line. The process is repeated until the patient is able to read a line. For best results, several 20/20 lines are used. The patient may be tricked into admitting better vision than initially claimed.

Near Card Test vision with a near card to bring out a discrepancy between near and distance visions not explained by media opacity or refractive error.

Reading Bar Test Place a tongue depressor vertically, ~6 inches in front of the patient's face with reading material positioned 10–14 inches behind. If vision is good in both eyes, the patient will be able to read continuously. If vision is truly poor in one eye, the patient will soon reach a point in the text where the good eye is occluded by the tongue depressor, impairing the ability to read continuously.

PAM Test Tell the patient you will perform a special test of "best potential vision" that actually bypasses the current problem, allowing you to know what the patient's vision would be if he or she did not have the current problem. A significant improvement in visual acuity in the absence of media opacity or retinal pathology unmasks nonorganic dysfunction.

Diagnostic "Refraction" Test Fog the normal eye with high "+" power and place a lens with minimal power over the affected eye. Have the patient read the chart with both eyes. The patient may be tricked into reading with the affected eye.

Paired Cylinder Refraction Test Based on similar principles, "+" and "−" cylinders of the same power and with their axes parallel are placed in a trial frame in front of the good eye. The patient is asked to use both eyes to read a line that was read previously with the good eye but not with the affected eye. As the patient begins to read, blur the vision in the good eye by rotating the axis of one of the cylinders about 10–15 degrees. If the patient

keeps reading or is able to read the line again when asked, he is obviously using the affected eye.

Red–Green Duochrome Chart Test The patient is given red–green glasses with the red lens over the affected eye. The patient is asked to read the red–green duochrome chart with both eyes. The eye behind the red lens will see both sides of the chart, but the eye behind the green lens will be able to see only the green side of the chart. If the patient is able to read the whole chart, he must be using the affected eye.

Mydriatic Test The patient is asked to read both a near card and the distance chart with both eyes. Next, anesthetic is instilled into both eyes prior to the IOP check. Tropicamide is also instilled into the good eye without the patient's knowledge. After 30 minutes, the patient is asked to read at distance and near with both eyes. Because accommodation has been selectively paralyzed in the good eye, successful near reading indicates good vision in the affected eye.

Dissociation with Prisms Test Explain to the patient that you are going to test eye movement and alignment and that the test will produce double vision. Place a loose prism (4 prism diopters) base down in front of the normal eye while a "−" prism diopter prism is placed over the affected eye (base in any direction). Project a 20/20 or larger Snellen letter in the distance, asking the patient whether he can detect double vision. If the patient admits to double vision, ask whether the two letters are of equal quality or sharpness. A reasonable assessment of visual acuity can be made.

Titmus Stereopsis Test Correct identification of nine out of nine circles indicates 20 seconds of arc stereo acuity, which correlates with 20/20 visual acuity. A reliable correlation between Titmus score and visual acuity has been demonstrated.[24]

Size Consistency Test The patient reads the Snellen chart at half the testing distance. At half the distance, the patient should be able to read letters a least half the size of the letters read at the full testing distance. If the visual acuity is worse than expected, the visual loss is most likely nonorganic.

American Optical Polarizing Test The projected letters on this specially polarized chart are seen alternately by each eye when polarizing glasses are worn. One letter may be visible to both eyes, the next by the right eye, the next by the left eye etc. The patient can be tricked into admitting better visual acuity in the affected eye.

Techniques for Patients Claiming Loss of Peripheral Vision[22,23]

Saccade Test   Ask the patient to follow an object as it is moved in various directions, then to perform saccades from central gaze to eccentric target objects. Move the target from one area to another, asking the patient to look straight ahead, usually at the examiner's nose, then to the target. A successful saccade into the area of claimed visual field loss indicates nonorganic disease.

Monocular and Binocular Visual Field Testing   If the field defect is present in only one eye on monocular testing but is still present on binocular testing, the defect is nonorganic (the test cannot be used in patients claiming bilateral field loss).

Visual Field Test with a Goldmann Perimeter or Tangent Screen   If the visual field becomes smaller and smaller as the target is moved circumferentially, creating a so-called spiraling field, a nonorganic deficit exists.

• A patient claiming nonorganic field loss may be encouraged or coaxed into seeing a larger field during testing. The examiner compliments the patient, adding that instead of waiting until he is absolutely sure of seeing the target, he should respond right at the moment the light stimulus is just barely detected.

• Tangent screen field testing is performed at different distances while maintaining the same ratio of target size to testing distance. For example, the size of the test object used at a distance of 1 m is doubled when used at a testing distance of 2 m. The patient with organic field constriction will show an increase in the absolute size of the visual field when tested at 2 m. In contrast, the patient with nonorganic field loss is more likely to show no change at all in the absolute size of the field.

SUMMARY

Without proper evaluation, it is impossible to provide complete and maximal treatment for the patient with eye injury. The basic thought processes underlying the various diagnostic steps are shown in Figure 9–22.

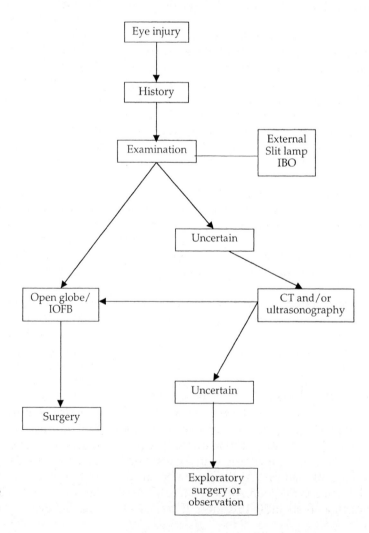

FIGURE 9–22   Flowchart for the evaluation of possible open globe injury.

REFERENCES

1. Pieramici DJ, MacCumber MW, Humayun MU, et al. Open-globe injury. Update on types of injuries and visual results. *Ophthalmology*. 1996;103:1798–1803.
2. Kuhn F, Morris R, Witherspoon CD, et al. A standardized classification of ocular trauma. *Ophthalmology*. 1996;103:240–243.
3. Pieramici DJ, Sternberg P Jr., Aaberg TM Sr, et al. A system for classifying mechanical injuries of the eye (globe). The ocular trauma classification group. *Am J Ophthalmol*. 1997;123:820–831.
4. Boldt HC, Pulido JS, Blodi CF, et al. Rural endophthalmitis. *Ophthalmology*. 1989;96:1722–1726.
5. Rubsamen PE, Cousins SW, Winward KE, Byrne DF. Diagnostic ultrasound and pars plana vitrectomy in penetrating ocular trauma. *Ophthalmology*. 1994;101:809–814.
6. Deramo VA, Shah GK, Baumol CR, et al. Ultrasound biomicroscopy as a tool for detecting and localizing occult foreign bodies after ocular trauma. *Ophthalmology*. 1999;106:301–305.
7. McNicholas MMJ, Brophy DP, Power WJ, Griffin JF. Ocular trauma: evaluation with US. *Radiology*. 1995;195:423–427.
8. Kwong JS, Munk PL, Lin DT, et al. Real-time ultrasonography in ocular trauma. *Am J Radiol*. 1992;158:179–182.
9. Koornneef L, Zonneveld F. The role of direct multiplanar high resolution CT in the assessment and management of orbital trauma. *Radiol Clin North Am*. 1987;25:753–766.
10. Mafee MF, Peyman GA. Retinal and choroidal detachments: role of magnetic resonance imaging and computed tomography. *Radiol Clin North Am*. 1987;25:487–507.
11. Joseph DP, Pieramici DJ, Beauchamp NJ. Computed tomography (CT) in the diagnosis and prognosis of open globe injuries. *Ophthalmology*. 2000;107:1899–1906.
12. LoBue TD , Deutsch TA, Lobick J, Turner DA. Detection and localization of nonmetallic intraocular foreign bodies by magnetic resonance imaging. *Arch Ophthalmol*. 1988;106:260–261.
13. Green BF, Kraft SP, Carter KD, et al. Intraorbital wood. Detection by magnetic resonance imaging. *Ophthalmology*. 1990;97:608–611.
14. Bilaniuk LT, Atlas SW, Zimmerman RA. Magnetic resonance imaging of the orbit. *Radiol Clin North Am*. 1987;25:509–528.
15. Lagouros PA, Langer BG, Peyman GA, et al. Magnetic resonance imaging and intraocular foreign bodies. *Arch Ophthalmol*. 1987;105:551–553.
16. Otto PM, Otto RA, Virapongse C, et al. Screening test for detection of metallic foreign objects in the orbit before magnetic resonance imaging. *Invest Radiol*. 1992;27:308–311.
17. Summanen P. Vitrectomy for diabetic eye disease. The prognostic value of preoperative electroretinography and visual evoked potentials. *Ophthalmologica*. 1989;199:60–71.
18. Mandelbaum S, Cleary PE, Ryan SJ, Ogden TE. Bright-flash electroretinography and vitreous hemorrhage. An experimental study in primates. *Arch Ophthalmol*. 1980;98:1823–1828.
19. Neubauer H. Ocular metallosis. *Trans Ophthalmol Soc UK*. 1979;99:502–510.
20. Weiss MJ, Hofeldt AJ, Behrens M, Fisher K. Ocular siderosis. Diagnosis and management. *Retina*. 1997;17:105–108.
21. Rosenthal AR, Marmor MF, Leuenberger P, Hopkins JL. Chalcosis: a study of natural history. *Ophthalmology*. 1979;86:1956–1972.
22. Miller NR. *Walsh and Hoyt's Clinical Neuro-Ophthalmology*. 4th ed. Part 2. Baltimore: Williams & Wilkins; 1995:4541–4563.
23. Kramer KK, La Piana FG, Appleton B. Ocular malingering and hysteria: diagnosis and management. *Surv Ophthalmol*. 1979;24:89–96.
24. Levy NS, Glick EB. Stereoscopic perception and Snellen visual acuity. *Am J Ophthalmol*. 1974;78:722–724.

SECTION II

EMERGENCY MANAGEMENT

MANAGEMENT OF PATIENTS WITH POLYTRAUMA

Joel A. Pearlman and Dante J. Pieramici

 Treating polytraumatized patients can be extremely challenging, requiring rapid and efficient collaboration of multiple specialists and paramedical personnel (e.g., nurses, technicians, emergency physicians, surgeons, radiologists, anesthesiologists, operating room personnel, even interpreters).

> **PEARL...** Emergency medical technicians, police, and fire fighters often provide critical details of the injury and past medical history. They also help to preserve the integrity of evidence that might later be used in court.

In the initial phase of emergency medical care, the visual system commonly has low priority, but loss of vision can significantly diminish the quality of life for the otherwise rehabilitated patient and may result in the most devastating long-term disability.[1]

EPIDEMIOLOGY

A retrospective analysis[1] of 1119 cases from a major hospital over a 7-year period (Fig. 10–1) found the following:

- age ranged from 15 to 90 years;
- 80% of the patients were male;
- 16% suffered ocular or adnexal injuries and 23% of these patients died;

- 29% had facial injuries, of which 55% were ocular injuries; and
- 1.2% of injuries resulted in vision less than 20/200.

Significant eye injury was statistically associated with the following:

- driving a motor vehicle;
- age younger than 50 years;
- male sex;
- associated basal skull fracture;
- orbital fracture; and
- lid laceration or superficial eye injury.

Of the patients with the most severe injuries:

- 0.8% had open globe injuries;
- 1.9% had optic nerve trauma, half of whom had vision less than 20/200; and
- 9.2% had orbital fracture.

In another study, among 6313 patients with major injuries admitted to a level I trauma facility over a 4-year period, 14% were found to have concomitant eye injury, most commonly eye/adnexa contusion (67%), adnexal lacerations (27%), and open globe injury (4%).[2]

INITIAL ASSESSMENT

The initial steps are based on the general principles of advanced trauma life support.[a]

---

[a] Ensuring the patency of the airway and establishing breathing and cardiovascular stability (ABC).

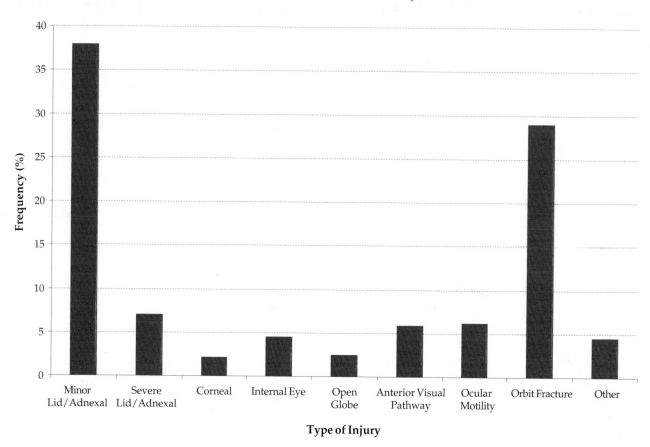

FIGURE 10–1 Ocular injuries associated with major trauma. (Adapted from Poon A, McCluskey PJ, Hill DA. Eye injuries in patients with major trauma. *J Trauma*. 1999;46:494–499. Reprinted by permission from Lippincott Williams & Wilkins.)

PEARL... In many cases, it is helpful for the ophthalmologist to be present in the ER or trauma room to try to protect the eyes during manipulations of the mouth, nose, and trachea. Emergency ocular problems (e.g., chemical burn, central retinal artery occlusion, open globes, retrobulbar hemorrhage) must also be addressed early.

PEARL... In patients with severe intracranial injuries in whom changes in pupil size and reactivity may presage impending herniation and the need for immediate neurosurgical intervention, the integrity of the pupil (i.e., no pharmacologic dilation) is more important than the information provided by dilated-pupil IBO.

When possible, an initial assessment of the vision should be performed, although altered mental status as a result of intracranial trauma or the use of analgesia or anesthesia may prevent this. The miotic effect of narcotic agents can hinder the examination of the pupils and the retina.

Finally, urgent ophthalmic problems should be assessed; in most cases, the initial triage is possible using only a penlight examination. The eye's repair often has to be coordinated with other surgical interventions (e.g., an open globe should be closed before orbital surgery is performed; see Chapter 12).

EMERGENCY INTERVENTION

Ocular conditions requiring *immediate* evaluation and/or intervention include:

- chemical burn (see Chapter 11) and, to a lesser extent,
- retrobulbar hemorrhage (see Chapter 12) and
- open globe injury (see Chapter 9).

OPEN GLOBE INJURY AND THE NONOPHTHALMOLOGIST

Signs that suggest the presence or possibility of open globe trauma include:

- obvious open wound;
- collapsed or severely distorted eye;
- prolapsed uveal tissue;
- peaked pupil;
- subconjunctival hemorrhage with shallowing or deepening of the AC; and/or
- ocular hypotony with or without subconjunctival hemorrhage.

RADIOLOGIC EVALUATION

The eyes, orbits, and surrounding bones are best visualized with a noncontrast CT scan, which can usually be obtained concurrently with the imaging of the brain, thorax, and abdomen typically necessary in the evaluation of these patients (see Chapter 9).

SPECIAL CONSIDERATIONS

Children

In children with polytrauma, there are unique legal implications because of abuse. Abuse annually involves approximately 900,000 children in the United States[3] (see also Chapters 9, 30, and 33). More than 80% of shaken babies have ocular manifestations; therefore, an appropriate ophthalmic evaluation is critical.[4] Bilateral findings are present in 85% of affected children, and one fifth of surviving children have permanently poor vision.[4] There may be a correlation between the severity of retinal hemorrhage and neurologic outcome.[5] Perimacular retinal folds may be pathognomic.[6]

> **PEARL...** Although retinal hemorrhage has occasionally been noted to occur after CPR, a prospective study failed to find a causal relationship in nontraumatized patients.[7]

Examination of traumatized children can be difficult, even dangerous. Monitored sedation with ketamine, Fentanyl, and/or Versed can be helpful if administered by an experienced ER physician or anesthesiologist. Bradyarrhythmias and episodic apnea are common in neonates and are best managed by experienced neonatologists. Photographic documentation and/or careful drawings are important for both medical and legal reasons (see Chapter 8).

Patients with Psychiatric Disease

The injury mechanism in psychiatric patients is often dramatic, historical details are inaccurate, and consent is impossible. Early recognition of the psychiatric disturbance and appropriate consultation are key to successful management.

- *Oedipism* (autoenucleation) is a medical emergency requiring ophthalmic and psychiatric treatment. Both eyes may be injured or enucleated. Retrobulbar hemorrhage (see Chapter 12) can ensue, for which lateral canthotomy, cantholysis, and intravenous steroids may be useful; with treatment, even NLP initial vision can improve dramatically.[8] One should always consider concomitant illicit drug use and obtain a toxicology screen.
- *Dementia* or *delirium* should always be suspected in an elderly patient who suffers eye injury in a fall. Such patients need neurologic and musculoskeletal evaluations as well as close observation to reduce the risk of repeated injury.

Occult Ocular Trauma

Despite a lack of obvious signs, eye injury may be present in the polytraumatized patient; see Chapter 9 for risk factors and diagnosis.

Major Disasters in Peace and War

Terrorism-related eye injury appears to be an increasing threat (see the chapter on *The patient's perspective*), and the eye is commonly involved. In the Oklahoma City bombing[9] nearly 10% of survivors suffered ocular injury, most commonly corneal abrasions, lid and brow lacerations, open globe injuries, and conjunctivitis; 4% of eyes harbored IOFBs; and patients with eye injury had a higher risk of more severe systemic injuries.

In the bombing of the U.S. Air Force compound in Dahran, Saudi Arabia,[10] 11% of the victims had severe ocular injury.

In the 1973 Yom Kippur and 1982 Lebanon wars, almost 7% of all injuries in the Israeli Defense Force involved the eye.[11]

Concurrent Ocular and Orbital Injury

The timing of surgery for one injury in cases of ocular polytrauma may affect the timing of another (e.g., orbital fracture repair is deferred until the risk of rebleeding in hyphema is diminished; a "trap-door" fracture's otherwise urgent repair[12] is delayed because the globe's rupture must be closed first; see also Chapter 8).

Ophthalmic Conditions as a Result of Systemic Injuries

Traumatic Optic Neuropathy

Early identification of TON is very important. High-dose corticosteroids[13] or other interventions, rather than observation,[14] should be considered (see Chapter 37), although the results are not conclusive.[15]

Cranial Neuropathies

Acute palsy of a cranial nerve occasionally develops.

> **PEARL…** An oculomotor nerve palsy should raise concern about a ruptured aneurysm, best imaged by digital subtraction angiography or MRI and angiography if the patient is otherwise stable. With a 25 to 50% mortality rate and severe neurologic impairment in half of the survivors, a ruptured intracranial aneurysm requires early recognition and treatment.[16] The ophthalmologist's diagnostic input can be critical.

Purtscher's Retinopathy

Purtscher's retinopathy is discussed in Chapter 33.

> **PEARL…** Rapid identification of the problems and early, coordinated treatment can reduce morbidity and increase the quality of life for the polytraumatized patient.

Summary

Perhaps the most important roles of the nonophthalmologist are early recognition of eye injury in the polytraumatized patient and appropriate early consultation. The outcome can be optimized by effective communication and planning by all specialists involved in the case. Coordinating surgeries will spare the patient the risks of multiple general anesthesias and lessen the chance of iatrogenic injury.

References

1. Poon A, McCluskey PJ, Hill DA. Eye injuries in patients with major trauma. *J Trauma*. 1999;46:494–499.

2. Sastry SM, Paul BK, Bain L, Champion HR. Ocular trauma among major trauma victims in a regional trauma center. *J Trauma*. 1993;34:223–226.

3. United States Department of Health and Human Services. *Child Maltreatment 1998: Reports from the States to the National Child Abuse and Neglect Reporting System*. Washington, DC: US Government Printing Office; 2000.

4. Odom A, Christ E, Kerr N, et al. Prevalence of retinal hemorrhages in pediatric patients after in-hospital cardiopulmonary resuscitation: a prospective study. *Pediatrics*. 1997;99:E3.

5. Wilkinson WS, Han DP, Rappley MD, Owings CL. Retinal hemorrhage predicts neurologic injury in the shaken baby syndrome. *Arch Ophthalmol*. 1989;107:1472–1474.

6. Massicotte SJ, Folberg R, Torczynski E, Gilliland MG, Luckenbach MW. Vitreoretinal traction and perimacular retinal folds in the eyes of deliberately traumatized children. *Ophthalmology*. 1991;98:1124–1127.

7. Kivlin JD, Simons KB, Lazoritz S, Ruttum MS. Shaken baby syndrome. *Ophthalmology*. 2000;107:1246–1254.

8. Wolff RS, Wright MM, Walsh AW. Attempted autoenucleation. *Am J Ophthalmol*. 1996;121:726–728.

9. Mines M, Thach A, Mallonee S, Hildebrand L, Shariat S. Ocular injuries sustained by survivors of the Oklahoma City bombing. *Ophthalmology*. 2000;107:837–843.

10. Thach AB, Ward TP, Hollifield RD, Cockerham K, Birdsong R, Kramer KK. Eye injuries in a terrorist bombing: Dhahran, Saudi Arabia, June 25, 1996. *Ophthalmology*. 2000;107:844–847.

11. Belkin M, Treister G, Dotan S. Eye injuries and ocular protection in the Lebanon War, 1982. *Isr J Med Sci*. 1984; 20:333–338.

12. Blanc JL, Cheynet F, Lagier JP, Lachard J. Trap-door fractures of the orbit floor. Apropos of 8 cases. *Rev Stomatol Chir Maxillofac*. 1988;89:199–203.

13. Bracken MB, Shepard MJ, Collins WF, et al. A randomized, controlled trial of methylprednisolone or naloxone in the treatment of acute spinal-cord injury. Results of the Second National Acute Spinal Cord Injury Study. *N Engl J Med*. 1990;322:1405–1411.

14. Cook MW, Levin LA, Joseph MP, Pinczower EF. Traumatic optic neuropathy. A meta-analysis. *Arch Otolaryngol Head Neck Surg*. 1996;122:389–392.

15. Levin LA, Beck RW, Joseph MP, Seiff S, Kraker R. The treatment of traumatic optic neuropathy: the International Optic Nerve Trauma Study. *Ophthalmology*. 1999;106:1268–1277.

16. Hop JW, Rinkel GJ, Algra A, van Gijn J. Case-fatality rates and functional outcome after subarachnoid hemorrhage: a systematic review. *Stroke*. 1997;28: 660–664.

Chapter 11

CHEMICAL INJURIES: EMERGENCY INTERVENTION

Michael D. Wagoner and Kenneth R. Kenyon

 Chemical injuries of the eye may produce extensive damage to the ocular surface and thus lead to visual impairment.[1-4] In addition to causing ocular surface injury, alkalies (Fig. 11–1) readily penetrate into the eye, damaging the corneal stroma and endothelium as well as other anterior segment structures (e.g., iris, lens, ciliary body). Most acids (Fig. 11–2) tend to remain confined to the ocular surface. The important agents involved in chemical injuries of the eye are summarized in Table 11–1.[2,3]

> **PEARL...** Strong acids, such as hydrofluoric acid, may penetrate as readily as alkalies do, producing the same spectrum of ocular injury.[2]

ETIOLOGY

The most common *alkalis* causing injury[4] are:

- ammonia (NH_3; a common ingredient in many household cleaning agents and causing the most serious injury);
- lye (NaOH; a common ingredient in drain cleaners and causing the most serious injury);
- potassium hydroxide (KOH);
- magnesium hydroxide ($Mg[OH]_2$); and
- lime ($Ca[OH]_2$; the most common cause, which fortunately does not inflict as much damage as rapidly penetrating alkalies do).

The most common *acids* causing injury[4] are:

- sulfuric (H_2SO_4; the most common cause: an ingredient in automobile batteries[2]);
- sulfurous (H_2SO_3);
- hydrofluoric (HF; rapidly penetrating and causing the most serious injuries[2]);
- acetic (CH_3COOH);
- chromic (Cr_2O_3); and
- hydrochloric (HCl).

EPIDEMIOLOGY AND PROGNOSIS

In the USEIR, 3.6% of all serious injuries are chemical burns. In one study[5]:

- most victims were young (usually between 16 and 25 years of age) and male (76%);
- the most common sites of accidental injury were industrial premises (63%) and the home (33%);
- criminal assault was rather frequent (11%);
- alkali injuries were nearly twice as common as acid injuries; and
- only 8% of patients required hospitalization, and less than 1% suffered severe, permanent visual loss.

In another study[6]:

- 70% of patients were adult males, 23% were adult females, and 7% were children;
- most patients were between 16 and 45 years of age;
- industrial accidents accounted for 61% of the injuries; 37% were due to household accidents; and
- 88% of the injuries were classified as mild.

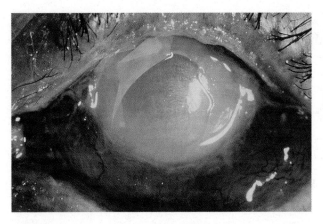

FIGURE 11–1   Severe alkali injury. The entire epithelium is either absent or devitalized. Because of stromal and intraocular penetration, the corneal stroma is cloudy, in contrast to the appearance in Figure 11–2. (From Wagoner MD. Chemical injuries of the eye: current concepts in pathophysiology and therapy. *Surv Ophthalmol.* 1997;41:275–313, Reprinted by permission from Elsevier Science.)

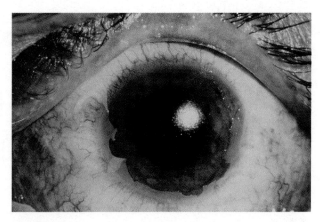

FIGURE 11–2   Acid injury caused by exploding car battery. A 100% epithelial defect is present. Following débridement of necrotic epithelium (some remaining peripherally), the stroma is remarkably clear because of the function of the epithelium as a barrier to acid penetration. (From Mandel ER, Wagoner MD. *Atlas of Corneal Disease.* Philadelphia: WB Saunders; 1989:71. Reprinted by permission from WB Saunders.)

TABLE 11–1   COMMON CAUSES OF CHEMICAL INJURY[3]

Class	Compound	Common Source/Use	Comments
Alkali	Ammonia	Fertilizers, refrigerants; cleaning agents (7% solution)	Combines with H_2O to form NH_4OH fumes; very rapid penetration
	Lye	Drain cleaners; caustic potash	Penetrates almost as rapidly as ammonia; severity similar to that of lye
	Magnesium hydroxide	Sparklers	Produces combined thermal and alkali injury
	Lime	Plaster; mortar; cement; whitewash	Most common work-related chemical injury; toxicity increased by retained particulate matter
Acid	Sulfuric	Industrial cleaners; batteries	Combines with H_2O to produce thermal injury; have may corneal/conjunctival foreign body
	Sulfurous	Fruit/vegetable preservatives; bleach refrigerants	Combines with corneal H_2O to form sulfur; penetrates more easily than most other acids
	Hydrofluoric	Glass polishing/frosting; mineral refining; gasoline alkylation; silicone production	Penetrates easily; produces severe injury
	Acetic	Vinegar (4–10%); essence of vinegar (80%); glacial acetic acid (90%)	Mild injury with <10% concentration; severe injury with higher
	Chromic	Chrome plating industry	Chronic exposure produces brown conjunctival discoloration
	Hydrochloric	31–38% solution	Severe injury only with high concentration and prolonged exposure

Although the majority of chemical injuries are without serious sequelae, the prognosis for eyes that present with severe injuries is guarded; in one series,[7] only 15% achieved adequate visual recovery.

PATHOPHYSIOLOGY

The severity of ocular injury after chemical exposure is related to:

- surface area of contact;
- depth of penetration; and
- degree of limbal stem cell injury.

Surface Area of Contact

Both alkalies and acids cause the ocular surface epithelial cells to die upon contact. The surface area of contact can be assessed by examination of the fluorescein-staining pattern of the corneal or conjunctival epithelium.

> **PEARL...** It is important to remember that retained particulate matter in the superior fornix (e.g., in case of lime plaster injury) can be a source of continued exposure of the ocular surface to additional damage.

Depth of Penetration

> **PEARL...** In general, alkalies tend to penetrate more effectively than acids.[1–4]

Penetration of alkalies and acids into the corneal stroma may result in keratocyte death and hydration of the ground substance with loss of stromal clarity.[8,9] Hydration of collagen fibrils results in thickening and shortening with distortion of the trabecular meshwork and potential increase in IOP.[7,8]

The time to penetration into the AC varies from almost immediate after ammonia injury to 3 to 5 minutes after sodium hydroxide injury.[10,11] Penetration into the AC can result in secondary glaucoma[a] and cataract.[7] Irreversible damage to the ciliary body with hypotony and phthisis may follow prolonged aqueous pH levels above 11.5.[11]

If the external pH is restored to normal, the aqueous pH levels return to normal within 30 minutes to 3 hours, depending upon the amount of penetration.[11]

Limbal Stem Cell Injury

> **PEARL...** Following corneal epithelial injury, recovery is dependent upon the most proximal, viable epithelium.[12,13]

- Complete corneal epithelial injury requires epithelium from the limbus,[14–20] where the stem cells of the corneal epithelium reside (see Chapter 32).
- With extensive corneal and limbal epithelial injury, the surrounding conjunctival epithelium provides the only source for epithelial regeneration.[21]

The clinical course of reepithelialization and its impact upon therapeutic decision making are discussed in Chapter 32.

THERAPEUTIC PRINCIPLES

A modification of our three-step approach to sterile corneal ulceration is applicable for treating the chemically injured eye from the outset.[22,23]

Step 1: Promote ocular surface epithelial recovery with proper phenotypic transdifferentiation.

> **PEARL...** The recovery of an intact and phenotypically normal corneal epithelium is the most important determinant of a favorable outcome following chemical injury.

---

[a]See Chapter 20 for the treatment of glaucoma in chemical injuries.

- *Débridement of necrotic epithelium* (Fig. 11–2) allows subsequent migration of adjacent viable epithelium into the denuded area.

- *Nonpreserved topical lubricants* may facilitate reepi-thelialization in older patients with aqueous tear deficiency. In young patients with adequate tear production, tear supplementation is not necessary.

- *Pressure patching* and/or *bandage soft contact lens* therapy does not improve the rate of reepithelialization but may provide pain relief.

Subsequent medical and surgical interventions to enhance corneal epithelial recovery are discussed in Chapter 32.

Step 2: Apply supportive repair (augment collagen production and/or minimize collagenase activity)

Aqueous levels of *ascorbate*[b] may be depleted following chemical injuries with intraocular penetration, due to impaired secretion by the ciliary body epithelium.[24–26]

The beneficial effects of supplemental topical and systemic ascorbate in facilitating collagen synthesis and reducing the risk of corneal ulceration due to excessive collagenolysis are achieved with *early* supplementation; when corneal ulceration begins, supplemental ascorbate is of limited benefit in halting its progression.[24–26]

Collagenase inhibitors were used earlier[27] but, being ineffective, have been abandoned.

The efficacy of *tetracycline derivatives* in preventing corneal ulceration after chemical injury is maximized with *early* administration. They have been shown to be efficacious in:

- reducing collagenase activity;[28]

- inhibiting polymorphonuclear leukocyte activity;[29] and

- inhibiting corneal ulceration[30] in experimental alkali injuries.

---

[b]A cofactor in the rate-limiting step of collagen synthesis; its deficiency may contribute to the impairment of corneal repair after chemical injury.

PEARL... **Therapeutic strategies that exclude polymorphonuclear and mononuclear leukocytes from the stroma contribute to prevention and arrest of corneal ulceration.**[31,32]

Step 3: Control inflammation

Citrate,[c] a naturally occurring vitamin, reduces leukocyte infiltration into the stroma and the incidence of corneal ulceration experimentally—provided that it is administered early.[26,35,d]

Corticosteroids reduce inflammatory cell infiltration and stabilize polymorphonuclear leukocyte cytoplasmic and lysosomal membranes.[36] The key to successful use of corticosteroids is to maximize their anti-inflammatory effect *during the first week*, when the risk-benefit ratio is favorable. There is little risk[37] of sterile ulceration in the first week following severe chemical injury whether or not corticosteroids are used. Corticosteroids interfere with stromal wound repair by impairing both keratocyte migration into the area of injury and collagen synthesis,[38–40] but their deleterious side effect does not become apparent until corneal repair processes begin after 10 to 14 days.[e]

Modifications of topical inflammatory therapy after the first week are discussed in Chapter 32.

Sᴘᴇᴄɪꜰɪᴄ Tʜᴇʀᴀᴘʏ

The specific therapeutic strategies employed immediately after injury focus upon:

- elimination of residual alkali or acid from the eye;

---

[c]A calcium chelator that decreases the membrane and intracellular calcium levels of polymorphonuclear leukocytes, with resultant impaired chemotaxis, phagocytosis, adherence, and release of lysosomal enzymes.[33,34]

[d]Similarly to ascorbate, it has no effect on the progression of *established* corneal ulceration.

[e]After 7 to 10 days, the suppression of keratocyte collagen production by corticosteroids may offset the advantages of their effect on inflammatory cell suppression and collagenase inhibition, resulting in a net shift of corneal repair toward ulceration.

- débridement of necrotic corneal epithelium and conjunctiva; and

- institution of topical and systemic medical therapy to minimize adverse sequelae.

Subsequent medical therapy and surgical intervention are discussed in Chapter 32.

SPECIAL CONSIDERATION

Chemical injury is an absolute *emergency* in which literally every second counts. Intervention must precede the steps of a traditional examination such as detailed history taking or even recording the visual acuity (see Chapter 9).

Irrigation

PEARL... The physician must assume that any previous irrigation was inadequate and thus copious irrigation should be resumed immediately.

One of the main determinants of the ultimate outcome following chemical injury is the duration of contact between the chemical agent and the eye. Because of the deep location and relatively protected site of the limbal stem cells, their injury may be averted with prompt irrigation. Follow these steps given below.

1. Irrigate copiously
   - No therapeutic differences have been identified between normal saline, normal saline with bicarbonate, lactated Ringer's, balanced salt solution (BSS), and BSS-plus.[41]
   - Try to use other *neutral* fluids.[f]
   - As it is impossible to "overirrigate" a chemically injured eye, irrigation for 15 to 30 minutes is recommended.

2. Evert the upper lid (see Chapter 13 for the technique) and irrigate the fornices.

PEARL... Use of topical anesthetics and lid retractors is very helpful; use of an intravenous infusion set provides convenience.

3. Check the pH a few minutes after irrigation; continue irrigating until the pH reaches 7.0.

4. Remove remnants of the agent (e.g., plaster) from the fornices mechanically with a moistened cotton-tipped[g] applicator or a jeweler's forceps. Double eversion (see Chapter 13) provides the best access to the upper fornix.

The benefit of *paracentesis and irrigation of the AC* following a severe chemical injury is uncertain.[42]

Débridement
Necrotic corneal epithelium should be débrided to allow proper migration of adjacent, viable epithelium.

Devitalized conjunctival epithelium should also be débrided to remove a nidus of persistent inflammation, which can also retard corneal reepithelialization.[43]

Medical Therapy
See the preceding rationale for the subsequent use of topical and systemic medications; the specific recommended dosages are listed in Table 11–2. Topical

TABLE 11–2 TOPICAL AND SYSTEMIC MEDICATIONS TO BE USED AT THE OUTSET IN THE TREATMENT OF MODERATE AND SEVERE CHEMICAL INJURIES

Drug	Dosage
Topical corticosteroids	Every 1 to 4 hours
Topical sodium ascorbate	Every 2 to 4 hours
Topical sodium citrate 10%	Every 2 to 4 hours
Topical tetracycline	4x daily
Sodium ascorbate 2 g	2x daily p. os
Doxycycline 100 mg	2x daily p. os
Glaucoma medications	As needed
Cycloplegics	As needed

[f]For example, do not use an acid to offset an alkaline agent.

[g]10% EDTA solution makes it easier to remove lime particles.

sodium ascorbate and citrate are not available commercially but can be prepared by most pharmacy departments.

SUMMARY

Chemical injuries of the eye are true ocular emergency. The most important aspect in the management of these injuries is to begin prompt and copious irrigation of the eye. Following this, the management is less emergent and focuses on the promotion of ocular surface recovery and ocular repair. The ultimate outcome of these injuries is determined, in large part, by the nature of the chemical agent and the duration of contact between that noxious agent and the eye.

REFERENCES

1. Hughes WF. Alkali burns of the cornea. I. Review of the literature and summary of present knowledge. *Arch Ophthalmol.* 1946;35:423–426.

2. McCulley JP. Chemical injuries. In: Smolin G, Thoft RA, eds. *The Cornea: Scientific Foundation and Clinical Practice.* 2nd ed. Boston: Little, Brown; 1987:527–542.

3. Wagoner MD, Kenyon KR. Chemical injuries of the eye. In: Albert DM, Jakobiec FA, eds. *Principles and Practice of Ophthalmology: Clinical Practice.* Vol 1. Philadelphia: WB Saunders; 1994:234–245.

4. Wagoner MD. Chemical injuries of the eye: current concepts in pathophysiology and therapy. *Surv Ophthalmol.* 1997;41:275–313.

5. Morgan SJ. Chemical burns of the eye: causes and management. *Br J Ophthalmol.* 1987;71:854–857.

6. Kuckelkorn R, Luft I, Kotteck AA, et al. Chemical and thermal eye burns in the residential area of RWTH Aachen. Analysis of accidents in 1 year using a new automated documentation of findings. *Klin Monatsbl Augenheilkd.* 1993;203:34–42.

7. Kuckelkorn R, Makropoulos W, Kotteck A, Reim M. Retrospective study of severe alkali burns of the eye. *Klin Monatsbl Augenheilkd.* 1993;203:397–402.

8. Matsuda H, Smelser GK. Epithelium and stroma in alkali-burned corneas. *Arch Ophthalmol.* 1973;89:396–401.

9. Matsuda H, Smelser GK. Endothelial cells in alkali-burned corneas; ultrastructural alterations. *Arch Ophthalmol.* 1973;89:402–409.

10. Grant WM. Experimental investigation of paracentesis in the treatment of ocular ammonia burns. *Arch Ophthalmol.* 1950;44:399–404.

11. Paterson CA, Pfister RR, Levinson RA. Aqueous humor pH changes after experimental alkali burns. *Am J Ophthalmol.* 1975;79:414–419.

12. Friedenwald JS, Buschke W. Some factors concerned in the mitotic and wound-healing activities of the corneal epithelium. *Trans Am Ophthalmol Soc.* 1944;42:371–383.

13. Kuwabara T, Perkins DG, Cogan DG. Sliding of the epithelium in experimental corneal wounds. *Invest Ophthalmol.* 1976;15:4–14.

14. Davanger M, Evensen A. Role of the pericorneal papillary structure in renewal of corneal epithelium. *Nature.* 1971;229:560–561.

15. Friend J, Thoft RA. Functional competence of regenerating ocular surface epithelium. *Invest Ophthalmol Vis Sci.* 1978;17:134–139.

16. Thoft RA, Friend J, The X, Y, Z hypothesis of corneal epithelial maintenance. *Invest Ophthalmol Vis Sci.* 1983;24:1442–1443.

17. Buck RC. Measurement of centripetal migration of normal corneal epithelial cells in the mouse. *Invest Ophthalmol Vis Sci.* 1985;26:1296–1299.

18. Schermer A, Galvin S, Sun TT. Differentiation-related expression of a major 64K corneal keratin in vivo and in culture suggests limbal location of corneal epithelial stem cells. *J Cell Biol.* 1986;103:49–62.

19. Zieske JD, Bukusoglu G, Yankauckas MA. Characterization of a potential marker of corneal epithelial stem cells. *Invest Ophthalmol Vis Sci.* 1992;33:143–152.

20. Thoft RA, Wiley LA, Sundarraj N. The multipotential cells of the limbus. *Eye.* 1989;3(2):109–113.

21. Shapiro MS, Friend J, Thoft RA. Corneal re-epithelialization from the conjunctiva. *Invest Ophthalmol Vis Sci.* 1981;21:135–142.

22. Kenyon KR. Decision making in the therapy of external eye disease: noninfected corneal ulcers. *Ophthalmology.* 1982;89:44–51.

23. Wagoner MD, Kenyon KR. Noninfected corneal ulceration. In: *Focal Points: Clinical Modules for Ophthalmologists.* Vol 3. San Francisco: American Academy of Ophthalmology; 1985:7.

24. Pfister RR, Paterson CA. Additional clinical and morphological observations on the favorable effect of ascorbate in experimental ocular alkali burns. *Invest Ophthalmol Vis Sci.* 1977;16:478–487.

25. Pfister RR, Paterson CA. Ascorbic acid in the treatment of alkali burns of the eye. *Ophthalmology.* 1980;87: 1050–1057.

26. Pfister RR, Haddox JL, Lank KM. Citrate or ascorbate-citrate treatment of established corneal ulcers in the alkali injured rabbit eye. *Invest Ophthalmol Vis Sci.* 1988;29:1110–1115.

27. Brown SI, Hook CW. Treatment of corneal destruction with collagenase inhibitors. *Trans Am Acad Ophthalmol Otolaryngol.* 1971;75:1199–1207.

28. Golub LM, McNamara TF, D'Angelo G, Greenwald RA. A nonantibacterial chemically-modified tetracycline inhibits mammalian collagenase activity. *J Dent Res.* 1987;66:1310–1314.

29. Gabler WL, Creamer HR. Suppression of human neutrophil functions by tetracyclines. *J Periodont Res.* 1991;26:52–58.

30. Perry HD, Hodes LW, Seedor JA, et al. Effect of doxycycline hyclate on corneal epithelial wound healing in the rabbit alkali-burn model. Preliminary observations. *Cornea.* 1993;12:379–382.

31. Kenyon KR. Inflammatory mechanisms in corneal ulceration. *Trans Am Ophthalmol Soc.* 1985;83:610–663.

32. Kenyon KR, Berman M, Rose J, Gage J. Prevention of stromal ulceration in the alkali-burned rabbit cornea by glued-on contact lens. Evidence for the role of polymorphonuclear leukocytes in collagen degradation. *Invest Ophthalmol Vis Sci.* 1979;18:570–587.

33. Paterson CA, Williams RN, Parker AW. Characteristics of polymorphonuclear leukocyte infiltration into the alkali-burned eye and influence of sodium citrate. *Exp Eye Res.* 1984;39:701–708.

34. Pfister RR, Haddox JL, Dodson RW, Deshazo WF. Polymorphonuclear leukocyte inhibition by citrate, other heavy metal chelators, and trifluoperazine: evidence to support calcium binding protein involvement. *Invest Ophthalmol Vis Sci.* 1984;25:955–970.

35. Haddox JL, Pfister RR, Yuille-Barr D. The efficacy of topical citrate after alkali injury is dependent on the period of time it is administered. *Invest Ophthalmol Vis Sci.* 1989;30:1062–1068.

36. Basu PK, Avaria M, Jankie R. Effect of hydrocortisone on the mobilisation of leucocytes in corneal wounds. *Br J Ophthalmol.* 1981;65:694–698.

37. Donshik PC, Berman MB, Dohlman CH, et al. Effect of topical corticosteroids on ulceration in alkali-burned corneas. *Arch Ophthalmol.* 1978;96:2117–2120.

38. Beams R, Linabery L, Grayson M. Effect of topical corticosteroids on corneal wound strength. *Am J Ophthalmol.* 1968;66:1131–1133.

39. Gasset AR, Lorenzetti DW, Ellison EM, Kaufman HE. Quantitative corticosteroid effect on corneal wound healing. *Arch Ophthalmol.* 1969;81:589–591.

40. Phillips K, Arffa R, Cintron C, et al. Effects of prednisolone and medroxyprogesterone on corneal wound healing, ulceration, and neovascularization. *Arch Ophthalmol.* 1983;101:640–643.

41. Herr RD, White GL Jr, Bernhisel K, et al. Clinical comparison of ocular irrigation fluids following chemical injury. *Am J Emerg Med.* 1991;9:228–231.

42. Burns RP, Hikes CE. Irrigation of the anterior chamber for the treatment of alkali burns. *Am J Ophthalmol.* 1979;88:119–120.

43. Wagoner MD, Kenyon KR, Gipson IK, et al. Polymorphonuclear neutrophils delay corneal epithelial wound healing in vitro. *Invest Ophthalmol Vis Sci.* 1984;25: 1217–1220.

Chapter 12

Nonglobe Injuries: Emergency (Room) Management

John A. Long and Thomas M. Tann

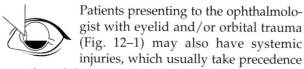 Patients presenting to the ophthalmologist with eyelid and/or orbital trauma (Fig. 12–1) may also have systemic injuries, which usually take precedence over the ophthalmic evaluation (see Chapters 9 and 10).

EVALUATION

Assessment of the orbit and the adnexa begins with a focused ophthalmic history; the mechanism by which the injury was inflicted helps direct the physical examination.

PEARL... Injuries caused by high-speed missiles or metal-on-metal contact increase the likelihood of an eyelid or intraorbital foreign body. Blows to the orbit by large objects can lead to orbital bone fractures. Dog bite injuries in the medial canthus are often associated with canalicular lacerations.

Evaluation of the adnexa begins with the eyelid and canalicular systems; and usually precedes detailed examination of the eyes.

PEARL... Evidence of laceration in the medial canthal area requires nasolacrimal duct probing and irrigation. Failure to diagnose the *canalicular laceration* can lead to lifelong tearing.[1] Remember that canalicular lacerations can result from a deceptively small *eyelid laceration*.

Assessing the eyelid position and function in the ER requires measurement and documentation of lid position and excursions. Lid lacerations may cause a dramatic ptosis, but lid function may dictate the method of repair. Traumatic ptosis may be present without eyelid laceration. Eyelid edema, burns, and preseptal cellulitis all compromise eyelid function, and their documentation is important.

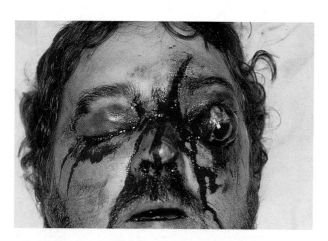

FIGURE 12–1 Dramatic ocular injury following a horse kick. Associated injuries include multiple bone fractures.

Extraocular muscle function is assessed to evaluate the presence of restricted movement. Restricted muscle function is a hallmark of:

- blowout fracture;
- orbital cellulitis; or
- orbital foreign body.

Progressive orbital signs and symptoms require expedited radiographic examination.[a] A CT scan with axial and coronal cuts best demonstrates the relationship between orbital bones and soft tissue.

EMERGENCY CONDITIONS AND THEIR MANAGEMENT

The repair of full-thickness eyewall injury always takes precedence over the repair of periocular trauma; repair of orbital bone damage can usually be delayed for weeks.[2]

PITFALL

The repair of a blowout fracture at the time of open globe repair is contraindicated.

True orbital or periocular emergencies are life or vision threatening. Fortunately, they are infrequent and include:

- expanding orbital hemorrhage;
- orbital abscess; and
- certain types of orbital foreign bodies (e.g., pressing on the optic nerve, protruding) (Fig. 12–2).

---

[a]Not required in case of a straightforward orbital blowout fracture.

Orbital hemorrhages are often iatrogenic, caused by retrobulbar injections or eyelid surgery. Depending on the severity of the condition, signs include:

- sudden proptosis;
- hemorrhagic chemosis;
- vision loss;
- elevated IOP/reduced or absent retinal perfusion;
- restricted extraocular muscle movements;
- APD; and
- asymmetrical color vision.

Medical treatment (for less severe cases) includes:

- mannitol;
- steroids; and
- antiglaucoma drops.

The *surgical* management options are:

- lateral cantholysis;
- evacuation of hemorrhage;
- paracentesis; and
- bony orbital decompression.

Orbital abscess is most frequently caused by spread of a preexisting sinus infection (Fig. 12–3). In severe cases, vision may be compromised. Classic signs[3] include:

- proptosis;
- restricted extraocular muscle movement;
- fever; and
- malaise.

The surgical planning for drainage of an orbital abscess requires a radiological examination; a CT scan with axial and coronal cuts is the first choice and contrast material often aids in the identification of the orbital abscess (Fig. 12–4). MRI is a second choice. The treatment involves surgical drainage and systemic antibiotics.

Orbital foreign bodies do not always require (emergency) removal. Metallic objects (e.g., BB, shotgun

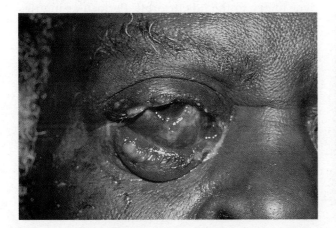

FIGURE 12–2 Retained wooden orbital foreign body.

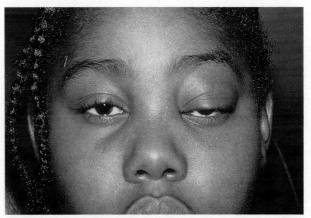

FIGURE 12–3 Orbital abscess associated with proptosis, restricted extraocular muscle movement, fever, and malaise.

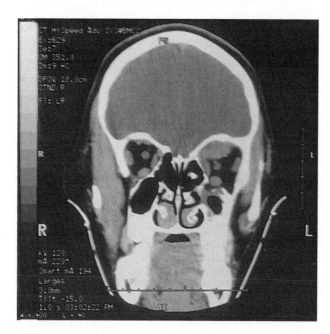

FIGURE 12–4 Superior orbital abscess, left side.

pellet) or glass buried deep in the orbit not only may be safely left in place, but their aggressive removal can lead to complications. Conversely, immediate removal is required for:

- protruding foreign bodies[b]; and
- objects pressing on the optic nerve.

Periocular Damage

These injuries rarely require urgent intervention; they must be adequately assessed and a treatment plan designed. It is usually possible to treat in the ER[c]:

---

[b]Do not simply pull out a protruding foreign body in the ER; it is usually wiser to remove the object in the well-equipped operating room.

[c]The inability of the patient to cooperate, the lack of equipment, and the technically challenged physician are reasons to consider repairing eyelid lacerations in the operating room instead.

- eyelid lacerations;
- puncture wounds; and
- abrasions.

> **PEARL...** Eyelid margin lacerations and canalicular lacerations require meticulous repair. If they can be safely protected, the treatment may be delayed for 48 hours or less because they are best repaired in the operating room. Clean eyelid and canalicular lacerations can be pressure patched over an antibiotic ointment, and reliable patients may be discharged until definitive repair later in the hospital. For patients with poor reliability, admission to the hospital is recommended. Antibiotics should be given if surgery is delayed; tetanus prophylaxis should also be considered (see **Chapter 8** and the **Appendix**).

Repair of Pediatric Eyelid Trauma

Children are best treated in the operating room, not in the ER: eyelid margin repair requires accurate, precise, suture placement. The close proximity of the globe makes needle passes dangerous if restraints have to be used for lack of cooperation.

SUMMARY

Blunt and sharp forces can lead to severe periocular injuries. It is important to rule out concomitant ocular injury, particularly open globe injury, since management of injury to the globe often takes precedence over injury to the lids or orbit. Periocular injuries rarely require urgent repair, but instead should be adequately assessed and a plan designed.

REFERENCES

1. Baylis HI, Axelrod R. Repair of the lacerated canaliculus. *Ophthalmology.* 1978;84:1271–1276.
2. Hawes MJ, Dortzbach RK. Surgery on orbital floor fractures. Influence of time of repair and fracture size. *Ophthalmology.* 1983;90:1066–1070.
3. Korhel GB, Krauss HR, Winnik J. Orbital abscess: presentation, diagnosis, therapy and sequelae. *Ophthalmology.* 1982;89:492–498.

SECTION III

MECHANICAL GLOBE INJURIES

Chapter 13

CONJUNCTIVA

M. Bowes Hamill

The conjunctiva, as the most superficial layer of the eye and inner eyelids, is frequently involved in ocular injuries. Although it has little intrinsic structural strength, it does provide significant protection against low-momentum foreign bodies (see Chapter 24) and chemical agents; careful examination of its entire surface should therefore always be a part of the examination.

EXAMINATION

Penlight

The penlight is used first to inspect the bulbar and palpebral conjunctiva; before opening the lids, ensure that no open globe injury is present (see Chapter 8). Follow the steps outlined below:

- With the patient looking upward, gently evert the lower lid and evaluate the lower bulbar/palpebral surfaces and the inferior fornix.

- With the patient looking downward, raise the upper lids and[a] inspect the superior bulbar surface.

To examine the superior tarsal conjunctiva, the upper lid needs to be everted:

- grasp the lashes gently;
- place a small instrument (e.g., cotton-tipped applicator) on the skin of the upper lid at the location of the lid crease;
- with gentle posterior pressure from the applicator handle and anterior traction on the lashes, the lid can be everted and the applicator handle removed; this results in more patient comfort and in a flatter palpebral surface (see Fig. 13–1).

---

[a]Press against bone, not the eye ball, when elevating the upper lid.

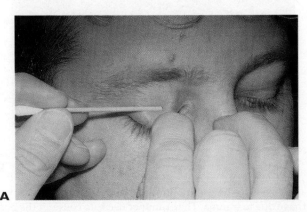
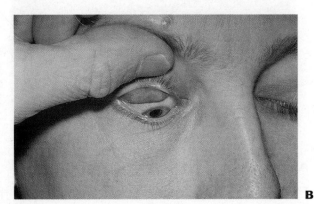

FIGURE 13–1 (**A** and **B**) Eversion of the upper lid (see the text for details).

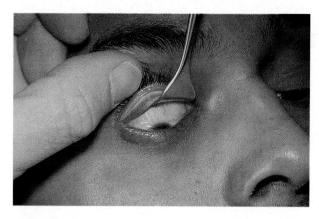

FIGURE 13–2   Double eversion of the upper lid. To visualize the fornix, the everted upper lid must be further lifted away from the globe. Here a Desmarres lid speculum is inserted behind the tarsal plate to allow inspection of the superior fornix and bulbar conjunctiva.

To inspect the superior fornix move the upper lid anteriorly, away from the globe, with an instrument (double eversion, see Fig. 13–2). A small dental mirror may be helpful.[1]

> **PEARL...**   Double eversion of the upper lid is required to inspect the superior fornix.

Slit-lamp

Slit-lamp evaluation of the conjunctiva proceeds similarly to the penlight inspection. Using medium-power magnification, the entire conjunctival surface should be examined for foreign bodies, lacerations, or areas of epithelial loss. The upper lid should be everted and the superior palpebral surface also inspected.

> **PEARL...**   The conjunctival surface can be stained with *fluorescein* dye to detect epithelial denudation. *Rose bengal* staining can help in detecting small foreign bodies lodged in the fornix or adherent to the palpebral conjunctiva.

SPECIFIC INJURIES

Subconjunctival Hemorrhage

It appears as a bright red patch of conjunctival tissue with distinct or feathered borders (Fig. 13–3A). If it is severe, the conjunctiva may become elevated and prolapse through the palpebral fissure; the entire bulbar conjunctiva may be involved (Fig. 13–3B). Generally resolving spontaneously in 7 to 10 days, its color evolves from bright red to yellow green. Occasionally, when the hemorrhage involves the perilimbal conjunctiva, blood breakdown products can be seen in the anterior peripheral corneal stroma as a greenish discoloration.

Hemorrhage under or into the conjunctiva can occur:

- as a result of even minor ocular *trauma*;
- *spontaneously*; or
- in association with a variety of *conditions* including Valsalva maneuvers (see Chapter 33), primary conjunctival amyloidosis,[3] inverted positioning,[4] dancing;[5] and, by far the most common, systemic hypertension.[b]

The management of a traumatic subconjunctival hemorrhage is hopeful expectancy, although it must

---

[b]The subconjunctival hemorrhage may be the first sign of hypertension[2]; consequently, the blood pressure should be checked in all patients with spontaneous subconjunctival hemorrhage.

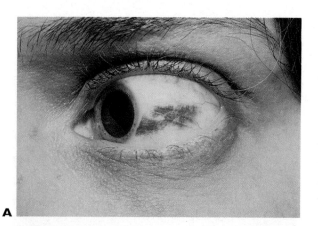

A

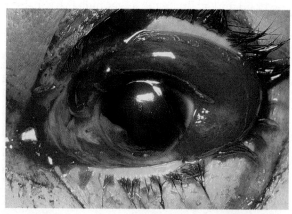

B

FIGURE 13–3   **(A)** Subconjunctival hemorrhage may be spontaneous or the result of trauma. In this patient, the hemorrhage was spontaneous. **(B)** Extensive subconjunctival hemorrhage due to trauma. The examiner needs to consider the possibility of globe rupture or laceration.

be ensured that the hemorrhage does not indicate or conceal a deeper or more extensive injury.

PITFALL

The presence of subconjunctival pigmentation in association with a hemorrhage is very suspicious of occult scleral rupture. The examiner must obtain a complete ocular history and perform an examination on all patients presenting with traumatic subconjunctival hemorrhage to rule out occult scleral wound or laceration with or without an IOFB (see Chapters 9 and 24).

Foreign Bodies

Conjunctival foreign bodies are common (Fig. 13–4). Because they may also indicate the possibility of deeper, more invasive injury, this must always be ruled out.[c] Most conjunctival foreign bodies can easily be removed with either a cotton-tipped applicator or a 30-gauge needle.

> **PEARL…** Removal of foreign bodies from the upper lid's conjunctival surface is a great relief for the patient as these objects scratch the cornea (twice) with each blinking.[d]

- Fine forceps (e.g., jeweler's) are helpful if the object is tightly adherent to the conjunctival surface or is slightly imbedded.
- If the foreign body is deeply imbedded, the overlying conjunctiva may need to be opened to facilitate removal. Following removal, a topical antibiotic ointment should be applied.

Some small nonreactive particulate objects can be left in place without complications, while certain deeply embedded foreign bodies (e.g., small metallic or glass fragments) will work themselves out with time.

> **PEARL…** Not all conjunctival foreign bodies are a result of involuntary trauma (e.g., self-introduction of foreign material into the fornix as a form of Munchausen syndrome[6]).

Lacerations

Lacerations may be isolated injuries or signal deeper trauma. It is imperative that all patients with conjunctival laceration have a thorough and extensive examination (including dilated fundus evaluation) to rule out conclusively an open globe injury. In case of true IOFBs, the findings may be subtle and limited to a barely visible conjunctival lesion.

---

[c] The foreign body may be partially intraocular (see Fig. 13–5).

[d] It is pathognomical so see vertical lines of epithelial defect on the cornea.

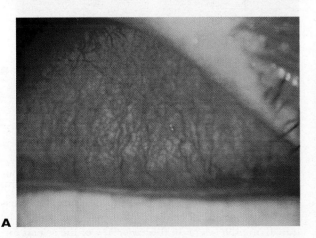 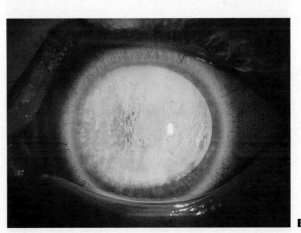

FIGURE 13–4   Small metallic foreign bodies have a predilection for the superior tarsal conjunctival surface. In this patient a small fragment of metal is adherent to the conjunctiva **(A)**, giving rise to typical vertical linear corneal abrasions resulting from the blinking action of the lid **(B)**.

> **PEARL...** The scleral wound rarely lies directly underneath the conjunctival deficit (see Fig. 13–5): in most cases, the patient is not in primary gaze at the time of injury. The scleral defect may even be at a significant distance from the site of the conjunctival lesion. Examining the eye in a variety of gazes and gently moving the anesthetized conjunctiva with a moistened cotton-tipped applicator help make the diagnosis; caution should be taken not to put pressure on the globe. If necessary, exploration should be performed under local anesthesia; if a scleral wound is appreciated or strongly suspected, this should be attempted only in the operating room.

Treatment of small lacerations involves only antibiotic ointment. Larger lacerations may require closure. Rapidly absorbable suture materials (e.g., chromic or plain gut) are adequate for most cases. Tissue healing is rapid and rarely is there sufficient tension on the conjunctiva during closure to require anything more than simple wound edge apposition.

Chemosis

Swelling of the conjunctiva is a primary dysfunction of its vascular endothelium, signaling a common response to a variety of injuries or noxious stimuli:

- inflammation;
- increased orbital pressure as in orbital congestion from contusion; or
- increased venous pressure in the setting of carotid cavernous fistula.

Although some chemosis is present in most cases of ocular trauma, its degree at the time of the initial evaluation is not a good indicator of the severity of the trauma; for example, severe alkali injuries may cause only minimal chemosis initially.

> **PITFALL**
>
> In contusions with orbital congestion, especially when associated with subconjunctival hemorrhage, the resultant conjunctival chemosis may be sufficient to obscure the examiner's view of the globe.

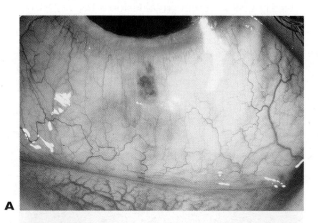

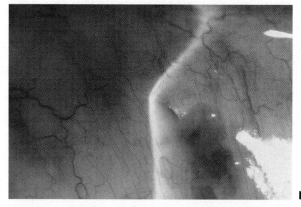

FIGURE 13–5 Scleral foreign body. **(A)** The obvious finding is a small subconjunctival hemorrhage. **(B)** With higher magnification and a slit illumination, the brass fragment from a .22 caliber bullet casing is seen to be transfixing the sclera. In this case, 90% of the scleral foreign body was *inside* the globe. The conjunctival laceration/hemorrhage did not overlie the scleral defect, a common situation in combined wounds of the conjunctiva and sclera. **(C)** The removed foreign body.

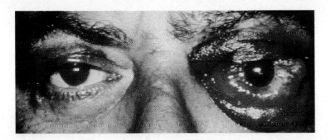

FIGURE 13–6 Conjunctival emphysema. Individual air bubbles may be visible and the conjunctiva is frequently regionally involved.

PROGNOSIS AND OUTCOME

The prognosis for the vast majority of conjunctival injuries is excellent. The conjunctiva heals rapidly and, due to its rich blood supply, infections are rare. Prognosis is more guarded for chemical injuries, however, as destruction of the conjunctival vascular supply and the corneal limbal stem cells may result in permanent ocular surface changes with corneal ulceration and long-term scarring and vascularization (see Chapters 11 and 32). In addition, destruction of the specialized cellular components of the conjunctival surface may permanently change the composition of the preocular tear film with unfortunate sequelae for the corneal surface.

Emphysema

Emphysema occurs when free air gets trapped under or in the conjunctiva (Fig. 13–6). The air can be from an internal source (endogenous) or an external source (exogenous). Endogenous emphysema is much more common, occurring in the setting of orbital fracture: an access route from the paranasal sinuses to the orbit is created. With nose blowing, coughing, or other forced exhalation, air is driven into the orbit and dissects anteriorly under and into the conjunctiva. This may result in conjunctival emphysema with very sudden and impressive exophthalmos.[7] Explosion is the most common source of exogenous emphysema.

THE NONOPHTHALMOLOGIST'S ROLE

Most of the minor conjunctival injuries can be managed by the nonophthalmologist.

> **PEARL...** The most important caveat is to recognize when the seemingly innocuous subconjunctival hemorrhage conceals a deeper injury. A complete evaluation of the eye and adnexa must be performed to ensure that the full extent of the injury is recognized and appropriate testing and treatment are undertaken.

> **PEARL...** Patients with orbital fractures should be cautioned against nose blowing or sneezing with a closed mouth so as to avoid orbital and subconjunctival emphysema.

In exogenous emphysema,[8–11] unless the stream of air is under very high pressure or associated with high-pressure fluid, the proptosis is a less prominent component than with endogenous emphysema. Conjunctival defects or lacerations are extremely uncommon in this setting.[11]

SUMMARY

The conjunctiva is a frequently injured ocular structure. If the injury is isolated to the conjunctiva the prognosis is often excellent and rarely requires surgical intervention. The most important aspect of conjunctival injury is that it may signal the presence of more serious ocular trauma.

REFERENCES

1. Duke-Elder S. *System of Ophthalmology*. Vol VII. St. Louis: CV Mosby; 1962:239.

2. Fukuyama JI, Hayasaka S, Yamada K, Setogawa T. Causes of subconjunctival hemorrhage. *Ophthalmologica*. 1990;200:63–67.

3. Lee HM, Naor J, DeAngelis D, Rootman DS. Primary localized conjunctival amyloidosis presenting with recurrence of subconjunctival hemorrhage. *Am J Ophthalmol*. 2000;129:245–247.

4. Caspari RF. A "new wave" of subconjunctival hemorrhage [letter]? *N Engl J Med*. 1980;303:1420.

5. Friberg TR, Weinreb RN. Ocular manifestations of gravity inversion. *JAMA*. 1985;253:1755–1757.

6. Cruciani F, Santino G, Trudu R, Balacco Gabrieli C. Ocular Munchausen syndrome characterized by self introduction of chalk concretions into the conjunctival fornix. *Eye*. 1999;13(pt 4):598–599.

7. Hunts JH, Patrinely JR, Anderson RL. Orbital emphysema. Staging and acute management. *Ophthalmology*. 1994;101:960–966.

8. Biger Y, Abulafia C. Subconjunctival emphysema due to trauma by compressed air. *Br J Ophthalmol*. 1986;70:227–228.

9. Li T, Mafee MF, Edward DP. Bilateral orbital emphysema from compressed air injury. *Am J Ophthalmol*. 1999;128:103–104.

10. Hitchings R, McGill J. Compressed air injury of the eye. *Br J Ophthalmol*. 1970;54:634–635.

11. King YY. Ocular changes following air-blast injury. *Arch Ophthalmol*. 1971;86:125–126.

Chapter 14

CORNEA

M. Bowes Hamill

 The cornea is frequently involved in facial and ocular trauma. As it provides most of the eye's refractive power, recognition and management of corneal injuries is critical for vision; even small irregularities in the corneal contour may result in significant functional morbidity. This chapter reviews the evaluation and management of corneal injuries.

EPIDEMIOLOGY AND PREVENTION

Excluding corneoscleral injuries, the cornea is involved in 51% of all serious ocular trauma in the USEIR; additional information from this database follows.

Age (years):
- range: 0–101;
- mean: 30;
- ≤15: 26%;
- ≥60: 8%.

Sex: 83% male.
Place:
- 41% home;
- 18% work;
- 9% street and highway.

Cause:
- 27% sharp object;
- 20% blunt object;
- 6% MVC;
- 3% fall.

Rate of various diagnoses among all corneal injuries:
- laceration, full-thickness: 52%;
- laceration, partial-thickness: 1%;
- rupture: 18%;
- chemical burn: 5%;
- edema: 5%.

Rate of corneal ruptures among all ruptures: 29%.
Rate of corneal lacerations among all lacerations: 59%.
Rate of iris prolapse among corneal ruptures: 38%.
Rate of in-the-visual-axis iris prolapse among ruptures: 19%.
Rate of iris prolapse among lacerations: 30%.
Rate of in-the-visual-axis iris prolapse among corneal prolapses in lacerations: 19%.

The vast majority of these injuries are preventable with appropriate eye protection[1] (see Chapters 4 and 27).

PATHOPHYSIOLOGY

The cornea is a five-layered tissue.

1. *Epithelium*, the most superficial layer, is 50 μm thick and consists of five to seven layers of cells. It is a highly active, rapidly reproducing tissue; when injured, the epithelium heals rapidly and without scarring, unless Bowman's layer is involved. Under

the epithelium and attached to the basal epithelial cells by an adhesion complex[a] is a basement membrane overlying Bowman's layer.

2. *Bowman's layer*[b] is not a true membrane but a condensation of the superficial stromal collagen.

3. The *stroma* makes up most of the corneal thickness and is composed of multiple lamellae of collagen fibers[c] packed in glycosaminoglycans. The collagen is produced by keratocytes, interspersed among the lamellae. These cells are similar to fibroblasts and can live up to 3 years.

4. *Descemet's membrane* lines the posterior surface of the stroma, representing the basement membrane of the corneal endothelium.

5. *Endothelium*, the most posterior layer, is a single layer of hexagonal cells, which are responsible for pumping water out of the corneal stroma, thus maintaining corneal deturgesence. Endothelial cells are derived from neural crest origins, capable of only limited reproduction; they are extremely delicate and are easily damaged by hydrostatic, thermal, contusive, or concussive insults as well as by direct mechanical trauma. When a sufficient number of cells are incapacitated (death, loss, or dysfunction[d]) and the endothelial density drops below a critical level, edema ensues: the cornea becomes swollen and cloudy.

See Chapter 27 for the strength of a healed wound.

EXAMINATION

History

The history frequently directs the course of subsequent laboratory and diagnostic testing. The event's description by the patient or witnesses allows the examiner to understand the circumstances of the injury, predicting the injury severity/type, the structures likely to be involved, and the risk of occult trauma. Specific questions to be asked concern:

- foreign bodies;
- chemical exposure; and
- previous corneal surgery[2-6] (see Chapter 27).

---

[a]Hemidesmosomes linked to anchoring filaments extending into the lamina of the basement membrane.

[b]Also called Bowman's membrane.

[c]Accounting for ≥70% of the corneal dry weight.

[d]Surrounding cells enlarge and fill in the defect, attempting to take over the pump function.

Inspection

Naked-eye

Corneal trauma is frequently visible by naked-eye inspection in room illumination or with a *penlight* (Fig. 14–1).

- Elevate the upper and depress the lower eyelid to view the entire cornea.
- Examine the cornea while swinging the penlight through a variety of angles.[e] This maneuver permits examination of the corneal surface and highlights abnormalities such as foreign bodies and lacerations, especially with tangential illumination or illumination near the limbus.

PEARL...   Epithelial defects can be visualized by looking at the light reflex from the corneal surface. The normal cornea has a high luster with a smooth reflective surface. Irregularities in the light reflex may indicate loss or denudation of the epithelium and possibly stroma.

---

[e]Helpful because the cornea is transparent.

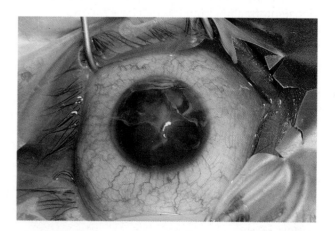

FIGURE 14–1   Corneal trauma can frequently be visualized with a penlight. In this photograph of a young boy with a corneal laceration, the edges of the laceration can be appreciated both by direct visualization and by the light reflex from the wound edge. Note also the opacified lens behind the laceration, indicating an injury involving deeper structures.

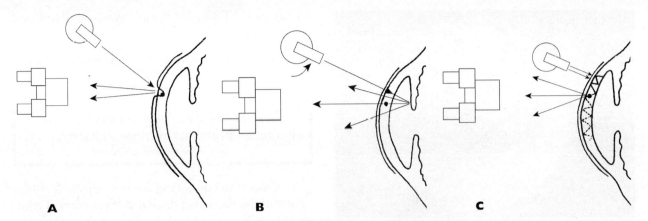

FIGURE 14–2   Diagrammatic representation of various slit-lamp illumination techniques helpful in visualizing corneal trauma. **(A)** *Direct illumination*: the cornea is illuminated directly with the slit beam. The lesion is seen by light scattering from its anterior surface. **(B)** *Retroillumination*: the light source is rotated off axis and the iris is illuminated. The examiner inspects the overlying cornea via light reflected from behind. This technique is especially useful for clear foreign bodies or wounds. The source of posterior illumination can also be the fundus red reflex. **(C)** *Sclerotic scatter* utilizes the total internal reflection of light within the cornea. Rotating the slit turret, the light beam is directed at the limbus. The cornea is inspected for discontinuities in the stroma. This technique is helpful when searching for partial-thickness foreign bodies or lacerations.

The most valuable examining tool is the *slit lamp* (Fig. 14–2).[f]

- With *direct illumination*, the object is viewed via light scattered from its anterior surface. Unfortunately, due to the complex optical nature of the cornea and the multiple interactive surfaces, clear foreign bodies (e.g., glass, plastic) and even lacerations may be difficult to appreciate.

- Under *retroillumination*, the object is illuminated from behind; the light can be reflected from the iris or the fundus, providing backlit relief of corneal lesions.

> **PEARL...** Retroillumination can be very useful in detecting light transmission anomalies such as those caused by corneal lacerations: light is scattered in the area of the laceration, which appears either highlighted or backlighted.

- *Sclerotic scatter* takes advantage of internal reflection. Light entering the cornea from the limbus is totally internally reflected from the epithelial and endothelial surfaces; any interruption in the light path results in anterior and posterior light scattering. This is very helpful in detecting corneal foreign bodies as well as structural abnormalities: interfaces between broken/cut stromal lamellae show up bright or dark.

Stains

Stains such as fluorescein and rose bengal provide additional help.

- *Rose bengal* is rapidly taken up by abnormal or damaged cells, making these red stained.
- *Fluorescein* rarely stains healthy cells, although the disruption of cell barriers or denudation of the epithelial basement membrane also results in fluorescein uptake. Fluorescein is able to show whether aqueous is leaking from a full-thickness wound (Seidel test; see Fig. 14–3 and Chapters 9 and 19). A cobalt blue filter enhances fluorescein detection.

> **PEARL...** The cornea must be examined within seconds of fluorescein instillation as the dye rapidly diffuses into the tissue: 3 to 5 minutes after instillation, the area of uptake is blurred, the edges are diffuse, and the test's value is significantly decreased.

---

[f]The slit lamp is a binocular microscope mounted horizontally with an illumination system capable of delivering a thin, well-focused slit. Using different lighting techniques, the slit allows estimation in the clear cornea of the location of opacities in the anteroposterior axis (see Fig. 14–2).

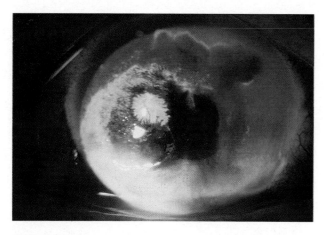

FIGURE 14–3   Seidel's test. Seidel's testing utilizes the characteristic of fluorescein to quench fluorescence in high concentrations. In the photograph, the area of corneal injury was coated with a high concentration of fluorescein from a dampened strip. The aqueous leakage diluted the dye and allowed fluorescence to occur, thus indicating the presence of a full-thickness wound.

Specific Injuries

Abrasion

Epidemiology

One of the most common globe injuries is corneal abrasion: 10% of new patient visits to an ophthalmic ER in one study were due to epithelial cell loss.[7] Corneal abrasion frequently accompanies deeper/more extensive ocular trauma.

Pathophysiology

As discussed earlier, the corneal basal epithelial cells rest on a secreted basement membrane and are held in position by hemidesmosomal attachments. If the basal epithelial cells are removed from the basement membrane, corneal abrasion results. The abrasion can be partial or full thickness, and as long as Bowman's layer is not disturbed, healing generally follows without scarring.

Healing of the abraded epithelium occurs in several stages:

1. initially, there is a *migration of peripheral cells* onto the area of denuded basement membrane;
2. this is followed by *proliferation of the epithelial cells* to restore epithelial thickness;
3. the process ends with the *formation of hemidesmosomal attachments* to the underlying basement membrane.

It should be appreciated that corneal epithelial cells are in a constant state of reproduction, migration, and shedding. The source of restoration is felt to be the

limbal stem cell located at the corneoscleral junction (see Chapter 11).[8]

PITFALL

Damage to the limbal stem cells can result in significant problems in corneal healing.[9]

Because of the density of the sensory nerve innervation of the corneal epithelial surface, corneal abrasions cause:

- intense *pain* (which is instantaneous); generally associated with significant
- *photophobia*, and
- *lacrimation*.

Patients with epithelial loss may have symptoms that appear to be out of proportion to the severity of the injury. Because of the overwhelming pain associated with corneal abrasion,[8] patients are able to tell the ophthalmologist the exact time and circumstance of the injury.

PEARL...   An exception to the immediate occurrence of symptoms caused by epithelial damage is photokeratitis (e.g., a welder's burn due to UV light-induced damage to the cornea), in which the symptoms typically follow the exposure by 6–12 hours.[h]

Examination

Examination of patients with corneal abrasion may be difficult because of the discomfort, lacrimation, and photophobia. A drop of topical anesthetic (e.g., proparacaine 0.5%) can be of great benefit, permitting proper evaluation.

- The first step is an overall inspection of the patient's face for associated damage. This is followed by the examination of the cornea itself.
- A penlight is frequently helpful in detecting the irregular corneal light reflex, which may indicate the presence of an abrasion.

---

[8]The density of the unmyelinated nerve endings—terminating within the epithelium—is several hundred times higher than that in the epidermis.

[h]See also Chapter 34.

- A slit-lamp examination of the same area will reveal a denudation of the epithelium with a generally intact basement membrane and Bowman's layer. Occasionally, loose flaps or folds of the epithelium can be seen. In patients with abnormalities of epithelial basement membrane attachments (e.g., those with *map-dot-fingerprint dystrophy*), the surrounding epithelium may be thrown into folds while still attached to the corneal surface.
- Fluorescein staining makes epithelial denudation readily apparent (see Fig. 14–4).
- The underlying stroma must be examined carefully for deeper injury.

PITFALL

It is extremely important to rule out an occult open globe injury in the evaluation of patients with corneal abrasions.

In most cases of acute corneal abrasion, the underlying corneal stroma is clear, although white cell recruitment giving a granular appearance may occur 12–24 hours after epithelial absence. Stromal edema can be seen if the epithelial defect persists.

Management
The corneal epithelium represents the first line of defense against invading microorganisms; consequently, efforts should be directed at achieving corneal epithelial coverage as soon as possible. This is accomplished by:

- protecting the newly healing corneal epithelial surface from toxic insults (e.g., medications such as topical anesthetics) and
- sheltering the migrating cells.

PITFALL

Tight pressure patching of eyes with corneal abrasion was once a mainstay of therapy. It is now understood that this may be counterproductive to corneal healing by reducing the oxygen supply to the healing epithelium. Patching also increases the corneal temperature, increasing the risk of infection by facilitating microorganism replication in the preocular tear film under the patch.[10] Treatment without patching (with concurrent use of *antibiotics* and *cycloplegics*) may result in faster healing than with patching.[11]

If necessary, the healing corneal epithelium can be protected with the use of a *bandage soft contact lens*. The contact lens offers distinct advantages:

- the lens acts as a patch to protect and cover the epithelium but
  - does not prevent oxygen penetration or
  - result in temperature elevation; in addition,
- the patient is able to see with the affected eye during the healing process.

PITFALL

Patient compliance is a significant issue during treatment for corneal abrasion. In one study, 40% of patients removed their patch because of discomfort.[11] Soft contact lenses are generally beneficial but they may slow the healing process.[12]

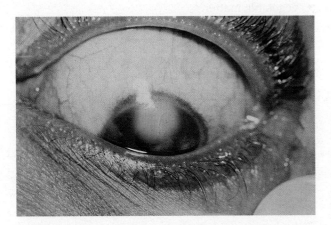

FIGURE 14–4 Fluorescein staining of an epithelial defect. As discussed in the text, fluorescein diffuses rapidly into the stroma bordering an epithelial defect. For this reason, it is important to inspect the cornea immediately after fluorescein instillation.

Patient comfort can be significantly increased with the use of topical cycloplegics.

PEARL... It is important to match the duration of the cycloplegic agent with the severity of the corneal abrasion; for example, a long-acting agent such as atropine is "overkill" for a corneal abrasion that is expected to heal within 24 hours. For most situations, a moderately long-acting cycloplegic agent, such as cyclopentolate 0.5%/1% or scopolamine hydrobromide 0.25%, is sufficient.

All medications, including topical antibiotics, are toxic.[13,14,i] An agent that does not interfere with epithelial healing has not been identified yet.

CONTROVERSY

The benefit of topical antibiotic agents in the treatment of routine corneal abrasions is questionable, given the drugs' potential epithelial toxicity. Conversely, loss of the epithelial covering is a risk factor for infection.

The decision whether to use antibiotics is an individual one. Most clinicians utilize topical antibiotics to treat corneal abrasions; broad-spectrum coverage seems to have theoretical advantages. Once the integrity of a healthy epithelial surface has been reestablished, there is no further need for topical antibiotics.

PITFALL

Under no circumstances should the patient be prescribed or given a *topical anesthetic.* Extended use of topical anesthetics results in corneal hyposensitivity and significantly interferes with corneal immunity.

Patients using topical anesthesia on an "ad hoc" basis generally present several days or weeks later with the classic appearance of a large epithelial defect overlying a white granular corneal opacity that is anesthetic, even though the lesion is intensely painful. Frequently these corneas become infected, which may be difficult to eradicate.

In most cases, corneal epithelial abrasions heal rapidly,[j] although large abrasions may take several days. The classic appearance of a healing abrasion is of advancing convex edges of epithelium, which eventually meet in an epithelial healing line.

PEARL... The healing line in corneal epithelial abrasions may be branching and appear very similar to a dendrite; for this reason, a history of epithelial abrasion is very helpful in differentiating this lesion from herpes simplex keratitis.

Fluorescein staining frequently reveals pooling of the dye in the thinned zone of the advancing epithelial edge for several days to a week after healing.

Recurrent Erosion

Although most corneal abrasions heal without sequelae, recurrent erosion occurs in 7 to 8% of eyes,[15,16] presumably from abnormal adhesion complex formation in the base of epithelial defect. This results in delayed sloughing of the healed epithelial surface and is especially common if the trauma is caused by:

- fingernail[k]
- paper cut; or
- vegetable matter.

Diagnosis

The diagnosis is straightforward: the patient usually has a classic history.

PEARL... Typically, the patient with a recurrent erosion reports a sudden, very painful foreign body sensation with lacrimation and photophobia, which started immediately upon *awakening in the morning.*

[i]Gentamicin sulfate 0.3%, chloramphenicol 0.5%, and tobramycin 0.3% were all associated with healing delay. This may be due to the preservative in the medication rather than to the drug itself. Epithelial healing is less impaired with "fortified" than with "off-the-shelf" gentamicin; the preservative (benzalkonium chloride) is found in higher concentration in the commercially available preparation.[14]

[j]The healing process may be much slower in diabetic patients.

[k]A common example is a mother whose eye was injured by the fingernail of her small child.

The symptoms exist for several hours, generally resolving by midday to late afternoon. If the erosion is large, the symptoms may persist for days. The patient commonly presents only after healing has occurred and the cornea appears normal. In some cases, small gray areas in the epithelium or intraepithelial cysts can be seen.

Treatment

Treatment is aimed at maintaining epithelial stability and integrity until the adhesion complex can form and hemidesmosomal anchoring fibers extend into the basement membrane to secure the epithelium firmly in place. The staged management process is outlined in Figure 14–5.

1. The initial step is a *topical hyperosmotic agent* (e.g., 5% sodium chloride ointment) applied nightly, immediately before retiring. In the majority of cases, a topical hyperosmotic agent applied nightly for 8 weeks results in resolution of the condition.[1]

---

[1]The need to utilize the nightly agent for at least 8 weeks should be stressed to the patient: this is the *minimal* time required for the formation of the adhesion complex (some authors feel that the agent needs to be used even longer).

PEARL... Theoretically, with prolonged lid closure (i.e., during sleep) the tear film becomes hypotonic due to lack of the evaporation that takes place when the lids are open. With tear hypotonicity, the corneal epithelium becomes slightly edematous and easily damaged with the first blinks upon awaking. Application of a hyperosmotic agent is thought to reduce the corneal epithelial edema and thus sloughing.

PITFALL

If a "breakthrough" erosion occurs during treatment, the clock must be reset to zero and an additional 8 weeks of treatment is required.

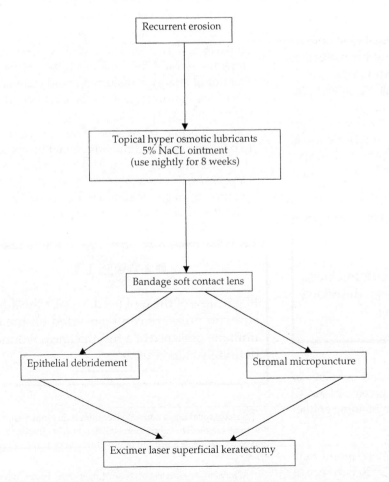

FIGURE 14–5 Treatment algorithm for recurrent erosion.

2. If the patient does not respond to topical hyperosmotics, the next step is an *extended-wear bandage contact lens*. The lens (changed every 2 weeks) should be worn full time (waking *and* sleeping) for a minimum of 6 to 8 weeks.

3. *Surgical treatment* is required. In some patients, the symptoms persist despite conservative therapy. There are several options.

Débridement   can be performed either with a:

* cotton-tipped applicator, removing all of the loose epithelium and scrubbing the basement membrane; or a

* blade in the operating room. Bowman's layer should be gently roughened but not damaged. Scraping should be done with the blade held parallel to the surface or at a slight angle to avoid inadvertent penetration into the corneal stroma. If these measures fail to result in healing, another surgical option is:

Stromal micropuncture[17]   The rationale for this treatment is that, due to inadequate adhesion, the epithelium is not anchored to its foundation. The micropunctures are aimed at attaching the epithelium by taking advantage of the normal scarring following injuries to Bowman's layer.

* First, the area of epithelial abnormality should be well identified. Fluorescein should be instilled to enable the examiner to follow his progress.

* The micropunctures are laid down in a grid pattern and should include margins of normal tissue. A straight 20-gauge needle is used to create a partial-thickness penetration of the anterior corneal stroma. To prevent deep corneal penetration, special needles have been developed.[18]

PITFALL

Despite careful manipulations, full-thickness penetration of the cornea has been described during stromal micropuncturing.[18]

---

* Postoperatively, *topical antibiotic* and *nonsteroidal anti-inflammatory drops* should be given. A *bandage soft contact lens* can be helpful in maintaining epithelium that is still loose.

Excimer Laser,   ablating the basement membrane and the superficial Bowman's layer.[19,20] Recurrence of the erosion has been reported.[21,22]

Lacerations and Ruptures

Corneal lacerations typically involve the stroma, partial- or full-thickness.[m] Most lacerations and all ruptures are full thickness (i.e., involving all five layers of the cornea) and commonly associated with facial, periorbital, or intraocular trauma.

PEARL...   One of the most important tasks in dealing with full-thickness corneal wounds is confirming or ruling out the presence of intraocular pathology.

Epidemiology

In one study of open globe injuries of children, the cornea was involved in 92%.[23] Ruptures due to falls are rather common in the elderly. Previous eye surgery makes the cornea even more vulnerable (see Chapter 27).

Evaluation

An appropriately taken *history* helps to estimate the risks of deep penetration (IOFB) and injuries to intraocular structures. In certain cases (e.g., explosion), the possibility of chemical contamination also needs to be considered (see Chapter 11).

The *physical examination* begins with an

* *external inspection* for evidence of foreign material on the face, skin, or eyelashes and for other obvious signs that would help the examiner estimate the amount of energy transferred and the characteristics of the injuring agent if it is unknown. It is frequently helpful to utilize a *penlight*.

* The eyelids may be swollen. If the patient is unable to open the eyes and the lids cannot be opened by the ophthalmologist's fingers,[n] *lid retractors* (e.g., Desmarres; if unavailable, retractors can be manufactured from paper clips, see Fig. 14–6) should be carefully inserted under the upper and lower lids.

PITFALL

Regardless of the tool used to open the lid fissure, no pressure can be exerted on the eye until the presence of a full-thickness wound is definitely ruled out.

---

[m] Strictly speaking, a corneal laceration is any injury that breaks Bowman's layer. This definition is different from the BETT definition (see Chapter 1) since the tissue of reference is the *cornea* here, *not the globe.*

[n] Always make sure to keep your fingers over bones, never over the eye, if extra effort to separate the lids is necessary.

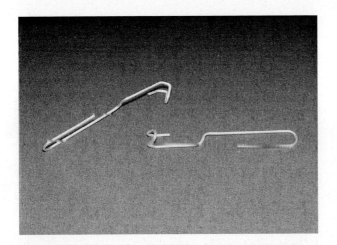

FIGURE 14–6   Always inspect the entire surface of the eye if injury is suspected. Should Desmarres lid retractors be unavailable, retractors can be manufactured from paper clips.

PEARL...   Topical anesthetic is helpful in overcoming the patient's resistance to lid opening, but the examiner should first determine whether the anesthetic contains preservative; its use is contraindicated in an open globe injury.[o]

All patients with suspected corneal injury should also be evaluated with the *slit lamp*.

• Although the majority of corneal wounds are easily seen, they can be subtle and difficult to detect. All illumination techniques (see earlier) should be utilized to identify small, self-sealing corneal lacerations, which may indicate deeper injury or the presence of an IOFB. Seidel testing can demonstrate whether the wound is leaking.

• Careful gonioscopy with a Zeiss lens under no-preservative topical anesthesia can be performed if the wound is self-sealing.

• The AC should be inspected for local shallowing/deepening.

• Iris transillumination defects may indicate occult penetration (see Chapter 24).

• Light transmission anomalies in the lens can alert the examiner to the possibility of deep injury/IOFB.

---

[o]If larger quantities of anesthetics somehow become intraocular, they may anesthetize the retina, leading to NLP vision. One of the editors (FK) witnessed this as a consultant when lidocaine was accidentally injected into the eye; within 30 minutes, vision returned to normal and no consequence occurred other than the scare to both patient and surgeon.

Management

The history and evaluation should help answer three questions, which determine the management steps to be taken:

1. Is there a (partial- or full-thickness) corneal wound?
2. Is the wound self-sealing?
3. Is the wound large or small?

There are several wound types.

• For a *small, self-sealing corneal laceration*, only prophylactic antibiotics may be required. Lack of surgical intervention is preferred for both short-term (speed of recovery) and long-term (refraction) reasons.[p]

• For *larger self-sealing lacerations*, a bandage contact lens or cyanoacrylate tissue glue is usually sufficient.

• *Flaps* may be in place or displaced.

PEARL...   If the flap in a partial-thickness injury is not displaced, suturing is counterproductive: it will induce astigmatism and no benefit. A bandage soft contact lens usually suffices.

○ A displaced flap needs to be repositioned and secured with suture(s), placed partial thickness through the surrounding stroma and tight enough only to hold the flap in place.

○ If, due to the elapsed time between injury and examination, epithelium has grown underneath the flap, the flap may need to be débrided.

○ With deturgesence, especially in the presence of a contact lens, most corneal flaps return to their normal anatomical position with excellent optical clarity.

PITFALL

Surgical closure is necessary for large self-sealing lacerations if the risk of wound reopening is high (e.g., rubbing or inadvertent bumping of the eye might occur during healing). Care should be taken to minimize suture-induced astigmatism.

---

[p]Also take into consideration that subsequent reopening of such wounds (e.g., because of external pressure) may lead to contamination and late endophthalmitis development.

- *Full-thickness non-self-sealing corneal wounds* generally require repair in the operating room with 10-0 or 11-0 nylon sutures. The knots should be buried to improve the patient's comfort and reduce the risk of corneal neovascularization (see the Appendix for details).

Timing

The open corneal wound should be closed in the operating room as soon as possible because with delay, the risk of infection and/or ECH increases (see Chapter 8).

> **PEARL...** **Minimize tissue handling to reduce tissue maceration and edema of the wound's edge that make good anatomic closure more difficult.**

Complications

Most corneal wounds heal well; significant postoperative complications are rare.

Scarring   While depending largely on the anatomy of the original injury, scarring can be minimized by meticulous, anatomically correct closure, and aggressive treatment of intraocular inflammation (see Chapter 8).

> **PEARL...** **Even with the most meticulous closure of a stellate laceration, some scarring is inevitable, with refractive and visual sequelae. Astigmatism induced by tight sutures is reversible with suture removal, whereas astigmatism induced by misapposition or misalignment of the wound edges is permanent. For this reason, every effort should be made to restore the preexisting anatomy carefully.**

Loss of Corneal Tissue   This is extremely rare, and in most cases the "missing" edges or flaps can be found.[q]

Wound Leak   This occurs mostly following repair of stellate lacerations. If the cornea is not watertight at the conclusion of the primary closure, the surgeon has several choices.

- *Additional sutures.* Each added suture, however, compounds the problem of corneal flattening and distorts the corneal architecture.
- *Cyanoacrylate tissue adhesive.* A good alternative; every effort should be made not to apply the glue over suture material, as the glue–suture bond is permanent, in contrast to the glue–tissue bond, which is temporary (duration: days to weeks). When applying the glue, make sure that the surface is dry; otherwise no bond develops.
- *Bandage soft contact lens.*
- *Patch grafting.*
- *PK.*

In the *first postoperative days* and most commonly with large, complex stellate lacerations, leaking despite apparently good surgical closure occasionally develops as the edema of the wound edges decreases.

- If the wound leak is small, it can be managed conservatively with hypotensive agents (reducing aqueous production) and bandage soft contact lenses. Withdrawing or decreasing topical corticosteroids during this period allows the buildup of a moderate intraocular inflammatory response, which aids in the sealing process.
- Occasionally, patients may require tissue glue or even a return to the operating room, but the decision to intervene can usually be delayed for several days.

Infection   Following corneal wound repair infection is rare. The clinician should always be alert for the development of keratitis or endophthalmitis.[r]

Postoperative Medical Management

Most physicians treating patients with full-thickness corneal wounds use both topical and systemic antibiotics; no data are available to recommend one group or type of antibiotic over another. We treat patients with a penetrating eye injury for 3 days with oral antibiotics, followed by intensive topical treatment for up to 3 weeks. In addition, cycloplegic agents and topical corticosteroids are helpful to improve the patient's comfort and diminish ocular inflammation/scarring.

> **PITFALL**
>
> No "best" regimen has yet been universally accepted as the topical antibiotic/corticosteroid regimen of choice.

---

[q]Turned under into the AC or slid aside from their normal anatomical location.

[r]Much less common in ruptures than in lacerations.

Prognosis

The visual outcome following injuries limited to the cornea is good,[s] though grafting may be required. The type and extent of damage to other ocular structures are decisive in more complex cases.

Summary

Lacerating trauma is the most common of the serious corneal injuries; ruptures are much less frequent. The examination should also be directed toward the detection of (occult) deeper intraocular trauma, including IOFBs. Whereas small self-sealing lacerations can be treated conservatively with contact lens or corneal glue, larger lacerations and ruptures generally require surgical intervention. The goal of the surgery is restoration of the normal anatomy and reconstruction of a watertight anterior segment. Postoperative management is directed at minimizing scarring and infection.

Role of the Nonophthalmologist

Corneal laceration/rupture is an injury that can usually be recognized by the nonophthalmologist.

- Protect the eye with a rigid cover[t] (not with a patch!) to prevent any inadvertent pressure on the eye that would lead to the extrusion of intraocular contents (Fig. 14–7).
- Refer the patient to, or request a consultation by, an ophthalmologist.

---

[s]Provided the normal corneal anatomy has been restored.

[t]A specially manufactured eye shield or one of opportunity (e.g., a Styrofoam coffee cup, see Fig. 14–7).

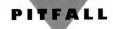

PITFALL

Under no circumstances should a patient with a corneal laceration/rupture have any medications instilled into the eye prior to evaluation by an ophthalmologist.

Foreign Bodies

Corneal foreign bodies may involve minor trauma (e.g., small particles embedded in the epithelium) or major trauma (e.g., a fishhook embedded in the globe and protruding through the lids). One of the most important aspects of the management of corneal foreign bodies is to ensure detection of any material that has become intraocular.

Epidemiology

Corneal foreign bodies are the second most common form of eye trauma, representing 40% of eye injuries in one study.[24]

Most injuries are mild, without significant visual morbidity or loss of work: in one report, only 7.3% of patients lost more than 12 hours of work.[25] The majority of corneal foreign bodies are amenable to prevention with appropriate eyewear. This is especially important when the patient is involved in activities known to be high-risk (e.g., welding, hammering, drilling, grinding). One study found that 1.8% of all injuries seen in an ER were ocular foreign bodies; only 60% of patients had eye protection, even though they were involved in high-risk activity.[26]

In Desert Shield/Storm, 17% of all ocular injuries were corneal foreign bodies and only 3% of those

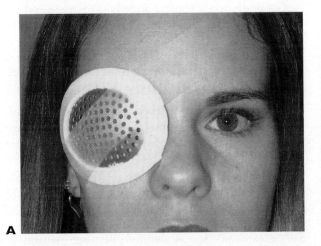
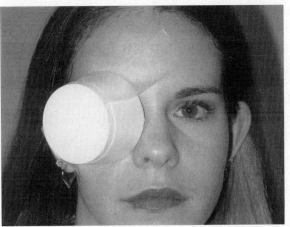

FIGURE 14–7   Protecting the eye with a rigid cover is indicated in patients with an open globe injury (see the text for details).

injured had protective eyewear (even though all Army personnel had been issued goggles on deployment).[27]

Evaluation

Because of the sensitivity of the corneal surface, most foreign bodies are immediately noticed by the patient.

> **PEARL…** The symptoms caused by corneal foreign bodies are frequently out of proportion to the severity of the injury. Individuals with foreign bodies remaining on the corneal surface can be highly symptomatic; conversely, high-speed objects that are embedded in or pass completely through the cornea (i.e., becoming an IOFB) may give rise to no or only minimal symptoms.[a]

The patient should be *examined* initially with a penlight, looking for foreign material on the skin or conjunctiva, which alerts the examiner to the possibility of a corneal foreign body. The *slit lamp*, however, remains the most effective detection method.

> **PEARL…** It is important to use various illumination techniques at the slit lamp; this is especially true if the foreign body is transparent (e.g., glass, plastic). These can be very difficult to find under direct illumination but stand out quite clearly with retroillumination or sclerotic scatter. The benefit of the slit lamp over diffuse illumination devices such as the penlight becomes obvious when examining intrastromal foreign bodies: the slit illumination allows the localization of foreign material within the transparent cornea (see Fig. 14–8).

Fluorescein can identify breaks in the epithelium and therefore show an entrance wound.

Management

Superficial Foreign Bodies   These are usually easily removed with a:

- cotton-tipped applicator or
- small sharp instrument, such as a 30-gauge needle on an insulin syringe.

---

[a]The relationship between injury severity and symptoms is almost inverse.

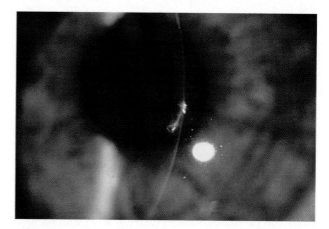

FIGURE 14–8   A corneal foreign body imbedded in the midcorneal stroma. The slit illumination aids greatly in the appreciation of the depth of the foreign body.

The material should be gently lifted from the surface, causing as little disturbance to the surrounding tissue as possible.

> ▼ **PITFALL**
>
> Under no circumstances should removal of a foreign body be attempted if its depth within the corneal stroma is unknown. Not infrequently, foreign material, which appears to be on the surface, can be quite deep; significant corneal trauma and scarring can follow an ill-advised attempt to "dig out" the foreign object. There is even a risk of dislodging the foreign material into the AC.

Generally, only topical anesthesia is required for removal of superficial foreign bodies; afterwards, the cornea can be managed as for an abrasion.

Deep-Seated Foreign Bodies   Material located deep in the corneal stroma requires a different approach.

- If the material is not large/antigenic/toxic/contaminated and causes no pain or visual complains, it can be left in place (e.g., glass splinter following an MVC).
- Vegetable matter should be retrieved if possible due to the risk of an antigenic response and of (especially fungal) infection.

SURGICAL REMOVAL   A slender grasping instrument (e.g., a very fine-tipped tying forceps) may be used to ease the object out through the same track in which it entered. This is especially helpful when removing foreign bodies with tangential entry (e.g., a plant splinter).

More difficult is the foreign body embedded through a shelving or direct laceration. Occasionally, these can be extracted at the slit lamp, but in more difficult cases, removal in the operating room is recommended.

SPECIAL CONSIDERATION

Although the operating microscope and regional/general anesthesia may facilitate removal, stereopsis through the microscope compared with the slit lamp and the lack of a tangential slit illuminator may make depth perception more difficult. Careful drawings, therefore, should be made before going to the operating room to document the depth, location, and entrance tracks of all intracorneal foreign bodies. Never attempt corneal foreign body removal if the depth of the object is not accurately determined. "Digging" for a retained foreign body in the cornea will cause additional corneal injury, leading to more extensive scarring than necessary.

In eyes with deep ferrous foreign bodies, a strong permanent intraocular magnet (see Chapter 24) can help retrieve the object through its entrance track.

Complications
Complications following corneal foreign body removal are rare and limited to those following any laceration: scarring and infection. With deep-seated, especially large, foreign bodies, removal can result in aqueous leak, which the clinician should be prepared to treat as necessary (see earlier). Unless there is tissue loss, most wounds are self-sealing, although occasionally the utilization of bandage soft contact lenses or a corneal glue can be helpful.

Special Issues of Importance
Ferrous foreign bodies deserve special mention as they oxidize, forming *rust* deposits in the cornea. Rusting can occur as early as 3 hours after injury.[28] Because rust can retard wound healing,[29] its removal by scraping or by a specially designed, rapidly rotating burr is recommended.

PEARL... In a rabbit model, rust removal utilizing a burr resulted in smaller epithelial defects and more rapid healing than removal by scraping the area with a needle.[30]

There are other, albeit less common, corneal foreign materials deserving special mention, such as animal *hair*.

- The abdominal hairs of *tarantulas*[v] present a defense mechanism for this arachnid; when threatened, the animal rubs its hind legs across its abdomen, releasing a cloud of hairs. The type III tarantula hair is thin and long (between 0.3 to 1.2 mm), with sharp points and multiple barbs. These hairs are capable of penetrating the skin[31] or the cornea and becoming embedded. They cause itching and intense irritation and can migrate into the deep stroma, even into the AC. Treatment is directed at reducing the inflammatory response and removing any hairs that protrude from the surface of the cornea. Completely embedded hairs have been reported to resorb.[32]
- *Caterpillar* setae (hairs) may cause a similar reaction.[33,34]

Role of the Nonophthalmologist
Most superficial corneal foreign bodies can be managed by the nonophthalmologist, provided that a slit lamp or other magnifying device is employed to ensure that the foreign material is in fact located on the surface and not embedded within the cornea and that there is no occult corneal wound. These objects can be removed utilizing a moist cotton tip or a needle and the patient managed as having a corneal abrasion. Because of the risk of an occult corneal wound or more extensive injury, any foreign body suspected of being underneath Bowman's layer or embedded deep in the stroma should be managed by an ophthalmologist.

Injuries without Wounds
Such injuries are less common than those already listed but still represent a significant portion of ocular trauma. They may occur via two mechanisms.

- *Concussion* is due to rapid acceleration, deceleration, or oscillation of the cornea and surrounding tissues, following energy transfer from the direct impact of a blunt object or from the hydrostatic shock waves generated by the impact.

---

[v]The Mexican red knee tarantula (*Brachypelma smithi*) is a popular pet.

- *Contusion* results directly from the blunt object and may lead to bruising or other types of tissue destruction.

Pathophysiology and Evaluation

Damage from a blunt object depends upon several variables:

- the physical characteristics of the agent;
- the area over which the impact is applied;
- the time over which the energy transfer occurs; and
- the amount of force applied.

The characteristics of the traumatizing object are important (see also Chapter 1) as they determine the area over which the force is applied as well as the amount of energy transferred:

- energy transfer over a small area (i.e., sharp object) typically results in tissue penetration;
- the same force applied over a large area (i.e., blunt object) results in contusion, concussion, or rupture;
- similar force applied over a shorter, rather than longer, period of time is generally associated with increasing injury severity (both surface and deeper) because the likelihood of generating significant hydrostatic shockwaves increases.

An effort should be made to determine these variables during history taking.

> **PEARL...   A blunt object with sufficient force to cause corneal changes is frequently associated with intraocular damage. The examination, therefore, needs to be directed at determining the full extent of the injury.**

Specific Injuries

Blunt objects frequently cause *abrasion* when they directly strike the cornea. Unless the force applied is great or particularly rapid, the stroma is rarely involved.[w]

Very rapid energy transfer can result in *stromal fractures (ruptures)*, although this condition is rare and requires substantial force.[35] Stromal fractures may be limited to Bowman's layer or the anterior stroma but may also involve the deeper stromal layers. This type of injury is becoming increasingly important as the number of individuals with prior refractive surgery increases: the corneal incisions never truly heal to the

strength of the surrounding tissue. Although individuals have been reported to sustain significant injury without rupture,[36,37] ophthalmologists and patients should realize that refractive surgery represents an increased risk in case of eye trauma (see Chapter 27).

If Descemet's membrane or the endothelium is involved, *corneal edema* will be a prominent clinical feature. This is rather common following trauma by a blunt object. Endothelial injury results in two types of clinical presentation.

- *Diffuse endotheliopathy* occurs when sufficient energy transfer is accomplished so that posterior displacement, corneal infolding, or a hydrostatic shock wave propagating from the blow damages the endothelium. Although in some cases the corneal epithelium actually strikes the iris and lens, in many cases the endothelium is injured without direct contusive contact. These injuries classically occur following a high-speed, high-energy transfer (e.g., injuries from bungee cords, BB pellet). Probably because these injuries occur in younger individuals, recovery is usually complete, although permanent endothelial cell loss has also been reported.[38,39] The acute clinical picture typically shows regional, zonal, or occasionally total corneal edema; cells and flare in the AC; angle recession; and iris sphincter tears.
- *Corneal endothelial rings.* Localized corneal edema can result from endothelial concussive injury following impact with high-speed foreign bodies.[40–42] It is postulated[43,44] that the rings result from the transmission of foreign body impact-induced hydrostatic shock waves from the corneal surface to the endothelium. In humans, specular microscopy and slit-lamp photography demonstrated that the ring was the result of endothelial swelling. These lesions resolve spontaneously without detectable abnormalities.[44]

SUMMARY

Injury to the cornea is relatively common, although most injuries are superficial and not sight-threatening. Because the corneal surface and clarity are critical to good vision, appropriate management of (especially full-thickness) corneal injuries is of utmost importance for achieving the best possible outcome. It should be appreciated that while corneal injury may be the most obvious consequence of the trauma, significant intraocular damage can also occur. The eye with an injured cornea requires a *complete* examination and appropriate treatment of all lesions (see Chapter 8). The Appendix provides details of proper closure of corneal wounds.

---

[w]Secondary complications may occur due to endothelial damage.

REFERENCES

1. Simmons ST, Krohel GB, Hay PB. Prevention of ocular gunshot injuries using polycarbonate lenses. *Ophthalmology*. 1984;91:977–983.

2. Peacock LW, Slade SG, Martiz J, Chuang A, Yee RW. Ocular integrity after refractive procedures. *Ophthalmology*. 1997;104:1079–1083.

3. Schmitt-Bernard CF, Villain M, Beaufrere L, Arnaud B. Trauma after radial keratotomy and photorefractive keratectomy. *J Cataract Refract Surg*. 1997;23: 803–804.

4. Eggleston RJ. Surgical repair of multiple ruptures of radial and transverse incisions under topical anesthesia. *J Cataract Refract Surg*. 1996;22:1394.

5. Leung ATS, Rao SK, Lam DSC. Traumatic partial unfolding of laser in situ keratomileusis flap with severe epithelial ingrowth. *J Cataract Refract Surg*. 2000; 26: 135–139.

6. Lemley HL, Chodosh J, Wolf TC, Bogie CP, Hawkins TC. Partial dislocation of laser in situ keratomileusis flap by air bag injury. *J Refract Surg*. 2000;16:373–374.

7. Chiapella AP, Rosenthal AR. One year in eye casualty. *Br J Ophthalmol*. 1985;69:865–870.

8. Davanger M, Evens A. Role of the pericorneal papillary structure in the renewal of corneal epithelium. *Nature*. 1971;229:560–561.

9. Chen JJ, Iseng CG. Corneal epithelial wound healing and partial limbal deficiency. *Invest Ophthalmol Vis Sci*. 1990;31:1301–1314.

10. Parris CM, Chandler JW. Corneal trauma. In: Kaufman HE, et al, eds. *Non-Perforating Mechanical Injuries. The Cornea*. New York: Churchill Livingstone; 1988.

11. Kirkpatrick JNP, Hoh HB, Cook SD. No eye pad for corneal abrasion. *Eye*. 1993;7:468–471.

12. Ali Z, Insler MS. A comparison of bandage lenses, tarsorrhaphy, and antibiotic and hypertonic saline on corneal wound healing. *Ann Ophthalmol*. 1986;18: 22–24.

13. Pfister RR, Burnstein NL. The effects of ophthalmic drugs, vehicles, and preservatives on corneal epithelium: a scanning electron microscope study. *Invest Ophthalmol Vis Sci*. 1976;15:246–259.

14. Stern GA, Schemmer GB, Farber RD, et al. Effect of topical antibiotic solutions on corneal epithelial wound healing. *Arch Ophthalmol*. 1983;101:644–647.

15. Weene LE. Recurrent corneal erosion after trauma: a statistical study. *Ann Ophthalmol*. 1985;17:521–524.

16. Kenyon KR. Recurrent corneal erosion: pathogenesis and therapy. *Int Ophthalmol Clin*. 1979;19:169–195.

17. McLean, EN, MacRae, SM, Rich LF. Recurrent erosion: treatment by anterior stromal puncture. *Ophthalmology*. 1986;93:784–788.

18. Rubinfeld RS, Laibson PR, Cohen EJ, et al. Anterior stromal puncture for recurrent erosion: further experience and new instrumentation. *Ophthalmic Surg*. 1990; 21:318–326.

19. Dausch D, Landesz M, Klein R, et al. Phototherapeutic keratectomy in recurrent corneal epithelial erosion. *Refract Corneal Surg*. 1993;9:419–424.

20. John ME, Van der Karr MA, Noblitt RL, et al. Excimer laser phototherapeutic keratectomy for treatment of recurrent corneal erosion. *J Cataract Refract Surg*. 1994;20:179–181.

21. Fountain TR, de la Cruz Z, Green WR, et al. Reassembly of corneal epithelial adhesion structures after excimer laser keratectomy in humans. *Arch Ophthalmol*. 1994;112:967–972.

22. Busin M, Meller D. Corneal epithelial dots following excimer laser photorefractive keratectomy. *Refract Corneal Surg*. 1994;10:357–359.

23. Rostomian K, Thach AB, Isfahani A, Pakkar A, Pakkar R, Borchert MJ. Open globe injuries in children. *JAAPOS*. 1998;2(4):234–238.

24. Mönestam E, Björnstig U. Eye injuries in Northern Sweden. *Acta Ophthalmol*. 1991;69:1–5.

25. Alexander MM, MacLeod JD, Hall NF, et al. More than meets the eye: a study of time lost from work by patients who incurred injuries from corneal foreign bodies. *Br J Ophthalmol*. 1991;75:740–742.

26. Banerjee A. Effectiveness of eye protection in the metal working industry. *BMJ*. 1990;301:645–646.

27. Heier JS, Enzenauer RW, Wintermeyer SF, et al. Ocular injuries and disease at a combat supported hospital in support of Operations Desert Shield and Desert Storm. *Arch Ophthalmol*. 1993;111;795–798.

28. Zuckerman B, Lieberman TW. Corneal rust ring. *Arch Ophthalmol*. 1960;63:254–264.

29. Jayamanne DGR, Bell RW. Non-penetrating corneal foreign body injuries: factors affecting delay in rehabilitation of patients. *J Accid Emerg Med*. 1994;11: 195–197.

30. Liston RL, Olson RJ, Mamalis N. A comparison of rust-ring removal methods in a rabbit model: small-gauge hypodermic needle versus electric drill. *Ann Ophthalmol*. 1991;23:24–27.

31. Cooke JA, Miller FH, Grover RW, et al. Urticaria caused by tarantula hairs. *Am J Trop Med Hyg*. 1973;22:130–133.

32. Chang PCT, Soong HK, Barnett JM. Corneal penetrations by tarantula hairs [letter]. *Br J Ophthalmol*. 1991; 75;253–254.

33. Teske SA, Hirst LW, Gibson BH, et al. Caterpillar-induced keratitis. *Cornea*. 1991;10:317–321.

34. Haluska FG, et al. Experimental gypsy moth (*Lymantria dispar*) ophthalmia nodosa. *Arch Ophthalmol.* 1983; 101:799–801.

35. Duke-Elder S, MacFaul PA. Lacerations of the cornea. In: Duke-Elder S, ed. *System of Ophthalmology.* Vol XIV. Part 1. St. Louis: Mosby; 1972.

36. John ME, Schmitt TE. Traumatic hyphema after radial keratotomy. *Ann Ophthalmol.* 1988;15:930–932.

37. Spivack LE. Case report: radial keratotomy incisions remain intact despite facial trauma from plane crash. *J Refract Surg.* 1987;4:59–60.

38. Slingsby JG, Forstot SL. Effect of blunt trauma on the corneal endothelium. *Arch Ophthalmol.* 1981;99:1041–1043.

39. Roper-Hall MJ, Wilson RS, Thompson SM. Changes in endothelial cell density following accidental trauma. *Br J Ophthalmol.* 1982;66:518–519.

40. Löwenstein A. Überlegungen zu einem Fall von traumatischer Hornhautquellung nebst Bemerkungen über die Bedeutung des Hornhautendothels. *Graefes Arch Clin Ophthalmol.* 1931;127:598–605.

41. Payrau P, Raynaud G. Lésions de la cornée par souggle: corps étrangers perforants microscopiques; anneaux veloutés postérieurs. *Ann Ocul.* 1965;198:1057–1074.

42. Forstot SL, Gasset AR. Transient traumatic posterior annular keratopathy of Payrau. *Arch Ophthalmol.* 1974; 92:527–528.

43. Cibis GW, Weingeist TA, Krachmer JH. Traumatic corneal endothelial rings. *Arch Ophthalmol.* 1978;96: 485–488.

44. Maloney WF, Colvard M, Bourne WM, et al. Specular microscopy of traumatic posterior annular keratopathy. *Arch Ophthalmol.* 1979;97:1647–1650.

Chapter **15**

SCLERAL AND CORNEOSCLERAL INJURIES

Jennifer L. Lindsey and M. Bowes Hamill

 Trauma is a common cause of corneoscleral and scleral defects in the young, otherwise healthy patient. Traumatic corneoscleral defects may take two forms:

1. those resulting acutely in the context of closed or open trauma; and
2. those occurring secondarily from tissue necrosis as a result of post-traumatic inflammation or infection.

Although the acute consequences can generally be repaired primarily, those occurring late often require repair by patching. When faced with the penetrating type of corneo/scleral[a] trauma, the clinician must rule out conclusively the presence of IOFBs and must evaluate and attend to intraocular damage.

Goals in the management of corneo/scleral injury include[1]:

- restoration of the integrity of the globe;
- avoidance of further injury to ocular tissues; and
- prevention of corneal[b] scarring and astigmatism.

Small, isolated scleral defects without uveal prolapse may respond to conservative management with observation and appropriate prophylactic antibiotic therapy. Larger wounds or areas of scleral thinning may require surgical repair, either by primary closure or by patch grafting.

---

[a]For simplicity, the term "corneo/scleral" substitutes for "corneoscleral and scleral" in this chapter.

[b]Treatment of isolated corneal injuries is discussed in Chapter 14.

> **PEARL...** Successful surgical management of traumatic corneo/scleral defects requires identification of, and tailoring of the surgical approach to, the underlying mechanism of injury.

EPIDEMIOLOGY

The following information is from the USEIR database.

Incidence:
- rate of corneoscleral involvement among eyes with serious injuries: 10%;
- rate of purely scleral involvement among eyes with serious injuries: 30%.

Age (years):
- range: 0–101;
- mean: 32;
- ≤15: 22%;
- 20 to 39: 38%;
- ≥60: 11%.

Sex:
- males: 82%;
- among those aged 0 to 59 years, males outnumber females nearly 5 times;
- among those aged 60 to 69 years, males outnumber females 1.5 times;

111

- in the ≥70-year-old population, females outnumber males nearly 1.5 times.

Place:

- 44% home;
- 17% street and highway;
- 11% work.

Cause:

- 33% blunt object;
- 13% sharp object;
- 12% MVC;
- 12% fall.

Injury type (purely scleral, not corneoscleral injuries):

- rate of scleral ruptures among all scleral injuries: 28%;
- rate of scleral lacerations among all scleral injuries: 28%;
- rate of scleral ruptures among all ruptures: 54%;
- rate of scleral lacerations among all lacerations: 59%.

> **PEARL...** Trauma inflicted by blunt objects plays a major role in corneo/scleral injury. The clinician must be alert for this type of injury in patients involved in MVCs and in falls (particularly among the elderly).

EVALUATION

History

A detailed history regarding the mechanism of injury directs the manner in which evaluation and repair will proceed. The clinician should address the following critical questions.

- Are there other life-threatening injuries that need to be addressed before repair of the ocular injury (see Chapters 9 and 10)?
- What was the exact mechanism of injury?
- If the injury resulted from an IOFB, what was the composition of the object, at what speed was it traveling, and what was the angle of impact to the eye/orbit (see Chapter 24)?

Surgical repair of corneo/scleral wounds may need to be delayed if other life-threatening injuries are present. Wound closure should take place, however, as soon as possible to avoid adverse sequelae such as infection. The mechanism of injury alerts the clinician

to the possibility of occult scleral injuries, intraocular damage, and IOFBs.

Physical Examination

- Gentle separation of the eyelids may be required; avoid pressure on the globe (see Chapters 8, 9, and 14).
- Assess the visual acuity; and, using "naked" inspection and the slit lamp, assess (see Chapters 9, 12, and 14):
  - periocular structures;
  - conjunctiva;
  - cornea;
  - sclera;
  - pupil(s) and other anterior segment structures.
- Ophthalmoscopy should also be attempted in the setting of obvious open globe injury and especially with uveal or vitreous prolapse. Dilating drops should not be used. In such cases, the remainder of the examination should be deferred to the more controlled operating room setting (see Chapter 8).

Preoperative findings associated with scleral rupture include[2]:

- visual acuity of light perception or NLP;
- chemosis;
- 360-degree subconjunctival hemorrhage;
- hyphema;
- IOP <10 mm Hg;
- peaked pupil (the apex of the peak is often aligned with the meridian of the rupture); and
- relative displacement of the lens–iris diaphragm (asymmetry of AC depths).

> **PITFALL**
>
> Scleral rupture may be occult and posterior. The clinician who pays attention to the (often subtle) signs of scleral rupture will not miss these injuries.

Careful preoperative examination of the patient with attention to the size and location of the corneo/scleral defect and the condition of the surrounding tissues allows the surgeon to plan the steps of exploration and repair. If a retinal tear/detachment or an IOFB is discovered preoperatively, involvement of a retinal surgeon in the primary repair is recommended.

Ancillary Studies

Appropriate imaging studies of the orbits may have to be obtained preoperatively (see Chapter 9).

- Ultrasound is useful in the setting of small wounds where the risk of extrusion of intraocular contents is minimal.
- If CT scans are indicated, fine (<1.5 mm) cuts through the entire orbit, with axial and coronal images, are required so that small IOFBs will not be missed (see Chapter 24).

Other Issues

When a patient has concomitant systemic disease, the clinician must be alert to the possibility of an underlying inflammatory or infectious process that may predispose the patient to the formation of a scleral wound (see Chapter 20).

Inflammation: In a study[3] of patients with autoimmune disease treated with scleral homografting for necrotizing scleritis, rapid graft melting occurred in those who did not receive chemotherapy before, or concomitant with, surgical intervention. The grafts remained stable, however, in those who received chemotherapy concomitant with surgery.[c]

Infection: Post-traumatic bacterial or fungal scleritis may cause scleral thinning and rupture/perforation. Surgery is often an important adjunct to antimicrobial therapy in these cases. Weakened sclera can be reinforced with a patch following débridement of devitalized tissue and harvest of material for culture. A readily vascularized patch provides optimal healing in this setting.

> ### P I T F A L L
>
> Lack of attention to, or treatment of, underlying infection or inflammation increases the risk of failure of the scleral repair.

Summary

The exact mechanism of scleral wound formation cannot always be determined preoperatively, particularly in acute cases or in patients with concomitant systemic disease. However, to achieve the optimal outcome for each patient, the surgeon should:

- establish the causative factors;
- institute medical therapy if indicated;

- carefully assess the extent of injury;
- exclude or confirm the presence of IOFBs; and
- plan a stepwise surgical approach.

See Chapter 27 for the strength of a healed wound.

ANESTHESIA

General Anesthesia

It is the preferred method for repair of corneo/scleral injuries because it:

- provides the dual benefit of excellent anesthesia and akinesia with minimal increase in intraocular/intraorbital pressure (see Chapter 8); and
- allows operative intervention at multiple sites for the harvest of fascia lata and other autologous graft material if and as necessary for the patching of large tissue defects.

General anesthesia may be inappropriate in patients who are:

- systemically ill;
- elderly; and/or
- debilitated.

Topical Anesthesia

It is suitable for small, anterior defects; but such defects are rare. Of all types of anesthesia available to the surgeon, the topical approach may carry the lowest risk of systemic stress and inadvertent injury to the globe. Topical anesthesia alone, however, is inadequate for the extensive dissection of conjunctiva and Tenon's capsule required for repair of large or posteriorly located areas of scleral thinning or wound.

Retrobulbar Anesthesia

It provides excellent local anesthesia and akinesia with minimal cardiac and respiratory stress. However, injection of a retrobulbar anesthetic agent increases the intraorbital, and consequently the intraocular, pressure.

> ### P I T F A L L
>
> Retrobulbar anesthesia may put undue pressure on the traumatized globe, leading to prolapse of intraocular contents.

This anesthetic technique is most appropriate for the repair of defects too extensive for topical anesthesia or for patients in whom general anesthesia poses an unacceptable systemic risk (see Chapter 8).

---

[c] Although these patients did not suffer ocular trauma, the cases illustrate the importance of attention to underlying predisposing factors.

Techniques of Operative Repair

Depending on the size of the defect and the nature of the underlying disease, various techniques are available for the closure of scleral defects.

> **PEARL...** A Jaffe-style lid speculum avoids undue pressure on traumatized tissues by lifting the palpebral circle off the globe via the force of the elastic bands.[4]

Tissue Adhesive

Tissue adhesive[d] is:

- generally reserved for small, puncture-type wounds in which the overall integrity of the globe is not compromised; and
- useful in very small or partial-thickness corneo/scleral lacerations.

Primary Closure

Scleral Wound

Figure 15–1 illustrates the technique of globe exploration and primary closure.

> **PEARL...** Scleral ruptures most commonly involve weak or thin areas of the sclera such as at the limbus, just behind muscle insertions, and at the insertion of optic nerve.

If an occult scleral wound is suspected, globe exploration is required.

- A 360° peritomy is made and Tenon's capsule is retracted posteriorly to reveal the underlying sclera.
- The extraocular muscle insertions and the areas in between insertions are directly visualized. If necessary, a traction suture[e] may be carefully introduced under the muscle under meticulous direct observation.[5]

For wound closure, the following points have to be remembered.

- Scleral wounds are closed from anterior to posterior, beginning at a recognizable landmark such as

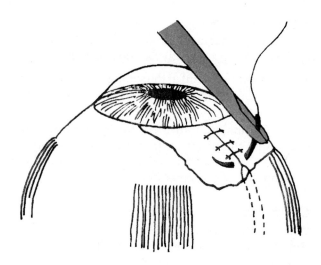

FIGURE 15–1 The "close-as-you-go" technique for exploration and primary closure of a scleral wound. The conjunctiva and Tenon's capsule are opened enough only to visualize the next suture site. In this manner, the periorbita maintains pressure on the scleral defect, thus keeping the intraocular contents stabilized until the lips of the scleral wound are apposed.

the limbus or the apex of the laceration. Tight closure prevents fibrovascular proliferation through an open scleral wound.

> **PEARL...** If the scleral wound is large, the surgeon must close the visible/accessible portion *before* further exploration is performed posteriorly. This stabilizes and enhances the integrity of the globe, allowing a higher safety margin during subsequent manipulations.

- Interrupted sutures, passing through deep sclera[f] while avoiding damage to the underlying choroid, are used.
- Most scleral lacerations can be closed using 8-0 or 9-0 nylon, silk, or Dacron.
- Small wounds with significant gaping forces may require thicker sutures.
- Nonabsorbable suture material should be used for all but the smallest scleral defects.
- Prolapsed uveal tissue is gently reposited to avoid incarceration in the wound. An assistant can use a cyclodialysis spatula to accomplish this while the

---

[d]See Chapter 14 for the technique of tissue adhesive application.

[e]4-0 silk.

[f]75–80% scleral thickness.

surgeon places the overlying sutures (zipper technique; see Chapter 16 for this and other tissue prolapses).

- If vitreous is present in the wound, it should be amputated at the scleral surface.
- Prolapsed retinal tissue is gently reposited if possible (see Chapter 5, Fig. 5–2). Incarceration is nevertheless likely, requiring vitreoretinal consultation/ intervention.

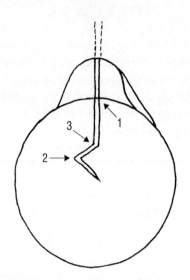

- If the scleral wound (usually rupture) extends under the insertion of a rectus muscle, the involved muscle may be temporarily disinserted.
  - ○ The standard technique with 6-0 double-armed Vicryl suture is used, avoiding undue traction on the globe.
  - ○ After closure of the scleral defect, the muscle is reinserted near its normal anatomic insertion.

> ## PITFALL
>
> Wounds extending posterior to the equator should be closed very carefully. If the full extent of the wound cannot be safely visualized, the best treatment may be to leave the most posterior portion unsutured.

Corneoscleral Wounds

Figure 15–2 illustrates the primary closure of a corneoscleral laceration.

> **PEARL...** Complicated corneoscleral wounds can be intimidating. Starting at a landmark, such as the limbus, provides the foundation for an anatomically correct repair.

For closure of the corneoscleral laceration:

- begin with placement of an interrupted 9-0 or 10-0 nylon, 90–100% depth, suture at the *limbus*;
- continue with repair of the *corneal* aspect (see Chapter 14 and Appendix);
- address the *scleral* portion of the defect as described earlier.

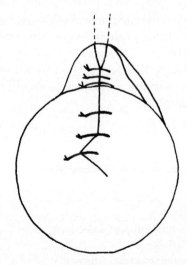

FIGURE 15–2 Illustration of primary closure of a corneoscleral wound. The first step is to identify the anatomic landmarks. (Top) the landmarks are the limbus (1) and angles in the wound (2, 3). Unless the conjunctiva is extensively involved, the corneal closure should be completed prior to the scleral wound. (Bottom) As discussed in relation to Figure 15–1, the closure of scleral wound should proceed posteriorly, opening and exploring enough only to visualize a part of the wound to avoid tissue extrusion.

> ## PITFALL
>
> When dealing with corneoscleral wounds, the surgeon should be alert for concurrent (while avoiding iatrogenic) damage to the iris, ciliary body, or lens. These and deeper structures should be carefully examined and any damage appropriately addressed (see Chapters 8, 9, and 17 through 24).

Scleral Patch Repair

Severe trauma to the globe may result in scleral defects that cannot be closed primarily. Staphyloma formation and rupture in this area may occur in eyes sustaining trauma by a blunt object.

Scleral thinning is rather common in case of:

- infection;
- inflammation; and/or
- high myopia.

In these cases, repair using a scleral patch is indicated. The surgical technique depends primarily on the type of graft material used (see Table 15–1).

> **PEARL...** Choosing the right graft material is critical to the success of scleral patch grafting. Before entering the operating room, the surgeon should consider the underlying process in each case and make an informed choice of graft material.

Homologous Sclera

Homologous sclera is the most commonly used graft material; it is stored in glycerin or alcohol or frozen in antibiotic solution until needed.[6]

- Frozen sclera can be used for up to 3 months from the date of preservation. Slow thawing at room temperature or in a warm (37°C) water bath with gentle shaking is recommended. Once thawed, the material should be refrigerated at 2–6°C until used (within 24 hours).

- Glycerin-dehydrated sclera may be used for up to 1 year from the date of preservation. Thorough rinsing and soaking in balanced salt solution for 30 minutes with a change to fresh solution at 15 minutes is recommended.

- Alcohol-fixed sclera is stored in absolute ethanol and can be used for up to 1 year after preservation. It should be rinsed and soaked as described for glycerin-preserved sclera.

> **PITFALL**
>
> Bacteria, including *Streptococcus pneumoniae*, *Pseudomonas aeruginosa*, and *Staphylococcus aureus*, have been recovered from sclera preserved in glycerin but not from alcohol-fixed sclera, suggesting that ethanol may be the superior preservative.[7]

When the surgeon is ready to use the donor material, the following steps are performed.

- Residual episcleral and choroidal tissues are carefully removed.
- The scleral defect is exposed in its entirety by performing a conjunctival peritomy and dissection.
- If necessary, the conjunctival edges are tagged with colored sutures to aid in reapproximation of multiple edges.
- The recipient bed is prepared by removal of all necrotic or suppurative sclera to identify good tissue margins.

TABLE 15–1   THE APPROPRIATE USE OF GRAFT MATERIALS

Material	Useful In:
Homologous sclera	Large defects requiring structural support
Conjunctiva/Tenon's capsule	Small defects with little need for structural support; infectious etiologies (vascularized graft preferred)
Tarsoconjunctival flap	Moderately sized defects requiring some structural support; infectious etiologies
Autologous sclera	Small to large defects requiring support
Fascia lata or periosteum	Small to large defects requiring support; severe disease with diffuse scleral involvement; patients able to tolerate multiple incision sites and general anesthesia
Split-thickness dermal graft	Severe ocular surface (epithelial) disruption; patients able to tolerate multiple incision sites and general anesthesia

- Solid, uninvolved, architecturally stable sclera is used to anchor the graft.
- Care is taken not to injure the choroid, which may bulge into the scleral defect.

PITFALL

Choroid often prolapses through the scleral defect and can easily be injured during exploration and repair.

A piece of plastic operative drape or similar material can be used to make a template of the size and shape of the needed patch.

PEARL... The graft must be oversized several millimeters beyond the defect to allow adequate suture bites into, and tissue apposition with, normal sclera to promote healing.

Once cut, the donor sclera is placed over the area of the defect and sutured using any of a variety of suture materials.

- Rapidly absorbing sutures are not recommended, as prolonged healing is often required for scleral stability.
- Permanent sutures such as silk and Dacron offer ease of manipulation and prolonged wound support.
- Sutures at the perimeter of the graft may be 6-0 to 10-0, depending on the condition of the recipient bed.
- When the graft abuts the limbus, 10-0 nylon sutures are recommended for the anterior sutures and for all sutures extending into the cornea.

PEARL... The use of interrupted sutures provides excellent edge apposition and allows the patch to be tightened in a controlled manner to reposit prolapsing uvea in case of a staphyloma.

Homologous sclera can be stored for an extended time without the need for specialized technology and is therefore widely available. The storage of whole scleral shells allows an adequate tissue supply for any patient. The material is flexible, easy to use, and well tolerated. Disadvantages include:

- the potential for inciting an inflammatory reaction; and
- a brighter white color, which often is not as cosmetically appealing as the more natural color of autologous sclera.

In addition to closure of scleral defects resulting from trauma, homologous scleral patch grafting has been used successfully for other indications.[g]

Conjunctiva/Tenon's Capsule

Although conjunctiva, with or without attached Tenon's capsule, is not a good choice in situations requiring structural strength, this graft material is useful in small scleral defects and exposed orbital implants. The technique is straightforward.

- The area of scleral defect is identified and necrotic tissue carefully débrided.
- In an adjacent, uninvolved area, the conjunctiva is mobilized with or without adherent Tenon's capsule.
- The graft is utilized as a free patch or as a pedicle graft, and the conjunctiva is sutured over the defect using interrupted sutures.

Advantages of this technique include the ready availability of the tissue and the technical ease of the procedure. The vascularized nature of the graft makes it especially useful for small wounds resulting from infection.

PITFALL

The conjunctiva does not provide significant structural rigidity against extrusion of intraocular contents (i.e., large defects, elevated IOP).

---

[g]Revision of trabeculectomy[8]; repair of scleral fistula after cataract surgery[9]; coverage of exposed hydroxyapatite implants.[10]

Conjunctival flaps (with or without adherent Tenon's capsule) have been used successfully for other indications.[h]

Tarsoconjunctival Flap

Tarsoconjunctival flap, offering more rigidity than conjunctiva alone and some structural support, is use-

---

[h]To repair a leaking filtering bleb following trabeculectomy[11]; to cover an exposed hydroxyapatite orbital implant after scleral patch grafting had been unsuccessful[12]; to close a perilimbal scleral defect in scleromalacia perforans.[13]

ful in cases of significant scleral thinning or moderate uveal prolapse.

- After dissection of the bulbar conjunctiva near the scleral defect and débridement of necrotic tissue, a pedicle flap with tarsus and overlying conjunctiva is created.
- The flap is then mobilized and sutured to cover the defect (Fig. 15–3).

This graft material retains the advantages of the well-vascularized, self-epithelialized conjunctival tis-

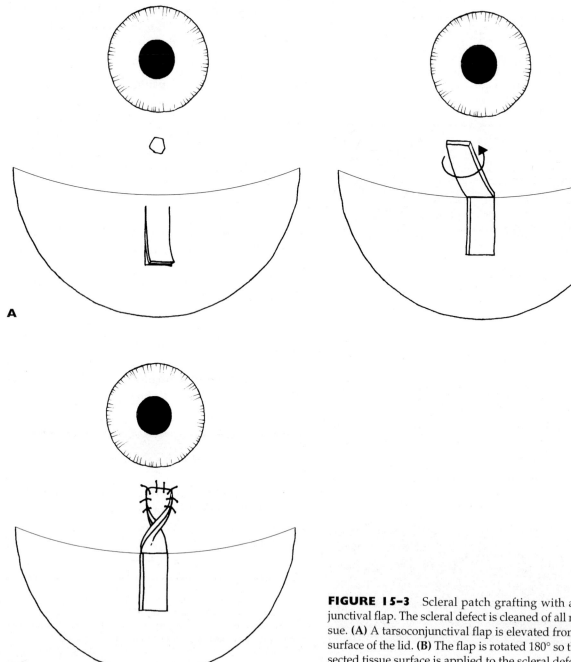

FIGURE 15–3 Scleral patch grafting with a tarsoconjunctival flap. The scleral defect is cleaned of all necrotic tissue. **(A)** A tarsoconjunctival flap is elevated from the tarsal surface of the lid. **(B)** The flap is rotated 180° so that the dissected tissue surface is applied to the scleral defect. **(C)** The flap is sutured into position.

sue and has the added benefit of the increased structural rigidity of the tarsus. Even scleral wounds caused by chemical injury have been repaired successfully using this technique.[14]

Autologous Sclera

Patient-derived sclera is commonly applied as a graft material in the patching of scleral defects. This method is appropriate for patients with scleral defects requiring structural support in the presence of adequate areas of healthy, uninvolved sclera available for use in patching.

The use of the patient's own tissue has two distinct benefits:

- it eliminates the risk of inciting an inflammatory reaction; and
- it has superior cosmesis because of the normal color of the patch.

Disadvantages include the following:

- in individuals with underlying autoimmune disease, this tissue may be more prone to involvement by the primary disease process than would unrelated donor tissue and
- there may not be sufficient healthy tissue available in patients with severe disease.

Depending on the lesion's size, there are two surgical options.

- For small defects, a partial-thickness, *hinged (trapdoor) scleral flap* is created immediately adjacent to the defect, reflected over the defect, and sutured into place (Fig. 15–4).
- For larger defects, a *free patch* is often required. This technique involves creation of a partial-thickness scleral patch from uninvolved sclera of the affected or from the fellow eye. The patch is placed over the area of scleral defect and sutured into position.

Scleral autografts have been used successfully for various etiologies.[i]

Fascia Lata

Fascia lata is an alternative autologous tissue and is useful when structural support is needed but inadequate uninvolved sclera is available for use as a patch. Fascia lata is generally used as an overlay graft using a technique similar to that described before for scleral homografts.

This tissue offers the advantages of strength, ease of harvest, and flexibility. It is thin and conforms well to the contour of the globe. Fascia lata is harvested at the same time as the patching procedure, requiring a second incision site and the use of general anesthesia.

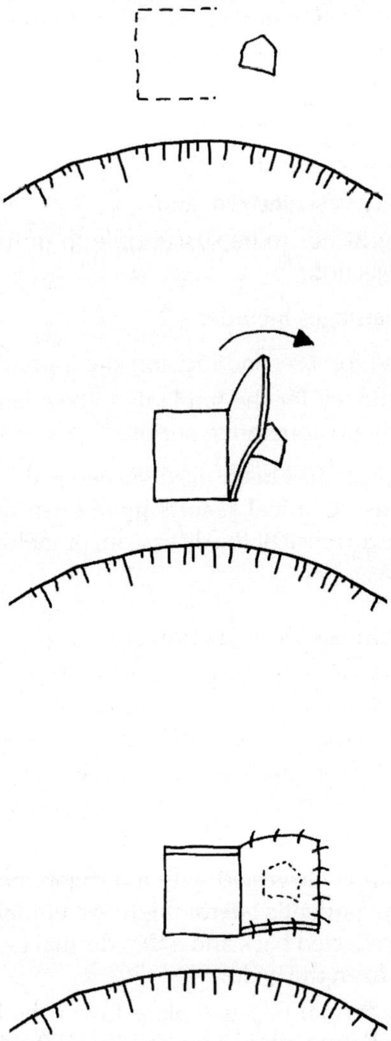

FIGURE 15–4 The trap-door scleral flap. The scleral defect is cleaned of all necrotic tissue. For this technique to be successful, the surrounding sclera must be normal. (Top) The area of the trap door is marked. (Middle) The flap is then created and reflected over the scleral defect. (Bottom) The flap is sutured into place.

If the tissue is not covered with epithelium or conjunctiva, it may undergo necrosis.[17]

Fascia lata grafts have also been used successfully for other indications.[j]

Periosteum

Periosteum is an autologous graft tissue harvested by making an incision along the anterior tibial crest and dissecting the preperiosteal tissues. The periosteum is

---

[i]Perilimbal scleromalacia[15]; idiopathic; postoperative (removal of limbal squamous cell carcinoma); and post-traumatic.[16]

[j]Scleromalacia perforans[18–23]; adjunct to glaucoma tube shunt surgery.[24]

then incised and lifted free of its underlying attachments with a periosteal elevator. The tissue should be kept moist in sterile saline until used.

Advantages include:

- tissue is easily harvested;
- has good tensile strength;
- is readily vascularized; and
- is thought not to be susceptible to immunologic graft rejection.[25,26]

Disadvantages include:

- the need for a second incision site for harvest; and
- the tendency for the implants to be edematous in the early postoperative period.[25]

Periosteum has been used successfully for other indications.[k] Clinical results have been favorable, without recurrence of the disease in, or melting of, the graft tissue.

Split-Thickness Dermal Graft

Dermal tissue is capable of self-epithelialization. Derived from the skin appendages within the graft, the epithelium is nonkeratinized and lacks adnexal structures.[17] The graft has been successfully used for the repair of corneal and scleral defects of various etiologies.[29]

- The graft is harvested with a dermatome, usually from the patient's lateral thigh. An epidermal flap is first reflected back and a thin dermal graft is harvested from the bed.
- The epidermal flap is replaced over the bed after fenestration to allow egress of tissue fluids.
- The recipient site is prepared as for other graft materials and the graft is sewn in place over the defect, taking care to maintain the appropriate orientation of the graft tissue.

> **PEARL...** The capacity for epithelialization makes split-thickness dermal graft tissue desirable when the patient lacks normal epithelium or has severe ocular surface disruption, for example, after chemical injury.

Other Materials

Other materials have been used with various degrees of success:

- cadaveric aortic tissue[30];
- lyophilized dura (with sutures and fibrin glue)[31];
- cornea[32]; and
- synthetic material.[l]

Postoperative Considerations

The resected tissue should undergo laboratory evaluation. If the underlying etiology is unknown or if systemic inflammatory disease is suspected, histological and immunopathological evaluation is useful. If an infectious etiology is suspected, a portion of the tissue should be sent to the microbiology laboratory for special stains and cultures. This will allow institution of specific, directed antibiotic therapy.

Summary

When faced with corneo/scleral injury, the clinician must:

- discover the mechanism of injury and be aware of its implications for the type and extent of ocular damage likely to be present;
- examine the patient carefully, with attention to signs of occult ocular injury;
- note the location and extent of injury;
- perform appropriate ancillary studies to detect all intraocular injuries/IOFBs;
- plan surgical exploration and repair, weigh the risks and benefits of primary closure versus patch graft, and decide on the appropriate graft material if necessary;
- perform proper surgical repair with the goals of restoring globe integrity, avoiding further trauma to ocular tissues, and minimizing corneal scarring and astigmatism;
- request the assistance of a vitreoretinal surgeon, if necessary;
- institute appropriate prophylactic antibiotic therapy as well as therapy for underlying conditions that may have predisposed the eye to injury; and
- monitor for postoperative complications such as retinal detachment, cataract, and endophthalmitis.

Figure 15–5 provides an overview of the thought process in treating eyes with corneo/scleral wounds.

---

[k]Necrotizing scleritis with staphyloma[27]; scleromalacia with impending scleral perforation[28]; repair of corneoscleral wound dehiscence.[25]

[l]Polytetrafluoroethylene, Gore-Tex; although successful experimentally,[33,34] its use is not recommended as a patch material in humans.[35]

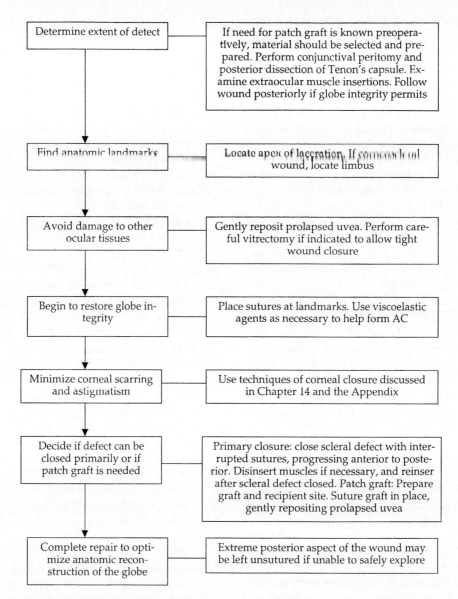

FIGURE 15-5 Outline of the important steps in the closure of corneo/scleral wounds.

REFERENCES

1. Koster HR, Kenyon KR. Complications of surgery associated with ocular trauma. *Int Ophthalmol Clin*. 1992;32: 157–178.

2. Navon SE. Management of the ruptured globe. *Int Ophthalmol Clin*. 1995;35:71–91.

3. Sainz de al Maza M, Tauber J, Foster CS. Scleral grafting for necrotizing scleritis. *Ophthalmology*. 1989;96: 306–310.

4. Hamill MB. Management of scleral perforation. In: Krachmer JH, Mannis MJ, Holland EJ, eds. *Cornea, Surgery of the Cornea and Conjunctiva*. St. Louis: Mosby; 1997.

5. Beatty RF, Beatty RL. The repair of corneal and corneoscleral lacerations. *Semin Ophthalmol*. 1994;9:165–176.

6. Nguyen QD, Foster CS. Scleral patch graft in the management of necrotizing scleritis. *Int Ophthalmol Clin*. 1999;39:109–131.

7. Dailey JR, Rosenwasser GO. Viability of bacteria in glycerin and ethanol preserved sclera. *Refract Corneal Surg*. 1994;10:38–40.

8. Laroche D, McGowan B, Greenfield D, et al. Late hypotony after cataract extraction due to a scleral fistula: a technique for surgical correction. *Ophthalmic Surg Lasers*. 1998;29:140–143.

9. Shields CL, Shields JA, De Potter P, et al. Problems with the hydroxyapatite orbital implant: experience with 250 consecutive cases. *Br J Ophthalmol*. 1994;78:702–706.

10. Clune MJ, Shin DH, Olivier MM, et al. Partial-thickness scleral-patch graft in revision of trabeculectomy. *Am J Ophthalmol*. 1993;115: 818–820.

11. Morris DA, Ramocki JM, Shin DH, et al. Use of autologous Tenon's capsule and scleral patch grafts for repair of excessively draining fistulas with leaking filtering blebs. *J Glaucoma*. 1998;7:417–419.

12. Oestreicher JH. Treatment of exposed coral implant after failed scleral patch graft. *Ophthal Plast Reconstr Surg*. 1994;10:110–113.

13. Van der Hoeven J. Scleromalacia perforans. *Arch Ophthalmol*. 1934;11:112–118.

14. Rootman DS, Insler MS, Kaufman HE. Rotational tarsal conjunctival flap in the treatment of scleral necrosis. *Ophthalmic Surg*. 1988;19:808–810.

15. Cappin JM, Allen DW. Paralimbic scleromalacia. *Br J Ophthalmol*. 1973;57:871–872.

16. Gopal L, Badrinath SS. Autoscleral flap grafting: a technique of scleral repair. *Ophthalmic Surg*. 1995;26:44–48.

17. Mauriello JA Jr, Fiore PM, Pokorny KS, et al. Use of split-thickness dermal graft in the surgical treatment of corneal and scleral defects. *Am J Ophthalmol*. 1988;105:244–247.

18. Torchia RT, Dunn RE, Pease PJ. Fascia lata grafting in scleromalacia perforans. *Am J Ophthalmol*. 1968;66: 705–709.

19. Bick MW. Surgical treatment of scleromalacia perforans. *Arch Ophthalmol*. 1959;61:907–917.

20. Armstrong K, McGovern VJ. Scleromalacia perforans with repair grafting. *Trans Ophthalmol Soc Aust*. 1955;15:110–121.

21. Taffet S, Carter GZ. The use of fascia lata graft in the treatment of scleromalacia perforans. *Am J Ophthalmol*. 1961;52:693–696.

22. Blum FG, Salamoun SG. Scleromalacia perforans. *Arch Ophthalmol*. 1963;69:287–289.

23. Zer I, Machtey I, Kurz O. Combined treatment of scleromalacia perforans in rheumatoid arthritis with penicillamine and plastic surgery. *Ophthalmologica*. 1973; 166:293–300.

24. Tanji TM, Lundy DC, Minckler DS, et al. Fascia lata patch graft in glaucoma tube surgery. *Ophthalmology*. 1996;103:1309–1312.

25. Koenig SB, Sanitato JJ, Kaufman HE. Long-term follow-up study of scleroplasty using autogenous periosteum. *Cornea*. 1990;9:139–143.

26. Koenig SB, Kaufman HE. The treatment of necrotizing scleritis with an autogenous periosteal graft. *Ophthalmic Surg*. 1983;14:1029–1032.

27. Breslin CW, Katz JI, Kaufman HE. Surgical management of necrotizing scleritis. *Arch Ophthalmol*. 1977;95: 2038–2040.

28. Rao GN, Aquavella JV, Palumbo AJ. Periosteal graft in scleromalacia. *Ophthalmic Surg*. 1977;8:86–92.

29. Mauriello JA, Pokorny K. Use of split-thickness dermal grafts to repair corneal and scleral defects—a study of 10 patients. *Br J Ophthalmol*. 1993;77:327–331.

30. Merz EH. Scleral reinforcement with aortic tissue. *Am J Ophthalmol*. 1964;57:766–770.

31. Mori S, Komatsu H, Watari H. Spontaneous posterior bulbar perforation of congenital scleral coloboma and its surgical treatment. *Ophthalmic Surg*. 1985;16:433–436.

32. Bernauer W, Allan BD, Dart JK. Successful management of *Aspergillus* scleritis by medical and surgical treatment. *Eye*. 1998;12:311–316.

33. Tawakol ME, Peyman GA, Liu KR, et al. Gore-Tex soft tissue bands as scleral explants in rabbits: a preliminary histologic study. *Ophthalmic Surg*. 1989;20:199–201.

34. Whitmore WG, Harrison W, Curtin BJ. Scleral reinforcement in rabbits using synthetic graft materials. *Ophthalmic Surg*. 1990;21:327–330.

35. Huang WJ, Hu FR, Chang SW. Clinicopathologic study of Gore-Tex patch graft in corneoscleral surgery. *Cornea*. 1994;13:82–86.

Chapter 16

Extrabulbar Tissue Prolapse

José Dalma-Weiszhausz

 The primary objective in managing injured eyes is to reestablish the original anatomy and function.[1,2] Proper handling of prolapsed tissues is essential to achieving a good outcome.[3] In this chapter we provide guidelines regarding the indications and techniques of treating tissue prolapse, a common finding in open globe trauma. The incidence of tissue prolapse is:

- 42% (USEIR) to 45% (México City, 1991[a]) in open globe injuries; and
- significantly higher in ruptures (70%) than in lacerations (49%; USEIR).

Definition and History

Tissue prolapse is defined as extrusion of intraocular content outside its normal compartment, whether intrabulbar (e.g., vitreous in the AC) or extrabulbar (e.g., expulsed lens).

Before the early 20th century, iris prolapse[b] through a corneal wound was considered a severe complication because of:

- fear of infection;
- fear of SO; and
- technical difficulties in management.

When topical eserine and bright light were not sufficient to return the iris to the AC, the wound was simply covered by a conjunctival flap with a purse-string suture and left to heal. Scleral wounds were treated similarly, with no intent of closure by sutures. Leeches were recommended to deal with the "congested uvea" associated with trauma.[4] It was accepted that wounds involving the retina or choroid would be followed by retinal detachment and phthisis.[4] Enucleation was routinely performed in cases of prolapsed ciliary body, choroid, retina, or vitreous.[5,6] The vitreous was thought to hold the retina in place; consequently, its removal was prohibited.[5] Even when wounds finally began to be sutured, corneal scarring and retinal detachment commonly resulted in poor visual results, which started improving only after the 1950s, with the advent of microsurgery, antibiotics, and steroids. The functional outcomes still leave room for improvement.[5,7–9]

Pathophysiology

Tissue extruded in the context of open globe injury is usually perceived as:

- a condition complicating the initial repair; and
- a risk factor for a less favorable anatomical/visual outcome.

With the formation of a full-thickness wound, the globe's sudden decompression may force the iris/choroid/vitreous/retina into the wound. Because of their inside-out mechanism (see Chapter 1), ruptures have a worse prognosis than lacerations: due to the increased IOP,[10–12] tissue loss is not only more common but also more severe.[8,13] Other acute and chronic aggravating factors include:

- orbital and intraocular bleeding/inflammation/injection;

---

[a] Unpublished data of the author.

[b] Especially if older than 24–48 hours.

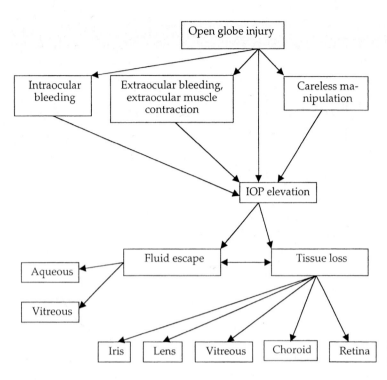

FIGURE 16–1   The pathomechanism of acute tissue prolapse.

- extraocular muscle spasm;
- choroidal edema;
- lens swelling; and
- excessive manipulations during evaluation (Fig. 16–1).

PEARL...   Tissue incarceration eventually plugs the wound, reestablishes the IOP, and tamponades the bleeding, helping to preserve the eye's anatomy.[11]

The trapped prolapsed tissue is subsequently secured by fibrin formation within a few hours and fibrosis within a few days[1,14] (Fig. 16–2). This may lead to:

- inadequate wound healing;
- leakage of aqueous;
- hypotension;
- endophthalmitis;
- epithelial ingrowth;
- chronic inflammation;
- corneal decompensation;
- dense, vascularized corneal scars;
- synechia formation;
- CME[1,15]; and
- retinal detachment.

EVALUATION

PEARL...   Intraocular tissue prolapse should be suspected in all open globe injuries. Remember that the wound may remain hidden (e.g., occult rupture).

Unless the wound is posterior and underneath a congested, edematous conjunctiva or blood-stained Tenon's capsule (see Chapters 13 and 15), the tissue prolapse is usually visible upon careful inspection. The clinician should look for the following signs:

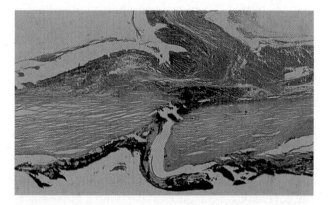

FIGURE 16–2   Photomicrograph. Uveal tissue incarcerated in scleral wound prevents adequate wound apposition and healing. (Courtesy of Dr. Alfredo Gomez-Leal, Asocoación para Evitar la Ceguera en México.)

- full-thickness eyewall defect;
- subconjunctival melanic pigment or blood;
- chemosis;
- peaked or irregular pupil;
- APD;
- hyphema;
- vitreous traction strands (best seen in the retrolental space at the slit lamp);
- vitreous hemorrhage; and
- low IOP.

PITFALL

Tissue prolapse may occur during transportation or be due to poor patient instruction and restriction and/or lack of eye shielding. As soon as an open globe injury is suspected, further diagnostic manipulations should be kept to a minimum (see Chapter 8).

PEARL... The nonophthalmologist should shield the eye and consult an ophthalmologist regarding transportation, systemic antibiotics, and pain medication.

Preoperative echography and CT scan may show tissue prolapse in case of a posterior scleral break. Although these techniques are seldom necessary when deciding whether to explore the globe, they may aid in planning the surgery.[16,17]

MANAGEMENT

Heavy topical and systemic corticosteroid therapy is essential to minimize inflammation (see Chapter 8). The rules of culturing and antibiotic therapy[10,18] follow the general principles for open globe trauma (see Chapter 28 and the Appendix). The implications, instrumentation, and technique of management vary with each tissue (see below and Fig. 16–3). All tissue prolapses should be addressed at the time of wound repair (Fig. 16–4).

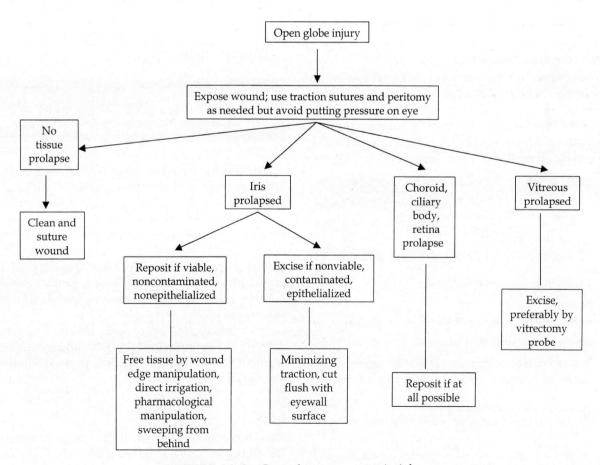

FIGURE 16–3   General management principles.

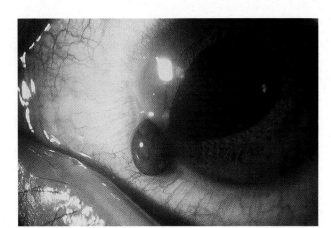

FIGURE 16–4 Iris prolapse through limbal wound.

PITFALL

Leaving tissue prolapsed may lead to severe complications such as SO and is acceptable only if severe bleeding occurs (ECH/SCH; see Chapter 22).

Iris[c] (see also Chapter 18)

Conventional wisdom dictated that iris exposed for more than 24 hours should be excised for fear of introducing infected material or epithelial cells into the eye.[2,10,19] With improved surgical techniques, technology, and pharmaceuticals, the surgeon should not be dogmatic about this 24-hour deadline.[15]

PEARL... The pupillary margin is more susceptible to ischemia than the root of the iris.

Excision[d] is recommended for:

• necrotic;
• nonviable (macerated, depigmented, feathery); or
• severely contaminated iris.

If excision is required, maximal iris preservation is the goal for cosmesis and to minimize glare by pre-

---

[c]The other parts of the uvea (i.e., ciliary body and uvea) are virtually never excised.

[d]When excising iris tissue incarcerated in wound, remember that more iris is drawn from the central iris than from the root area.

serving pupillary function. Traction should be minimized and suturing of the defect is recommended (see Chapter 18).

The removed material can be cultured. Epithelial cells can usually be removed by mechanical (abrasion), chemical (alcohol), or thermal (cryotherapy) means.

Reposit the prolapsed iris if it is:

• viable;
• free from epithelial overgrowth; and
• free from bacterial contamination

Prior antibiotic irrigation may prevent endophthalmitis. The repositioning technique varies by the extent, location, and duration of the prolapse. Approaching the commonly atonic and floppy, difficult-to-manipulate[2] iris at the original wound seldom works and may cause further damage to the iris and/or cornea. Usually, one or a combination of the following is attempted:

• gentle sweeping/pulling with a spatula through a limbal paracentesis;
• viscoelastics;
• miotics[20] (if the peripheral iris is entrapped);
• mydriatics[10] (if the central iris is involved); and
• in a more chronic injury with the iris "glued" to the wound edges by fibrin, careful dissection using fine, atraumatic forceps.

PEARL... Repositioning the iris is easier by pulling than by pushing.

Whether the iris is incised or repositioned, it is crucial to prevent postoperative synechia formation by using pharmacological agents, air, or viscoelastics.

Prolapse of the ciliary body and the choroid is much less common. As mentioned, they are rarely excised for fear of bleeding, inflammation with cyclitic membrane formation, and phthisis. They are usually reposited using the *zipper* technique, gently pushing/holding the uveal tissue back with a spatula while the sutures are placed.

Postoperatively, aggressive anti-inflammatory therapy is recommended. Any secondary anterior segment reconstruction is usually performed after a few months.[2]

Lens

No intervention is needed if the lens is completely lost. Subconjunctival lens/remnants require removal. Rarely, lens particles may be entrapped in the wound.

These must be removed; simultaneous vitreous prolapse is common (see Chapter 21).

Vitreous

Poor management of prolapsed vitreous is a rather common and avoidable source of late complications such as:

- corneal decompensation;
- chronic inflammation;
- CME;
- tractional retinal detachment; and
- phthisis.[9,19]

> **PEARL...** Vitreous prolapse is not simply the target of a surgical manipulation: by doubling the risk of retinal detachment development in case of open globe injury (30% vs. 14%, USEIR), it has prognostic significance.

The incidence of retinal detachment is higher with wounds at the ora serrata than at the equator (78% vs. 16%), due to the involvement of the vitreous base.[21] Removal of the prolapsed vitreous:

- permits orderly wound healing;
- gets rid of the matrix for fibrous ingrowth and/or proliferation[22];
- prevents traction on the vitreous base and retina[1]; and thus
- prevents the formation of retinal breaks and detachment.

> **PEARL...** Damage to the zonules must have occurred if vitreous prolapses into the AC.[e] Retinal injury exists if vitreous prolapse occurs through a scleral wound posterior to the insertion of extraocular muscles.[11]

Retinal breaks, including giant tears, are most commonly found either just posterior to the scleral wound or 180° away, and are caused by direct traction (Fig. 16–5).

> **PEARL...** The vitreous responsible for complications is not what has been removed but what remains behind.[11]

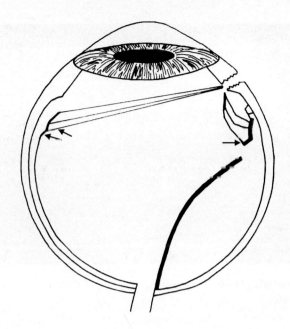

FIGURE 16–5 Vitreous prolapse often leads to traction and retinal tears, either in the vicinity of the prolapse (arrow) or 180° away (double arrow).

Vitreous prolapsed into the AC or into the lens must be removed. Several techniques increase the chance of recognizing that there are vitreous remnants in the AC[19]:

- air;
- viscoelastics (less effective than air; see Chapter 17);
- miotics;
- tangential light shone externally with the endoilluminator from the limbus; and
- pupillary deformation caused by vitreous strands.

To minimize traction, the vitrectomy probe is preferred to cellulose sponges and scissors for removing vitreous from the wound. This is especially crucial when the wound is scleral and the expulsed vitreous is mixed with blood.

> **PEARL...** Vitreous gel may remain attached to the interior aspect of the wound, especially over the sclera. The surgeon must attempt to remove it as completely as is consistent with safety, without causing globe collapse or retinal injury.

The vitreous may be incarcerated in the posterior exit wound of a perforating injury (Fig. 16–6). These rapidly self-sealing wounds usually do not permit external tissue excision. The surgeon may be forced

---

[e]Rare exception: vitreous prolapse through an in situ lens.

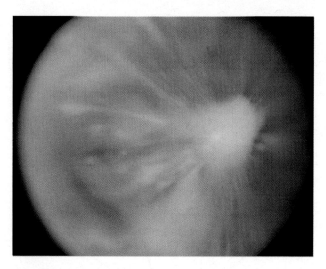

FIGURE 16–6   Vitreous incarcerated in posterior scleral wound.

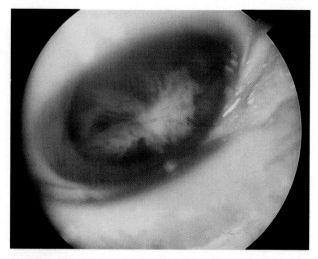

FIGURE 16–7   Retina incarcerated at the pars plana.

to limit the intervention to internal trimming of the trapped vitreous (see Chapter 26).

PITFALL

Too early intervention for posterior vitreous prolapse may result in wound reopening with disastrous consequences.

Vitreous prolapse often leads to retinal traction along the vitreous base.[22] Prophylactic encircling bands are nevertheless controversial. We prefer their use if:

- the wound involves an area near the vitreous base;
- vitreous removal is suboptimal; and
- secondary reconstruction is unlikely to be performed (e.g., systemic reasons, poor patient compliance[9]).

Retina

Of all prolapses, that of the retina has by far the poorest prognosis.

PEARL... Proper management of incarcerated vitreous is of utmost importance to prevent retinal entrapment in the wound and subsequent retinal detachment.

Retinal extrusion usually occurs in cases of large posterior ruptures, commonly associated with severe ECH. Vitreous is almost always present and its loss often substantial (Fig. 16–7).

If possible, the retina should be gently pushed back into the eye, using viscoelastics if necessary (see Chapter 5, Fig. 5–2). The wound should then be sutured and the retinal lesion and the injury's consequences dealt with during a second procedure.

Subsequent fibrous ingrowth may entrap the retina if it is caught in between the lips of the scleral wound. Typically, retinal detachment with folds radiating from the incarceration site develops within weeks. In more severe cases, the whole anterior aspect of the retina is drawn to the wound. Echography is useful in case of media opacity. Because these detachments are difficult to treat[1] and the PVR[23] rate is high, prophylaxis of retinal incarceration is preferred by excising all extruded vitreous, gently pushing the retina back and using the zipper technique to close the wound.

PITFALL

Because it increases inflammation and stimulates PVR development, it is best to avoid prophylactic cryotherapy of the scleral wound.[24,25]

If retinal incarceration occurs, secondary reconstruction must almost always be performed,[7] typically involving a scleral buckle[7] and vitrectomy. We perform it 10 to 14 days after the injury, when inflammation is under control and the intraocular anatomic status has been assessed adequately. A wide-angle viewing system is invaluable to optimize the surgical tactics when the vitreous hemorrhage and residual vitreous have been removed (see Chapter 8).

- Small anterior retinal entrapments may be left without excision if supported by a scleral buckle, but the risk of secondary detachment is high.
- Larger and posterior folds may require both buckles[15] and retinotomy.[26]
- If the incarceration is near the equator, an exoplant may be added to relieve the traction.[7,23]
- If retinotomy is necessary, the surgeon's initial instinct is to minimize the size of the resulting retinal defect, but "small" is usually less effective than "large." Enough space should be left between the freed retinal edge and the remaining scar tissue to prevent a secondary retinal detachment.

PEARL... Retinotomies usually need to be larger than originally anticipated.

- The retinotomy should be performed only after the vitreous, including the posterior hyaloid, and all proliferative tissues have been removed.
- The retina is cauterized and cut by scissors, rather than by the vitrectomy probe,[26] to increase accuracy.
- Removal of the peripheral retina in cases of anterior incarceration is important to prevent subsequent neovascular proliferation.

- Subretinal membranes can be extracted through the same retinotomy. Use of PFCL helps keep the retina stable while these maneuvers are performed.
- Although long-acting gases may also be used for tamponade, silicone oil is usually preferred if large retinotomies are required.[27]

Vitrectomy has improved the anatomic success rates in the past 30 years (from 52[13] to 73%[7]), but the visual outcome in eyes with retinal prolapse/incarceration is still disappointing: only 40% achieve >5/200[7] vision because of severe PVR and macular damage at the time of the original injury.

SUMMARY

Proper management of all tissue prolapses is essential to achieve good visual and anatomic results in the traumatized eye. The preservation of as much viable and noninfected uveal tissue as possible is important. Although the surgeon performing the initial repair is commonly required to remove prolapsed tissue from the wound, this procedure has received surprisingly little attention in the literature. Observation of the rules outlined here should help reduce complications, whether caused by the injury or inflicted by inadequate tissue handling.

REFERENCES

1. Conway BP, Michels RG. Vitrectomy techniques in the management of selected penetrating ocular injuries. *Ophthalmology.* 1978;85:560–583.
2. Colby K. Management of open globe injuries. *Int Ophthalmol Clin.* 1999;39:59–69.
3. Brinton GS, Aaberg TM, Reeser FH, et al. Surgical results in ocular trauma involving the posterior segment. *Am J Ophthalmol.* 1982;93:271–278.
4. Ramsey AM. *Eye Injuries and Their Treatment.* Glasgow: Maclehose; 1907:65–69.
5. Callahan A. *Surgery of the Eye: Injuries.* Springfield, IL: Charles C Thomas; 1950.
6. Spaeth EB. *Principles and Practice of Ophthalmic Surgery.* 4th ed. Philadelphia: Lea & Febiger; 1948.
7. Han DP, Mieler WF, Abrams GW, et al. Vitrectomy for traumatic retinal incarceration. *Arch Ophthalmol.* 1988;106:640–645.
8. Russel SR, Olsen KR, Folk JC. Predictors of scleral rupture and the role of vitrectomy in severe blunt ocular trauma. *Am J Ophthalmol.* 1988;105:253–257.
9. Ahmadieh H, Soheilian M, Sajjiadi H, et al. Vitrectomy in ocular trauma. Factors influencing final visual outcome. *Retina.* 1993;13:107–113.
10. Navon SE. Management of the ruptured globe. *Int Ophthalmol Clin.* 1995;35:71–91.
11. Kuhn F, Mester V. Anterior open globe injuries with vitreous prolapse and/or incarceration. In: Stirpe M, ed. *Anterior and Posterior Segment Surgery: Mutual Problems and Common Interests.* New York: Ophthalmic Communications Society; 1998:252–257.
12. Freitag SK, Eagle RC, Jaeger EA, et al. An epidemiologic and pathologic study of globes enucleated following trauma. *Ophthalmic Surg.* 1992;23:409–413.
13. Meredith TA, Gordon PA. Pars plana vitrectomy for severe penetrating injury with posterior segment involvement. *Am J Ophthalmol.* 1987;103:549–554.
14. Winthrop SR, Cleary PE, Minckler DS, Ryan SJ. Penetrating eye injuries: a histopathological review. *Br J Ophthalmol.* 1980;64:809–817.

15. Orlin SE, Farber MG, Brucker AJ, et al. The unexpected guest: problem of iris reposition. *Surv Ophthalmol.* 1990;35:59–66.

16. Benjamin L, Wormald R. CT scan diagnosis of scleral rupture. *Eye.* 1987;1:757.

17. Coleman DJ, Jack RL, Franzen LA. Ultrasonography in ocular trauma. *Am J Ophthalmol.* 1973;75:279–288.

18. Rubsamen PE, Cousins SW, Martinez JA. Impact of cultures on the management decisions following surgical repair of penetrating ocular trauma. *Ophthalmic Surg Lasers.* 1997;28:43–49.

19. Hudson HL, Thomas EL, Novack RL, et al. Primary surgical management of penetrating eye injuries. In: Alfaro DV, Liggett PE. *Vitreoretinal Surgery of the Injured Eye.* Philadelphia: Lippincott-Raven; 1998: 71–85.

20. Getnick RA, Peterson WS. Pharmacologically assisted repair of iris prolapse. *Ophthalmic Surg.* 1995;29:89.

21. Hsu HT, Ryan SJ. Experimental retinal detachment in the rabbit. *Retina.* 1986;6:66–69.

22. Cleary PE, Ryan SJ. Method of production and natural history of the experimental posterior penetrating eye injury in the rhesus monkey. *Am J Ophthalmol.* 1979; 88:212–220.

23. Michels RG, Thompson JT, Rice TA, et al. Effect of scleral buckling on vector forces caused by epiretinal membranes. *Am J Ophthalmol.* 1986;102:449–451.

24. Campochiaro PA, Gaskin HC, Vinores SA. Retinal cryopexy stimulates traction retinal detachment formation in the presence of an ocular wound. *Arch Ophthalmol.* 1987;105:1567–1570.

25. Jaccoma EH, Conway BP, Campochiaro PA. Cryotherapy causes extensive breakdown of the blood-retinal barrier. *Arch Ophthalmol.* 1985;103:1728–1730.

26. Machemer R, McCuen BW, de Juan E. Relaxing retinotomies and retinectomies. *Am J Ophthalmol.* 1986;102: 7–12.

27. Liggett PE, Mani N, Green RE, et al. management of traumatic rupture of the globe in aphakic patients. *Retina Suppl.* 1990;10:S59–S64.

Chapter 17

ANTERIOR CHAMBER

Bradford J. Shingleton and Ferenc Kuhn

 The AC is the most anterior compartment of the eye; it is bordered by the cornea, the angle, the iris, and the lens and is filled with a completely transparent aqueous. Injury to the bordering structures and its implications are discussed in the appropriate chapters; here we cover issues related to synechiolysis and the removal from the AC of the following materials:

- blood;
- fibrin and inflammatory debris (including infectious organisms);
- lens (see also Chapter 21);
- vitreous;
- IOFBs (see also Chapter 24);
- air bubble(s); and
- viscous/viscoelastic material.

We also discuss methods of reformatting the AC.

SYNECHIALYSIS AND PUPILLARY MEMBRANES

Anterior synechiae represent iris tissue that is adherent to the cornea or the angle, typically to an area of a former traumatic or surgical wound. The synechia may interfere with vision, deform the pupil, even cause secondary glaucoma (see Chapter 20). Should such complications result, the synechia is best broken: it may be lysed by a sweeping motion using a spatula. Stronger connections require cutting by scissors or the vitrectomy probe. Viscoelastics are also useful. If the scar is vascularized, these may have to be diathermized first to avoid hemorrhage. Adequate attention

must also be paid to avoiding damage to the endothelium and Descemet's membrane. Especially following extensive injury, the scar may be too large and leaving it behind is preferable to causing iatrogenic damage. Rarely, a PK is required.

Posterior synechiae are usually the result of inflammation, "gluing" iris tissue onto the anterior lens capsule. This may cause pupil deformity and inability of the pupil to dilate; secondary glaucoma is much more common than in eyes with anterior adhesion.

> **PEARL...** When breaking posterior synechiae, special attention is required if the lens is clear to avoid breaching the anterior capsule. Strong adhesions between the iris and the anterior lens capsule are therefore better broken with a spatula before viscoelastics are injected, thus avoiding both capsular damage and the entrapment of viscoelastics behind the iris.

If posterior segment surgery is needed, iris retractors may be inserted[a] to keep the pupil open when all synechiae have been broken.

---

[a]When introducing iris retractors, aim with the preparatory needle path a little more central than what the appearance suggests: try somewhere midway between actual iris margin and desired iris position after insertion and pull-back because the retractor is too weak to bend. If the needle's angle is too steep, you cannot "catch" the iris margin; if the needle is too shallow, dilation will not be sufficient (or the iris will be lifted toward the cornea).

Pupillary membranes should be removed because they interfere with vision and may lead to secondary glaucoma. If they are mildly adherent, blunt dissection using a spatula suffices; otherwise, forceps and scissors have to be used. These membranes may be vascularized, requiring diathermy first.

HYPHEMA

Blood in the AC commonly accumulates in case of (closed as well as open) globe trauma. Consequences include IOP elevation, corneal blood staining, the formation of anterior/posterior synechiae, cataract, and a wide variety of indirectly related pathologic changes. Because traumatic hyphema may lead to a significant reduction in vision, all ophthalmologists must be comfortable with its diagnosis, evaluation, and management. We review the setting, pathophysiology, evaluation, and treatment of hyphema.[1]

Epidemiology and Prevention

- The estimated incidence rate in North American studies is 17–20/100,000 population/years.[2,3]
- The vast majority of patients are younger than 20 years of age.[4]
- The male/female ratio is approximately 3 to 1.
- The most common cause is a blunt object.[4-11]
- Sports are the source in 60% in the younger population.

The USEIR found that:

- 33% of all eyes with serious injury develop hyphema;
- the risk of hyphema is 31% in open globe and 35% in closed globe trauma;

- 46% of hyphemas occur in eyes with open globe trauma;
- 80% of those injured are males;
- the mean age of those injured is 29 years (median: 30 years).

Wearing proper eye protection (polycarbonate lenses with sturdy frames and posterior retaining lips) could significantly reduce traumatic hyphema.

Classification

Hyphema is graded according to the amount of blood in the AC (Table 17–1).[2,4,5,12]

Pathophysiology

Mechanism of Injury

Contusion causes anteroposterior globe compression with equatorial scleral expansion, limbal stretching, and posterior displacement of the lens/iris diaphragm. There is an acute IOP elevation, which may be associated with tissue damage in the angle (Fig. 17–1).[13] Bleeding generally occurs from tears in the:

- major arterial circle and branches of the ciliary body;
- choroidal arteries;
- ciliary body veins[13]; and/or (less commonly)
- iris vessels at the pupillary margin or in the angle.

Associated Clinical Findings

- *Angle recession.* Common following closed globe trauma, it represents a separation between the longitudinal and circular fibers of the ciliary muscle.[14]

TABLE 17–1   THE GRADING OF HYPHEMAS BASED ON HOW MUCH OF THE AC IS FILLED WITH BLOOD

Grade	Hyphema Size
I	<1/3
II	1/3–1/2
III	1/2–near total
IV	Total
Microscopic*	Circulating RBCs only; no gross collection of blood

*It is difficult to ascertain the true significance of microscopic hyphema because it is not always easy to differentiate it from traumatic iritis. However, as rebleeding may occur in approximately 7% of children with microscopic hyphema,[10,11] even small amounts of blood in the AC need to be taken seriously and the patient followed closely.

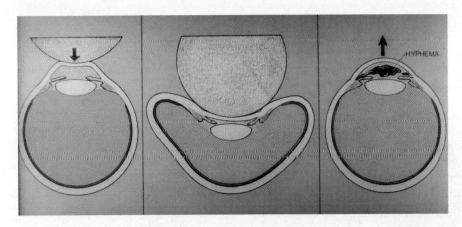

FIGURE 17–1 Mechanism of bleeding resulting from closed globe trauma to the eye: equatorial expansion with posterior displacement of lens/iris diaphragm and tearing of blood vessels. Adapted from Campbell DG. Traumatic glaucoma. In: Shingleton RJ, Hersh PS, Kenyon KR, eds. *Eye Trauma* St. Louis: Mosby Year Book; 1991: 118, by permission from Mosby.

Angle recession may occur in 85% of patients with traumatic hyphema[2,3,5] and be associated with early as well as late onset of glaucoma (see Chapter 20).

> **PEARL...** Angle recession may be significant even in eyes with small hyphemas and is not necessarily correlated with the degree of acute IOP elevation.

- *Cyclodialysis cleft*. An important cause of hypotony (see Chapter 19).
- *Traumatic iritis*, with inflammatory cells in the AC, always accompanies hyphema; the pigmentary changes may persist even after the blood has cleared. It is not uncommon to have focal zones of iris atrophy and pigment on the anterior capsule, sometimes in the form of a Vossius ring.[7]
- *Miosis*.
- *Mydriasis*. Occurs in approximately 10% of eyes.
- *Iridodialysis*. Occurs in approximately 10% of eyes.[2,7]
- *Corneal changes*. May range from minor abrasion to corneal endothelium damage and limbal rupture.
- *Cataract*. May be a late occurrence.
- *Lens subluxation*. Less common.
- Concentric rings of ocular tissues have been described as potentially damaged in closed globe trauma (Fig. 17–2).[15]
- The full spectrum of *posterior segment injuries*[b] (vitreous hemorrhage, retinal edema/hemorrhages/holes/tears, choroidal rupture etc.). Optic atrophy

may also occur, particularly in the setting of marked IOP elevation.[2,7] Even a marginal pressure increase may be associated with significant optic atrophy in patients with sickle disease or sickle trait.

Clot Formation and Dissolution

IOP elevation, vascular spasm, and formation of a fibrin/platelet clot facilitate cessation of the bleeding.[16,17] A pseudocapsule may develop with firm attachments to surrounding tissues. Blood may extend from the AC into the PC. Maximum clot integrity tends to occur 4–7 days after injury; fibroblastic activity is not seen at this stage.

> **PEARL...** The AC is fibrinolytically active.[18] Plasminogen (profibrinolysin) is converted to plasmin (fibrinolysin) by coagulation cascade activators. Plasmin, in turn, breaks down the fibrin, leading to clot dissolution. Clot degradation products, free blood cells, and inflammatory debris clear through trabecular meshwork outflow pathways and uveal scleral channels.[19] Only minimal direct absorption through the iris vasculature occurs.

Evaluation

History

In addition to details of the eye injury's occurrence, information should be sought on bleeding disorders, sickle cell disease, concurrent anticoagulant therapy, and systemic conditions such as pregnancy and kidney and liver disease, which may be affected by the medical treatment for hyphema. Always question the

---

[b]The HEIR found (V. Mester and F. Kuhn, 1999) that of contused eyes with hyphema, 61% had posterior segment pathology.

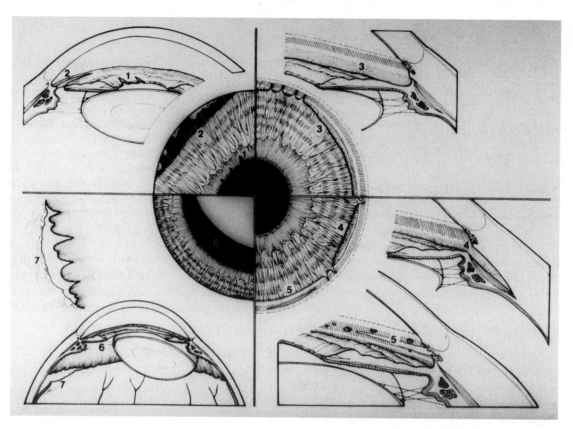

FIGURE 17–2   The seven typical anterior tears that occur following closed globe trauma to the eye. Clockwise from left: 1, Pupillary tears; 2, iridodialysis; 3, angle recession; 4, cyclodialysis; 5, meshwork tears; 6, ruptured zonules; 7, retinal dialysis. (From Campbell DG. Traumatic glaucoma. In: Shingleton RJ, Hersh PS, Kenyon KR, eds. *Eye Trauma*. St. Louis: Mosby Year Book; 1991:118. Reprinted by permission from Mosby.)

patient about preexisting ocular conditions (e.g., glaucoma) that may increase the risk of post-traumatic IOP elevation.

Clinical Examination

A complete eye examination is required for each case; suspect an open globe injury until confirmed otherwise. At all visits, the visual acuity, various tissue injuries, the hyphema's extent, and the IOP need to be documented.

- The slit lamp should be used to describe carefully all details of blood accumulation. The clot must be differentiated from free, circulating red blood cells. The hyphema's size may be described in three ways:
  - height (mm);
  - grade (see Table 17–1); or
  - clock-hour extent.

PEARL...   High magnification with a narrow slit-lamp beam is the most effective way to detect the presence of corneal blood staining by demonstrating yellow granular changes in the posterior corneal stroma and reduced definition of the posterior stromal fibular structure of the cornea.

CONTROVERSY

Gonioscopy can be performed at the time of the initial injury if important information can be gained, for example, to document a site of active bleeding.

PITFALL

It is important not to compress the eye and exacerbate the bleeding. Gonioscopy should be performed in all patients 1 month after injury.

- IBO is indicated but the blood may hamper the view. We favor deferring scleral depression until 1 month after the trauma.

Ultrasonography

The USEIR (2000) found a rate similar to the HEIR's: 57% of contused eyes with hyphema sustain damage to posterior segment structures. It is therefore crucial to evaluate the nature and extent of posterior segment injuries.

Laboratory Tests

All black and Hispanic patients with hyphema should have their sickle status examined[19]:

- sickle cell preparation;
- hemoglobin electrophoresis;
- bleeding tests (prothrombin time, partial thromboplastin time, platelet counts, and bleeding time); and
- kidney and liver functions (pending medical treatment decisions, e.g., whether systemic antifibrinolytics will be used).

PITFALL

Homozygotic patients (SS) and heterozygotic carriers (SA, SC) are predisposed to sickling and may be at significant risk.

Radiological Tests

Radiographic studies are not routinely obtained, although CT may be indicated if an IOFB, open globe injury, or orbital fracture is suspected.

Differential Diagnosis

Blood may collect in the AC even after trivial trauma in cases of:

- rubeosis iridis;
- malignant neoplasms;
- juvenile xanthogranuloma; or
- IOL (especially if AC or iris fixated).[1]

In addition to looking for abnormal clotting factors, occult (open globe) trauma must be considered in the differential diagnosis of "spontaneous" bleeding.

Treatment

Treatment Strategy

Medical and *supportive* treatment should be directed toward:

- reducing the rebleeding rate;
- clearing the hyphema;
- treating the associated tissue lesions; and
- minimizing the long-term sequelae.

Surgery is generally indicated for:

- IOP elevation not responding to medical treatment; and
- corneal blood staining.

The patient must be closely *followed*; sickle cell patients require more aggressive management and especially close observation.

The treatment protocols are highly varied and tend to be geographically and institutionally biased. It is important to avoid dogmatism and develop a reasonable, logical, and individualized approach.

Inpatient versus Outpatient Treatment

For the physician, there are advantages in hospitalization:

- ease of follow-up examination;
- increased compliance with medical therapy;
- a more "restful" environment; and
- earlier detection of complications.

Most patients, however, prefer treatment at home, which is also less expensive. In uncontrolled studies,[20,21] no significant differences in rebleeding rates and clinical outcomes were noted in patients treated at home versus in a hospital.

Regardless of the site of therapy, the responsibility for adherence to the treatment program and follow-up care remains with the treating physician. Guidelines for medical and surgical management of traumatic hyphema is provided in Table 17–2.

Supportive Care includes the following.

- *Moderate vs. strict bed rest*: most reports[22,23] found no significant outcome difference.

Table 17–2   Management Guidelines for Traumatic Hyphema

Supportive care	Moderate activity; may sit and walk
	Elevate head of bed to 30°
	Metal shield protection
Laboratory tests	CBC, PT, PTT, platelet count, BUN, creatinine, electrolytes, liver function tests as necessary
	Sickle cell prep, hemoglobin electrophoresis for patients at risk for sickle cell disease
Medications	Oral acetaminophen as needed
	No aspirin or NSAID
	Atropine 1% 2 × daily
	Prednisolone acetate 1% 1 drop 4 × daily; increase as necessary
	Oral aminocaproic acid 50 mg/kg 4 × daily up to 30 g/day for 5 days or prednisone 20 mg p. os 2 × daily for high-risk patients
Surgery	Paracentesis and AC washout for IOP not responsive to medical therapy within 24 hours
	Other types of surgery as needed

- *Bilateral vs. unilateral patching*: no difference in clinical results.[24]

- *Reading restrictions*: do not appear to be necessary.

- *Sedation*: rarely needed if activity is restricted to normal levels.

- *Metal shield protection*: usually indicated to prevent further damage to the eye in the first 5 days after injury.

- *Elevation of the head of the bed*: sedimentation of the blood facilitates posterior segment examination and visual recovery.

Medical Care   A wide range of medicines have been proposed. Some of these treatments appear contradictory (e.g., miotics vs. cycloplegics; antifibrinolytics vs. fibrinolytics). Only a few of the recommendations have stood the test of time; these are reviewed in the following.

- *Aspirin* use has been reported to increase the rebleeding rate significantly in some,[25–27] but not in other,[28,29] studies. Most clinicians favor avoiding the antiplatelet effect of aspirin and the subsequent prolongation of bleeding time. This may also be an issue for nonsteroidal anti-inflammatory agents.

- *Cycloplegics* may stabilize the blood–aqueous barrier, enhance patient comfort in case of traumatic iritis, and facilitate posterior segment evaluation. However, topical atropine was found not to have any beneficial effect on rebleeding, blood resorption, or vision.[30]

- *Miotics* are generally avoided because of their tendency to exacerbate inflammation and lead to synechia formation.

- *Antifibrinolytic agents* (e.g., aminocaproic acid, tranexamic acid) are used because they are fibrinolytically active and slow the rate of clot lysis.

PEARL... The efficacy of antifibrinolytic agents to reduce rebleeding has been confirmed.[29,31–35] The recommended dosage for aminocaproic acid is 50 mg/kg p. os every 4 hours up to a maximum of 30 g/day, for a total of 5 days.[29] Its use is contraindicated in cases of active intravascular clotting disorders, pregnancy, and certain cardiac, hepatic, and renal diseases.

PITFALL

Side effects include postural hypotension, nausea, and vomiting, which may require discontinuation of the antifibrinolytic agent,[31–35] potentially increasing the risk of rebleeding.[29] Rapid clot dissolution occurs in >30% hyphemas 1–2 days after cessation of aminocaproic acid,[36,c] possibly with a marked IOP elevation and a need for further medical or even surgical intervention.

---

[c]Although it is not FDA approved and is still under investigation, a significant antifibrinolytic effect can be achieved with topical administration of aminocaproic acid.[37–39]

• *Fibrinolytic agents* such as TPA,[40] injected intracamerally, may have a role in stagnant clots. The typical dosage is 10 μg.

• *Corticosteroids* are used topically to counter the associated traumatic iritis and to facilitate comfort. Systemic steroids are favored by some[41,42] but not by others.[13] Prednisone at 40 mg/day in divided doses was in some series effective in reducing the reblooding rate to a level comparable to that achieved with systemic aminocaproic acid.[44] Systemic steroids have serious side effects[45] but are generally well tolerated by the usually young and healthy patient.

Surgical Care   Surgical intervention is required in approximately 5% of eyes.[46] The *traditional indications*[47] included:

• IOP elevation >50 mm Hg for 5 days;

• IOP elevation >35 mm Hg for 7 days to avoid optic nerve damage;

• IOP elevation >25 mm Hg for 5 days in cases of total or near-total hyphema to prevent corneal blood staining; or

• large stagnant clots persisting for ≥10 days to prevent peripheral anterior synechia formation.

Currently, surgical intervention is recommended if:

• the IOP does not respond to intense medical therapy within 24 hours; and

• the patient has sickle cell disease or sickle trait.

The various techniques available are:

• *Paracentesis*[d]/*AC washout for liquid blood* is the simplest and safest method,[48] able to evacuate circulating red blood cells (Fig. 17–3). Advantages include:
   ○ ease of performance;
   ○ repeatability;
   ○ sparing of the conjunctiva for future filtration surgery;
   ○ providing for control of intraoperative bleeding; and
   ○ fast reduction of the IOP at the slit lamp.

Technical modifications such as injecting air[49] instead of irrigation with BBS and use of fibrinolytic agents[50–52] do not appear to offer advantages.

• *Expression and limbal delivery for clotted hyphema* require a large limbal incision and usually a violation of the conjunctiva. The ideal time for limbal expression is day 4–7[6,17] (maximal consolidation and retraction of the clot).[53] Careful manipulations are necessary to avoid damaging the corneal epithelium, iris, and lens. Use of the cryoprobe has been suggested to facilitate clot delivery.[54]

• Bimanual *cutting/aspiration*[e] *for clotted hyphema*, using the vitrectomy probe, is effective in removing

---

[d]Remember that the more peripheral your incision, the more likely that synechiae will form.

[e]Remember that instruments in the AC appear to be higher by 1 mm than they actually are; to be in the desired plane, aim a little higher.

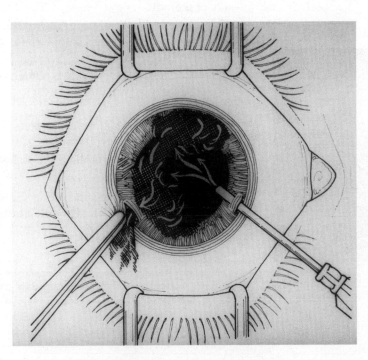

FIGURE 17–3 Paracentesis and AC washout for traumatic hyphema. Simultaneous balanced salt solution irrigation via one paracentesis and depression of posterior top of second paracentesis.

both loose blood cells and the clot,[55] typically through clear corneal incisions. By allowing tight control over intraocular bleeding via simultaneous infusion (e.g., using a needle or an AC maintainer; see later) and intraocular diathermy,[56] this technique offers definite advantages. It also allows anterior segment reconstruction such as lens and vitreous removal.

PITFALL

Vitrectomy techniques for hyphema evacuation in phakic eyes require considerable expertise and experience.

- Other surgical interventions that may become necessary include:
  - peripheral iridectomy and trabeculectomy for glaucoma;
  - peripheral iridectomy without[57] or with[58] trabeculectomy for pupillary block;
  - cyclodiathermy[59]; and
  - ultrasonic emulsification and aspiration.[60]

Complications

Rebleeding (Fig. 17–4) remains one of the greatest concerns following traumatic hyphema because it is associated with a higher complication rate (58%) than eyes that do not suffer rebleeding (22%).[61] The reported rate of rebleeding varies greatly: 3.5–38%.[2–6,12,13,26,29,31,32,34,35,61] The most critical time for rebleeding seems to be 2–5 days after injury when lysis and retraction of the clot occur.

Higher rebleeding rates are associated with:

- large hyphemas[2–5] (not confirmed in all studies);
- young patients;
- black patients;
- Hispanic patients;
- patients taking aspirin; and
- patients presenting more than 24 hours after injury.[2,3,5,29,46]

Glaucoma (see Chapter 20) can be an early or late complication. Approximately 25% of eyes develop acute IOP levels >25 mm Hg and 10% of eyes >35 mm Hg.[5] The acute IOP rise appears to be due to impaired aqueous egress through normal trabecular meshwork pathways because of outflow obstruction by red blood cells, fibrin/platelet aggregates, and degraded cell products. Contusion damage to the trabecular meshwork and inflammation aggravate the problem, as does topical or systemic steroid use.

The treatment of glaucoma following hyphema depends on the level of IOP elevation and whether or not the patient has sickle cell disease. We[f] generally favor initiating medical therapy for an IOP >30 mm Hg in the acute setting and for persistent elevation of IOP >25 mm Hg for 2 weeks or more.[1]

- Topical and oral *aqueous suppressants* are the mainstay of therapy.
- *Alpha agonists* may be appropriate to use, although concern has been raised about their sympathomimetic effect.
- The role of *prostaglandin agonists* remains to be elucidated but it appears that it is best to avoid them in inflamed eyes.
- Oral or intravenous *hyperosmotic agents* are helpful for acute/high IOP elevations.
- *Cycloplegics* in case of pupillary block; laser iridectomy may be needed.

More aggressive therapy, including surgical intervention, is indicated for patients with additional risk

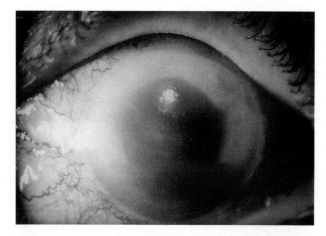

FIGURE 17–4   Rebleeding in patient with traumatic hyphema. Note fresh red blood layered over dark clot.

---

[f]Others favor starting treatment of hyphema patients at lower levels of IOP to avoid the complications caused by even minimal IOP spikes, especially in patients at risk (e.g., sickle cells).

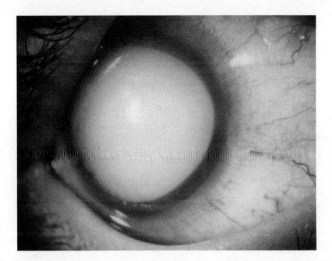

FIGURE 17–5 Corneal blood staining following traumatic hyphema.

(e.g., sickle cell disease, known glaucoma, optic nerve damage) and for eyes with large clots and/or corneal endothelial damage.

Late glaucoma developing weeks to years after the hyphema is generally due to angle recession, ghost cells, or the formation of peripheral anterior synechiae.

Corneal blood staining (Fig. 17–5) occurs in ≤5% of hyphema patients.[5,12,13,62] It is associated with

- larger hyphemas;
- rebleeding;
- prolonged clot duration;
- elevated IOP; and
- compromised endothelial function.[1,63]

> **PEARL...** Corneal blood staining is an indication for early surgical evacuation of the blood if the IOP is elevated because, once present, the staining tends to persist for months, even years. Patients rarely require PK, but those in the appropriate age group may be predisposed to amblyopia (see **Chapter 30**).

Special Issues of Importance

Sickle Cell Disease

Pathophysiology Sickle cell disease represents a unique problem for the ophthalmologist treating

patients with hyphema.[1,19] These cells are poorly tolerated in the AC.

> **PITFALL**
>
> A vicious circle quickly develops because sickle cells are highly resistant to clearance through normal trabecular meshwork pathways. Even with very small hyphemas, significant obstruction of the trabecular meshwork occurs, leading to marked IOP elevation, which causes hypoperfusion of the anterior segment and thus hypoxia, acidosis, and hypercarbia. Each factor in turn exacerbates sickling.

In addition, sickle cells can compromise the optic nerve even at marginally (mid-20 mm Hg) elevated IOP levels, requiring close monitoring and aggressive treatment.

Unique Issues in the Treatment

- More aggressive than usual intervention is required to normalize the IOP.
- *Epinephrine* derivatives should be avoided because of concerns regarding vasoconstriction that may increase hypoxia and vascular sludging.
- *Miotics* may increase inflammation and should be avoided.
- *CAIs* may lead to hemoconcentration, systemic acidosis, elevated ascorbic acid levels, and increase sickling. If systemic CAIs are needed, methylazolamide is theoretically preferable to acetazolamide (reduced acidosis).
- *Hyperosmotic agents*, whether intravenously or orally administered, may lead to hemoconcentration and thus exacerbate sickling.

> **PEARL...** Reduction of the IOP is usually more important than the medicine-associated risks. If medical therapy does not bring the IOP to at least the low 20 mm Hg promptly, we favor surgical intervention.[1,64]

Traumatic Hyphema in Children

The prognosis of hyphema may be worse in those younger than 6 years than in older patients.[65] Using antifibrinolytic agents is not contraindicated in children, and tranexamic acid[65] (unlike aminocaproic acid[66]) has been shown to reduce the rebleeding rate.

Prognosis and Outcome

- >75% of hyphema eyes have >20/50 final vision.[4,5,9,12,13,61]
- Although traditionally reported,[5,13] larger hyphemas do not necessarily have a poorer prognosis.
- Rebleeding is consistently associated with a higher incidence of elevated IOP, blood staining, the need for surgery, and poor final vision. However, vision reduction in patients with hyphema is related more to posterior segment pathology, particularly retinal damage, than to anterior segment problems.

PITFALL

All patients with hyphema, regardless of whether rebleeding occurs, must be considered to be at risk for visual compromise due to retinal damage.[5,12,61]

Controversies and Future Trends

For fear of potentially serious complications, the most widely debated issue is the supplementation of topical drugs with systemic medications to reduce the rebleeding rate.[67] Balancing risks and benefits, we use antifibrinolytic agents or systemic steroids only in those with high risk, such as:

- blacks (rebleeding rate in a predominately white population: 5%[46]; in an urban black population: 33%[29]);
- sickle cell patients[68];
- patients with coagulation abnormalities;
- patients who present >24 hours after injury[46];
- patients with <20/200 initial vision;
- patients with elevated IOP; and
- patients with hyphemas grade II or more.[69]

The Nonophthalmologist's Role

Triage evaluation by the nonophthalmologist is critical,[68] performed via a:

- careful history; and a
- simple penlight examination.

If blood is present in the AC, the patient should be treated as having an open globe injury, until proved otherwise, and requiring:

- shield protection (see Chapter 14); and
- urgent ophthalmologic consultation.

Only supportive care is required in the general ER or at the office:

- pain relief (avoid aspirin);
- activity restriction;
- NPO, should surgery be necessary; and
- elevation of the head.

REMOVAL OF OTHER MATERIALS

Fibrin

The decision tree includes answering the following questions:

- Is it truly fibrin?
- If it is fibrin, does it justify removal?
- If removal is justified, can the original wound be utilized or is a separate incision preferred?
- What is the best instrument for fibrin removal?

It may be difficult to confirm the presence of fibrin in case of a cataractous lens (see Chapter 21), especially if the cornea is not clear. Careful inspection of the iris, provided visibility permits, may help. In case of uncertainty, it may be safer not to attempt removal.

Small amounts of fibrin do not require intervention. Their effect can be neutralized by high doses of corticosteroids and keeping the pupil mobile.[g] Larger fibrin membranes should be removed because they can form pupillary membranes and, by blocking access to the angle, significantly raise the IOP. It is usually not possible to remove all of the fibrin, and occasionally it can reform very rapidly (we have seen fibrinous membranes reappear by the completion of wound closure).

If atraumatic fibrin removal is possible through the original wound, the surgeon may utilize this opening, although it is frequently less traumatic to prepare a paracentesis[h] in the temporal corneal periphery. As a general rule, corneal wounds in the visual axis should not be used because of the potential damage to the endothelium.

In cases of a large wound and a less adherent membrane, the fibrin may be wiped off the iris surface

---

[g] Use of short-acting dilating agents prevents the formation of posterior synechiae in the presence of a dilated pupil.

[h] An oblique needle path creates a valve; IOP elevation makes it even more watertight. However, if the wound is incongruent (as in most trauma cases) or if foreign material is caught in the wound lips (e.g., lens fibrin), leaking is inevitable because the valve cannot function as such.

using cellulose sponges. In other cases, it is best to use fine (e.g., iris) forceps.

> **PEARL...** The vitrectomy probe with its adjustable aspiration rate is very helpful for fibrin removal, but its port must be kept occluded at all times to prevent a sudden collapse of the AC.

Inflammatory Debris

Removal of inflammatory debris (e.g., white blood cells) is relatively easy. It is usually sufficient to irrigate the AC with BSS; occasionally, antibiotics and/or corticosteroids may also be used. Avoid using strong streams to prevent endothelial damage. It is best to use a cannula and introduce it through the original wound. If a needle has to be inserted in the corneal periphery and the eye is soft, try the insertion over the iris (e.g., temporally at 10 o'clock so that the tip of the needle points toward 8 o'clock in *right* eyes) to avoid damaging the lens. An oblique path ensures that it remains watertight.

Vitreous

The eye is a sphere filled with liquid; when subjected to extra pressure (whether it comes from the outside [injuring agent] or from the inside [hemorrhage]), certain intraocular tissues are prone to dislocate. In case of an open wound, fluid (aqueous) and tissues (e.g., uvea) tend to externalize until the IOP and the atmospheric pressure equalize; in closed globe injuries, tissues may dislocate but remain intraocular (e.g., lens in the vitreous).

As a result of open or closed globe trauma, vitreous may be present in the AC; in open globe trauma, the vitreous may also prolapse extraocularly.[70] It is not always easy to identify vitreous in the AC; an air bubble is extremely helpful because it is deformed by the gel.[70] Leaving substantial amounts of vitreous in the AC may lead to serious complications (see also Chapter 16), such as:

- chronic inflammation;
- corneal decompensation;
- iris/pupillary deformity;
- secondary glaucoma;
- vitreous traction on retina; and
- retinal complications such as CME, hemorrhage, tear, and detachment.

Subluxation or dislocation of the lens commonly accompanies the presence of vitreous in the AC in closed globe injuries (see Chapter 21).

Whether or not vitreous removal from the AC is recommended depends on the actual situation (Table 17–3).

The two instruments most commonly used for removal are the cellulose sponge/scissors and the vitrectomy probe (Table 17–4). We strongly advocate the use of the vitrectomy probe; the eye's condition determines whether an anterior or posterior approach is preferred (Table 17–5). In either case, however, it is crucial to maintain control over the IOP via one of the following:

- vitrectomy probe with infusion capability;
- AC maintainer;
- (butterfly) needle in the AC; or
- pars plana infusion.

Air

Air may get into the AC because of the injury or it may be introduced by the surgeon for diagnostic (see earlier) or therapeutic purposes. It is extremely rare, fortunately, but air may also form because of the presence of gas-producing bacteria[71] (see Chapter 8); resulting in a potentially life-threatening infection.

TABLE 17–3 VITREOUS PROLAPSE INTO THE AC

Condition	Recommended Treatment
Open globe injury with extraocular vitreous prolapse	Complete removal of the vitreous from the AC should be performed (see Chapter 16)
Open globe injury without extraocular vitreous prolapse	Complete removal of the vitreous from the AC should be performed
Closed globe injury with most of the AC filled with vitreous	Complete removal of the vitreous is recommended to prevent the development of additional complications (see text)
Closed globe injury with minimal vitreous prolapse into the AC	Removal usually not recommended unless complications occur or surgery is performed for other indications (e.g., lens dislocation); in these cases, remove the vitreous

TABLE 17-4   INSTRUMENTATION FOR THE REMOVAL OF VITREOUS FROM THE AC

	Cellulose Sponge and Scissors	*Vitrectomy Probe*
Advantages	Simple	Atraumatic
	Readily available	IOP under control
	Original wound may be utilized	As much of the vitreous as necessary can be removed
		Additional pathologies may be addressed (e.g., hyphema or lens removal)
Disadvantages	Cannot be used in closed globe injury	Special equipment needed
	Considerable traction on vitreous (and retina)	Expertise necessary, especially if pars plana approach is preferable
	Difficult to maintain and monitor the IOP	
	Complete vitreous removal rarely possible	
	May be traumatic to cornea	

TABLE 17-5   USE OF THE VITRECTOMY PROBE FOR VITREOUS REMOVAL FROM THE AC: DIFFERENT APPROACHES

	Original Wound	*Limbus*	*Pars Plana*
Advantages	New incision unnecessary	Less special training required	Unhindered visibility
	Able to address extra- and intrabulbar vitreous prolapse	Available option even if lens is present	Lens removal is easy to complete
		If lensectomy also performed, greater chance of preserving (posterior) lens capsule for subsequent IOL implantation	Further tissue prolapse/corneal damage easy to prevent by injecting viscoelastics in the AC
			Vitrectomy behind the iris is easy and safe
			Additional manipulations in the posterior segment are possible
Disadvantages	Impossible if wound is too small	Potentially more traumatic to cornea	Expertise in vitreoretinal techniques required
	May be traumatic	IOP control requires an assistant if only a butterfly needle is available	If lensectomy also performed, posterior lens capsule is difficult to preserve
	IOP control requires an assistant if only a butterfly needle is available	Limited potential for complete lens removal	
	Visibility may be hindered	Vitrectomy behind iris plane is difficult and potentially dangerous	

> **PEARL...** Small air bubbles have no useful function in the AC. Their removal is much easier if the surgeon first *injects* additional air so that a large, single bubble forms. Injection of BSS then easily pushes the air out of the AC.

Viscoelastics

Viscoelastics are usually not left behind in the AC because they may substantially raise the IOP.[i]

Injection of BSS is usually sufficient to push the viscoelastic material out through the wound; difficulty arises if the wound is too small. When injecting the fluid, start from as far in the AC as possible.

> **PEARL...** Never apply strong initial force with a fluid for viscoelastic removal because this will *prevent*, rather than facilitate, the viscoelastic material's flow from the eye by increasing its outflow resistance.[72] Air may facilitate removal of the viscoelastic material if BSS is injected first.[73]

[i]One notable exception is silicone oil prolapse in a phakic eye; the viscoelastic is used to prevent further oil prolapse when a silicone oil bubble is removed from the AC (see the Appendix).

REFORMATTING THE AC

Three materials are used for reformatting the AC:

- air;
- BSS; or
- viscoelastics.

Air reduces visibility in the postoperative period and may damage the endothelium; therefore, as a general rule, BSS is the most physiological option. Air's great advantage is that—unless it disappears too early—it can prevent anterior synechiae formation. Viscoelastics can also achieve this goal and maintain it for extended periods of time, but, as mentioned, they may drastically raise the IOP.

It is rarely necessary to measure the IOP when reformatting the AC; simply avoid overfilling. Aqueous formation will quickly restore the normal IOP even if the eye is left somewhat hypotonous.

SUMMARY

The AC is a frequent site of injury, particularly following severe contusion. The most common manifestation of AC structural damage is the presence of hyphema. In most cases, this blood will clear without sequele and the final visual prognosis will be determined by the associated ocular structures injured. The main goal in the management of hyphema is the prevention of rebleeding since this has been associated in some studies with worse outcomes and more ocular complications. In practice, the management of hyphema is quite variable amongst ophthalmologists in this country. However, most do use some combination of topical and/or systemic agents that help stabilize the AC clot and reduce intraocular inflammation. The future availability of a topical antifibrinolytic agent may increase the use of this type of medication in the management of traumatic hyphema.

REFERENCES

1. Shingleton BJ, Hersh PS. Traumatic hyphema. In: Shingleton BJ, Hersh PS, Kenyon KR, eds. *Eye Trauma*. St. Louis: Mosby–Year Book; 1991:104–116.
2. Kennedy RH, Brubaker RF. Traumatic hyphema in a defined population. *Am J Ophthalmol*. 1988;106:123–130.
3. Agapitos PJ, Noel LP, Clarke WN. Traumatic hyphema in children. *Ophthalmology*. 1987;94:1238–1241.
4. Edwards WC, Layden WF. Traumatic hyphema. *Am J Ophthalmol*. 1993;75:110–116.
5. Read J, Goldberg ME. Comparison of medical treatment for traumatic hyphema. *Trans Acad Ophthalmol Otolaryngol*. 1974;78:799–815.
6. Cassell GH, Jeffers JB, Jaeger EA. Wills Eye Hospital traumatic hyphema study. *Ophthalmic Surg*. 1984;16:441–443.
7. Thygeson P, Beard C. Observations on traumatic hyphema. *Am J Ophthalmol*. 1952;35:977–985.
8. Pilger IS. Medical treatment of traumatic hyphema. *Surv Ophthalmol*. 1975;20:28–34.

9. Rakusin W. Traumatic hyphema. *Am J Ophthalmol.* 1972;74:284–292.

10. Collet BI. Traumatic hyphema: a review. *Ann Ophthalmol.* 1982;14:52–56.

11. Schein OD, Hibberd PL, Shingleton BJ, et al. The spectrum and burden of ocular injury. *Ophthalmology.* 1988; 95:300–305.

12. Read J. Traumatic. hyphema: surgical vs medical management. *Ann Ophthalmol.* 1975;7:659–670.

13. Wilson FM. Traumatic hyphema: pathogenesis and management. *Ophthalmology.* 1980;87:910–919.

14. Wolfe SM, Zimmerman LE. Chronic secondary glaucoma associated with retrodisplacement of iris root and deepening of the AC angle secondary to contusion. *Am J Ophthalmol.* 1962;64:547–563.

15. Campbell DG. Traumatic glaucoma. In: Shingleton BJ, Hersh PS, Kenyon KR, eds. *Eye Trauma.* St. Louis: Mosby–Year Book; 1991:112–125.

16. Caprioli J, Sears ML. The histopathology of black ball hyphema: a report of two cases. *Ophthalmic Surg.* 1986; 15:491–495.

17. Wolter JR, Henderson JW, Talley TW. Histopathology of a black ball clot around four days after total hyphema. *J Pediatr Ophthalmol Strabismus.* 1971;8:15–17.

18. Pandolfi M, Nilsson IM, Martinsson G. Coagulation and fibrinolytic components in primary and plasmoid aqueous humor of rabbit. *Acta Ophthalmol.* 1964;42:820–825.

19. Goldberg MF. Sickled erythrocytes, hyphema and secondary glaucoma. *Ophthalmic Surg.* 1979;10:17–31.

20. Clever VG. Home care of hyphemas. *Ann Ophthalmol.* 1982;14:25–27.

21. Witteman GJ, Brubaker SJ, Johnson M, et al. The incidence of rebleeding in traumatic hyphema. *Ann Ophthalmol.* 1985;17:525–529.

22. Darr JL, Passmore JW. Management of traumatic hyphema. *Am J Ophthalmol.* 1967;63:134–136.

23. Wright KW, Sunal PM, Urrea P. Bedrest versus activity ad lib in the treatment of small hyphemas. *Ann Ophthalmol.* 1988;20:143–145.

24. Edwards WC, Layden WF. Monocular versus bilateral patching in traumatic hyphema. *Am J Ophthalmol.* 1973; 76:359–362.

25. Crawford JS. The effect of aspirin on rebleeding in traumatic hyphema. *Trans Am Ophthalmol Soc.* 1975;73:357–362.

26. Gorn RA. The detrimental effect of aspirin on hyphema rebleed. *Ann Ophthalmol.* 1979;11:351–355.

27. Ganley JP, Geiger JM, Clement JR, et al. Aspirin and recurrent hyphema after blunt ocular trauma. *Am J Ophthalmol.* 1983;96:797–801.

28. Marcus M, Biedner B, Lifshitz T, et al. Aspirin and secondary bleeding after traumatic hyphema. *Ann Ophthalmol.* 1988;20:157–158.

29. Palmer DJ, Goldberg MF, Frenkel M, et al. A comparison of two dose regimens of epsilon aminocaproic acid in the prevention and management of secondary traumatic hyphemas. *Ophthalmology.* 1986;93:102–108.

30. Gilbert HD, Jensen AD. Atropine in the treatment of traumatic hyphema. *Ann Ophthalmol.* 1973;5:1297–1300.

31. Crouch ER, Frenkel R. Aminocaproic acid in the treatment of traumatic hyphema. *Am J Ophthalmol.* 1976; 81:355–360.

32. McGetrick JJ, Jampol LM, Goldberg MF, et al. Aminocaproic acid decreases secondary hemorrhage after traumatic hyphema. *Arch Ophthalmol.* 1983;101: 1031–1033.

33. Kutner B, Fourman S, Brein K, et al. Aminocaproic acid reduces the risk of secondary hemorrhage in patients with traumatic hyphema. *Arch Ophthalmol.* 1987;105: 206–208.

34. Varnek L, Dalsgaard C, Hansen A, et al. The effect of tranexamic acid on secondary hemorrhage after traumatic hyphema. *Acta Ophthalmol.* 1980;58:787–792.

35. Vangsted P, Nielsen PJ. Tranexamic acid and traumatic hyphema. *Acta Ophthalmol.* 1983;61:447–453.

36. Dieste MC, Hersh PS, Kylstra JA, et al. Intraocular pressure increase associated with epsilon-aminocaproic acid therapy for traumatic hyphema. *Am J Ophthalmol.* 1988;106:383–390.

37. Crouch ER Jr, Williams PB, Gray MK, Crouch ER, Chames M. Topical aminocaproic acid in the treatment of traumatic hyphema. *Arch Ophthalmol.* 1997;115: 1106–1112.

38. Allingham RR, Williams PB, Crouch ER Jr, et al. Topically applied aminocaproic acid concentrates in the aqueous humor of the rabbit in therapeutic levels. *Arch Ophthalmol.* 1987;105:1421–1423.

39. Allingham RR, Crouch ER Jr, Williams PB, et al. Topical aminocaproic acid significantly reduces the incidence of secondary hemorrhage in traumatic hyphema in the rabbit model. *Arch Ophthalmol.* 1988;106: 1436–1438.

40. Lambrou FH, Snyder RW, Williams GA. Use of tissue plasminogen activator in experimental hyphema. *Arch Ophthalmol.* 1987;105:995–997.

41. Yasuna E. Management of traumatic hyphema. *Arch Ophthalmol.* 1974;91:190–191.

42. Rynne MV, Romano PE. Systemic corticosteroids in the treatment of traumatic hyphema. *J Pediatr Ophthalmol Strabismus.* 1980;17:141–143.

43. Spoor TC, Hammer M, Belloso H. Traumatic hyphema. Failure of steroids to alter its course: a double-blind prospective study. *Arch Ophthalmol.* 1980;98: 116–119.

44. Farber MD, Fiscellar, Goldberg MF. Aminocaproic acid versus prednisone for the treatment of traumatic hyphema. *Ophthalmology.* 1991;98:279–286.

45. Fujikawa LS, Meisler DM, Nozik LA. Hyperosmolar hyperglycemic nonketotic coma: a complication of short-term systemic corticosteroid use. *Ophthalmology.* 1983;90:1239–1242.

46. Volpe NJ, Larrison WI, Hersh PT, Kim T, Shingleton BJ. Secondary hemorrhage in traumatic hyphema. *Am J Ophthalmol.* 1991;112:507–513.

47. Deutsch TA, Feller DB. *Paton and Goldberg's Management of Ocular Injuries.* 2nd ed. Philadelphia: WB Saunders; 1985.

48. Belcher CD, Brown SVL, Simmons RJ. AC washout for traumatic hyphema. *Ophthalmic Surg.* 1985,16:475–479.

49. Wilson JM, et al. Air injection in the treatment of traumatic hyphema. *Am J Ophthalmol.* 1954;37:409–411.

50. Jukofsky SL. A new technique in the treatment of hyphema. *Am J Ophthalmol.* 1951;34:1692–1696.

51. Scheie HG, Ashley BJ, Burns DT. Treatment of total hyphema with fibrinolysin. *Arch Ophthalmol.* 1963;69:147–153.

52. Liebman SD, Pollen A, Podos SM. Treatment of experimental total hyphema with intraocular fibrinolytic agents. *Arch Ophthalmol.* 1962;68:72–78.

53. Sears ML. Surgical management of black ball hyphema. *Trans Am Acad Ophthalmol Otolaryngol.* 1970;74:820–827.

54. Hill K. Cryoextraction of total hyphema. *Arch Ophthalmol.* 1968;80:368–370.

55. McCuen BW, Fung WE. The role of vitrectomy instrumentation in the treatment of severe traumatic hyphema. *Am J Ophthalmol.* 1979;88:930–934.

56. Michels RG, Rice TA. Bimanual bipolar diathermy for treatment of bleeding from the AC angle. *Am J Ophthalmol.* 1977;84:873–874.

57. Parrish RK, Bernardino V. Iridectomy in the surgical management of eight ball hyphema. *Arch Ophthalmol.* 1982;100:435–437.

58. Weiss JS, Parrish RK, Anderson DR. Surgical therapy of traumatic hyphema. *Ophthalmic Surg.* 1983;14:343–345.

59. Gilbert HD, Smith RE. Traumatic hyphema: treatment of secondary hemorrhage with cyclodiathermy. *Ophthalmic Surg.* 1975;7:31–35.

60. Kelman CD, Brooks DL. Ultrasonic emulsification and aspiration of traumatic hyphema. A preliminary report. *Am J Ophthalmol.* 1971;71:1289–1291.

61. Thomas MA, Parrish RK, Feuer WJ. Rebleeding after traumatic hyphema. *Arch Ophthalmol.* 1986;104:206–210.

62. McDonnell PJ, Green WR, Stevens RE, et al. Blood staining of the cornea. Light microscopic and ultrastructural features. *Ophthalmology.* 1985;92:1668–1674.

63. Slingsby JG, Forstot SL. Effect of blunt trauma on the corneal endothelium. *Arch Ophthalmol.* 1981;99:1041–1043.

64. Deutsch TA, Weinreb RN, Goldberg MF. Indications for surgical management of hyphema in patients with sickle cell trait. *Arch Ophthalmol.* 1984;102:566–569.

65. Uusitalo RJ, Ranta-Kemppainen L, Tarkkanen A. Management of traumatic hyphema in children. *Arch Ophthalmol.* 1988;106:1207–1209.

66. Kraft SP, Christianson MD, Crawford JS, et al. Traumatic hyphema in children. Treatment with epsilon-aminocaproic acid. *Ophthalmology.* 1987;94:1232–1237.

67. Fong LP. Secondary hemorrhage in traumatic hyphema. *Ophthalmology.* 1994;101:1583–1588.

68. Nagrullah A, Kerr NC. Sickle cell trait as a risk factor for secondary hemorrhage in children with traumatic hyphema. *Am J Ophthalmol.* 1997;123:783–790.

69. Shingleton BJ, Mead MD. *Handbook of Eye Emergencies.* Thorofare, NJ: Slack; 1998.

70. Kuhn F, Mester V. Anterior globe injuries with vitreous prolapse and/or incarceration. In: Stirpe M, ed. *Anterior and Posterior Segment Surgery: Mutual Problems and Common Interests.* New York: Ophthalmic Communications Society; 1998:252–257.

71. Bhargava S, Chopdar A. Gas gangrene panophthalmitis. *Br J Ophthalmol.* 1971;55:136–138.

72. Eisner G. *Eye Surgery.* Berlin: Springer-Verlag; 1990:14.

73. Eisner G. *Eye Surgery.* Berlin: Springer-Verlag; 1990:47.

Chapter 18

IRIS

Bernd Kirchhof

 Injuries of the iris compromise its function as an optical aperture and a mechanical barrier between the AC and the posterior chamber/vitreous. The iris base, along with the ciliary body and angle, is especially sensitive to the shear stress caused by contusion. In open globe injuries, even total aniridia due to actual iris extrusion or subsequent iris retraction may occur.[1,2] Discussed separately below are the five major consequences of trauma to the iris:

1. mydriasis;
2. iatrogenic iris laceration;
3. prolapse;
4. iridiodialysis; and
5. aniridia.

MYDRIASIS

Pathophysiology

Mydriasis (see Tables 18–1 and 18–2) may be an immediate or late complication of contusion or laceration; it can also occur as a result of head trauma. Mydriasis may present early or late and may be uni- or bilateral. There are various causes of pupil dilatation.

- *Sphincter rupture/laceration* has been reported from rare sources (water jets, water balloons[19,20]) and accompanies cataract surgery in 1.3[21] to 2.3%[22] of eyes. It is irreversible, and secondary scarring further restricts pupil motility.

TABLE 18–1 DIFFERENTIAL DIAGNOSIS OF MYDRIASIS: ETIOLOGY UNRELATED TO TRAUMA

Iatrogenic pharmacological: scopolamine patches[3,4]

Nightshade[5]

Aniridia

Lack of cholinergic sensitivity

Aplasia of the pupillary sphincter and ciliary muscle[6,7]

Congenital[8]

Coloboma[9] (typical location: inferonasal)

Migraine[10,11]

Siderosis[12] (see Chapter 24)

Dysgenital disorders (progressive)

Iridocorneal endothelial syndrome (iris nevus [Cogan-Reese] syndrome, Chandler's syndrome, essential progressive iris atrophy[13]) with pain secondary to corneal edema or secondary angle closure glaucoma

TABLE 18–2 UNI- VERSUS BILATERAL CAUSES OF MYDRIASIS AFTER SEVERE EYE TRAUMA
AND HEAD INJURY

	Early	*Late*
Anisocoria	Sphincter rupture[14]	Anterior PVR[15,16]
	Ischemia/compression of the third cranial nerve	Siderosis[12]
	Iatrogenic pharmacological mydriasis	Aberrant cranial nerve regeneration[17,18]
Bilateral	Ischemia/compression of the third cranial nerve	
	Optic nerve injury[19]	
	Iatrogenic pharmacological mydriasis	

- *Third cranial nerve injury* may result from uncal herniation causing mechanical compression of the third nerve and subsequent brain stem compromise. A decrease in the brain stem blood flow is another frequent cause.[23]

- *Aberrant cranial nerve regeneration* can follow severe head trauma, even if the eye is uninjured. The pupil does not react to light or near but correlates with horizontal gaze. Constriction of the pupil reflects misdirected regeneration of abducens nerve neurons into the parasympathetic pathway of the oculomotor nerve.

- *Anterior PVR* involves fibrovascular membranes connecting the peripheral retina, ciliary body, and the peripheral iris. Membrane contraction and collagen deposition lead to iris retraction (see Chapter 19 and the Appendix).

> **PEARL...** It is difficult to free the iris from scar tissue during secondary reconstruction. A thorough primary anterior vitrectomy is much more effective in avoiding iris retraction and anterior PVR in combined anterior/posterior segment injury.

Therapy

If glare and visual deterioration persist, surgical reconstruction should be considered.

- *A single suture* (Fig. 18–1) constricts the pupil by apposing the sphincter muscle and pupillary margin to each other.[24]

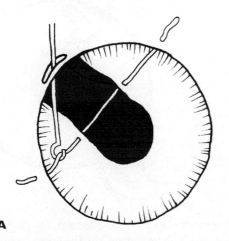
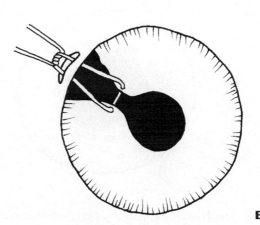

A   **B**

FIGURE 18-1 **(A and B)** Single iris suture **(A)**. A 9-0 Prolene suture is passed through the limbus and through the iris in line with the proposed suture tract. A bonds hook is introduced through a paracentesis and the two suture ends are drawn out through the wound. **(B)** A triple throw knot is placed externally and is pulled together with the iris into the corneal wound. The suture ends are cut externally and close to the knot. The sutured iris is pushed back into the AC.

- *A running suture* (Fig. 18–2) distributes the forces to the pupillary margin more evenly,[25] acting as an "encircling band." Surgical steps include:

  ○ limbal paracentesis in each quadrant;
  ○ loosening of posterior synechiae and mobilizing all iris remnants;

  ○ weaving of a transchamber needle through the iris margin in each quadrant;
  ○ continuing until the suture is passed through the pupillary margin in all quadrants;
  ○ exiting through the first paracentesis and preparing a knot; and
  ○ tightening the knot inside the AC.

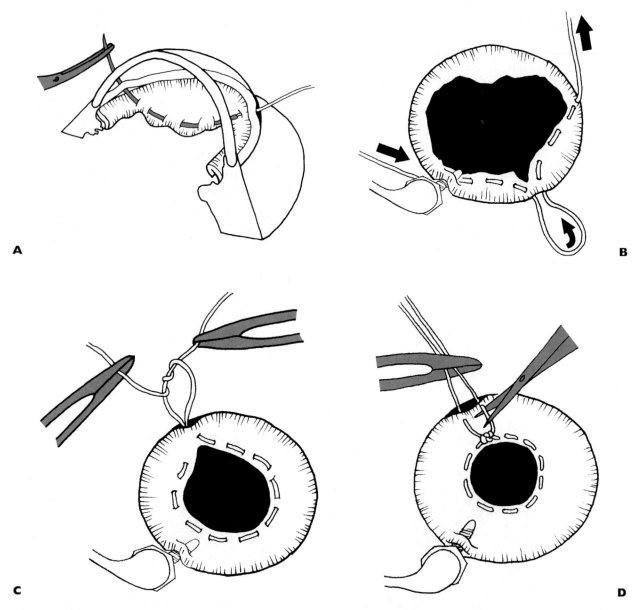

A   **B**   **C**   **D**

FIGURE 18–2   **(A–D)** Iris running suture. **(A)** One limbal paracentesis is placed in each quadrant. The AC is entered with a long, spatula-type, curved transchamber needle, double armed on 10-0 polypropylene. **(B)** The needle is passed through the iris margin weaving the suture through. After weaving through the iris margin about three to four times, the needle is pulled out through the next paracentesis without damaging the cornea. The needle is then grasped in the same fashion and reentered into the eye through the same incision, and weaving is continued toward the next paracentesis. **(C)** After exit through the last paracentesis, the knot is tied together, brought into the eye with a hook, and tightened. **(D)** Following tightening the cerclage suture, the knot is completed and the suture ends cut.

IATROGENIC IRIS LACERATION

This may occur during phacoemulsification, usually while sculpting anteriorly if the critical distance between the phaco tip and the iris is not maintained. Additional risk factors include atonia/atrophy of the iris, miosis, and high flow. The pigment epithelium or even the stroma may be injured. The consequences include:

- cosmetic problems;
- visual symptoms and peripheral synechia development due to deep sphincterectomy that tend to enlarge with time;
- iridodialysis[26]; or even
- complete aniridia.[a]

Therapy[b]

The need for and type of intervention depend on the lesion. A simple laceration may easily be sutured (McCannel method, see later in this Chapter) using a straight transchamber needle introduced at the limbus through the two iris flaps and out through the limbus on the other side. The needle is cut, and the suture is retrieved through a paracentesis, tightened, and released back into the AC.

PROLAPSE (SEE ALSO CHAPTER 16)

The consequences of prolapse include:

- adhesion to the corneal wound;
- intraocular infection;
- ischemia/necrosis/atrophy;
- goniosynechia and secondary glaucoma (with prolapses at or near the limbus);
- surface epithelization (this starts immediately following the injury,[27–29] although epithelial downgrowth into the AC, which can be modulated,[30] is rare); and
- monocular diplopia (likely to occur when an area of extensive iris resection with an intact pupillary margin is exposed to the palpebral fissure; usually requires suturing).

Therapy

Reposition early to prevent intraocular infection[31]; in addition to spatula sweeping from the AC, use viscoelastics (see Chapter 16).[32] A peripheral iridectomy is

advised whenever it is impossible to reposition the iris and to free the angle.

> **PEARL...** Necrosis and surface epithelization are indications for iris resection. This causes less complications than preserving poorly repositioned and nonviable iris tissue. The resulting defect can usually be sutured.[24,33]

IRIDODIALYSIS

Pathophysiology

Iridodialysis represents a rupture of the iris at its root: the peripheral portion is torn off the ciliary spur. It is typically a consequence of contusion, stretching the iris at and from its insertion. The complaints (glare, monocular double vision) depend on the size of the defect and its position relative to the lid fissure.

Treatment

The most widely used technique is based on the principles of the McCannel[34,35] suture. A scleral incision is prepared as a fixation site. Using a double-armed straight transchamber polypropylene suture, the torn iris is brought out through the incision so that one loop is in front of the iris and the other underneath it (Fig. 18–3). The knot is either internalized or buried by a scleral flap. For a large iridodialysis, two or more sutures may be required. Complications of the procedure include:

- epithelial downgrowth with secondary glaucoma[36]; and
- late suture erosion in eyes with less resistant sclera (e.g., children or high myopia)—this can be prevented by use of a scleral tunnel incision.[37]

ANIRIDIA

Pathophysiology

See Table 18–3 for differential diagnosis.

Complete loss of the iris may occur in ruptured eyes with wounds near the limbus.[1,2] Structural weakness in this region (e.g., Elliot's trepanation,[39] ICCE and ECCE incisions, or, to a lesser extent, corneoscleral tunnel incisions[40]) is a risk factor (see Chapter 27).

Treatment

Aniridia results in serious subjective and objective consequences and should be addressed.

---

[a]W. Konen, personal communication, 2000.

[b]The treatment is the same if the laceration is caused by noniatrogenic trauma.

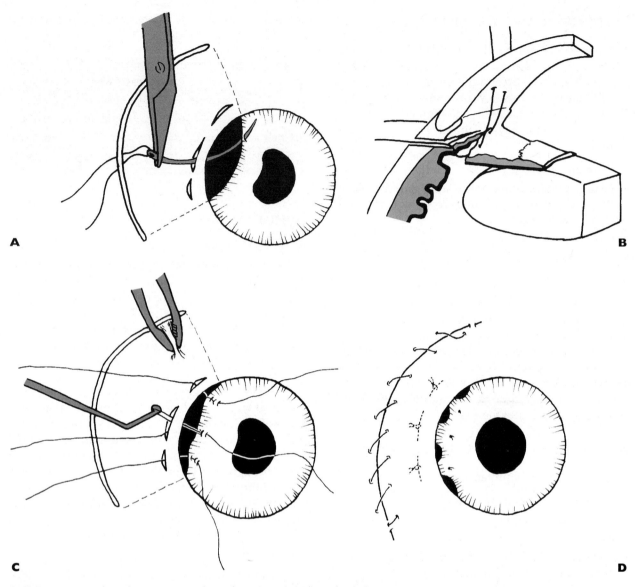

FIGURE 18–3 **(A–D)** Jameson-McCannel sutures. **(A)** Three limbal paracenteses are placed. The suture needle passes through the lower rim of the scleral paracentesis into the PC and through the iris root. The needle leaves the AC through the peripheral cornea. **(B)** Cross-section of the anterior segment of the eye showing the needle track across sclera, iris, and cornea. **(C)** A hook draws the free end of the sutures back and out through the paracentesis wound. **(D)** The three sutures pull the iris root to its original insertion. The knots are buried within the paracentesis. Each paracentesis is sutured.

TABLE 18–3   DIFFERENTIAL DIAGNOSIS OF ANIRIDIA

	Bilateral Congenital	*Unilateral Traumatic*
Visual disturbances	Foveal aplasia	Glare and light scatter
	Associated pendular nystagmus	
	Photophobia	
Glaucoma	Angle closure secondary to posterior synechia formation	Damage to ciliary body and zonules
	Dysgenesis of trabecular meshwork[38]	Ghost cell
		Angle recession (if exceeding 180°)

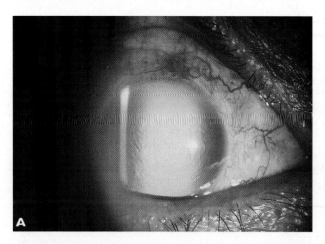 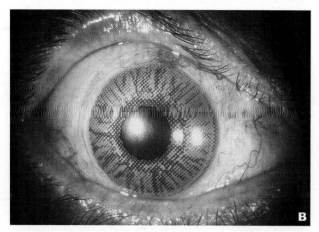

FIGURE 18–4 **(A)** Aniridia as a result of severe contusion injury. **(B)** Iris print contact lens with good cosmesis. (Courtesy of R. Morris, MD, and F. Kuhn, MD.)

> **PEARL...** Several options are available for patients with aniridia to fight the cosmetic and optical consequences. Implants[41,42] have the advantage of maintaining two ocular compartments.

Iris print contact lenses (e.g., Hema contact lens) give the appearance of iris tissue. They are also helpful for albinism, iris coloboma, essential iris atrophy, and leukoma corneae.[43] These lenses (Fig. 18–4) diminish glare but may also reduce visual acuity and contrast sensitivity[44] and are therefore most useful in blind eyes.

Corneal tattooing is cost-effective and involves localized staining of the corneal stroma, corresponding to the iris defects. Originally described for leukoma, it has recently been proposed for iris defects.[45–47] Different techniques are available.

- Lamellar corneal preparation is created at 50% depth of the stroma, from
  - limbal incisions[45] or from a
  - central half-depth 4-mm trephination[46] (this is especially suitable for complete aniridia, when complete staining is required).
- For smaller iris defects (Fig. 18–5), the pigment is applied in a punctuated fashion.[47]

The pigment used for skin tattooing seems to be sufficiently inert for intracorneal application. It is usually possible to achieve the desired color because the pigment is available in different shades. Side effects such as inflammation, epithelial irregularities, or stromal vascularization have not yet been noted.

> **PITFALL**
>
> Long-term results for pigment stability and tolerance by the corneal stroma are unavailable. Currently, corneal tattooing is best recommended for cosmesis in blind eyes.

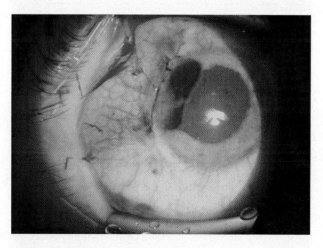

FIGURE 18–5 Corneal tattoo of about three clock hours. The dye is based on candle soot. Its black color contrasts with the light blue iris color. Soot particles are appropriate for dark irises.

TABLE 18–4   INDICATIONS FOR AND TYPES OF OPTICAL IRIS DIAPHRAGMS*

	Coloboma or Small Defects	Aniridia
Capsular tension rings as artificial iris diaphragm	Black PMMA, Morcher, Germany Type 96G, 2.5 mm width, covers 90°	Black PMMA, Type 50C,[†] seven diaphragms at 46.5° (1.5 × 2 mm); green, brown, or blue PMMA,[‡] a central ring defines the size of the artificial pupil; two other rings are fixed onto this ring, each containing several centrifugally oriented small diaphragms
Intraocular lens as artificial iris diaphragm		Black PMMA periphery and haptic; variable size of the clear optical zone (2.5–5 mm),[†] Type 67a-s and Type 94[48,49]; frosted iris lens[50]

*Most of these devices lack FDA approval.
[†]Morcher, Germany.
[‡]Ophtec, Netherlands.

Stained intraocular optical diaphragms (see Table 18–4) are implanted during or after cataract extraction.[51] If attached to a capsular tension ring, an intact capsular bag is required. In eyes without (firm) capsular bags, transscleral fixation of a stained IOL is recommended. Because of the size and the stiffness of such PMMA devices, 180° corneoscleral incisions are required. Chronic low-grade inflammation may ensue.

> **PEARL...**   In phakic eyes with aniridia, the surgeon may perform lens removal with an atypically large capsulorrhexis, followed by IOL implantation. If the rim of the lens capsule attaches to the IOL's equator, subsequent capsular fibrosis will opacify the peripheral capsular bag and will at least cosmetically imitate *light* iris tissue.

Clear intraocular mechanical (Heimann) diaphragms (see Tables 18–5 and 18–6) were designed because severely injured eyes commonly need permanent sili-

TABLE 18–5   SPECIFICATIONS OF THE HEIMANN DIAPHRAGMS*

Open	PMMA, transparent, stiff, inferior indentation simulating an Ando iridectomy[52] (Fig. 18–6). A slot on both sides allowed for attachment of sutures. Diameters from 9 to 13 mm, thickness 0.35 mm. Optimal diameter: 2 mm larger than the horizontal corneal diameter.
Closed	Highly purified silicone coutchouc, transparent, flexible (Fig. 18–7). Diameters from 9.5 to 14 mm, thickness 0.4 mm.

*Acritec, Glienicke, Germany.

cone oil tamponade (see the Appendix) to fight aqueous production insufficiency and eventual phthisis.[41,42,53] These eyes are usually aphakic and have a compromised iris; the artificial iris diaphragm prevents corneal touch by the silicone oil and thus band keratopathy. Two types of diaphragm are available:

1. The *open* (stiff) diaphragm is designed for eyes with normal IOP. Success (i.e., silicone oil retained behind the diaphragm) has been reported in 40% of eyes during a mean follow-up of 579 days.[41,42] Causes of failure include:
   - closure of the Ando iridectomy (35%);
   - tractional retinal redetachment (5%); and
   - permanent ocular hypotony (25%).

TABLE 18–6   TECHNIQUE OF IMPLANTATION OF THE CLOSED TYPE OF HEIMANN DIAPHRAGM

Vitrectomy with membrane peeling if necessary

PFCL to reattach the retina and stabilize the eye

Sclerotomies 4 mm from the limbus to keep the instruments clear from the position of the later diaphragm near the ciliary sulcus

Four scleral flaps 2 mm posterior to the limbus to cover the fixation sutures subsequently

A clear corneal incision or a corneoscleral tunnel in the superior circumference

Four sutures attached to the diaphragm at the same distance from each other (looped 9-0 Prolene with 15-mm-long needles*)

The two inferior sutures, then the diaphragm itself, then the two superior sutures placed into the eye. The diaphragm can be folded to narrow the size of the tunnel

AC stabilized by viscoelastic

PFCL–silicone oil exchange and IOP normalization (Fig. 18–8)

*Ethicon, Norderstedt, Germany.

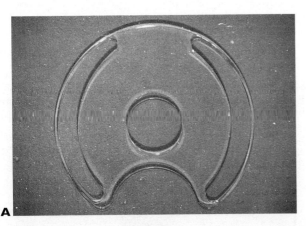
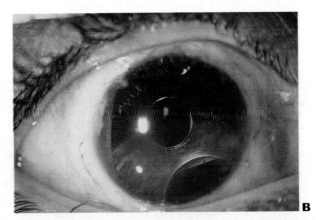

FIGURE 18–6 **(A)** Iris diaphragm, open type. The diaphragm imitates the natural iris by a central "pupil" complemented by an inferior indentation functioning as an Ando iridectomy. The implant is made of transparent, unstained PMMA. A slot on both sides allows attachment of sutures. **(B)** Near-complete aniridia with implanted open-type iris diaphragm. The "inferior iridectomy" is somewhat tilted to 5 o'clock.

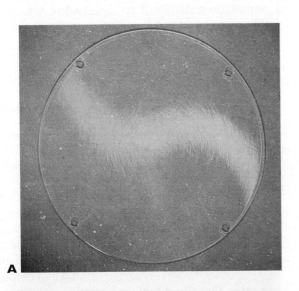

FIGURE 18–7 **(A)** Iris diaphragm, closed type. The diaphragm consists of a flexible round plate of silicone coutchouc. Four holes near the rim allow the attachment of sutures. Partial aniridia with closed iris diaphragm implanted. The diaphragm can hardly be discerned from the silicone oil. **(B)** Implanted diaphragm shown by retroillumination. **(C)** A silicone bubble is spreading on the diaphragm's anterior surface between 11 and 1 o'clock.

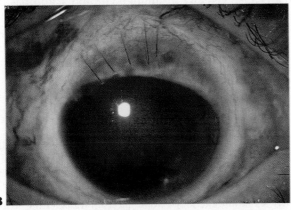
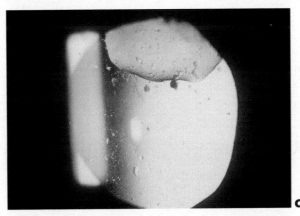

2. The *closed* (flexible) diaphragm is designed for eyes with low IOP, whether from primary damage to the ciliary body or from secondary fibrous overgrowth (PVR, uveitis, endophthalmitis, advanced proliferative diabetic retinopathy).[42,54] It may be used, however, in eyes with normal IOP because the aqueous does tend to penetrate the barrier.

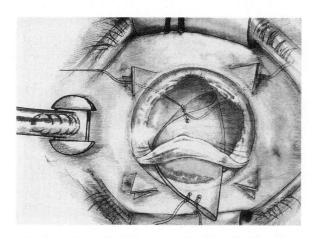

FIGURE 18-8 Implantation of a flexible closed iris diaphragm through a clear corneal incision with four fixation sutures.

PEARL... Today we implant only the closed diaphragm; the success rate is 50%. In addition, although the IOP is below 10 mm Hg in 75% of eyes, the silicone oil prevented or delayed phthisis in two thirds of cases.

PEARL... Diaphragm implantation in trauma-related aniridia must be performed at the time of secondary reconstruction to prevent fibrous overgrowth of the implant.

Failure to retain the silicone oil behind the closed diaphragm is independent of the IOP. The reason for failure is commonly (46%) unknown; a valve mechanism may develop from unavoidable gaps between the diaphragm and the eyewall, with clefts inevitably developing between them as a result of traumatic scars. Finally, the diaphragm may be of inadequate size or outside the ciliary sulcus.

Wrapping or stretching must be avoided by accurate intraoperative fitting. The four scleral fixations must closely correspond to the holes of the implant. When silicone oil moves anteriorly despite more than two revisions, further revisions do not appear to be effective.

P I T F A L L

Because silicone oil and the silicone diaphragm have the same refractive index, it is sometimes difficult to determine whether there is oil in the AC. An abnormal glistening reflex from the anterior surface of the iris and a lack of fluorescein penetration into the AC indicate the presence of silicone oil in the AC.

Summary

Damage to the iris is a common manifestation of severe open and closed globe injuries. In most cases, the damage to the iris is without major consequences other than that its presence should alarm the clinician to the possibility of damage to other ocular structures. In some cases, however, partial or total loss of the iris can cause visually disabling symptoms, and has the potential of causing secondary complications if silicone oil use is required. For such eyes various surgical treatments are available typically requiring referral to a specialist.

References

1. Rossa V, Sundmacher R. Kontusionsinduzierte traumatische Aniridie. *Klin Monatsbl Augenheilkd.* 1991;199: 444–445.
2. Conrads H, Dakkak H. Komplette Aniridie. Ein Problem bei Bulbusruptur. *Klin Monatsbl Augenheilkd.* 1981; 178:377–378.
3. Rosen NB. Accidental mydriasis from scopolamine patches. *J Am Optom Assoc.* 1986;57:541–542.
4. Chiaramonte JS. Cycloplegia from transdermal scopolamine. *N Engl J Med.* 1982;306:174.
5. Rubinfeld RS, Currie JN. Accidental mydriasis from blue nightshade "lipstick". *J Clin Neuroophthalmol.* 1987;7:34–37.

6. Graf M. Bilateral congenital mydriasis with accommodation failure. *Ophthalmologe*. 1996;93:377–379.

7. Richardson P, Schulenburg WE. Bilateral congenital mydriasis. *Br J Ophthalmol*. 1992;76:632–633.

8. Suzuki T, Obara Y, Fujita T, Shoji E. Unilateral congenital mydriasis. *Br J Ophthalmol*. 1994;78:420.

9. Pagon RA. Ocular coloboma. *Surv Ophthalmol*. 1981;25:223–236.

10. Van Engelen BG, Renier WO, Gabreels FJ, Cruysberg HR. Bilateral episodic mydriasis as a migraine equivalent in childhood: a case. *Headache*. 1991;31:375–377.

11. Sarkies NJ, Sanders MD, Gautier-Smith PC. Episodic unilateral mydriasis and migraine. *Am J Ophthalmol*. 1985;99:217–218.

12. Monteiro ML, Coppeto JR, Milani JA. Iron mydriasis. Pupillary paresis from occult intraocular foreign body. *J Clin Neuroophthalmol*. 1993;13:254–257.

13. Yanoff M. In discussion of Shields MB, McCracken JS, Klintworth GK, Campbell DG. Corneal edema in essential iris atrophy. *Ophthalmology*. 1979;86:1549–1555.

14. Landau D, Berson D. High-pressure directed water jets as a cause of severe bilateral intraocular injuries. *Am J Ophthalmol*. 1995;120:542–543.

15. Elner SG, Elner VM, Diaz-Rohena R, Freeman HM, Tolentino FI, Albert DM. Anterior proliferative vitreoretinopathy. Clinicopathologic, light microscopic, and ultrastructural findings. *Ophthalmology*. 1988;95:1349–1357.

16. Stefani FH. Phthisis bulbi—an intraocular fluoride proliferative reaction. *Dev Ophthalmol*. 1985;10:78–160.

17. Sebag J, Sadun AA. Aberrant regeneration of the third nerve following orbital trauma. Synkinesis of the iris sphincter. *Arch Neurol*. 1983;40:762–764.

18. Pfeiffer N, Simonsz HJ, Kommerell G. Misdirected regeneration of abducens nerve neurons into the parasympathetic pupillary pathway. *Graefes Arch Clin Exp Ophthalmol*. 1992;230:150–153.

19. Michiels J, Waterschoot MP. Optic nerve tract injuries. *J Fr Ophtalmol*. 1982;5:273–281.

20. Bullock JD, Ballal DR, Johnson DA, Bullock RJ. Ocular and orbital trauma from water balloon slingshots. A clinical, epidemiologic, and experimental study. *Ophthalmology*. 1997;104:878–887.

21. Teodoru A. Intraoperative complications in extracapsular extraction with a posterior-chamber lens implant. Medical record data. *Oftalmologia*. 1996;40:307–311.

22. Wollensak J, Pham DT, Kraffel U. Intraoperative complications in cataract surgery. A prospective study. *Ophthalmologe*. 1992;89:274–277.

23. Ritter AM, Muizelaar JP, Barnes T, et al. Brain stem blood flow, pupillary response, and outcome in patients with severe head injuries. *Neurosurgery*. 1999;44:941–948.

24. Shin DH. Repair of sector iris coloboma. *Arch Ophthalmol*. 1982;100:460–461.

25. Ogawa GS. The iris cerclage suture for permanent mydriasis: a running suture technique. *Ophthalmic Surg Lasers*. 1998;29:1001–1009. Published erratum appears in *Ophthalmic Surg Lasers*. 1999;30:412.

26. Oshika T, Amano S, Kato S. Severe iridodialysis from phacoemulsification tip suction. *J Cataract Refract Surg*. 1999;25:873–875.

27. Härting F, Jochheim A. Perforierende Verletzung mit Irisprolaps. Ein Beitrag zur Frage der Resektion oder Reposition. *Fortschr Ophthalmol*. 1984;81:40–42.

28. Riedel K, Stefani FH, Jehle P. Der posttraumatische Irisprolaps und seine Bedeutung für das intraokulare Epithelwachstum. *Fortschr Ophthalmol*. 1984;81:46–49.

29. Stefani FH. Irisprolaps: Abtragen oder Rücklagern? Zur intraoperativen Prophylaxe der Epithelimplantation. *Fortschr Ophthalmol*. 1984;81:43–45.

30. Yanoff M, Cameron JD. Human cornea organ cultures. Epithelial endothelial interactions. *Invest Ophthalmol*. 1977;16:269–273.

31. Orlin SE, Farber MG, Brucker AJ, Frayer WC. The unexpected guest: problem of iris reposition. *Surv Ophthalmol*. 1990;35:59–66.

32. Neubauer H. Healon als Nothilfe. *Klin Monatsbl Augenheilkd*. 1983;182:269–271.

33. Siepser SB. The closed chamber slipping suture technique for iris repair. *Ann Ophthalmol*. 1994;26:71–72.

34. McCannel MA. A retrievable suture idea for anterior uveal problems. *Ophthalmic Surg*. 1976;7:98–103.

35. Jameson PC. Reattachment in iridodialysis: a method which does not incarcerate the iris. *Arch Ophthalmol*. 1909;38:391.

36. Abbott RL, Spencer WH. Epithelialization of the anterior chamber after transcorneal (McCannel) suture. *Arch Ophthalmol*. 1978;96:482–484.

37. Brown SM. A technique for repair of iridodialysis in children. *JAAPOS*. 1998;2:380–382.

38. Berlin HS, Ritch R. The treatment of glaucoma secondary aniridia. *Mt Sinai J Med*. 1981;48:111–115.

39. Burger M, Mackensen G. Aniridia caused by contusion-related rupture of a bleb following Elliot's trepanation. *Klin Monatsbl Augenheilkd*. 1982;181:123–124.

40. Pham DT, Anders N, Wollensak J. Wund Ruptur ein Jahr nach Kataraktoperation mit einem 7mm skleralen Tunnel (no-stitch technique). *Klin Monatsbl Augenheilkd*. 1996;208:124–126.

41. Heimann K, Konen W. Künstliches Irisdiphragma für die Silikonölchirurgie. *Fortschr Ophthalmol*. 1990;87:329–330.

42. Heimann K, Konen W. Artificial iris diaphragm and silicone oil surgery. *Retina*. 1992;35:90–94.

43. Schulze F. Iris reconstruction: surgery, laser or contact lenses with iris structure. *Fortschr Ophthalmol.* 1991;88: 30–34.

44. Spraul CW, Roth HJ, Baumert SE, Lang GK. Motif expressing soft print lenses. Effect on visual function. *Ophthalmologe.* 1999;96:30–33.

45. Burris TE, Holmes-Higgin DK, Silvertrini TA. Lamellar intrastromal corneal tattoo for treating iris defects. *Cornea.* 1998;17:169–173.

46. Beekhuis WH, Drost BH, van der Velden/Samderubun EM. A new treatment for photophobia in posttraumatic aniridia: a case report. *Cornea.* 1998;17:338–341.

47. Remky A, Redbrake C, Wenzel M. Intrastromal corneal tattooing for iris defects. *J Cataract Refract Surg.* 1998; 24:1285–1287.

48. Reinhard T, Engelhardt S, Sundmacher R. Black diaphragm aniridia intraocular lens for congenital aniridia: a long-term follow up. *J Cataract Refract Surg.* 2000; 26:375–381.

49. Reinhard T, Sundmacher R, Althaus C. Schwarze Irisdiaphragma Linsen zur Korrektur der traumatischen Aniridie. *Klin Monatsbl Augenheilkd.* 1994;205: 196–200.

50. Vajpayee RB, Majii AB, Taherian K, Honavar SG. Frosted-iris intraocular lens for traumatic aniridia with cataract. *Ophthalmic Surg.* 1994;25:730–734.

51. Osher RH, Burk SE. Cataract surgery combined with implantation of an artificial iris. *J Cataract Refract Surg.* 1999;25:1540–1547.

52. Ando F. Usefulness and limit of silicone in management of complicated retinal detachment. *Jpn J Ophthalmol.* 1987;31:138–146.

53. Wiedemann P, Konen W, Heimann K. Reconstruction of the anterior and posterior segment of the eye after massive injury. *Ger J Ophthalmol.* 1994;3:1–6.

54. Thumann G, Kirchhof B, Bartz-Schmidt KU, et al. The artificial iris diaphragm for vitreoretinal silicone oil surgery. *Retina.* 1997;17:330–337.

Chapter 19

CILIARY BODY

Derek Kuhl and William F. Mieler

 Normal functioning of the ciliary body has a pivotal role in the long-term health of the traumatized eye. Dysfunction of the ciliary body may result in loss of the normal IOP.

> **PEARL...** Frequently, the ultimate success or failure of the surgical or medical management of the traumatized eye rests on whether or not the eye can maintain a normal IOP.

Even after successful treatment of an open globe injury, which in many cases also includes repair of various corneal and AC pathologies as well as a complicated retinal detachment (see Chapter 25), it is not uncommon for eyes to become and remain hypotonous.

> **PITFALL**
>
> With the loss of IOP, phthisis invariably ensues, leading to a poor functional and cosmetic result.

> **PEARL...** Occasionally, abnormally high IOP is the long-term consequence of trauma-associated inflammation, but the mechanisms of treating elevated IOP are better developed (see Chapter 20).

This chapter discusses the causative mechanisms of hypotony along with management of the individual conditions.

DEFINITION

Hypotony has been defined statistically in the past as an IOP below 6.5 mm Hg,[1] but harmful effects on the eye are only rarely noted before the IOP falls and remains below 4 mm Hg.[2]

PATHOPHYSIOLOGY

IOPs that chronically remain below 4 mm Hg can result in a *prephthisical state* with:

- anterior and posterior segment infolding; and
- marked limitation of vision.

The causes of hypotony in the traumatized eye are varied and sometimes difficult to determine. They are generally divided into two classes.

1. The first class is *excessive filtration* secondary to:
    - wound leak;
    - ciliochoroidal detachment;
    - cyclodialysis cleft; or
    - retinal detachment.
2. The second class is *reduced aqueous production* as a result of:
    - intraocular inflammation;
    - anterior PVR; or
    - ciliary body ischemia and/or damage.

Dynamics of the Aqueous

Aqueous humor is *produced* by a combination of mechanisms in the pigmented and nonpigmented layers of the ciliary epithelium in the ciliary processes. In the human eye:

- aqueous is formed by the ciliary body at approximately 2.5 µL/min and
- 1% of the aqueous is turned over every minute.[3]

There are four pathways for the aqueous to *drain* from the eye:

1. through the trabecular mesh;
2. uveoscleral outflow;
3. through the vitreous; and
4. through a wound.

Most of the aqueous passes out through the *trabecular meshwork* as a result of a pressure gradient since the IOP in Schlemm's canal exceeds episcleral venous pressure.[a] This outflow is so pressure dependent that very little drainage occurs through Schlemm's canal when the IOP is less than the episcleral venous pressure.

> **PEARL...** When significant hypotony is present, the aqueous humor must leave the eye by some route other than Schlemm's canal.

Of the other pathways of aqueous drainage, the most important is the *uveoscleral outflow*,[5] leading from

- the AC through
- the intermuscular spaces of the ciliary muscle, into
- the suprachoroidal space and into
- the choroidal vessels or out through the sclera or emissarial channels.

The actual percentage of aqueous humor that exits via the uveoscleral route depends on the IOP. In humans with a normal IOP, approximately 10% of the aqueous passes along this route.

In addition to these two routes, aqueous may also escape either:

- posteriorly through the vitreous, *across the retina and choroid;* or
- in the presence of a *full-thickness wound.*

---

[a]The typical episcleral venous pressure is approximately 9 mm Hg.[4]

> **PEARL...** The magnitude of hypotony depends on the rate of aqueous production and the facility of extracanalicular outflow.

It is important to note that if no other parameter is altered, reduced aqueous humor production can account for hypotony only if it falls below 10% of its normal rate,[6] which is uncommon.

> **PEARL...** Generally, increased extracanalicular outflow and reduced aqueous production coexist to produce hypotony.

CLINICAL CONDITIONS: THE CAUSES OF HYPOTONY

Increased Filtration
Wound Leak

Wound leak is a common cause of hypotony after open globe injury, although it may occasionally be very difficult to recognize.

> **PITFALL**
>
> The only manifestation of a leaking wound may be a low and diffuse filtering bleb, which can be difficult to distinguish from postoperative chemosis.

Diagnosis   Occasionally, *subepithelial microcystic conjunctival* changes may signal leakage through the scleral wound. However, in cases of:

- a posterior wound (e.g., the exit wound in a perforating injury; see Chapter 26); or
- an occult wound (see Chapters 13 and 15), there may be no anterior signs of aqueous loss.

In selected cases, if the view is unobstructed, the posterior wound can be *directly visualized.*

> **PITFALL**
>
> On occasion, a posterior rupture may behave in a trap-door fashion: open only upon application of slight pressure on the globe.

An anterior wound fistula may be detected using the *Seidel test* (see Chapters 9 and 14). Failure to detect a positive result on the Seidel test is commonly due to one of two factors:

- use of diluted fluorescein; or
- inadequate pressure on the globe while inspecting the suspected area.

> **PEARL...** Use of a fluorescein-impregnated paper strip for the Seidel test is preferable to using a drop of fluorescein–topical anesthetic solution because in the latter case the concentration of fluorescein is often inadequate for detection of a subtle leak. Pressure on the globe is also important because the leak may be only intermittent if the IOP is very low.

B-scan ultrasonography is occasionally useful in identifying discontinuities in the posterior sclera (Fig. 19–1). However, care must be taken to avoid excessive pressure on a globe with an open wound to prevent extrusion of further intraocular contents.

> **PITFALL**
>
> There is no definitive test for finding a posterior wound fistula; its existence must frequently be diagnosed by indirect clinical findings based on a high index of suspicion.

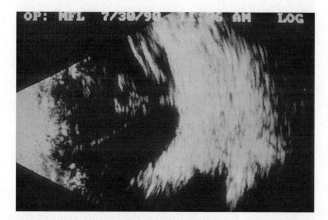

FIGURE 19–1 B-scan echogram documenting an occult posterior scleral rupture with incarcerated retinal tissue and localized choroidal detachment.

Management In general, leaking wounds must be surgically repaired because they:

- have a very low rate of spontaneous closure;[b] and
- represent a significant risk for endophthalmitis, despite a formed AC.

Common exceptions to this "close the full-thickness traumatic wound" rule include:

- a small (e.g., typically less than 2 mm long), linear, sharp, clean wound, which may close spontaneously with medical management alone; or
- a wound too posterior for safe closure (see Chapter 15).

Conservative treatment includes use of:

- pressure patch;
- CAIs; and
- topical beta-blocker(s).

These measures reduce the aqueous flow, potentially allowing the fistula to close. Devices that also may be helpful are a *bandage contact lens*[c] or *Simmons shell*, which tamponade the leak.

> **PEARL...** An inadvertent, small filtering bleb that develops after cataract surgery need not be repaired unless it is causing significant discomfort or visual impairment secondary to astigmatism or hypotony (Fig. 19–2). Closure of a scleral fistula often results in an initially marked IOP elevation until the trabecular meshwork begins to function normally again.

Cyclodialysis

Pathophysiology Separation of the ciliary body from the scleral spur can be seen after:

- anterior segment surgery;
- ocular trauma (especially contusion); or as the intended goal of
- glaucoma surgery.[d]

Cyclodialysis creates free communication between the AC and the suprachoroidal space.[8,e]

---

[b]Even leaks occurring through the conjunctiva at the limbus may not close spontaneously.

[c]A contact lens increases the risk of infection.[7]

[d]This surgery has been almost completely abandoned.

[e]In experimentally induced cyclodialysis, uveoscleral outflow is markedly enhanced in monkeys[9]; in rabbits, fluorescein moves more readily into the supraciliary space.[10]

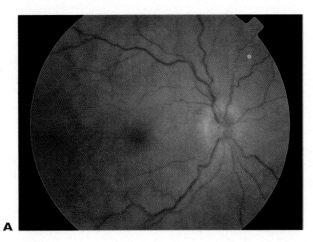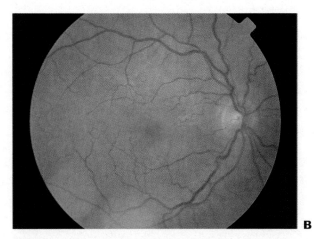

A   B

FIGURE 19–2 **(A)** Color photograph revealing optic disk congestion, vascular tortuosity, and chorioretinal folds in a patient with prolonged hypotony due to an inadvertent filtering bleb following repair of a corneoscleral laceration. The visual acuity was 20/200. **(B)** Color photograph 1 month following surgical closure of the filtering bleb, showing resolution of disk congestion and the chorioretinal folds. The IOP is now normal with visual acuity of 20/40.

It has been argued that cyclodialysis also results in reduced aqueous production.[11] However, aqueous flare is commonly present in eyes with an acute cyclodialysis, which prevents measurement of aqueous production. It has been found that eyes showing hypotony from chronic cyclodialysis but no aqueous flare have normal aqueous flow as measured by fluorophotometry.[6]

> **PEARL...** Hypotony associated with a cyclodialysis is due to increased fluid egress. If there is reduced aqueous production in an eye with acute cyclodialysis, it is the result of associated inflammation rather than the cyclodialysis itself.

> **PEARL...** The presence of a cyclodialysis cleft should be suspected in any hypotonous eye that had recent surgery or trauma (Fig. 19–3 A–C).

Cyclodialysis creates a rather unique clinical condition.

• If the cyclodialysis cleft suddenly closes, the IOP may rise to extreme levels.[12] This is analogous to the rapid rise in pressure that occurs after closure of a wound leak.
• If the cleft is reopened with miotics, the IOP may again fall rapidly.[13]

> **PEARL...** The size of the cyclodialysis cleft does not appear to correlate directly with the degree of hypotony.[11,14] Even a small cleft is capable of carrying the full amount of aqueous produced.

Diagnosis   The cleft between the ciliary body and the scleral spur can be directly identified by gonioscopy. With profound hypotony, visualization of the cleft may be difficult because of corneal deformation during gonioscopy.

> **PEARL...** A viscoelastic agent may be injected into the AC to facilitate the diagnosis; this can also aid in the treatment.[15–18]

Management   More than one treatment modality may be necessary to close the cleft.

> **PEARL...** The cleft may close spontaneously; observation prior to surgical intervention should be considered.

• If the cleft can be visualized, *argon laser photocoagulation* can be applied directly in and around the cleft to induce an inflammatory response. This is typically adequate to allow closure of the cleft.[15–18]

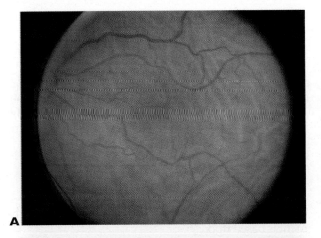
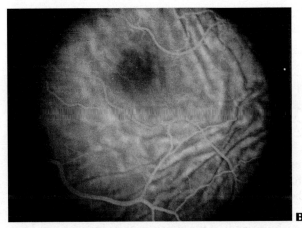
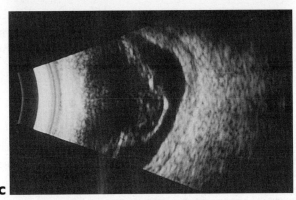

FIGURE 19-3 (A) Color photograph documenting the posterior segment manifestations of hypotony in an eye with a post-traumatic cyclodialysis cleft. Note the prominent chorioretinal folds. (B) Corresponding FA highlighting the chorioretinal folds. (C) B-scan echogram documenting diffuse thickening of the chorioretinal layer with an overlying posterior vitreous separation.

- Typical argon laser settings are 100 μm spot size, 0.1 to 0.2 second duration, and 0.5 to 1 watt of power, applied confluently to the cleft and the surrounding area.
- An IOP spike lasting several days is common after successful closure of the cleft.

Other techniques used to close the cyclodialysis cleft include:

- *external diathermy;*
- *cryotherapy*[19,20];
- ciliary body *suturing*[21,22]; and
- *external plumbage.*[23]

Occasionally, additional measures are necessary to identify a cyclodialysis cleft:

- exploratory surgery;
- fluorescein-stained BSS; if injected into the AC, the fluorescein-stained fluid will rapidly exit from a supraciliary sclerostomy[11]; or
- ultrasound biomicroscopy, a noninvasive technique.[24]

Surgical closure of the cleft involves:

- localization of the cleft with a diagnostic goniolens;
- marking the precise site on the sclera over the cleft;
- preparation of a partial-thickness scleral flap over the cleft, hinged at the limbus;
- passage of a 9-0 or 10-0 nylon suture deeply through the scleral bed to reattach the ciliary body;
- optional placement of cryotherapy or diathermy in the scleral bed to create an inflammatory response to secure the reattachment; and
- closure of the scleral flap.

Ciliochoroidal Detachment

Pathophysiology Ciliochoroidal detachment is commonly seen in the presence of hypotony. However, the relationship between the two is not fully understood.[25] It was originally believed that suprachoroidal fluid was derived from aqueous humor, which was responsible for creating the ciliochoroidal detachment. However, electrophoretic protein analysis of suprachoroidal fluid suggests that the fluid originates from the choroidal vessels with molecular sieving across the capillary endothelium.[26]

Human eyes with a ciliochoroidal detachment have been shown to have stagnation of aqueous flow, as estimated after systemic administration of fluorescein.[11,f]

P**EARL...** Uveoscleral outflow is enhanced as a result of the ciliochoroidal detachment and attendant ciliary body edema.

In most eyes with ciliochoroidal detachment, aqueous flare is also present,[28–30] and a breakdown of the blood–aqueous barrier may be responsible for the observed hyposecretion. Thus, the hyposecretion seen clinically in humans with ciliochoroidal detachment may be a result of the concurrent iridocyclitis and not the detachment of the ciliary body.

Most patients with ciliochoroidal detachment undergo spontaneous resorption of the suprachoroidal fluid. This may occur by absorption into choroidal vessels or by passage of fluid through the emissarial channels.[29,30]

PITFALL

Hypotony can induce a cycle: increasing transudation across the choroidal vessels and reducing the pressure drop across the sclera; the suprachoroidal fluid remains and contributes to continued hypotony.

---

[f]In a monkey model,[27] injection of silicone oil into the suprachoroidal space, which created large choroidal detachments, did not lower the IOP. This strongly suggests that mechanical detachment of the ciliary body does not cause hyposecretion. However, injection of Ringer's solution or autologous serum into the suprachoroidal space in the same model led to hypotony associated with a normal rate of aqueous humor flow.

Diagnosis   In most cases the diagnosis of ciliochoroidal detachment can be made by:

- *direct observation* of the retina (Fig. 19–4A and B); or by
- *B-scan echography* of the posterior segment (Fig. 19–5).[31]

Small anterior choroidal detachments or very shallow localized ciliochoroidal detachments can occasionally be missed. Useful diagnostic modalities for the detection of very anterior ciliochoroidal detachments include:

- *echographic biomicroscopy;* or
- *B-scan echography using an immersion mode.*

Management   Treatment of the ciliochoroidal detachment is based upon:

- maintenance of a normal anatomy; and
- breaking the vicious circle of *hypotony–suprachoroidal fluid transudation–ciliary body inflammation–aqueous hyposecretion–hypotony.*

Nonsurgical treatment includes the use of:

- cycloplegics;
- topical corticosteroids; and
- CAIs (e.g., acetazolamide, which may also speed up the absorption of suprachoroidal fluid, although the mechanism is poorly understood[32]).

P**EARL...** Cycloplegics are useful in deepening the AC and preventing corneal touch.

The maintenance of normal anatomy provided by cycloplegics is valuable even though they increase the uveoscleral outflow and may theoretically slightly worsen the degree of hypotony.

Topical corticosteroids are useful in decreasing ciliary body inflammation and normalizing aqueous

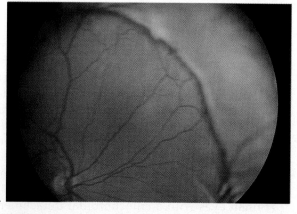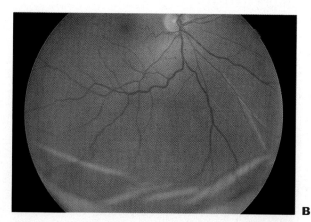

FIGURE 19–4   (A and B) Color photographs of a peripheral ciliochoroidal detachment in a patient following an open globe injury involving the anterior segment. With restoration of normal IOP, the ciliochoroidal detachment cleared spontaneously.

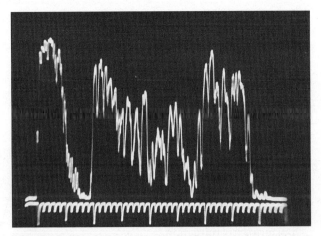 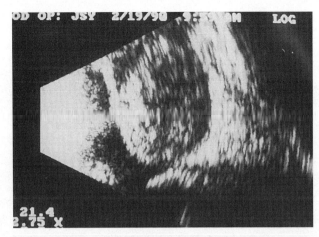

FIGURE 19–5 A- and B-scan echogram documenting a prominent, superiorly located choroidal detachment following an open globe injury. Dense cataract precluded viewing of the posterior segment. Following repair of the corneal laceration and removal of the cataract, the choroidal detachment cleared spontaneously.

humor production. Occasionally, systemic corticosteroids are used if the eye is unusually inflamed. Increased fluid intake may also increase the production of aqueous humor.

Surgical drainage of the suprachoroidal fluid is indicated if:

• the AC is flat with corneal decompensation; or

• peripheral anterior synechiae are forming (Fig. 19–6).[33]

> **PEARL...** Hypotony may improve after drainage of suprachoroidal fluid alone.[11]

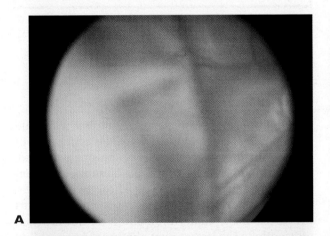 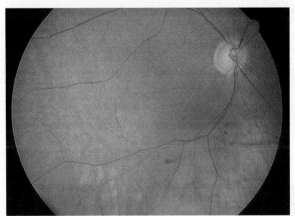

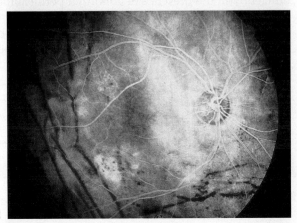

FIGURE 19–6 (A) Color photograph showing a prominent peripheral serous choroidal detachment, which led to flattening of the AC. Visual acuity was hand motions. (B) Color photograph showing the posterior segment 2 weeks following successful external drainage of the choroidal detachment. Note the intraretinal pigment lines throughout the periphery ("high-water marks"). The vision is now 5/200. (C) FA highlighting the intraretinal pigmentary deposition from the previous choroidal detachment.

To prevent recurrence of a flat AC:

- a viscoelastic agent may be injected into the AC[34,35]; or in more difficult/recurrent cases,
- suturing of the ciliary body to the sclera.[36]

Hypotony in *uveal effusion syndrome* may also be treated by injection of a viscoelastic agent into the AC.[37]

Retinal Detachment

Rhegmatogenous retinal detachment is most commonly associated with mild hypotony, although occasionally profound hypotony develops.[38]

> **P**EARL... **The level of hypotony is frequently related to the extent of the retinal detachment, even if not all detached eyes become hypotonous (Fig. 19–7).**

Pathophysiology   The etiology of the hypotony is controversial. Hypotony could be due to:

- decreased aqueous production; or
- increased filtration.

The production of aqueous humor in retinal detachment has been assessed in several studies.

- Aqueous flow was found to be reduced[39] as well as normal.[40]
- Decreased aqueous production may be caused by concurrent iridocyclitis.
- In eyes with more profound hypotony, reduced aqueous humor production alone cannot explain the low IOP.

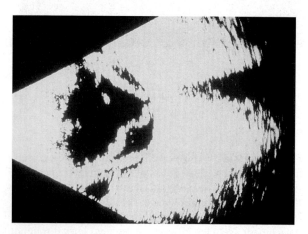

FIGURE 19–7 B-scan echogram documenting a retinal detachment with an underlying choroidal detachment in a patient who sustained an open globe injury.

- It was suggested that the aqueous may be shunted posteriorly through the vitreous, through the retinal hole, and across the RPE/choroid.[41,g]
- In experimental rhegmatogenous retinal detachment, fluorescein-labeled dextran injected into the vitreous moved into the subretinal space, where it was sequestered for many months.[42,43]
- Presumably, the rate of fluid removal in the vitreous cavity by the RPE exceeds the rate of aqueous production.
- Iris retraction syndrome also offers clinical evidence: in an eye with retinal detachment and a secluded pupil, administration of CAIs can cause posterior iris retraction.

> ## PITFALL
>
> Occasionally, the IOP becomes very elevated after retinal detachment repair, presumably as a consequence of aqueous hypersecretion compensating for increased filtration while the retina was attached. This typically normalizes within a few days with the application of the usual medications reducing aqueous production.

The diagnosis and management of retinal detachment are discussed in Chapter 23.

Decreased Aqueous Production

Iridocyclitis

Pathophysiology   Clinicians are familiar with mild hypotony that commonly accompanies acute anterior uveitis.[44] In these cases, the flow of aqueous is reduced, and the blood–aqueous barrier is abnormal, as manifested by aqueous flare.[39,45,46] These two observations may be interrelated because the transport processes of the ciliary epithelium do not function efficiently in the presence of abnormal permeability of the blood–aqueous barrier.[47]

If edema of the ciliary body exists, fluid would be expected to move more readily through the edematous tissue from the AC into the suprachoroidal space.[48,h]

---

[g]This posterior filtration could cause the extremely viscous nature of cronic subretinal fluid: protein-rich fluid continues to enter the subretinal space from the vitreous while only water is pumped through the RPE, leaving the protein behind

[h]In experimentally induced iridocyclitis and an edematous ciliary body, uveoscleral outflow is markedly increased.[45] In more profound cases of uveitis, ciliary body vasculitis may lead to vascular occlusion and reduced blood flow.[49]

Diagnosis The diagnosis of post-traumatic iridocyclitis causing hypotony is based upon the identification of intraocular inflammation. Cells and flare in the AC are the critical signs.

PITFALL

In the traumatized eye, recognizing inflammation in the AC is frequently not straightforward because corneal edema and intraocular pigment or hemorrhage may interfere with visualization.

The presence of keratic precipitates, ocular pain, and periocular vascular congestion may also be equivocal given the traumatized state of the eye. The diagnosis of iridocyclitis is frequently only presumed in a post-traumatic eye with hypotony.

Management The treatment of post-traumatic iridocyclitis is the same as that of iridocyclitis in the nontraumatized eye.

- Strong cycloplegics help reduce pain and relax the ciliary muscle. This helps break the inflammatory cycle of muscle spasm and inflammation.
- Topical corticosteroids (and occasionally systemic corticosteroids) directly reduce the amount of inflammation.

Anterior PVR

Pathophysiology The clinical findings of anterior PVR include:

- chronic hypotony after trauma or surgery (especially following lensectomy *and* concurrent vitrectomy);
- a fixed, widely dilated pupil; and
- a posteriorly displaced iris.[50]

PEARL... A posteriorly displaced iris indicates adhesions via a proliferative tissue between the posterior iris surface and the ciliary processes, remnants of the zonules/lens and the anterior insertion of the vitreous base, and/or the presence of secondary membranes in the retroiridal space.

Additional findings include the following.

- Eyes with anterior PVR have a high incidence of hypotony compared with eyes with only posterior PVR.[51]

- Frequently there is no evidence of suprachoroidal fluid or ciliochoroidal detachment; the hypotony must be secondary to another mechanism. Instead, there is an abnormal tissue covering and/or causing traction on the ciliary processes.
- Two basic patterns of fibrosis are recognized.[51]
  ○ In some eyes, there is a prominent, white, fibrotic ring of contracted tissue. It is slightly elevated from the ciliary body and causes traction on the ciliary processes via the remaining zonules. This tissue is thought to represent fibrosis and contracture of the remaining equatorial lens material and capsule. This causes decreased aqueous fluid production by detachment of the ciliary body and distortion of the normal architecture.[i]
  ○ In other eyes, there is a continuous sheet of fibrous-appearing material extending from the vitreous base to the posterior iris, completely covering the pars plicata ciliaris. The tissue originates from cellular invasion, and secretion and contraction of new collagen within the anterior cortical vitreous over the ciliary body. The membrane causes decreased aqueous production by physically obstructing outflow and distorting the anatomy of the ciliary body.

Diagnosis Clinical signs of anterior PVR include:

- dense anterior membranes;
- posterior synechiae; and
- posterior retraction of the iris.

PEARL... Anterior PVR as a cause of hypotony must always be considered in severely traumatized eyes.

This area is exceptionally difficult to visualize with the *IBO*, especially in the presence of a retracted and poorly functional iris. Traditional *B-scan ultrasound* could be utilized in an immersion mode. *Ultrasound biomicroscopy* could potentially have great utility in these cases to allow detailed visualization of the ciliary body.

The diagnosis is best confirmed via direct visualization during *vitrectomy*. Scleral depression and use of a wide-angle system are especially helpful. The *endoscope* offers unparalled advantages in such eyes (see the Appendix).

---

[i]This may be one reason why removal of the posterior lens capsule may be preferred to keeping it for the sake of IOL implantation (see Chapter 21).

Management   The mainstay of treatment for anterior PVR is pars plana vitrectomy with:

- radical vitreous base dissection; and
- careful removal of all fibrotic material from the ciliary body.

Hypotony may be reversed by:

- removal of the cyclitic membrane or epiciliary tissue, presumably as a result of canceling the tractional irritation on the ciliary epithelium[52]; and by
- releasing traction from a shrunken posterior capsule.[53–56] This may allow reattachment of the ciliary body and a reduction in uveoscleral outflow.

Upon removal of the fibrotic ring, it is not uncommon for a posterior shift of the ciliary body to be observed. In these cases with a flatly adherent sheet of scar over the ciliary body, incision of the membrane frequently leads to extrusion of the ciliary processes through the opening, implying compression of the ciliary body by the scar. In one report of patients undergoing meticulous surgical dissection of anterior scar tissue for anterior PVR with hypotony, resolution of the hypotony occurred in 64% of eyes.[51]

Panoramic endoscopic systems provide adequate visualization not only for diagnostic purposes but also for the surgical removal of any scar tissue that may contribute to ciliary body dysfunction (see the Appendix).

PEARL... Prevention of anterior PVR development is becoming a goal of lensectomy/vitrectomy procedures. Adequate removal of the peripheral vitreous (even in phakic eyes) and of the posterior capsule in selected cases (see Chapters 21 and 24) is crucial. The tremendous advantage of wide-angle viewing systems must again be emphasized in helping maneuvers at the vitreous base.

Ciliary Body Ischemia/Necrosis
Pathophysiology   In many severely injured eyes, blood flow to the ciliary body is compromised by damage to:

- the long posterior and anterior ciliary arteries; and
- the major arterial circle.

This damage can arise from:

- the original trauma; or from
- subsequent interventions during:
  - wound repair;
  - scleral buckling; and/or
  - cryotherapy.

In these eyes, ischemic necrosis of the ciliary body occurs and aqueous production falls to very low levels. The hypotony eventually proceeds to phthisis.

PEARL... Even with necrotic-appearing ciliary processes, aqueous production may be sufficient to prevent phthisis development.[51]

Diagnosis   The diagnosis of ciliary body ischemia is frequently a diagnosis of exclusion. It can be suspected at the time of pars plana vitrectomy when, upon direct inspection, the ciliary processes appear white. Scleral depression is typically employed to visualize the ciliary body under anesthesia. Endoscopic viewing systems allow visualization of the ciliary body without scleral depression (see the Appendix).

Management   After it has been established that it is the ciliary body itself that is damaged and thus simply cannot produce enough aqueous to prevent hypotony, management options revolve around the prevention of fluid egress or artificial maintenance of globe volume.

When the ciliary body is only temporarily nonfunctional as a result of inflammation, repeated fluid–gas exchanges have been utilized to keep the eye inflated temporarily.[56] This, however, is certainly not a long-term solution.

PEARL... In an eye with poor fluid turnover, clearance of the intraocular gas is much slower than usual (see the Appendix), and long-acting gases may keep the eye inflated for months.

MANAGEMENT OF THE PHTHISICAL EYE

It is increasingly common for ophthalmologists treating patients with severe eye injuries to observe during follow-up eyes that have an attached retina but are gradually becoming phthisical because of ciliary body nonfunction or dysfunction (see Chapter 25).

Whereas in the past these eyes were eventually lost, usually enucleated for reasons of cosmesis and convenience, our armamentarium today has at least one useful weapon.

- *Silicone oil* has been employed successfully (see Chapter 18) in an attempt to maintain the IOP and mechanically prevent the eye from shrinking.[57] This requires, however, that an adequate volume of silicone oil be infused into the eye (i.e., a *complete fill*; see Chapter 8) because there will be little contribution from aqueous production.

An additional option would be to reduce aqueous outflow by inducing scarring in the angle. Theoretically, argon laser photocoagulation to the ciliary body face in the angle could produce peripheral anterior synechiae and reduce uveoscleral outflow in eyes with hypotony.

SUMMARY

Hypotony after ocular trauma is a rather common occurrence and is frequently the major determinant of success versus failure. Diagnosis and treatment depend upon identification of sites of possible excessive filtration and maximization of aqueous fluid production. Sensitivity to all of the possible causes of hypotony in the traumatized eye will help in the identification of eyes in which hypotony can be treated successfully. Additional research is needed to find methods of preventing ciliary body ischemia and eventual necrosis after trauma; phthisis is not merely a cosmetic but a major functional problem.

REFERENCES

1. Leydhecker W. Zur Verbreitung des Glaucoma simplex in der Scheinbar gesunden, augenarztlich nicht behandelten Bevolkerung. *Doc Ophthalmol.* 1959;13:359.

2. Ormerod LD, Baerveldt G, Green RL. Cyclodialysis clefts: natural history, assessment, and management. In: Weinstein GW, ed. *Open-Angle Glaucoma: Contemporary Issues in Ophthalmology.* Vol 3. New York: Churchill Livingstone; 1986:314–337.

3. Brubaker RF. The physiology of aqueous humor formation. In: Drance SM, Neufeld AH, eds. *Glaucoma: Applied Pharmacology in Medical Treatment.* Orlando, FL: Grune & Stratton; 1984:27–40.

4. Stepanik J. Die Tonographie und der episklerale Venendruk. *Ophthalmologica.* 1957;133:397.

5. Bill A. The aqueous humor drainage mechanism in the cynomolgus monkey (*Macaca irus*) with evidence for unconventional routes. *Invest Ophthalmol.* 1965;4:1.

6. Pederson JE. Ocular hypotony. *Trans Ophthalmol Soc UK.* 1986;105:220.

7. Ritch R. Management of the leaking filtration bleb. *J Glaucoma.* 1993;2:114.

8. Bill A. The routes for bulk drainage of aqueous humour in rabbits with or without cyclodialysis. *Doc Ophthalmol.* 1966;20:157.

9. Suguro K, Toris CD, Pederson JE. Uveoscleral outflow following cyclodialysis in the monkey eye using a fluorescent tracer. *Invest Ophthalmol Vis Sci.* 1985;26:810.

10. Joo SH, Ko MK, Choe JK. Outflow of aqueous humor following cyclodialysis or ciliochoroidal detachment in rabbit. *Korean J Ophthalmol.* 1989;3:65.

11. Chandler PA, Maumenee AE. A major cause of hypotony. *Am J Ophthalmol.* 1961;52:609.

12. Kronfeld PC. The fluid exchange in the successfully cyclodialyzed eye. *Trans Am Ophthalmol Soc.* 1954; 52:249.

13. Shaffer RN, Weiss DI. Concerning cyclodialysis and hypotony. *Arch Ophthalmol.* 1962;68:25.

14. Viikari K, Tuovinen E. On cyclodialysis surgery in the light of follow-up examination. *Acta Ophthalmol (Copenh).* 1957;35:528.

15. Harbin TS Jr. Treatment of cyclodialysis clefts with argon laser photocoagulation. *Ophthalmology.* 1982; 89:1092.

16. Joondeph HC. Management of postoperative and posttraumatic cyclodialysis clefts with argon laser photocoagulation. *Ophthalmic Surg.* 1980;11:186.

17. Ormerod LD, Baerveldt G, Murad AS, Vekhof FT. Management of the hypotonous cyclodialysis cleft. *Ophthalmology.* 1991;98:1384.

18. Partamian LG. Treatment of a cyclodialysis cleft with argon laser photocoagulation in a patient with a shallow anterior chamber. *Am I Ophthalmol.* 1985;99:5.

19. Barasch K, Galin MA, Baras I. Postcyclodialysis hypotony. *Am I Ophthalmol.* 1969;68:644.

20. Castier PH, Asseman PH, Razemon L. Évolution d'une hypotonie posttraumatique après cyclopexie. *Bull Soc Ophthalmol Fr.* 1982;82:261.

21. Demeler U. Surgical management of ocular hypotony. *Eye.* 1988;2:77.

22. Zheng Y, Ji X. Reattachment of the detached ciliary body with suturing for treatment of contusional ocular hypotension. *Ophthalmic Surg.* 1991;22:360.

23. Portney GL, Purcell TW. Surgical repair of cyclodialysis induced by hypotony. *Ophthalmic Surg.* 1974;5:30.

24. Pavlin CJ, Harasiewicz K, Sherar MD, Foster FS. Clinical uses of ultrasound biomicroscopy. *Ophthalmology.* 1991;98:287.

25. Berkowitz RA, Klyce SD, Kaufman E. Aqueous hyposecretion after penetrating keratoplasty. *Ophthalmic Surg.* 1984;15:323.

26. Chylack LT Jr, Bellows AR. Molecular sieving in suprachoroidal fluid formation in man. *Invest Ophthalmol Vis Sci.* 1978;17:420.

27. Pederson JE, Gaasterland DE, MacLellan HM. Experimental ciliochoroidal detachment: effect on IOP and aqueous humor flow. *Arch Ophthalmol.* 1979;97:536.

28. Streeten BW, Belkowitz M. Experimental hypotony with Silastic. *Arch Ophthalmol.* 1967;78:503.

29. Bill A. Movement of albumin and dextran through the sclera. *Arch Ophthalmol.* 1965;74:248.

30. Inomata H, Bill A. Exit sites of uveoscleral flow of aqueous humor in cynomolgus monkey eyes. *Exp Eye Res.* 1977;25:113.

31. Gentile RC, Pavlin CJ, Liebmann JM, et al. Diagnosis of traumatic cyclodialysis by ultrasound biomicroscopy. *Ophthalmic Surg Lasers.* 1996;27:97–105.

32. Thorpe HE. Diamox in the treatment of nonleaking flat interior chamber after cataract extraction and associated with choroidal detachment. *Proceedings of the XVII International Congress of Ophthalmology.* Vol 3. Toronto: University of Toronto Press; 1955.

33. Bellows AR, Chylack LT Jr, Hutchinson BT. Choroidal detachment: clinical manifestation, therapy, and mechanism of formation. *Ophthalmology.* 1981;88:1107.

34. Cadera W, Willis NR. Sodium hyaluronate for postoperative aphakic choroidal detachment. *Can I Ophthalmol.* 1982;17:274–275.

35. Fisher YL, Turtz AI, Gold M, et al. Use of sodium hyaluronate in reformation and reconstruction of the persistent flat anterior chamber in the presence of severe hypotony. *Ophthalmic Surg.* 1982;13:819.

36. Shea M, Mednick EB. Ciliary body reattachment in ocular hypotony. *Arch Ophthalmol.* 1981;99:278.

37. Daniel S, Schepens CL. Can chronic bulbar hypotony be responsible for uveal effusion? Report of two cases. *Ophthalmic Surg.* 1989;20:872.

38. Burton TC, Arafat NT, Pheips CD. Intraocular pressure in retinal detachment. *Int Ophthalmol.* 1979;1:147.

39. O'Rourke J, Macri FJ. Studies in uveal physiology. II. Clinical studies of the anterior chamber clearance of isotopic tracers. *Arch Ophthalmol.* 1970;84:5.

40. Tulloh GG. The aqueous flow and permeability of the blood aqueous barrier in retinal detachment. *Trans Ophthalmol Soc UK.* 1972;92:585.

41. Beigelman MN. Acute hypotony in retinal detachment. *Arch Ophthalmol.* 1929;1:463.

42. Pederson JE. Experimental retinal detachment. V. Aqueous humor dynamics in rhegmatogenous retinal detachments. *Arch Ophthalmol.* 1984;102:136.

43. Tsuboi S, Pederson JE. Volume flow across the isolated retinal pigment epithelium of cynomolgus monkey eyes. *Invest Ophthalmol Vis Sci.* 1988;29:1652.

44. Aronson SB, Elliott JH. *Ocular Inflammation.* St. Louis: Mosby; 1972.

45. Toris CB, Pederson JE. Aqueous humor dynamics in experimental iridocyclitis. *Invest Ophthalmol Vis Sci.* 1987;28:477.

46. Weekers R, Delmarcelle Y. Hypotonie ocularie par réduction du débit de l'humeur aqueuse. *Ophthalmologica.* 1953;125:425.

47. Pederson JE, Green K. Solute permeability of the normal and prostaglandin-stimulated ciliary epithelium and the effect of ultrafiltration on active transport. *Exp Eye Res.* 1975;21:569.

48. Guyton AC, Scheel K, Murpree D. Interstitial fluid pressure. 3. Its effect on resistance to tissue fluid mobility. *Circ Res.* 1966;19:412.

49. Aronson SB, Howes EL, Jr, Fish MB, et al. Ocular blood flow in experimentally induced immunologic uveitis. *Arch Ophthalmol.* 1974;91:60.

50. Lewis H, Aaberg TM. Anterior proliferative vitreoretinopathy. *Am J Ophthalmol.* 1988;105:277–284.

51. Zarbin MA, Michels RG, Green WR. Dissection of epiciliary tissue to treat chronic hypotony after surgery from retinal detachment with proliferative vitreoretinopathy. *Retina.* 1991;11:208–213.

52. Burney EN, Quigley HA, Robin AL. Hypotony and choroidal detachment as late complications of trabeculectomy. *Am I Ophthalmol.* 1987;103:685.

53. Fritsch E, Bopp S, Lucke K, Laqua H. Resection of the lens capsule by a pars plana approach for the treatment of ocular hypotony resulting from capsular shrinkage with ciliary body detachment. *Fortschr Ophthalmol.* 1991;88:802.

54. Geyer O, Godel V, Lazar M. Hypotony as a late complication of extracapsular cataract extraction. *Am J Ophthalmol.* 1983;96:112.

55. Wollensak J, Seiler T. Hypotoniesyndrom durch geschrumpfte Linsenkapsel. *Klin Monatsbl Augenheilkd.* 1986;188:242.

56. Stallman JB, Meyers SM. Repeated fluid-gas exchange for hypotony after vitreoretinal surgery for proliferative vitreoretinopathy. *Am J Ophthalmol.* 1988;106:147.

57. Morse LS, McCuen BW. The use of silicone oil in uveitis and hypotony. *Retina.* 1991;11:399.

Chapter 20

GLAUCOMA

Kristin Hammersmith Matelis and Nathan Congdon

Ocular trauma is an important, usually preventable cause of glaucoma. Injury is an especially common etiology for elevated IOP in young patients. In one study, trauma was the cause of glaucoma in 36% of patients under the age of 30, whereas it was the etiology in only 1.3% of patients over 30 years of age.[1]

PITFALL

One reason why glaucoma is an important cause of trauma-related vision loss is that it frequently occurs late, after other problems have been treated or stabilized. Given its insidious nature, it is unsuspected by the physician or by the patient; opportunities to prevent permanent visual loss due to elevated IOP may have been missed.

In discussing trauma-associated glaucoma, it is useful to categorize the type of injury as open globe or closed globe because both the mechanisms and the management are unique.[a] It is also helpful to distinguish between glaucoma that develops immediately following trauma and that with a delayed onset[2] (Table 20–1). Finally, high IOP may result from non-mechanical factors.

---

[a]Some injuries (e.g., pellet gun trauma) have mixed mechanisms within the open globe category, see Chapter 2.

GLAUCOMA ASSOCIATED WITH CLOSED GLOBE TRAUMA

Epidemiology   Contusion is responsible for a large percentage of ocular trauma. Data derived from hospital discharge summaries in the United States between 1984 to 1987 revealed an annual ocular trauma rate of 13.2 per 100,000 population; 40% of these were coded as contusion of the eyeball, adnexa, or orbit.[3]

Pathophysiology   As an object strikes the eye, the force can result in ocular damage from two mechanisms:

- *direct transfer of energy:* impact by a blunt agent leads to the transference of force vectors radiating from the point of contact. If the force is significant, it can lead to necrosis of the tissue; and
- *secondary changes in ocular shape:* as the globe is compressed in the anterior-posterior direction, it elongates equatorially (Fig. 20–1). The central lens–iris diaphragm is forced posteriorly while at the same time the attachments of these structures are anchored to the eyewall, which is moving in a perpendicular direction. This leads to shearing forces that can tear these structures at their root.

> **PEARL...**   Acutely following contusion injury, some eyes have a temporary reduction in their IOP. This is thought to result from decreased aqueous production and possibly from increased outflow.

TABLE 20–1   Classification of Trauma-Related Glaucoma

Closed globe, earlier onset	traumatic uveitis	
	trabecular meshwork disruption	
	hemorrhage-associated	
	lens-associated	
Closed globe, later onset	angle recession	
	closure of cyclodialysis cleft	
	hemorrhage-associated	ghost cell
		hemolytic
		hemosiderotic
	lens-associated	subluxation
		phacomorphic
		particle
		uveitis
Open globe	inflammation	
	flat AC	
	epithelial downgrowth	
	intraocular hemorrhage	ghost cell
		hemolytic
		hemosiderotic
	IOFB	
Chemical		
Thermal		
Electrical		

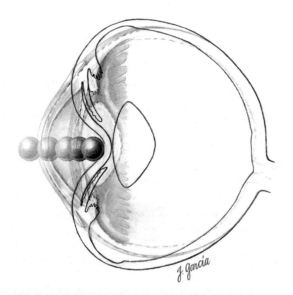

FIGURE 20–1   When a blunt object strikes the eye, it causes ocular shortening in the anteroposterior dimension and elongation of the globe equatorially. As this occurs, the lens-iris diaphragm is pushed posteriorly in its central aspect while the peripheral aspects of these structures are expanding with the equator of the globe. This leads to tearing of the structures in the anterior segment, particularly in the angle.

Early-Onset Glaucomas

Trabecular Meshwork Obstruction/Inflammation

Inflammatory cells obstruct the (inflamed) trabecular meshwork, decreasing outflow facility. This IOP elevation may be seen even without:

- hyphema;
- angle recession; or
- disruption of the trabecular meshwork.

Treatment   requires:

- close monitoring, as most cases are self-limited; and
- topical corticosteroids (typically necessary only for a short period).

Trabecular Disruption

Trauma-related changes in the trabecular meshwork have been documented with gonioscopy within 48 hours of injury.[4] Findings include:

- sharply demarcated hemorrhage into Schlemm's canal;
- full-thickness rupture of the trabecular meshwork; and, occasionally,

- a trabecular flap, hinged at the region of the scleral spur; or
- cyclodialysis (see also Chapter 19).[b]

Hyphema

It commonly results from contusion, which causes a tear in the ciliary body and bleeding from the small branches of the major arterial circle of the iris. Less commonly, bleeding may result from tears within the iris or trabecular meshwork.

Hyphema is an indicator of significant trauma and may lead to IOP elevation by several mechanisms:

- disruption of the trabecular meshwork;
- obstruction of the meshwork with RBCs; or
- obstruction of the meshwork with inflammatory cells and fibrin.

Treatment   If conservative management does not reduce the IOP, surgical intervention may be necessary (see Chapter 17).

Delayed-Onset Glaucomas

Angle Recession

PEARL... The term "angle recession glaucoma" is somewhat misleading, as the recessed angle, caused by contusion,[6] is not the cause of the glaucoma, but rather an *indicator* of significant trauma to the eye.[7]

Epidemiology   Angle recession is a common consequence of contusion. Among patients with a hyphema, angle recession has been observed in 71 to 100% of eyes.[8–11]

PEARL... Glaucoma is seen in only 7 to 9% of patients with angle recession.[8,10,12,13]

Some authors have sought to correlate the amount of angle recession with the risk of glaucoma development. An increased risk of glaucoma development was found if the angle recession exceeded 180[1] or 240[4] degrees.

It must be understood, however, that patients who develop glaucoma following trauma may have an underlying predisposition to reduced aqueous flow:

- these patients frequently have IOP elevation in the fellow eye[14–16]; and
- elderly patients more frequently develop postcontusion glaucoma.[17]

Pathophysiology   (Fig. 20–2) includes the following.

- Angle recession represents a tear between the longitudinal and circular fibers of the ciliary body.
- Acutely, iridodialysis (a tear of the peripheral iris attachment), which separates the iris from the ciliary body, may be also be present (see Chapter 18).
- Cyclodialysis (a separation of the ciliary body attachment to the scleral spur), may also be seen.
- Elevated IOP results not from the angle recession but from collateral damage and scarring of the trabecular meshwork. Following trauma, there are tears in the trabecular meshwork posterior to Schwalbe's line; this produces a flap of trabecular tissue that was hinged at the scleral spur. Scarring ensues and leads to chronic obstruction.[15]
- An additional mechanism for IOP elevation is the extension of an endothelial layer with a Descemet-like membrane from the cornea over the AC.[7,18,19,c]

Clinical Picture   Patients may present during the first year after injury or as late as more than 10 years after the trauma.[15] Typically, patients present several years following the injury.

The amount of angle recession affects the time of presentation. Patients with more than 270 degrees of recession usually present earlier.[15]

Evaluation   In patients with unilateral glaucoma, a careful history of the trauma must be obtained.

The slit-lamp/IBO examination may reveal:

- discrepancy of AC depth;
- difference in pigmentation between the two irises and in the angle;
- tears in the iris root or sphincter;
- increased peripheral anterior synechiae in the area of trauma;
- paralysis of the pupillary sphincter[20];
- Vossius ring or circular pattern of pigment deposition on the lens;
- zonular rupture with prolapse of vitreous into the AC (Fig. 20–3);
- iridodonesis and phacodonesis;
- cataract; and/or

---

[b]Remember that while cyclodialysis typically results in hypotony, closure of the cleft can acutely increase the IOP via reduced permeability of the trabecular meshwork.[4,5]

[c]It is unclear whether this membrane is the primary cause of glaucoma or represents a secondary change in the damaged trabecular meshwork.

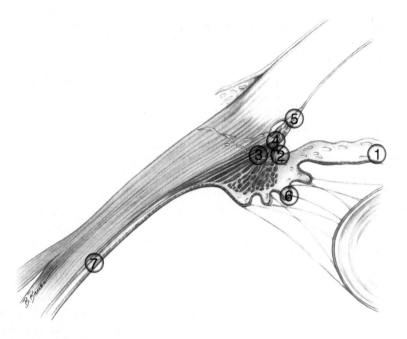

FIGURE 20-2 Seven commonly injured intraocular structures following contusion injury. 1, Iris sphincter. 2, Iris root (iridodialysis). 3, Between the longitudinal and circular muscles of the ciliary body (angle recession). 4, At the insertion of the ciliary body (cyclodialysis). 5, In the trabecular meshwork. 6, Lens zonules (subluxation or dislocation of lens). 7, Retinal tears or dialysis. (From Pieramici D, Parver LM. A mechanistic approach to ocular trauma. *Ophthalmol Clin North Am.* 1995;8:575. Reprinted by permission from WB Saunders.)

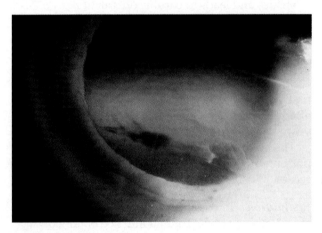

FIGURE 20-3 This patient experienced severe contusion to the phakic right eye a few years following radial keratotomy. Although the corneal incisions remained intact, bloody vitreous was seen in the AC, suggesting zonular dialysis.

- posterior signs of trauma (e.g., pigment in the vitreous, RPE hyperplasia, choroidal or retinal scars).

Common gonioscopic findings include:

- widened ciliary body;
- prominent scleral spur secondary to angle recession; and
- a gray to white membrane covering the angle.

> **PEARL...** Simultaneous, bilateral Koeppe gonioscopy is a useful technique to detect subtle angle recession.

Management   (Fig. 20–4) This includes medical therapy, laser therapy, and surgery.

MEDICAL THERAPY   Recommended agents include:

- beta-blockers;
- alpha agonists; and
- topical and oral CAIs.

  Agents *not* recommended include:

- pilocarpine (may cause a paradoxical IOP rise[d]); and
- prostaglandins (may increase the inflammation in the acute phase; should be considered in later onset cases).

LASER THERAPY   ALT yields disappointing results with only a 23 to 27% success rate.[22,23]

SURGERY   The following surgeries are performed.

- *Filtration surgery* is less successful in patients with angle recession than with open angle glaucoma. The success rate of trabeculectomy without antimetabolite therapy in one report was 74% at 1 year, 53% at 3 years, and 29% at 5 years.[24] Statistically improved success rates were found in patients with mitomycin C compared with those without an antimetabolite: the life-table success rates were 58% versus 39% at 1 year and 58% versus 26% at 2 years, respectively.[24]
- *Shunt surgery* with Molteno tube implantation has been disappointing with 56% 1-year, 41% 3-year, and 27% 5-year life-table success rates.[24]

---

[d]Decreased uveoscleral flow,[21] increased inflammation, and posterior and peripheral anterior synechiae may contribute to this phenomenon.

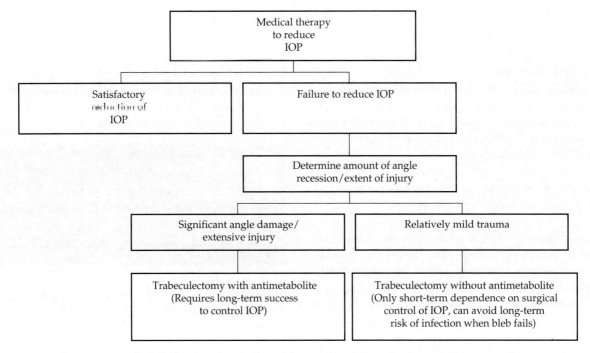

FIGURE 20–4   Flowchart for management of traumatic glaucoma.

• *Nd:YAG trabeculopuncture* has yielded mixed results. One series achieved success[e] in 42% of patients[23]; another series had a 12-month life-table success rate of 91%.[25]

Ghost Cell Glaucoma

Pathophysiology   Described in 1975,[26] this type of glaucoma requires two conditions to be present:

1. vitreous hemorrhage; and
2. a defect in the anterior hyaloid face.

> **PEARL...** Ghost cell glaucoma may occur after trauma, cataract extraction, or vitrectomy.

Characteristics of the ghost cell glaucoma include the following.

• The RBCs in the vitreous degenerate,[f] enter the aqueous cavity, and temporarily obstruct the aqueous outflow.
• The interval from the inciting event to the onset of glaucoma can vary from 2 weeks to 3 months.[27]

• The level of elevation in IOP depends on the number of ghost cells in the AC.

Evaluation   Patients often present with pain and corneal edema.

• On slit-lamp evaluation, characteristic khaki-colored cells are seen in the vitreous and on the corneal endothelium.
• A pseudohypopyon may be present. Occasionally, this may be associated with a layer of fresh RBCs (candy-stripe sign).
• Gonioscopy usually reveals a normal, open angle, although scant to heavy amounts of ghost cells may be seen.
• Diagnosis may be confirmed by evaluation of an aqueous aspirate, which revels thin-walled, hollow cells with clumps of denatured hemoglobin (Heinz bodies).

Differential Diagnosis   This includes:

• hemolytic glaucoma;
• hemosiderotic glaucoma;
• neovascular glaucoma; and
• inflammatory glaucoma.

Management   Conventional medical therapy, followed by surgical intervention in recalcitrant cases. In one study, fewer than half of patients responded to medical therapy alone.[27] Although AC lavage may be

---

[e]Defined as IOP ≤19 mm Hg.

[f]Transformed from biconcave, pliable cells to khaki-colored, less pliable spheres, referred to as erythroclasts or "ghost cells."

effective, many cases require vitrectomy for more complete removal of the supply of degenerating RBCs.

Hemolytic Glaucoma

Pathophysiology   The IOP increases within days to weeks after the hemorrhage. Hemolytic debris, including hemoglobin-filled macrophages, obstructs the trabecular meshwork, leading to IOP elevation[28] (Fig. 20–5).

Evaluation   Slit lamp examination may show reddish brown cells in the aqueous humor.

- Cytological evaluation of the aqueous, which may be used to establish the diagnosis, reveals macrophages containing golden brown pigment.[29]
- Ultrastructural study with hemolytic glaucoma reveals RBCs and macrophages with phagocytized pigment and RBCs in the trabecular spaces.[30]

Management   Hemolytic glaucoma is self-limiting and should be managed medically when possible. AC lavage or pars plana vitrectomy has been recommended for recalcitrant cases.[29]

Hemosiderotic Glaucoma

This is a rare and poorly understood condition, seen after a long-standing intraocular hemorrhage. Hemoglobin from lysed RBCs is phagocytized by endothelial cells in the trabecular meshwork. Iron from the hemoglobin is released and causes subsequent siderosis. It is believed that the siderosis leads to obstruc-

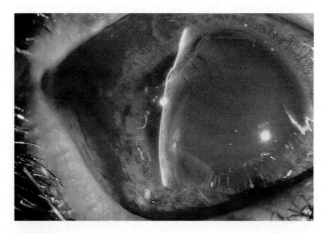

FIGURE 20–5   A few weeks following repair of open globe injury, the IOP is elevated with evidence of circulating RBCs and debris still present in the AC. Early blood staining of the cornea is also present.

tion of aqueous outflow, although this association has yet to be clearly established.[31]

Lens-Associated Glaucoma

Traumatic changes to the integrity or position of the lens (see also Chapter 21) may result in glaucoma through several distinct mechanisms.

> **PEARL...**   Lens subluxation and phacomorphic glaucoma lead to secondary closed angle closure, whereas phacolytic, lens particle, and lens-induced uveitic glaucomas share a secondary open angle mechanism.

Subluxation

Pathophysiology   of subluxation includes the following.

- It typically occurs if more than 25% of the zonular fibers are ruptured.[32]
- The lens causes pupillary block and subsequent angle closure when displaced anteriorly.[33]
- Pupillary block and angle closure may also result when the lens is dislocated posteriorly and vitreous blocks the pupil, although this is much less common.

Evaluation   Past history of trauma is essential in establishing the correct diagnosis, especially in differentiating it from primary angle closure glaucoma.
Findings include:

- reduced visual acuity;
- acquired myopia;
- acutely painful red eye;
- iridodonesis;
- asymmetry of the AC depth;
- closed angle on gonioscopy[g]; and
- visibly subluxated lens, although it may be difficult to recognize if subtle; the presence of vitreous prolapse helps establish the diagnosis (see Chapter 21).

Management   Management is directed at relieving the pupillary block with a peripheral iridectomy, either surgically or with the YAG laser. Removal of the subluxated lens (via ICCE or other techniques; see

---

[g]In differentiating lens subluxation from primary angle closure glaucoma, careful gonioscopy of the fellow eye is important, demonstrating a narrowed angle and peripheral synechiae in the affected eye.

Chapter 21 and the Appendix) may be required for IOP reduction or visual rehabilitation.

Phacomorphic Glaucoma

Pathophysiology Swelling of the lens may cause a secondary angle closure glaucoma in eyes with a traumatic (even age-related) cataract. Rapid lens swelling may result in pupillary block or forward displacement of the lens–iris diaphragm.[34] This phenomenon is especially common in children (see Chapter 30).

Evaluation A history of trauma and asymmetric shallowing of the AC are essential in making the diagnosis. A dense cataract will usually be evident on examination, with increased lens thickness compared with the contralateral eye on A scan ultrasonography.

Management options include:

- aqueous suppressants (e.g., topical beta-blockers, topical alpha agonists, and CAIs) initially;
- peripheral iridectomy if there is no need for cataract extraction; and
- cataract extraction as the definitive treatment of choice.

Lens Particle Glaucoma

Pathophysiology A secondary open angle glaucoma, this may occur days to years after trauma or cataract surgery. True disruption of the lens capsule allows the release of lens particles into the AC and causes obstruction of the trabecular meshwork.

Evaluation Patients may present with pain, redness, and decreased vision, although some have minimal symptoms.

- There are cells, flare, and white particles in the aqueous.
- Peripheral anterior and posterior synechiae may form when treatment is delayed.

Management This includes the following.

- Aqueous suppressants, cycloplegics, and topical corticosteroids.[h]

---

[h]Excessive use of steroids may delay absorption of the lens material.[35]

- Surgical removal of the lens material by irrigation or cataract extraction. Often necessary in cases in which the IOP cannot be controlled medically (see Chapter 21).

Phacolytic Glaucoma

Pathophysiology This open angle glaucoma, associated with a mature cataract, is thought to result from the leakage of lens proteins. The high-molecular-weight proteins are engulfed by macrophages and together they obstruct the trabecular meshwork.[36]

Evaluation The typical findings include:

- pain and redness;
- high IOP;
- diffuse corneal edema;
- open AC;
- prominent flare in the AC;
- iridescent particles in the AC;
- mature or hypermature cataract; and
- AC fluid revealing swollen macrophages.

Differential Diagnosis includes:

- acute angle closure;
- glaucoma secondary to uveitis;
- glaucoma secondary to intraocular hemorrhage; and
- lens particle glaucoma.

Management as an emergency is commonly necessary.

- Medical control of glaucoma may be attempted.
- The definitive treatment is removal of the lens.

> **P**EARL... If a lens causing phacolytic glaucoma is removed, it is best to lower the IOP first if possible.

Lens-Induced Uveitis ("Phacoanaphylactic Glaucoma"[37,38] or "Phacoantigenic Glaucoma")

Pathophysiology Lens protein may be liberated by trauma or spontaneously with lens aging, stimulating a granulomatous inflammation (lens-induced uveitis). Following exposure to the proteins, a latent period (during which time sensitization takes place) must occur. The exact sequence of events from the liberation of the antigens to the onset of the granulomatous uveitis is unknown.

Evaluation Patients with traumatic lens-induced uveitis usually present 1 to 14 days following the inciting event, although the time may range from hours to months.[39]

Clinically, AC inflammation is present with:

- mutton-fat keratic precipitates on the corneal endothelium; and, occasionally,
- a hypopyon.

Hypotony may be observed initially, but the formation of posterior synechiae or peripheral anterior synechiae may cause a secondary glaucoma.

Confirmation of the diagnosis may require a histopathologic specimen.

Differential Diagnosis   includes:

- endophthalmitis[34,40] (see Chapter 28); and
- SO (see Chapter 29); and

Management   in all cases includes surgical removal of any lens material.

GLAUCOMA ASSOCIATED WITH OPEN GLOBE TRAUMA

Epidemiology   In one analysis of patients with open globe injuries[41]:

- the injury was caused by a blunt object in 22%, a sharp object in 37%, and a missile in 41%;
- 86% of the patients were males; and
- the mean age was 26 years.

Several distinct mechanisms can lead to glaucoma in these patients (Fig. 20–6).

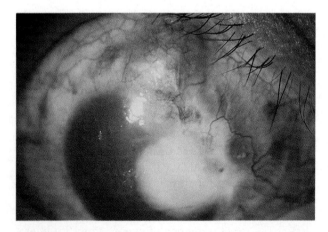

FIGURE 20–6 This patient presented with poor vision, chronic pain, and a history of an open globe eye injury of many years. The IOP was 45 mm Hg. There are a number of potential causes of the elevated IOP, including a flattened AC with a closed angle and lens-related glaucoma. The pressure rise in this case has been long-standing and insidious as evidenced by the staphylomatous changes and relative clarity of the temporal cornea.

Inflammation

All open globe injuries lead to significant inflammation in the acute setting. Inflammatory cells may obstruct the trabecular meshwork and cause an elevation of the IOP via:

- posterior synechia formation;
- pupillary block (iris bombans); and
- angle closure glaucoma.

Management   includes:

- reducing the inflammation with topical corticosteroids; and
- if pupillary seclusion occurs, laser iridotomy is recommended to avoid angle closure glaucoma.

Flat AC

Aqueous loss may result in a flat AC. When prolonged, especially in the presence of significant inflammation, peripheral anterior synechiae form and close the angle.

Management   Prevention is the best option via:

- meticulous wound closure (see Chapter 14);
- intraoperative reformation of the AC (see Chapter 17); and
- postoperative mydriasis and topical corticosteroids.

Postoperative topical steroids may reduce the chance of anterior synechia formation.

> **PEARL...** Following closure of a corneal wound, it is important to reform a flat AC to reduce the chance of permanent anterior synechia formation.

Epithelial Downgrowth

It may occur following open globe injuries in the presence of a patent eye wall fistula. Glaucoma is caused by epithelial or fibrous obliteration of the trabecular meshwork, resulting in a reduced outflow facility. Although fortunately rare, epithelial downgrowth has a poor prognosis. The clinician should be suspicious of this etiology in eyes that remain chronically irritated following open globe trauma (Fig. 20–7).

> **PEARL...** If suspected, epithelial downgrowth may be diagnosed by the blanching of the downgrowth membrane when involved ocular surfaces are treated with an argon laser. The management is surgical removal of the membranes.

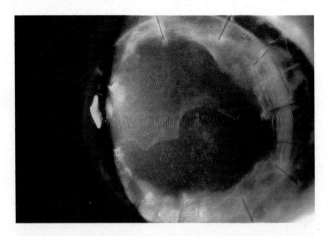

FIGURE 20–7 This patient presented 1 year following repair of a ruptured PK with 2/200 vision and elevated IOP. Cellular proliferation is present on the corneal endothelium, extending from the previous wound, consistent with epithelial downgrowth.

Intraocular Hemorrhage
See earlier in this Chapter and Chapter 17.

IOFB
- Retained ferrous IOFBs lead to glaucoma if siderosis develops; the released iron is toxic to epithelia, including that of the trabecular meshwork.
- Retained copper IOFBs may oxidize and lead to severe tissue damage. Glaucoma is less frequently observed with chalcosis than with siderosis, although retinal changes may result in visual field defects that mimic glaucoma.[42]

The specifics of IOFB diagnosis and management are discussed in Chapter 24.

CHEMICAL INJURIES

Chemical injuries may have a devastating effect on the eye and visual potential. Alkaline chemicals, which cause tissue saponification, may penetrate into the AC within seconds of contact and cause severe anterior segment ischemia.[43] In contrast, acidic chemicals cause coagulation of tissue proteins, which usually limits the penetration and resulting damage (see also Chapters 11 and 32).

Pathophysiology and Evaluation Following chemical exposure, a pattern of characteristic alterations in IOP may be seen:

- There is an initial rapid rise in IOP, followed by a return to normal or subnormal pressure and then a slower, sustained elevation of IOP.[44]
- The initial rise in IOP is hypothesized to be secondary to shrinkage of the cornea and sclera[45,46] and an increase in uveal blood flow, which may be prostaglandin mediated.[44]

Inflammation in the AC may also contribute to the IOP elevation. In cases of extensive damage to the ciliary body, hypotony may be observed.[47] An intermediate phase is seen within weeks to months of the exposure and is characterized by repair, scarring, and ongoing inflammation.[48]

Additional mechanisms of glaucoma include:

- pupillary block, as extensive posterior synechiae or iris bombans may form; and
- phacomorphic glaucoma from a cataractous lens.

In the late phase of chemical injury, responsible for the IOP increase[49] may be:

- trabecular damage; and
- peripheral anterior synechiae

Management is by immediate irrigation with copious fluids and removal of any retained material from the cornea or fornices (see Chapter 11).

The IOP may be managed with[i]:

- beta-blockers;
- alpha agonists;
- CAIs; and
- hyperosmotics.

PITFALL

Miotics, which may increase inflammation and the formation of peripheral anterior synechiae, should be avoided.

- Topical corticosteroids are useful initially to reduce inflammation.

SPECIAL CONSIDERATION

Topical corticosteroids may be used during the first few days without increasing the risk of corneal melting; the risk increases thereafter[50] (see Chapter 11).

- Adequate cycloplegia is important to minimize synechia formation.
- Late-onset glaucoma from alkali burns should be treated in the same manner as all forms of chronic glaucoma.

---

[i]Systemic formulations may be preferred in some instances because reepithelization can be hindered by topical medications.

Thermal Burns

Thermal injuries generally involve the external surfaces of the eye. The globe is usually spared, with the exception of corneal burns. In victims of severe thermal injury, administration of large quantities of iv fluids may lead to increased IOP from marked orbital congestion and periorbital swelling.[51] Lateral canthotomies may result in significant IOP reduction.[51]

Electrical Injury

IOP elevation has been reported after accidental and therapeutic electrical injuries.[52–54] The rise in IOP may be associated with:

- loss of iris pigment epithelium;
- venous dilation; and
- contraction of the extraocular muscles.

Since the increase in IOP is transient, treatment is seldom required.

Orbital Pressure Elevation

Accidental or surgical trauma to the orbit may result in retrobulbar hemorrhage, leading to acute elevation of the IOP (see Chapter 12). Emergent lateral canthotomy may be necessary.

Orbital emphysema may be seen in cases of orbital fracture involving the ethmoid and sphenoid sinuses, especially when there is vigorous nose blowing. Acute elevation of the IOP may also require timely lateral canthotomy.

Summary

Trauma, both open and closed globe, can cause elevated IOP and glaucoma due to a number of mechanisms. In most cases the rise in pressure is temporary and can be effectively managed with topical medication. In the more severe cases, surgical intervention is often necessary.

Despite the presence of normal IOP acutely following severe ocular injury, patients still need to understand that their lifetime risk of glaucoma is increased and they therefore require regular monitoring.

References

1. Sihota RN, Sood NN, Agarwal HC. Traumatic glaucoma. *Acta Ophthalmol Scand.* 1995;73:252–254.

2. Tingey DP, Shingleton BJ. Glaucoma associated with ocular trauma. In: Albert DM, Jakobiec FA, Azar DT, eds. *Principles and Practice of Ophthalmology.* Philadelphia, PA:WB Saunders. 2000:2752.

3. Klopfer J, Tielsch JM, Vitale S, et al. Ocular trauma in the Unites States. Eye injuries resulting in hospitalization, 1984 through 1987. *Arch Ophthalmol.* 1992;110: 838–842.

4. Alper MG. Contusion angle deformity and glaucoma: gonioscopic observations and clinical course. *Arch Ophthalmol.* 1963;69:455–467.

5. Goldmann H. Klinische Studien zum Glaucomproblem. *Ophthalmologica.* 1953;125:16.

6. Collins ET. On the pathological examination of three eyes lost from concussion. *Trans Ophthalmol Soc UK.* 1892;12:180–186.

7. Wolff SM, Zimmerman LE. Chronic secondary glaucoma: associated with retrodisplacement of iris root and deepening of the AC angle secondary to contusion. *Am J Ophthalmol.* 1962;54:547–563.

8. Blanton FM. Anterior chamber angle recession and secondary glaucoma. *Arch Ophthalmol.* 1964;72:39–43.

9. Tonjum AM. Intraocular pressure and facility of outflow late after ocular contusion. *Acta Ophthalmol.* 1968;46:886–908.

10. Monney D. Angle recession and secondary glaucoma. *Br J Ophthalmol.* 1973;57:608–612.

11. Canavan YM, Archer DB. Anterior segment consequences of blunt ocular injury. *Br J Ophthalmol.* 1982; 66:549–555.

12. Kaufman JH, Tolpin DW. Glaucoma after traumatic angle recession: a 10-year prospective study. *Am J Ophthalmol.* 1974;78:648–654.

13. Salmon JF, Mermoud A, Ivey A, et al. The detection of post-traumatic angle recession by gonioscopy in a population-based glaucoma survey. *Ophthalmology.* 1994; 101:1844–1850.

14. Spaeth GL. Traumatic hyphema, angle recession, dexamethasone hypertension, and glaucoma. *Arch Ophthalmol.* 1967;78:648–654.

15. Herschler J. Trabecular damage due to blunt anterior segment injury and its relationship to traumatic glaucoma. *Trans Am Acad Ophthalmol Otolaryngol.* 1977;83:239–248.

16. Tesluk GC, Spaeth GL. The occurrence of primary open-angle glaucoma in the fellow eye of patients with unilateral angle-cleavage glaucoma. *Ophthalmology.* 1985;92:904–911.

17. Thiel HJ, Aden G, Pulhorn G. Changes in the chamber angle following ocular contusions. *Klin Monatsbl Augenheilkd.* 1980;177:165–173.

18. Lauring L. Anterior chamber glass membranes. *Am J Ophthalmol.* 1969;68:308–312.

19. Iwamoto T, Witmer R, Landolt E. Light and electron microscopy in absolute glaucoma with pigment dispersion phenomena and contusion angle deformity. *Am J Ophthalmol.* 1971;72:420–434.

20. Tonjum AM. Gonioscopy in traumatic hyphema. *Acta Ophthalmol.* 1966;44:650–654.

21. Bleiman B, Schwartz AI. Paradoxical response to pilocarpine. *Arch Ophthalmol.* 1979;97:1305–1306.

22. Scharf B, Chi T, Grayson D, et al. Argon laser trabeculoplasty for angle-recession glaucoma. *Invest Ophthalmol Vis Sci.* 1992;33(suppl):1159.

23. Fukuchi T, Iwata K, Schoichi S, et al. Nd:YAG laser trabeculopuncture (YLT) for glaucoma with angle recession. *Graefes Arch Clin Exp Ophthalmol.* 1993;231:571–576.

24. Mermoud A, Salmon JF, Barron A, et al. Surgical management of post-traumatic angle recession glaucoma. *Ophthalmology.* 1993;100:634–642.

25. Melamed S, Ashkenazi I, Gutman I, et al. Nd:YAG laser trabeculopuncture in angle-recession glaucoma. *Ophthalmic Surg.* 1992;23:31–35.

26. Campbell DG, Grant WM. Alterations in red blood cells that prevent passage through the trabecular meshwork in human eyes. Read before the Association for Research in Vision and Ophthalmology, Sarasota, FL, April 29, 1975, ARVO Abstracts 1975:44.

27. Campbell DG. Ghost cell glaucoma following trauma. *Ophthalmology.* 1981;88:1151–1158.

28. Fenton RH, Hunter WS. Hemolytic glaucoma. *Surv Ophthalmol.* 1965;10:355–360.

29. Phelps CD, Watzke RC. Hemolytic glaucoma. *Am J Ophthalmol.* 1975;80:690–695.

30. Grierson I, Lee WR. Further observations on the process of haemophagocytosis in the human outflow system. *Graefes Arch Clin Exp Ophthalmol.* 1978;208:49–64.

31. Vannas S. Hemosiderosis in eyes with secondary glaucoma after delayed intraocular hemorrhages. *Acta Ophthalmol.* 1960;38:254.

32. Cullom RD, Chang B. *The Wills Eye Manual. Office and Emergency Room Diagnosis and Treatment of Eye Disease.* Philadelphia: JB Lippincott; 1994.

33. Higginbotham EJ, Lee D. *Management of Difficult Glaucoma.* Boston: Blackwell Scientific; 1994.

34. Epstein DL. Diagnosis and management of lens-induced glaucoma. *Ophthalmology.* 1982;89:227–230.

35. Epstein DL, Jedziniak JA, Grant WM. Obstruction of aqueous outflow by lens particles and by heavy-molecular weight soluble lens proteins. *Invest Ophthalmol Vis Sci.* 1978;17:272–277.

36. Zimmerman LE. Lens induced inflammation in human eyes. In: Maumenee AE, Silverstein AM, eds. *Immunopathology of Uveitis.* Baltimore: Williams & Wilkins; 1964:221–232.

37. Pelmann EM, Albert DM. Clinically unsuspected phacoanaphylaxis after ocular trauma. *Arch Ophthalmol.* 1977;95:244–246.

38. Rahi AHS, Misra RN, Morgan G. Immunopathology of the lens. III: Humoral and cellular immune responses to autologous lens antigens and their role in ocular inflammation. *Br J Ophthalmol.* 1977;61:371–379.

39. Meisler KM, Palestine AG, Vastine DW, et al. Chronic *Propionibacterium* endophthalmitis after cataract extraction and intraocular lens implantation. *Am J Ophthalmol.* 1986;102:733–739.

40. de Juan E Jr, Sternberg P, Jr, Michels RG. Penetrating ocular injuries. Types of injuries and visual results. *Ophthalmology.* 1983;90:1318–1322.

41. Rosenthal AR, Marmor MF, Leuenberger P, Hopkins JL. Chalcosis: a study of natural history. *Ophthalmology.* 1979;86:1956–1972.

42. Hughes WF. Alkali burns of the eye. I. Review of the literature and summary of the present knowledge. *Arch Ophthalmol.* 1946;35:423–449.

43. Green K, Paterson CA, Siddiqui A. Ocular blood flow after experimental alkali burns and prostaglandin administration. *Arch Ophthalmol.* 1985;103:569–571.

44. Paterson CA, Pfister RR. Intraocular pressure changes after alkali burns. *Arch Ophthalmol.* 1974;91:211–218.

45. Stein MR, Naidoff MA, Dawson CR. Intraocular pressure response to experimental alkali burns. *Am J Ophthalmol.* 1973;75:99–109.

46. Pfister RR, Friend J, Dohlman CH. The anterior segment of rabbits after alkali burn. Metabolic and histologic alterations. *Arch Ophthalmol.* 1971;86:189–193.

47. Mermoud A, Heuer DK. Glaucoma associated with trauma. In: Ritch R, Shields MB, Krupin T, eds. *The Glaucomas.* Vol 2. 2nd ed. St Louis: Mosby; 1996:1259.

48. Girard LJ, Alford WE, Feldman GR, et al. Severe alkali burns. *Trans Am Acad Ophthalmol Otolarygol.* 1970;74:788–803.

49. Donshik PC, Bemram MB, Dohlman CH, et al. Effect of topical corticosteroids on ulceration in alkali-burned corneas. *Arch Ophthalmol.* 1978;96:2117–2120.

50. Evans LS. Increased IOP in severely burned patients. *Am J Ophthalmol.* 1991;111:56–58.

51. Arstikaitis M, Hodgson H. The effect of lobotomy and electroshock on intraocular pressure. *Am J Ophthalmol.* 1952;35:1625.

52. Berger RO. Ocular complications of cardioversion. *Ann Ophthalmol.* 1978;10:161–164.

53. Berger RO. Ocular complications of electroconvulsive therapy. *Ann Ophthalmol.* 178;10:737–743.

54. Ottoson JO, Rendahl I. Intraocular pressure in electroconvulsive therapy. *Arch Ophthalmol.* 1963;70:462.

LENS

Viktória Mester and Ferenc Kuhn

 In the emmetropic human eye, the crystalline lens provides approximately one third of the refractive power necessary to project a focused image of the outside world on the retina. In younger individuals, the lens also changes its shape, maintaining a sharp view of the object even if it is close to the eye. To fulfill these requirements, the lens must maintain both clarity and position.

Although injury to the lens is rather common in serious eye trauma, it has received relatively little attention in the literature. Numerous publications discuss lens removal and IOL implantation in elective cases, but the number of reports dedicated to the same issues in the context of trauma is limited. Removing cataracts related to advanced age is the most commonly performed elective procedure in the human body, with very high rates of patient satisfaction once the eye's lost refractive power is restored. Management of mechanical lens injury, however, may involve a less favorable outcome while representing a much greater challenge. Several clinical dilemmas (see Table 21–1) need to be solved, and the most appropriate treatment option often remains elusive.

Removal of the injured lens is often complicated by:

- decreased visibility (e.g., corneal wound, hyphema, fibrin);
- injuries to adjacent structures;
- weakness of the lens zonules;
- injury to, and weakness of, the lens capsules;
- the potential for or presence of vitreous prolapse; and
- the attending surgeon's inexperience and lack of expertise in using vitrectomy instrumentation.

TABLE 21–1 BASIC MANAGEMENT QUESTIONS RELATED TO EYES WITH INJURY TO THE CRYSTALLINE LENS

Is the lens still in the eye?

If not, where is it?

Is the anterior lens capsule injured?

Is the lens cataractous?

If yes, does it hinder visualization of the retina?

If cataract is present but the posterior segment can be visualized, is the lens opacity likely to progress rapidly?

Is the posterior lens capsule injured?

Is the lens fragmented?

Is the lens swollen/swelling?

Is the lens firmly in its normal position?

Is vitreous prolapse present?

What is the condition of the vitreous and of the retina?

Is primary lens removal indicated?

If yes, what is the most appropriate method/technique?

Does the patient's age allow use of the vitrectomy probe?

If the vitrectomy probe is to be used, should a limbal or a pars plana approach be preferred?

In children, should posterior capsulectomy and anterior vitrectomy be performed?

Should an IOL be implanted at this time?

If yes, which type of IOL is the most ideal?

How should the IOL's refractive power be determined?

In this chapter we present a systematic approach to all of the important aspects of managing eyes with mechanical injury both to the lens and to IOLs (see Fig. 21–1).

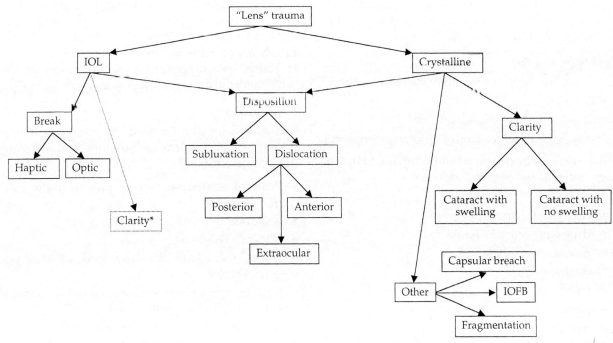

*Surface/s covered by material such as inflammatory debris or blood

FIGURE 21-1   Types of trauma involving the crystalline lens or IOL.

CRYSTALLINE LENS

Epidemiology and Selected Clinical Characteristics

Surprisingly little information is available on the epidemiology of lens involvement in the setting of serious eye injury.

Incidence: 23% *(USEIR[a])* to 50%[1] among serious eye injuries;

- 39% in open globe injuries;
- 11% in closed globe injuries (USEIR);
- 43[2] to 75% (HEIR) of traumatic cataracts occur in eyes with open globe injury.
- Incidence of trauma-related cataract among all cataract cases in children: 13 to 57%.[3–6]

Age:

- range: 0–97 years (USEIR) [HEIR: 5–81 years];
- average: 28 years (USEIR) [HEIR: 36 years];
- 53% of patients between 7 and 30 years (USEIR).

Sex: 84% male (USEIR, HEIR).

Source:

- 28% various sharp objects;
- 22% various blunt objects;
- 18% hammering/nail;
- 7% gunshot/BB/pellet guns;
- 6% fireworks (USEIR).

Place:

- 46% home;
- 18% industrial premises;
- 10% sports/recreation;
- 8% street and highway (USEIR).

Bystanders: 17% (USEIR).

Involved eye:

- 49% right;
- 3% bilateral (USEIR).

Injury type:

- 74% cataract (USEIR) [HEIR: 63%];
- 13% subluxation (USEIR) [HEIR: 23%];
- 13% dislocation (USEIR/HEIR); of these (HEIR): 61% complete loss (i.e., lens not found); 34% vitreous; 5% AC.

---

[a]Unless otherwise noted, all USEIR figures in this chapter relate to lens injury of any type; HEIR figures are based on an unpublished 1999 study on 196 eyes undergoing removal of a traumatic cataract.

A study from Kenya found different numbers: only 8% of patients were older than 30 years and 59% of injuries involved the right eye.[7]

Pathophysiology

The two basic types of trauma-related lens abnormality are:

1. loss of transparency (cataract); and
2. loss of position (subluxation or dislocation [luxation]).

The two may be combined and complicated by lens fragmentation and/or swelling.

Cataract can be caused by

- *nonmechanical factors* such as:
  - drugs (e.g., corticosteroids);
  - diseases (e.g., diabetes);
  - electricity[8];
  - laser[9];
  - microwave;
  - thermal, and UV energy; or
  - lightning;[10,11] and
- *mechanical factors*
  - Surgical intervention (e.g., gas or silicone oil injection) may also result in temporary or permanent lens opacification.
  - In open globe injuries, the agent can breach the anterior (and posterior) capsules, although this may also occur in closed globe trauma.[12,13]
  - In contusion injuries, coup and contrecoup forces may lead to cataract formation without (visible) violation of the capsules, although posterior capsule damage transmitted by movements of Wieger's ligament has also been described.[14]

SPECIAL CONSIDERATION

The presence of posterior capsule injury determines the method of choice for lens removal. In addition, if lens particles are dislocated posteriorly, the cortex/vitreous admixture may increase the severity of postinjury inflammation.[15]

Opacification usually, but not necessarily,[16,17] occurs if the capsule is injured, and successful prevention of cataract formation using human fibrinogen tissue adhesive has been reported.[18] The lens may remain at least partially clear even if an intralenticular IOFB causing siderosis is present,[19] or the cataract progression may be very slow.[20]

Following globe rupture, the surgeon may find no lens at all or one that is dislocated subconjunctivally.[21]

Such lens extrusions have been reported even after iatrogenic trauma (globe "explosion" after inadvertent intraocular injection of peribulbar anesthetic).[22] In contused eyes, the lens may dislocate suprachoroidally (C. D. Witherspoon, personal communication), anteriorly,[23] and, most commonly, posteriorly.[24]

Evaluation

The *slit lamp* is by far the most important tool in diagnosing a traumatic lens abnormality. The following must be determined.

- What associated injuries are present in the anterior segment?
- Is the anterior lens capsule breached?
- Is there a lens opacity?
- Is the lens opacity likely to progress and, if yes, how rapidly?
- Is the lens subluxated or dislocated (luxated) and, if yes, where and to what extent?
- Are there lens fragments/particles in the AC?
- Is vitreous present in the AC?
- Is the posterior lens capsule breached?
- Has the vitreous prolapsed into the lens, or, conversely, are there lens particles in the vitreous (is lens–vitreous admixture present)?
- Is there an IOFB in the eye/lens?
- What associated injuries are present in the posterior segment?

Especially in eyes with a corneal wound, edema, and/or fibrin and blood in the AC, it may be difficult to determine the following characteristics of the lens:

- clarity;
- position;
- stability;
- anteroposterior diameter (i.e., swelling); and
- capsule(s) integrity.

Retroillumination (see Chapter 14) may be helpful to reveal lens opacity and position, but the pupil may not dilate and false-positive findings may result because of material in front of the lens; vitreous hemorrhage may also interfere. In addition, even if the presence of a lens injury is confirmed, its visual significance may be difficult to assess.[1] Slit-lamp findings in case of subluxation are listed later in this chapter.

Additional helpful diagnostic modalities include:

- *IBO*;
- *ultrasound/biomicroscopy*[25] (although it may be ineffective in detecting posterior capsule damage[26,27]);[b]

---

[b]If the clinician performs ultrasonography on an open globe, extreme caution is necessary to avoid tissue extrusion.

• *CT*, showing lens damage in 38% of eyes that were diagnosed as clinically having an intact lens.[28]

PITFALL

Although CT has been reported to predict whether the lens in an injured eye will become cataractous over time,[28] it is not infallible and may fail to image an injured lens inside the eye.[29]

The question of whether the posterior lens capsule is intact is of crucial importance. The preoperative evaluation, even if carefully performed, may give a false-negative answer. In the HEIR, posterior capsule injury was found in:

• 23% preoperatively (another 10% was questionable);
• 45% postoperatively (another 8% was still questionable).

PEARL... The clinician must be cautioned against attempting overaggressive preoperative evaluation. In cases of closed globe injury, rarely is there a need for emergency intervention; in eyes with an open globe injury, an opportunity for a (much more) accurate evaluation will arise in the operating room (see Chapter 8).

Cataract

Strategy

There are two basic questions to answer:

1. whether primary or secondary cataract removal should be performed; and
2. if intervention is decided, what the most proper technique is.

Primary versus Secondary Cataract Removal   The advantages and disadvantages of primary extraction of a cataractous lens are listed in Table 21–2. The benefits and risks of primary removal must be carefully considered.

• The greatest benefit of primary removal is the surgeon's ability to inspect the posterior segment otherwise blocked by lens opacity. Involvement of the posterior segment is rarely mentioned in published series; the reported rate is 13[30] to 36%.[31]
• In addition, the lens-induced inflammatory reaction can be reduced/prevented.

PITFALL

It is not always easy to determine whether lens removal is necessary: the surgeon on call is often not the one most experienced and the operating facility may not be adequately equipped.[1]

TABLE 21–2   ADVANTAGES AND DISADVANTAGES OF PRIMARY EXTRACTION OF A CATARACTOUS LENS

Advantages

Eliminates the source of inflammation resulting from lens particles floating in the AC* or vitreous
Eliminates one potential source of IOP elevation
Allows visualization of the posterior segment
Allows early visual rehabilitation of the patient, which is crucial in the amblyopic age[6]
Establishing a clear visual axis in patients less likely to return for follow-up (crucial problem in developing countries)[7,41]
May allow single (rather than repeated) surgical intervention

Disadvantages

Increased risk of ECH
Lens may not have been truly cataractous
Cataract might not have become visually significant
Surgery in itself is a source of inflammation
Surgeon commonly inexperienced[1]
Operating room not always prepared for primary lens removal (fatigued personnel, late hours, etc.)[1]

*Usually better tolerated in children than in adults.

PEARL... **Both the USEIR and the HEIR found that one half of eyes with lens injury also had some type of posterior segment trauma. In addition, lens involvement signals significantly higher rates of serious vitreoretinal trauma when compared to eyes without lens injury (see Table 21–3).**

In general, primary cataract removal is recommended if the lens is:

• fragmentized;
• swollen; or
• causing pupillary block.

The results with primary lens removal are encouraging.[7,32,33]

Techniques of Cataract Removal   The *instrumentation* of lens removal is primarily determined by:

• the condition of the posterior lens capsule; and
• the presence of vitreous prolapse.

In open globe injuries, a breach can be expected:

• in the anterior capsule in 71% of the eyes (HEIR);
• in the posterior capsule in 38[7] to 45% (HEIR) of eyes.

In the HEIR, vitreous prolapse was found to be present in 34% of eyes.

PITFALL

If vitreous prolapse is (likely to be) present, instruments that aspirate without cutting must not be used; see Table 21–4 for our recommendations.

To restore the eye's lost refractive power (see later in this Chapter), preserving posterior capsular support for (simultaneous or subsequent) IOL implantation, while generally preferred, is only one of several options. The eye's overall condition and long-term prosperity should be taken into account.

PEARL... **The goal of preserving the posterior capsule for IOL implantation must not be the single decisive factor in the selection of surgical technique.**

An additional factor to consider when the surgeon is contemplating instrument selection is whether vitreoretinal surgery is also needed: vitrectomy has been

Table 21–3   Posterior Segment Involvement in Eyes with Lens Injury*

Variable	Rate	*p; risk ratio; confidence interval (95%)*
Posterior segment injury rate among eyes with any type of lens injury	48[†] to 51%	
Retinal detachment among eyes with lens injury of any type	14%	<0.0001; *2.11;*
Retinal detachment among eyes without lens injury of any type	7%	1.85/2.40
Vitreous hemorrhage among eyes with lens injury of any type	42%	<0.0001; *1.89;*
Vitreous hemorrhage among eyes without lens injury of any type	23%	1.77/2.00
Retinal detachment among eyes with cataract	12%	<0.0001; *1.64;*
Retinal detachment among eyes without cataract	7%	1.42/1.89
Vitreous hemorrhage among eyes with cataract	39%	<0.0001; *1.58;*
Vitreous hemorrhage among eyes without cataract	25%	1.47/1.69

*In the HEIR, 308 out of 705 eyes had lens injury of any type; in the USEIR, 2447 out of 10,450 eyes.

†Indicates information from the HEIR, all other data are from the USEIR.

Table 21–4   General Instrument/Technique Recommendations for Removing Traumatic Cataracts

Eye's Condition	Recommendation
Intact posterior lens capsule, no vitreous prolapse	Phacoemulsification (ECCE)
Posterior lens capsule's condition questionable, no vitreous prolapse	Careful phacoemulsification (ECCE); switch to vitrectomy if vitreous detected
Small posterior lens capsule lesion, no vitreous prolapse*	Careful phacoemulsification (ECCE); switch to vitrectomy immediately if vitreous prolapses; viscoelastics may help keep vitreous back
Large posterior lens capsule lesion, no vitreous prolapse	Vitrectomy
Vitreous prolapse	Vitrectomy, regardless of posterior lens capsule's condition

*Watch for lens capsule lesion's enlargement.

performed in 18% (HEIR) to 24% (USEIR) of eyes; one study[31] reported a 57% rate.

CONTROVERSY

If there is a need for posterior segment surgery during cataract removal, the surgeon may elect vitrectomy techniques,[c] rather than phacoemulsification, for lens removal.

The *incision site* for cataract extraction may be clear corneal,[34] limbal,[35] scleral,[36] or pars plana.[37] The selection is determined by several factors, including:

- site of the original wound (usually less traumatic if a new incision away from the wound is created);
- additional anterior segment injuries (e.g., avoid further compromising the cornea);
- the extraction technique applied and the need for vitrectomy equipment; and
- the surgeon's experience.

[c]That is, lensectomy.

If the *vitrectomy probe* is used, the surgeon can choose between various (original wound, limbal, and pars plana) approaches; Table 21–5 provides an overview of their advantages and disadvantages. Certain authors[38] prefer the pars plana approach, whereas others[39] found no difference. In the HEIR, the pars plana was used in 76% of eyes and the limbal route in 23%; only in 1% of the cases was the original wound utilized. The vitrectomy probe can be used in most patients up to 45–50 years old; beyond this age the nucleus usually proves to be too hard. In such eyes, careful combination of the vitrectomy probe to remove all prolapsed vitreous and pars plana phacofragmentation or vectis removal of the nucleus is recommended.

In children,[d] a unique problem is the high rate (39–92%[6,30,40–42]) of posterior capsule opacification. Because subsequent Nd:YAG laser capsulectomies have limited success,[43] it appears that performing primary posterior capsulectomy *and* anterior vitrectomy offers better long-term results.[7,37]

Another issue more common in children than in adults is the development of extraocular muscle

[d]See also in Chapter 30.

Table 21–5   Advantages and Disadvantages of Various Entries Using the Vitrectomy Probe for Removal of Traumatic Cataracts

	For	Against
Original wound	May be convenient	Corneal decompensation almost always increases
		Access is commonly limited, even within the AC
Limbal	Convenient Anterior lens capsule may be preserved	Corneal decompensation may increase Vitrectomy behind iris plane is impossible to complete
Pars plana	Corneal clarity maintained Full access to anterior and posterior abnormalities	Requires expertise, experience, and equipment Posterior lens capsule may be impossible to preserve centrally

deviation. It has been suggested that in such cases muscle surgery should be deferred for a year after cataract removal and IOL implantation.[44] Figure 21–2 provides an overview of the decision-making process.

Management

In virtually all cases, atraumatic closure of the corneal wound (see the Appendix) is the first step. *Not* using the original wound for cataract extraction avoids inflicting additional damage on the endothelium and Descemet's membrane. Any material (e.g., fibrin, blood) in the AC that hinders visualization of the deeper structures should be removed (see Chapter 17). Iris retractors have to be utilized if necessary to dilate the pupil sufficiently.

> **PEARL...**   If the anterior capsule is ruptured, use of scissors, rather than performing capsulorrhexis, is usually safer to achieve a capsulectomy because the zonules may also be torn. A capsule's rupture results in loss of the normal tension; therefore the incision is always smaller than intended/expected.

If no large posterior capsule lesion[e] and/or vitreous prolapse is present, phacoemulsification offers certain advantages over other methods of cataract removal, although the danger of a small capsular tear's intraoperative enlargement must be kept in mind. An AC maintainer or a butterfly needle-connected infusion is helpful in case SCH develops (see Chapter 22).

> **PITFALL**
>
> If vitrectomy behind the iris plane is performed from an anterior approach, an AC infusion is preferred to using an infusion sleeve over the vitrectomy probe. The fluid may otherwise get behind the vitreous gel, forcing more vitreous forward and possibly exerting additional traction.

---

[e]Remember that posterior capsule lesion may occur in an eye with closed globe (i.e., contusion) injury.

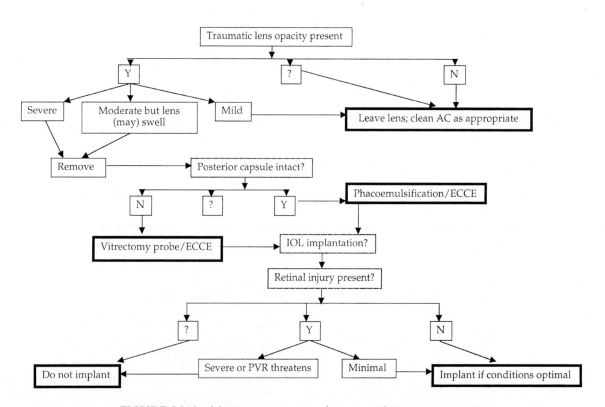

FIGURE 21–2   Management strategy for eyes with traumatic cataract.

The techniques of phacoemulsification, ECCE, or ICCE are not substantially different from those in elective cases. If the vitrectomy probe through a limbal approach is used and no vitreous prolapse is present, high suction and low cutting are recommended to remove a hard nucleus. Conversely, if vitreous prolapse is suspected, the suction rate must not exceed 200 mm Hg. Should the vitrectomy probe be introduced through the pars plana, it is difficult to preserve a sufficiently strong (i.e., supportive) posterior capsule.

PEARL... If the surgeon carefully polishes the anterior capsule,[36] the risk of capsule opacification is reduced and the anterior capsule will provide firm support for an IOL. Alternatively, an anterior capsulectomy may be performed.

Every effort should be made to:

- preserve as much of the posterior capsule as possible;
- preserve as much of the anterior capsule as possible if lensectomy is performed;[f]
- preserve as much of the capsule's zonular support as possible.

It is very helpful if the surgeon applies a bimanual technique for lensectomy. The vitrectomy probe should be introduced from the temporal side, even if this requires use of the surgeon's hand with less dexterity. Through the nasal pars plana incision, the surgeon inserts a conveniently bent 20-gauge needle[g] connected to the infusion line. Keeping this infusion inside the lens while the lens material is being aspirated prevents collapse of the lens capsules, which would lead to capsular injury with loss of lens material into the vitreous. The needle also acts as a second instrument, cracking larger pieces into smaller ones to allow their entry into the probe's port; by infusing the lens, recognition and removal of cortical material not yet cataractous also become easier.

If the nucleus is hard, an MVR blade may be helpful initially to break the nucleus into smaller pieces, but in older patients (see Table 21–6) ultrasonic energy is necessary.

PEARL... The technique of pars plana phacofragmentation is different from that in phacoemulsification. The goal is not to crack the nucleus in half but to maintain constant contact between nuclear material and the aspiration port by taking small bites along an advancing line ("nibbling"). This avoids a collapse of the lens capsule(s).

Filling the AC with viscoelastic material helps maintain its depth and prevent endothelial damage should the anterior capsule be breached.

PEARL... If the surgeon feels that the risk of (anterior) PVR is significant, removal of both lens capsules should be considered as an attempt at prophylaxis (see also Chapter 19): by removing the capsule, there is less surface ("scaffold") for the cells on which to proliferate and cause traction.

In young individuals with strong connections between the posterior capsule and the anterior hyaloid, anterior vitrectomy[h] has to be performed first; chemical zonulolysis should also be considered (alpha-chymotrypsin 1:5000/10,000). The capsule is then grasped with forceps[i] and removed; the probe is also helpful if the zonules are too strong. Table 21–7 provides a summary of the various extraction techniques.

SPECIAL CONSIDERATION

If an IOFB is lodged inside the lens (Fig. 21–3), siderosis development remains a threat[45,46] but cataract development is not inevitable.[17] If lens- and IOFB removal is decided, the surgeon must prevent the IOFB from falling back into the vitreous (e.g., using an IOM, see Chapter 24).

---

[f] As an alternative, both capsules may be preserved, see Chapter 25.

[g] The pars plana infusion should not be turned on until its correct position can be visually confirmed, that is, until the cataract has been reduced/removed.

[h] In general, sufficient anterior vitrectomy is recommended if vitreous is encountered in front of the posterior lens capsule's plane (see Chapter 17).

[i] A capsulectomy with the vitrectomy probe may have to be created first to provide a free edge.

TABLE 21-6   ADVANTAGES AND DISADVANTAGES OF VARIOUS TECHNIQUES FOR REMOVAL OF TRAUMATIC CATARACTS

Technique	For	Against
ICCE	Simple	Traction exerted on vitreous base/retinal periphery in patient young and if vitreous prolapse present
		Barrier between AC and vitreous gone
		Large incision required
		Significant ECH threat
		IOL implantation: limited options
ECCE	Relatively simple	Cornea may be further traumatized
	ECH threat somewhat smaller (smaller wound)	Traction exerted on vitreous in eyes with vitreous prolapse
		Relatively large incision required
Phacoemulsification	Relatively simple Small incision required	Traction exerted on vitreous in eyes with vitreous prolapse
	ECH threat much smaller (closed system)	Lens particles more likely to fall into vitreous if posterior capsule breached
	Early rehabilitation	Equipment required
Vitrectomy probe*	Corneal clarity maintained Vitreous prolapse/retinal pathology can be treated properly	Equipment/experience required Capsule preservation may be more difficult
	Small incision required	
	ECH threat minimized	

*See Figure 21–4.

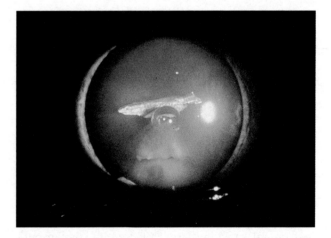

FIGURE 21-3   Intralenticular IOFB causing minimal cataract that has not shown progression over several months. The ERG does not show any sign of siderosis.

TABLE 21-7   SELECTION OF LENSECTOMY INSTRUMENTATION BASED ON THE PATIENTS'S AGES*

Age	Instrument and Technique
<20	Vitrectomy probe; aspiration without cutting usually suffices
20–45	Vitrectomy probe; cutting usually necessary[†]
45–55	Vitrectomy probe sometimes sufficient but use of another tool to crack to nucleus (MVR blade, needle) commonly necessary
>55	Phacofragmentor

*The years are approximate and individual variations exist.

[†]For example, lens removal in eyes that had or have silicone oil is difficult: the nucleus is hard and the posterior capsule not only opacified but so resistant that it is difficult to open it with a YAG laser; (see the Appendix.) A second instrument (e.g., a needle that also provides infusion) is helpful in fragmenting the lens and feeding it into the vitrectomy probe's port.

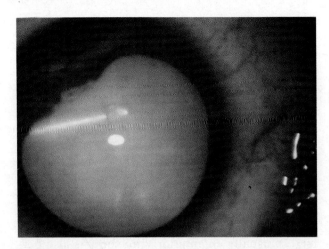

FIGURE 21–4 A 6-year-old boy sustained an ocular contusion from a bottle rocket. Because a posterior capsule rupture was suspected, the lens is removed with the vitrectomy probe; an iridodialysis is also present.

Complications

It may be difficult to differentiate tissue lesions caused by the intervention from those caused by the original trauma. *Intraoperative* complications include the following.

• Corneal decompensation commonly accompanies ICCE and ECCE but may also occur with phacoemulsification.

• If the IOP is too high and the wound is inappropriately closed, leakage may occur.

• A posterior capsule break may be caused/enlarged,[j] and lens particles may be lost into the vitreous.

• Hemorrhage (AC, vitreous, choroidal, even ECH) may occur if the IOP is too low.

• If a noncutting instrument (e.g., cryoprobe, phaco probe) engages the vitreous, traction ensues with severe complications (i.e., retinal tear along the vitreous base with subsequent development of retinal detachment).

Postoperative complications include the following.

• Anterior capsule opacification if it has not been polished adequately.

• Posterior capsule opacification in children, requiring surgical/YAG laser intervention in up to 100%

of eyes.[41,42,48] Primary posterior capsulectomy[k] (and anterior vitrectomy) reduces, but does not eliminate, this risk.[40]

• (Fibrinous) uveitis.[47]

• Anterior and posterior synechiae (see Chapter 17).

• Hypotony because of ciliary body detachment caused by contraction of the lens capsule, especially in young patients (see Chapter 19).

• Retinal detachment and CME[l] if vitreous traction persists.

PITFALL

Unless the posterior segment's condition was known before surgery, certain retinal complications (e.g., peripheral tear) may be conveniently but incorrectly attributed to the *injury* rather than to the surgeon's choice of an *improper cataract removal technique* (e.g., phacoemulsification instead of lensectomy).

In preventing/treating the complications, the most important factors are the following.

• Carefully selected type of and atraumatically performed surgery.[m]

• Generous use of topical (occasionally systemic) corticosteroids.

Prognosis

The visual prognosis of eyes with an isolated traumatic cataract is excellent;[n] in one study on closed globe injuries, 79% of eyes achieved ≥ 20/100 final visual acuity.[32] However, involvement of the posterior segment is a poor prognostic indicator.[30,35] In the USEIR, 28% of eyes achieved ≥ 20/40 final vision if the posterior segment was involved, compared with 47% if there was no vitreoretinal involvement ($p <0.0001$).

---

[j]Diagnosed in 42% of eyes in one study.[47]

[k]Commonly and incorrectly referred to as "capsulotomy"; the latter term should be used only when the capsule is incised rather than removed.

[l]Commonly caused by lens remnants hidden behind the iris.

[m]No difference was found in the retinal detachment rate when comparing three techniques: (1) lensectomy/anterior vitrectomy, (2) ECCE/IOL, and (3) ECCE/IOL/anterior vitrectomy/posterior capsulectomy.[37]

[n]So much so that it appeared as a "protective factor" during statistical analyses for the OTS project.

Subluxation

Partial dislocation of the lens typically occurs in closed globe injuries: as the globe's diameter in the frontal plane increases (see Chapter 17, Fig. 17–1), the zonules holding the lens in place may rupture. Along the rupture, the lens will tilt anteriorly or posteriorly; vitreous prolapse can also occur through the zonular breakage.

Symptoms do not necessarily develop but may include:

- deterioration of visual acuity;
- monocular diplopia;
- astigmatism;
- glare; and
- myopic shift.[o]

Findings include:

- inflammation;
- irregular AC depth in different meridians of the same eye;
- difference in AC depths between the two eyes;
- irido- and/or phacodonesis (best noticed if the pupil is undilated);
- visible lens edge (best noticed in retroillumination if the pupil is dilated);
- vitreous prolapse; in addition,
- iridodialysis; and
- elevated IOP are sometimes present.

The decision regarding which of the management options should be selected is primarily determined by the patient's complaints (unless IOP elevation is present; see Chapter 20):

- no intervention is necessary if the complaints are minimal;
- conservative treatment such as a contact lens may be attempted if the lens does become cataractous;
- miotics are not recommended;
- mydriatics are ineffective; and
- surgery is recommended if cataract is also present. IOL implantation is usually also performed (see later in this Chapter).

The *technique of lens removal* depends on the area of no zonular support and whether there is vitreous prolapse.[p] Iris retractors may be very useful if the pupil does not dilate.[49]

- ICCE: usually not recommended for fear of vitreo-retinal traction[50];

- ECCE and phacoemulsification: acceptable if no vitreous prolapse is present and if the area of zonulodialysis is small;
- lensectomy preferred if:
  - presence of vitreous prolapse is confirmed/cannot be excluded; or
  - there is extensive loss of zonular support.

Techniques described as helpful in lens removal include:

- use of a glide for hydroexpression[51]; and
- viscoelastics for lenses subluxated into the vitreous.[q]

Any vitreous prolapse must be removed (see Chapter 17); usually an anterior vitrectomy is also performed, and 360° scleral indentation (or endoscope use, see the Appendix) is necessary to ensure that no cortical lens material is left behind.

The rules of IOL implantation do not substantially differ from those described later in this Chapter. If the capsular support is only mildly affected, a capsular tension ring may be used,[52,53] but it must be understood that this puts additional stress on the remaining, potentially also weakened zonules. If there is substantial loss of zonular support, it is best to remove the capsules completely.

> **PEARL...** After removal of a subluxated lens, the fundus must always be carefully inspected for retinal injuries.

Dislocation

A lens whose zonular support has been completely severed, can be dislocated:

- *internally* (usually in contusion injuries):
  - in the AC[23];
  - suprachoroidally[54]; or
  - intravitreally;[24, r] or
- *externally* (typically in the context of globe rupture):
  - completely lost; or
  - subconjunctivally.[21]

The leading symptom is visual loss as a result of aphakia, combined with those of accompanying injuries and in case of an intravitreally dislocated lens, a positive scotoma that is mobile. An externally lost lens requires no special attention as it causes no further complications; a lens dislocated into the AC

---

[o]The lens takes on a more spherical shape.

[p]Posterior lens capsule rupture does not need not be present for vitreous prolapse to have occurred.

[q]R. Sorcinelly, Ocular Surgery News, March 15, 2000, pp. 70–71.

[r]A source of PVR development; see Chapter 23.

may cause severe corneal edema and IOP elevation, requiring urgent removal. The consequences[s] of lens dislocation into the vitreous (the most common type) include[55]:

- corneal edema (33–85%);
- inflammation (56–86%);
- IOP elevation (30–100%) (the various types of glaucoma caused by lens trauma are discussed in Chapter 20);
- vitreous hemorrhage (9–54%);
- CME (4–12%);
- retinal detachment (≤27%).

Left untreated, the condition is associated with an extremely poor visual prognosis. The rate and severity of complications increase if the lens is also ruptured or fragmented. The best treatment is lens removal during complete pars plana vitrectomy. The lens is extracted using one of these tools/ techniques:

- vitrectomy probe;
- phacofragmentation;
- limbal removal with the help of a vectis; and
- limbal removal with the help of an intraocular cryoprobe.

If the lens is fragmented and aspirated in the vitreous cavity, a pic fiberoptic or an endocryoprobe[56] may help stabilize it during the process. Nevertheless, the lens is likely to become fragmented with particles falling back onto the retinal surface.

> **PEARL...** During intravitreal phacofragmentation, never turn on the ultrasonic energy until the lens particle is first elevated, using suction only, into the midvitreous cavity. In one study, the rate of retinal detachment doubled to 24% in eyes with intravitreal phacofragmentation use.[57] PFCL[58] (see the Appendix) may be used to keep the lens at a safe distance from the retina (viscoelastics provide additional help; see Fig. 21–5).

The timing of vitrectomy[t] is still controversial, as some authors found no difference[59] whether the intervention was early or delayed. Most authors,[60–62] however, found much lower rates of complications and a significantly better outcome if the intervention was performed during the first week. In the context of trauma, this recommendation is probably even more true.

> **PEARL...** If the lens is traumatically dislocated into the vitreous, heavy topical, even systemic, corticosteroid therapy should be administered in the first few days, followed by surgical removal of the lens within a week after injury.

---

[s]The incidence figures are from nontraumatic cases.

[t]Based on nontraumatic cases.

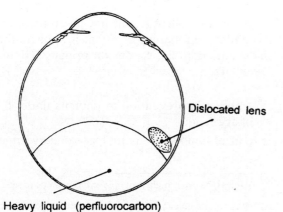

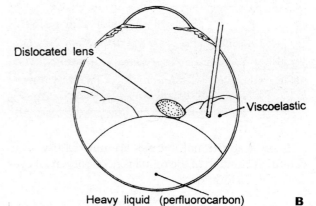

FIGURE 21–5   **(A)** If PFCL is used to elevate a dislocated lens (or IOL) from the retinal surface, the bubble tends to take on a spherical shape, and the lens slides sideways. **(B)** If a viscoelastic is injected circumferentially, the lens is kept centrally, making intravitreal manipulations much easier. (Courtesy of José Dalma-Weiszhausz, MD.)

IOL

Subluxation

In most eyes, it is possible to reposition and fixate the IOL by:

- simple rotating;
- positioning one loop in front of the remaining anterior capsule;
- suturing one or both haptics to the iris[63]; or
- suture-fixating one haptic to the sclera.

Dislocation

Trauma may dislodge an IOL anteriorly,[64,65] posteriorly,[66] or even subconjunctivally (see Chapter 27); in most cases, however, the IOL is found in the vitreous.[67]

The consequences of intravitreally dislocated IOLs include:

- decreased or, due to IOL movements, fluctuating visual acuity;
- monocular diplopia;
- halo phenomenon;
- inflammation;
- CME (17%);
- retinal erosion; and
- retinal detachment (6%).[66]

It is almost always recommended to remove the IOL, although it may also be retained and suture-fixated in the sulcus. Following a complete vitrectomy, the IOL is brought anteriorly using snares, standard or specially designed intravitreal forceps,[68] or PFCL.[69] A limbal extraction incision is preferred to a large pars plana wound.

> **PEARL...** Use of PFCL is especially helpful in the presence of retinal detachment and may also allow easier refixation of the IOL, although this is much less commonly advocated than in nontraumatic cases.[70]

Even if additional injuries are not readily seen, careful evaluation of the retina is necessary in all eyes with IOL dislocation.

Implantation

In eyes that had the injured lens removed, the following questions need to be answered: Is it necessary to implant an IOL? If yes, when? Which type?

Indication and Timing The aphakic eye's lost refractive power has to be restored.[u] In most cases, the IOL is the best option (see subsequently for alternatives to IOL implantation).

The initial question is whether the IOL should be placed at the time of primary reconstruction or whether its placement should be deferred. Primary IOL implantation remains a controversial issue. Although in selected cases primary implantation has been performed successfully,[1,7,31,34] the risk of complications following a combined procedure[v] is difficult to ignore:

- fibrinous uveitis in 25[71] to 100%[72];
- pupillary capture in ≤37%[71];
- synechia formation in 75%[73];
- lenticular precipitate formation in 75%[73];
- various posterior segment complications in 50%[74];
- retinal detachment in 18[75] to 20%.[34]

> ### SPECIAL CONSIDERATION
>
> **Primary implantation of an IOL introduces an additional source of inflammation and causes difficulties in case of subsequent vitreoretinal surgery by interfering with visualization (e.g., the edge of the IOL; inflammatory material accumulating on the IOL's surface; adherence to the IOL of intravitreal materials such as fluid in case of fluid-gas exchange[w] or silicone oil to silicone lenses). Table 21–8 lists conditions in which primary IOL implantation is *not* recommended.**

Because excellent results have been reported with secondary implantation,[3,47,73,77] it appears that the most important indications for primary IOL implantation are:

- amblyopia prevention in patients under 8 years of age[78]; and
- patients unlikely to return for secondary surgery.[7,41]

---

[u]Unless the eye is highly myopic or has no hope of seeing.

[v]It is not possible to determine what percentage of the complications are due to the original trauma.

[w]Silicone lens should *never* be used during primary IOL implantation if posterior segment involvement is present.[76] Viscoelastics may be used to remove fluid condensation from the IOL surface in a gas-filled eye.

TABLE 21-8 CONDITIONS IN WHICH PRIMARY IOL IMPLANTATION IS USUALLY *NOT* RECOMMENDED

Children <1 year of age

Patient at risk of being retraumatized in the near future

Severe inflammation/endophthalmitis present

High-risk injury (for endophthalmitis)

Significant corneal damage

Scleral wound[31]

Risk of AC re/bleeding (e.g., patients with sickle cell disease)

Significant iris loss

Inadequate zonular support for the remaining capsule

Inadequate/no capsular support and contraindications to AC IOL use

Posterior segment cannot be visualized

Serious posterior segment injury[7]

Increased risk of PVR

IOL power impossible to predict/calculate (e.g., anisometropia)*

Eye may not require correction (i.e., highly myopic)

---

*Although keratometry and knowledge of the fellow eye's axial length help in most cases.[31]

CONTROVERSY

IOL implantation appears to be the most effective method to fight amblyopia for some authors[79] but not for others[35,80] (see later in this Chapter). The age at which the procedure is safe is also debated; as early as 8 months has been recommended.[81] In addition, myopic shift because of IOL implantation in pediatric patients has been found by some[82] but not by others.[72,x]

Surgical Technique   In general, it is preferable to use a

- *PC IOL* and place it in the bag,[83] although no adverse affects are expected with sulcus-placed[6] or sulcus-fixated IOLs.[84,85]

Additional options include:

- *iris-fixated*, or
- open-loop, flexible *AC IOLs*.[86]

Additional findings to consider when the surgeon makes the individual decision regarding IOL placement are listed below.

- A PC IOL is more resistant to dislocation in a subsequent trauma than AC IOLs or iris-fixated IOLs.[87]
- Tilt and decentration are more likely to occur with sulcus-fixated IOLs.[88]
- Myopic shift is a greater risk with sulcus-fixated and out-of-the-bag than with in-the-bag IOLs.[88]
- If the IOL is placed in the sulcus and onto the anterior capsule, it is recommended to polish or centrally remove the capsule.[31]
- Improved techniques for suturing IOLs in the sulcus have been reported, minimizing the technique's inconveniences and complications.[84,85,89–91]
- If aniridia is also present, a specially designed black-diaphragm IOL[y] is available to counter the effects of iris loss (see Chapter 18).[92]

Alternative Methods to Restore the Eye's Refractive Power   In eyes in which IOL implantation is contraindicated:

- epikeratophakia[80]; or a
- contact lens[35] should be considered.

SUMMARY

Lens injury is common in eyes with serious trauma, although its presence may be difficult to confirm during the initial repair. If the surgeon is able to determine that cataract is present and it hinders visualization of the posterior segment, primary lens removal should be considered because vitreoretinal injuries are expected in approximately one half of eyes and an early retinal examination is mandatory in all eyes with lens trauma. Because of the high rate of posterior capsule injury, vitrectomy methods of lens removal are commonly required. Preservation of the posterior capsule is less important than avoiding traction on the anterior vitreous because alternative methods of IOL placement (e.g., onto the anterior capsule, iris- or sulcus-fixated, AC) offer similar functional results. Primary IOL implantation should be considered in eyes with no or minimal posterior segment injury and especially in children for amblyopia prophylaxis. In all other cases, there are strong arguments to delay the implantation.

---

[x] At the 2000 meeting of the American Academy of Ophthalmology in Dallas, Texas, an "accommodative IOL" was presented (HumanOptics, Germany); the device is not FDA approved and is still under investigation.

---

[y] Manufacturer: Morcher, Germany.

References

1. Lamkin JC, Azar DT, Mead MD, Volpe N. Simultaneous corneal laceration repair, cataract removal, and posterior chamber intraocular lens implantation. *Am J Ophthalmol*. 1992;113:626–631.

2. Blum M, Tetz M, Greiner C, Voelcker H. Treatment of traumatic cataracts. *J Cataract Refract Surg*. 1996;22: 342–346.

3. DeVaro JM, Buckley EG, Awner S, Seaber J. Secondary posterior chamber intraocular lens implantation in pediatric patients. *Am J Ophthalmol*. 1997;123:24–30.

4. Eckstein M, Vijayalakshmi P, Killedar M, Gilbert C, Foster A. Aetiology of childhood cataract in south India. *Br J Ophthalmol*. 1996;80:628–632.

5. Knight-Nanan D, O'Keefe M, Bowell R. Outcome and complications of intraocular lenses in children with cataract. *J Cataract Refract Surg*. 1996;22:730–736.

6. Zwaan J, Mullaney PB, Awad A, al-Mesfer S, Wheeler D. Pediatric intraocular lens implantation. Surgical results and complications in more than 300 patients. *Ophthalmology*. 1998;105:112–118, discussion 118–119.

7. Bowman R, Yorston D, Wood M, Gilbert C, Foster A. Primary intraocular lens implantation for penetrating lens trauma in Africa. *Ophthalmology*. 1998;105: 1770–1774.

8. Reddy S. Electric cataract: a case report and review of the literature. *Eur J Ophthalmol*. 1999;9:134–138.

9. Wollensak G, Eberwein P, Funk J. Perforation rosette of the lens after Nd:YAG laser iridotomy. *Am J Ophthalmol*. 1997;123:555–557.

10. Espaillet A, Janigian RJ, To K. Cataracts, bilateral macular holes, and rhegmatogenous retinal detachment induced by lightning. *Am J Ophthalmol*. 1999;127: 216–217.

11. Lagreze W, Bomer T, Aiello L. Lightning-induced ocular injury. *Arch Ophthalmol*. 1995;113:1076–1077.

12. Saika S, Kin K, Ohmi S, Ohnishi Y. Posterior capsule rupture by blunt ocular trauma. *J Cataract Refract Surg*. 1997;23:139–140.

13. Thomas R. Posterior capsule rupture after blunt trauma. *J Cataract Refract Surg*. 1998;24:283–284.

14. Campanella PC, Aminlari A, DeMaio R. Traumatic cataract and Wieger's ligament. *Ophthalmic Surg Lasers*. 1997;28:422–423.

15. Wallace R, McNamara J, Brown G, et al. The use of perfluorophenanthrene in the removal of intravitreal lens fragments. *Am J Ophthalmol*. 1993;116:196–200.

16. Hartnett ME, Coles WH. Lens clarity after vitrectomy in traumatic lens perforation and vitreous penetration. *Am J Ophthalmol*. 1993;116:250–251.

17. Pieramici D, Capone AJ, Rubsamen P, Roseman R. Lens preservation after intraocular foreign body injuries. *Ophthalmology*. 1996;103:1563–1567.

18. Buschmann W. Microsurgical treatment of lens capsule perforations. *Ophthalmic Surg*. 1987;18:276–282.

19. O'Duffy D, Salmon J. Siderosis bulbi resulting from an intralenticular foreign body. *Am J Ophthalmol*. 1999; 127:218–219.

20. Lee L, Briner A. Intralenticular metallic foreign body. *Aust N Z J Ophthalmol*. 1996;24:361–363.

21. Sathish S, Chakrabarti A, Prajna V. Traumatic subconjunctival dislocation of the crystalline lens and its surgical management. *Ophthalmic Surg Lasers*. 1999;30: 684–686.

22. Bullock J, Warwar R, Green W. Ocular explosion during cataract surgery: a clinical, histopathological, experimental, and biophysical study. *Trans Am Ophthalmol Soc*. 1998;96:243–276; discussion 276–281.

23. Netland K, Martinez J, LaCour OR, Netland P. Traumatic anterior lens dislocation: a case report. *J Emerg Med*. 1999;17:637–639.

24. Lam D, Chua J, Kwok A. Combined surgery for severe eye trauma with extensive iridodialysis, posterior lens dislocation, and intractable glaucoma. *J Cataract Refract Surg*. 1999;25:285–288.

25. Berinstein D, Gentile R, Sidoti P, et al. Ultrasound biomicroscopy in anterior ocular trauma. *Ophthalmic Surg Lasers*. 1997;28:201–207.

26. Clemens S, Kroll P, Busse H. Echographie der linsenhinterkapsel vor implantation einer kunstlinse. *Klin Monatsbl Augenheilkd*. 1987;191:110–112.

27. McElvanney A, Talbot E. Posterior chamber lens implantation combined with pars plana vitrectomy. *J Cataract Refract Surg*. 1997;23:106–110.

28. Boorstein JM, Titelbaum DS, Patel Y, Wong K, Grossman R. CT diagnosis of unsuspected traumatic cataracts in patients with complicated eye injuries: significance of attenuation value of the lens. *AJR*. 1995;164:181–184.

29. Almog Y, Reider-Groswasser I, Goldstein M, Lazar M, Segev Y, Geyer O. "The disappearing lens": failure of CT to image the lens in traumatic intumescent cataract. *J Comput Assist Tomogr*. 1999;23:354–356.

30. Krishnamachary M, Rathi V, Gupta S. Management of traumatic cataract in children. *J Cataract Refract Surg*. 1997;23:681–687.

31. Rubsamen PE, Irvin WD, McCuen BW, Smiddy W, Bowman C. Primary intraocular lens implantation in the setting of penetrating ocular trauma. *Ophthalmology*. 1995;102:101–107.

32. Chaundry N, Belfort A, Flynn HJ, Tabandeh H, Smiddy W, Murray T. Combined lensectomy, vitrectomy and scleral fixation of intraocular lens implant after closed-globe injury. *Ophthalmic Surg Lasers*. 1999;30:375–381.

33. Lam D, Tham C, Kwok A, Gopal L. Combined phacoemulsification, pars plana vitrectomy, removal of intraocular foreign body (IOFB), and primary intraocular lens implantation for patients with IOFB and traumatic cataract. *Eye*. 1998;12:395–398.

34. Pavlovic S. Primary intraocular lens implantation during pars plana vitrectomy and intraretinal foreign body removal. *Retina.* 1999;19:430–436.

35. Gelfand Y, Pikkel J, Miller B. Prognostic factors and surgical results in traumatic cataract. *Harefuah.* 1997; 132;18–21.

36. Ryan EJ, Gilbert H. Lensectomy, vitrectomy indications, and techniques in cataract surgery. *Curr Opin Ophthalmol.* 1996;7:69–74.

37. Basti S, Ravishankar U, Gupta S. Results of a prospective evaluation of three methods of management of pediatric cataracts. *Ophthalmology.* 1996;103:713–720.

38. Lucy S, Samir S, Ahmed Y. Pars plana versus limbal lensectomy in soft cataract. *Metab Pediatr Syst Ophthalmol.* 1992;15:60–63.

39. Ahmadieh H, Javadi M, Ahmady M, et al. Primary capsulectomy, anterior vitrectomy, lensectomy, and posterior chamber lens implantation in children: limbal versus pars plana. *J Cataract Refract Surg.* 1999;25: 768–775.

40. Anwar M, Bleik J, von Noorden G, el-Maghraby A, Attia F. Posterior chamber lens implantation for primary repair of corneal lacerations and traumatic cataracts in children. *J Pediatr Ophthalmol Strabismus.* 1994;31:157–161.

41. Eckstein M, Vijayalakshmi P, Killedar M, et al. Use of intraocular lenses in children with traumatic cataract in south India. *Br J Ophthalmol.* 1998;82:911–915.

42. Malukiewicz-Wisniewska G, Kaluzny J, Lesiewska-Junk H, Eliks I. Intraocular lens implantation in children and youth. *J Pediatr Ophthalmol Strabismus.* 1999; 36:129–133.

43. Buckley E, Klombers L, Seaber J, Scalise-Gordy A, Minzter R. Management of the posterior capsule during pediatric intraocular lens implantation. *Am J Ophthalmol.* 1993;116:656–657.

44. Alpar J. Monocular traumatic cataract, extraocular muscle deviation, and intraocular lens implantation. *Ophthalmic Surg.* 1992;23:166–169.

45. Keeney AH. Intralenticular foreign bodies. *Arch Ophthalmol.* 1971;86:499–501.

46. Klemen UM, Freyer H. Siderosis lentis et bulbi durch ein intralentales Rostpartikel. *Klin Monatsbl Augenheilkd.* 1978;172:258–261.

47. Bustos FR, Zepeda LC, Cota O. Intraocular lens implantation in children with traumatic cataract. *Ann Ophthalmol.* 1996;28:153–157.

48. Plager D, Lipsky S, Snyder S. Capsular management and refractive error in pediatric intraocular lenses. *Ophthalmology.* 1997;104:600–607.

49. Merriam J, Zheng L. Iris hooks for phacoemulsification of the subluxed lens. *J Cataract Refract Surg.* 1997;23: 1295–1297.

50. Aaberg TJ, Rubsamen P, Flynn H. Giant retinal tear as a complication of attempted removal of intravitreal lens fragments during cataract surgery. *Am J Ophthalmol.* 1997;124:222–226.

51. Blumenthal M, Kurtz S, Assia EI. Hydroexpression of subluxated lenses using a glide [Comment in Ophthalmic Surg 1994;25:657–658]. *Ophthalmic Surg.* 1994; 25:34–37.

52. Cionni RJ, Osher RH. Endocapsular ring approach to the subluxed cataractous lens. *J Cataract Refract Surg.* 1995;21:245–249.

53. Gimbel HV, Sun R, Heston JP. Management of zonular dialysis in phacoemulsification and IOL implantation using the capsular tension ring. *Ophthalmic Surg Lasers.* 1997;28:273–281.

54. Sneed S, Weingeist T. Suprachoroidal dislocation of a posterior chamber intraocular lens. *Am J Ophthalmol.* 1990;109:731–732.

55. Monshizadeh R, Samiy N, Haimovici R. Management of retained intravitreal lens fragments after cataract surgery. *Surv Ophthalmol.* 1999;43:397–404.

56. Rossi PL, Castiglioni C, Soldati MR, Monaco M. Cryofixation in the management of intravitreal luxated nucleus. 1998; *Ophthalmol Times.* 1998;June 15:67–69.

57. Borne MJ, Tasman W, Regillo C, Malecha M, Sarin L. Outcomes of vitrectomy for retained lens fragments. *Ophthalmology.* 1996;103:971–976.

58. Peyman GA, Schulman JA, Sullivan B. Perfluorocarbon liquids in ophthalmology. *Surv Ophthalmol.* 1995;39: 375–395.

59. Gilliland GD, Hutton WL, Fuller DG. Retained intravitreal lens fragments after cataract surgery. *Ophthalmology.* 1992;99:1263–1267.

60. Kim JE, Flynn HW, Smiddy WE, et al. Retained lens fragments after phacoemulsification. *Ophthalmology.* 1994;101:1827–1832.

61. Lambrou FH, Stewart MW. Management of dislocated lens fragments during phacoemulsification. *Ophthalmology.* 1992;99:1260–1262.

62. Yeo LMW, Charteris DG, Luthert PJ, Gregor ZJ. Anterior and posterior segment surgery: mutual problems and common interests. In: *Acta of the Fifth International Congress on Vitreoretinal Surgery.* Rome: Ophthalmic Communications Society; 1998:89–92.

63. McCannel M. A retrievable suture for anterior uveal problems. *Ophthalmic Surg.* 1976;7:98–103.

64. Khokhar S, Dhingra N. Anterior dislocation of foldable silicone lens. *Indian J Ophthalmol.* 1998;46:252–253.

65. Superstein R, Gans M. Anterior dislocation of a posterior chamber intraocular lens after blunt trauma. *J Cataract Refract Surg.* 1999;25:1418–1419.

66. Mello MO, Scott IU, Smiddy WE, et al. Surgical management and outcomes of dislocated intraocular lenses. *Ophthalmology.* 2000;107:62–67.

67. Bene C, Kranias G. Subconjunctival dislocation of a posterior chamber intraocular lens. *Am J Ophthalmol.* 1985;99:85–86.

68. Chang S, Coll G. Surgical techniques for repositioning a dislocated intraocular lens, repair of iridodialysis, and secondary intraocular lens implantation using innovative 25-gauge forceps. *Am J Ophthalmol.* 1995;119: 165–174.

69. Lewis H, Sanchez G. The use of perfluorocarbon liquids in the repositioning of posteriorly dislocated intraocular lenses. *Ophthalmology*. 1993;100:1055–1059.

70. Shakin EP, Carty JBJ. Clinical management of posterior chamber intraocular lens implants dislocated in the vitreous cavity. *Ophthalmic Surg Lasers*. 1995;26:529–534.

71. Vats D, Banerji A. IOL implantation in pediatric age group. *Afro-Asian J Ophthalmol*. 1993;12:338–341.

72. Thouvenin D, Lesueur L, Arne J. Intercapsular implantation in the management of cataract in children. Study of 87 cases and comparison to 88 cases without implantation. *J Fr Ophtalmol*. 1995;18:678–687.

73. Koenig S, Ruttum M, Lewandowski M, Schultz R. Pseudophakia for traumatic cataracts in children. *Ophthalmology*. 1993;100:1218–1224.

74. Tyagi A, Kheterpal S, Callear A, Kirkby G, Price N. Simultaneous posterior chamber intraocular lens implant combined with vitreoretinal surgery for intraocular foreign body injuries. *Eye*. 1998;12:230–233.

75. Chan T, Mackintosh G, Yeoh R, Lim A. Primary posterior chamber IOL implantation in penetrating ocular trauma. *Int Ophthalmol*. 1993;17:137–141.

76. Khawly JA, Lambert RJ, Jaffe GJ. Intraocular lens changes after short- and long-term exposure to intraocular silicone oil. *Ophthalmology*. 1998;105:1227–1233.

77. Mietz H, Konen W, Heimann K. Visual outcome of secondary lens implantation after trauma or complicated retinal detachment surgery. *Retina*. 1994;14:212–218.

78. Baxter R, Hodgkins P, Calder I, Morrell A, Vardy S, Elkington A. Visual outcome of childhood anterior perforating eye injuries: prognostic indicators. *Eye*. 1994;8:349–352.

79. Ben Ezra D, Cohen E, Rose L. Traumatic cataract in children: correction of aphakia by contact lens or intraocular lens. *Am J Ophthalmol*. 1997;123:773–782.

80. Uusiatalo RUH. Traumatic aphakia treated with an iris prosthesis/intraocular lens or epikeratophakia. *J Refract Surg*. 1997;13:382–387.

81. Lesuer L, Thouvenin D, Arne J. [Visual and sensory results of surgical treatment of cataract in children. Apropos of 135 cases]. *J Fr Ophtalmol*. 1995;18:667–677.

82. Kora Y, Shimizu K, Inatomi M, Fukado Y, Ozawa T. Eye growth after cataract extraction and intraocular lens implantation in children. *Ophthalmic Surg*. 1993; 24:467–475.

83. Pandey S, Ram J, Werner L, et al. Visual results and postoperative complications of capsular bag and ciliary sulcus fixation of posterior chamber intraocular lenses in children with traumatic cataracts. *J Cataract Refract Surg*. 1999;25:1576–1584.

84. Smiddy WE, Sawusch MR, O'Brien TP, Scott DR, Huang SS. Implantation of scleral-fixed posterior chamber intraocular lenses. *J Cataract Refract Surg*. 1990; 16:691–696.

85. Stark WJ, Goodman G, Goodman D, Gottsch J. Posterior chamber intraocular lens implantation in the absence of posterior capsular support. *Ophthalmic Surg*. 1988;19:240–243.

86. Mittra R, Connor T, Han D, Koenig S, Mieler W, Pulido J. Removal of dislocated intraocular lenses using pars plana vitrectomy with placement of an open-loop, flexible anterior chamber lens. *Ophthalmology*. 1998;105: 1011–1014.

87. Assia E, Legler U, Apple D. The capsular bag after short- and long-term fixation of intraocular lenses. *Ophthalmology*. 1995;102:1151–1157.

88. Hayashi K, Hayashi H, Fuminori N, Hayashi F. Intraocular lens tilt and decentration, anterior chamber depth, and refractive error after trans-scleral suture fixation surgery. *Ophthalmology*. 1999;106:878–882.

89. Akduman L. Transscleral fixation of a dislocated silicone plate haptic intraocular lens via the pars plana. *Ophthalmic Surg Lasers*. 1998;29:519–521.

90. Lewis J. Ab externo sulcus fixation. *Ophthalmic Surg*. 1991;22:692–695.

91. Uthoff D, Teichmann KD. Secondary implantation of scleral-fixed intraocular lenses. *J Cataract Refract Surg*. 1998;24:945–950.

92. Sundmacher R, Reinhard T, Althaus C. Black-diaphragm intraocular lens for correction of aniridia. *Ophthalmic Surg*. 1994;25:180–185.

Chapter 22

CHOROID

Nicholas E. Engelbrecht and Paul Sternberg, Jr.

 Two important trauma-related conditions involve the posterior uvea: choroidal rupture and SCH. The universally used term *choroidal rupture* is inaccurate because in addition to the rupture of Bruch's membrane, there is associated injury to the adjacent choriocapillaris and a break in the overlying RPE. It may lead to legal blindness if the fovea is involved. In *SCH*,[a] blood accumulates external to the choroid; the diagnosis may be difficult initially because of the presence of associated tissue injuries. SCH may develop/rebleed intraoperatively and result in the expulsion of intraocular contents with total blindness. Choroidal rupture is rather common[1] in contused eyes; SCH is less frequently recognized than its true incidence.

CHOROIDAL RUPTURE

Etiology and Diagnosis

Choroidal ruptures have been classified[2,3] as:

- *direct*, occurring at the site of impact, most commonly anteriorly and parallel with the limbus; or
- *indirect*, occurring away from the site of impact, usually in the posterior pole concentric to the optic disk or through the fovea (Fig. 22–1).

Choroidal rupture must always be ruled out in contused eyes; the lower (indirect) incidence figure[b]

---

[a] Also called ECH (see ref. 33); although the latter term suggests loss of intraocular contents, SCH and ECH are not clearly distinguished in the literature. SCH is the term used throughout this chapter.

[b] In the HEIR, the incidence of choroidal rupture is 10% among contused eyes and 1% among ruptured eyes (V. Mester and F. Kuhn, 1999).

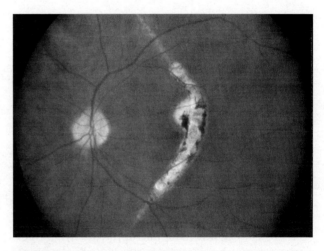

FIGURE 22–1 Fundus photograph showing a choroidal rupture through the center of the fovea.

in rupture injuries is probably due to the diffusion of the expansile forces and to the eyewall defect acting as a vent to release the force of the impact. The choroidal rupture in contusion trauma is probably caused by a rapid shortening of the globe's anteroposterior diameter and its expansion in the frontal plane. The relatively rigid sclera and the relatively distensible choriocapillaris and sensory retina are more resistant and thus less likely to rupture than Bruch's membrane. The crescent shape of indirect choroidal ruptures may be secondary to a "tethering" effect of the optic nerve.[4]

The diagnosis of an indirect choroidal rupture is easily made with the IBO; if obscured by overlying subretinal and/or vitreous hemorrhage,[4–7] the rupture remains invisible until the blood resolves, also limiting the usefulness of FA in earlier detection.[5–8] ICG imaging appears more helpful.[7,9,10] Studies of associated visual field defects have been inconsistent, but usually there is no direct correlation between the perimetry findings and the location of the rupture.[8]

> **PEARL...** Early identification of a transfoveal choroidal rupture assists the clinician in providing the patient with a more realistic prediction regarding the visual outcome.

Prognosis

The injured eye's vision can vary with time: it may be initially poor due to overlying hemorrhage but improve as the hemorrhage resolves. A more realistic prognostic indicator is the location of the rupture in relation to the fovea[4,11]; in patients with:

- *subfoveal* rupture, the vision tends to remain poor;
- *extrafoveal* rupture, the vision may remain excellent until and unless CNV develops;
- *contusion maculopathy*, the visual potential is limited (Fig. 22–2).

The development of CNV is a late (even 37 years after injury[16]) cause of vision loss[12–16] (Fig. 22–3). CNV presumably occurs from choroidal capillaries growing through the breaks in Bruch's membrane. Ruptures closer to the fovea and with greater length may have an increased risk of subsequently developing CNV.[11]

Treatment

- There is no treatment for the rupture itself, although surgery may be indicated for the subretinal or vitre-

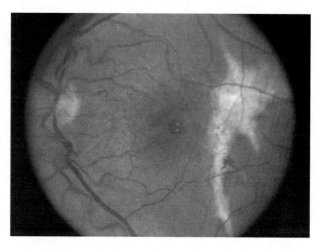

FIGURE 22–2   Choroidal rupture temporal to the fovea with associated traumatic macular hole.

ous hemorrhages (see Chapter 23). The CNV commonly regresses spontaneously[2] or may not progress, for which the relatively healthy RPE surrounding the lesions may be responsible.[16,c] Photocoagulation, even though shown to prevent the recurrence of CNV in association with choroidal rupture,[12,13] should therefore be used with caution.

> **PEARL...** CNV associated with choroidal rupture, usually responding poorly to laser photocoagulation, often involutes spontaneously, leaving a relatively small scotoma.

---

[c] Normal RPE cells have been shown to inhibit angiogenesis.[17]

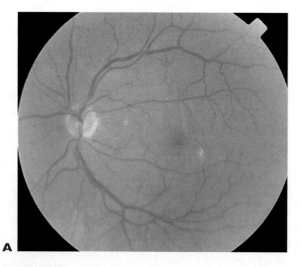

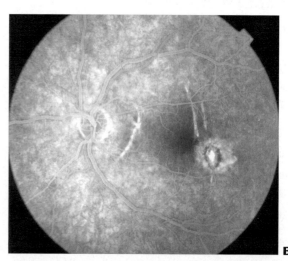

FIGURE 22–3   Choroidal rupture with associated choroidal neovascular membrane temporal to the fovea. **(A)** Clinical appearance. **(B)** Corresponding FA.

- *Extrafoveal* CNVs may be photocoagulated.
- *Subfoveal* and *juxtafoveal* lesions are usually observed, although successful surgical removal of subfoveal choroidal neovascular membranes in eyes with previously good vision has been reported.[18] Surgical results may nevertheless be limited by a high recurrence rate.

Photodynamic therapy may eventually become a treatment option; however, to date, there is no datum or even anecdotal clinical report regarding this treatment.

SCH[d]

Anatomy and Pathophysiology

The suprachoroidal space is a potential one between the choroid and the sclera, containing only approximately 10 μL of fluid.[19] The choroid is attached to the sclera at the edge of the optic nerve, at the scleral spur, and at the ampullae of the vortex veins. The arterial supply of the choroid comes mainly through the short posterior ciliary arteries[20] (Fig. 22–4); the long posterior ciliary arteries, passing within the

suprachoroidal space, contribute by forming anastamoses with the short posterior ciliary arteries.

Many hypotheses have been proposed for SCH development.[21–24] It is probably caused by the rupture of a short/long posterior ciliary artery, rapidly filling the suprachoroidal space with blood.

- SCH in open globe injuries may be related to direct trauma to the vessels.
- Contusion may cause SCH via vessel rupture due to shearing forces (anteroposterior shortening and equatorial expansion of the globe).
- SCHs can be precipitated by hypotony, presumed to lead initially to choroidal effusion with subsequent expansion of the suprachoroidal space, causing stretching and rupture of the ciliary arteries and potential expulsion of intraocular contents through the wound.[23]

Etiology, Epidemiology, and Risk Factors

SCH may occur intraoperatively[20–22,24–27] with tissue extrusion (expulsive SCH, Fig. 22–5), postoperatively (delayed SCH), or even spontaneously.[28–31]

---

[d]Much of what is presented here is based on nontraumatic SCH; the literature on injury-related SCH is limited.

> **PEARL...** The incidence of SCH in trauma is not known but appears to be greatly underreported. Analyzing the *pathological* specimens of a series of 28 NLP eyes that underwent enucleation due to rupture, an incidence of 100% was found even though *clinically* not a single eye was described to have SCH.[33]

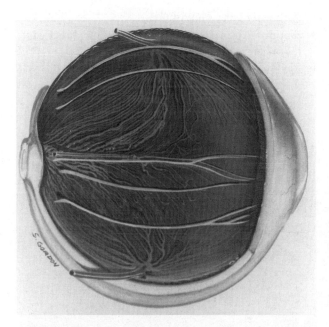

FIGURE 22–4 Drawing of dissected globe. Choroidal arteries that enter the suprachoroidal space by piercing the sclera surrounding the optic nerve can be seen radiating from the optic nerve (left). Two vortex veins are at the top and bottom. (From Tasman W, Jaeger EA, ed. *Duane's Foundations of Clinical Ophthalmology.* Philadelphia: Lippincott Williams & Wilkins, 1999:8, by permission from Lippincott Williams & Wilkins.)

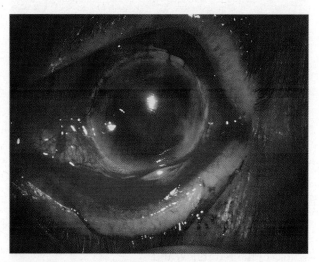

FIGURE 22–5 Clinical appearance of an intraoperative expulsive SCH (cataract extraction).

TABLE 22–1   RISK FACTORS FOR DEVELOPING (TRAUMATIC) SCH

Systemic	advanced age anticoagulation atherosclerotic disease blood dyscrasias diabetes mellitus hypertension
Ocular	aphakia/pseudophakia choroidal arteriolar sclerosis history of previous vitrectomy increased axial length increased preoperative IOP
Peri-/intraoperative	acute drop in IOP general anesthesia hypertension intraoperative tachycardia retrobulbar anesthesia without epinephrine Valsalva maneuvers vitreous loss
Postoperative	hypotony TPA use Valsalva maneuvers

TABLE 22–2   PROPHYLAXIS AGAINST (TRAUMATIC) SCH

Preoperatively	discontinue aspirin and anticoagulants when feasible lower the IOP if possible

Intraoperatively	use epinephrine if retrobulbar
	    anesthesia is applied
	maintain an intraoperative pulse rate
	    of less than 90
	avoid systemic hypertension
	avoid surgical trauma

Postoperatively	avoid Valsalva maneuvers avoid hypotony

Multiple risk factors for the development of non-traumatic SCH have been reported,[21,22,24–26,32,33] some of which may also play a role in the development of traumatic SCH (see Table 22–1). Few prophylactic measures to reduce the risk of SCH related to trauma are available (see Table 22–2).

> **PEARL...**   The surgeon must keep in mind that in eyes undergoing wound closure or secondary reconstruction following trauma, SCH may develop or rebleed with removal of the blood's tamponading effect when the eye is (re)opened. It is therefore crucial always to keep in mind that the time during which the eye is underpressurized (i.e., the wound is open) must be minimized.

Recognition and Management

Acute SCH

Common early signs of an intraoperative SCH include:

• shallowing of the AC;
• hardening of the globe (IOP elevation is likely to occur if tissue is being extruded);
• loss of the red reflex; and
• forward displacement of intraocular tissues/lens.

Late and poor prognostic signs include:

• tissue extrusion; and
• appearance of fresh blood.

> **PEARL...**   The most critical aspects in the management of an intraoperative SCH are early recognition and instantaneous restoration of the IOP.

To repressurize the eye immediately in case of an SCH (ECH), the surgeon has the following options:

• surgically close all wounds;
• reappose the wound lips by applying direct digital pressure; or
• use specialized tools (e.g., Byrne lens,[33] Fig. 22–6) if the wound is anterior and especially if it is large.

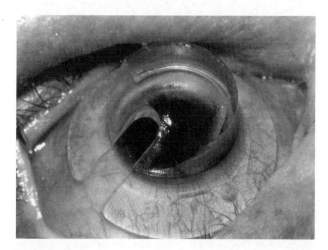

FIGURE 22–6   The Byrne lens, placed between the eyelids to maintain pressure on the globe while sutures are placed to close the surgical wound after an expulsive SCH.

> **PEARL...** Repositioning of prolapsed tissues in case of major intraocular bleeding is *not* a priority; tissue incarcerations may be best addressed secondarily.

Simultaneous drainage[34] is usually not advocated because of:

- poor initial drainage secondary to rapid clotting of the suprachoroidal blood;
- high incidence of reaccumulation of the hemorrhage;
- the threat of massive rebleeding if infusion is not (appropriately) used to maintain the IOP; and
- a lack of statistically significant improvement experimentally in the size or duration of the SCH.[22]

Delayed SCH

It is more common in patients with previous glaucoma filtering surgery, postoperative hypotony, or following Valsalva maneuvers, and is less severe than acute SCHs. Although expulsion of intraocular contents is rare, retinal apposition may occur. Delayed SCH may mimic the signs/symptoms of a retrobulbar hemorrhage[35] and usually causes severe ocular pain and loss of vision. The IOP may be elevated or low; in the latter case, it is crucial to restore the IOP as soon as possible.

Secondary Management

Systemic corticosteroids are thought to improve the prognosis.[33] A crucial question is whether drainage and/or vitrectomy should be performed. The two most important monitoring tools are the IBO and *ultrasound*[21,22,32,36]:

- A-scan shows clotted blood as a choroidal spike and a scleral spike with an intervening area of middle to low internal reflectivity, with liquefaction, the internal reflectivity becomes lower;
- B-scan shows clotted blood as a solid mass (Fig. 22–7); with liquefaction, the clot size decreases within a greater amount of fluid. Dynamic echography shows the movement of smaller clots within the liquefied blood.

> **PEARL...** Echography is helpful in determining the extent and consistency of SCH and, in patients with opaque media, identifying the presence of associated retinal detachment. It also assists in decision making (e.g., the need for, and timing of, secondary reconstruction).

Drainage indications include:

- uncontrollable pain[e]; and
- elevated IOP not adequately controlled with medical management.

---

[e]Believed to be secondary to stretching of the ciliary nerves within the suprachoroidal space.

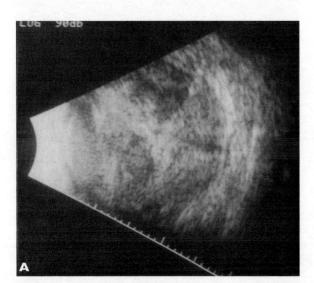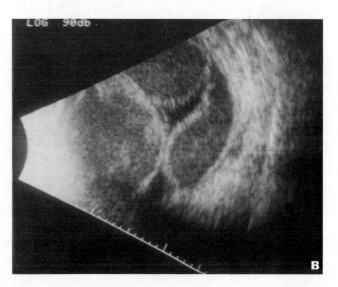

FIGURE 22–7   B-scan echography. **(A)** Initial appearance of SCH. Note the density of the clotted blood. **(B)** Same eye 10 days later. Note the decreased density of the liquefied blood.

Although time allows the clot to liquefy and the SCH may resorb spontaneously, vitrectomy offers an opportunity to drain the SCH even if it otherwise would not have been considered necessary. Ideally, however, drainage is not performed if the clot has not liquefied; this usually occurs in 7–14 days.

Early drainage may be unnecessary and:

- requires more skill; and
- has an increased risk.

If the clot is not liquefied, a surgeon experienced in vitreoretinal surgery may attempt "transscleral mechanical thrombectomy."[33]

Surgical steps of draining the suprachoroidal blood include the following.

- Determine the incision(s) site (IBO, ultrasonography).
- Introduce BSS infusion in the AC (if vitrectomy is also performed, an alternative is through the pars plana, using the 6-mm cannula; this infusion cannot be turned on until the cannula's tip becomes visible,[37] see Fig. 22–8); vitreous substitutes include:
  ○ BSS[38–40];
  ○ viscoelastics;
  ○ air (may interfere with visualization)[41];
  ○ silicone oil[42]; and
  ○ PFCL.[43]

- Create an axial posterior drainage sclerotomy.
- Apply gentle pressure (e.g., cotton-tipped applicator) or use careful manipulation (e.g., cyclodialysis spatula underneath the sclera) to release the blood. If the wound is too small, an L- or T-shaped incision is preferred.[33] The IOP must be monitored.

> **PEARL...** Even if the SCH involves all quadrants, one or two sclerotomies may be sufficient to drain most of the liquefied blood. Conversely, even vigorous efforts rarely allow complete removal of the SCH.

Vitreoretinal Surgery is usually performed in the presence of:

- incarceration of the vitreous and/or retina in the surgical wound;
- persistent vitreous hemorrhage;
- retinal detachment; and
- crystalline lens fragments in the vitreous (see Chapter 21).

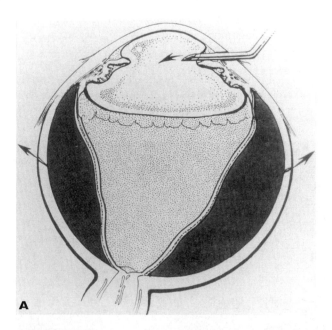 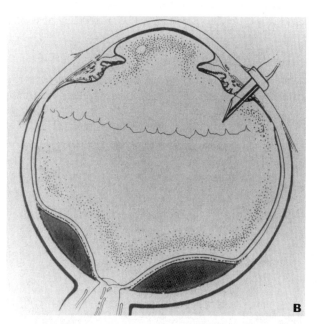

A   B

FIGURE 22–8 Surgical management of traumatic SCH with associated vitreous hemorrhage. **(A)** Scleral incisions to drain choroidal blood while a *limbal* infusion cannula is inserted to maintain the IOP. **(B)** After drainage, a 6-mm pars plana infusion cannula is inserted and infusion started only when the cannula can be visualized within the vitreous cavity. (From Sternberg P Jr. Trauma. Principles and techniques of treatment. In: Ryan SJ, ed. *Retina*. 2nd ed. St. Louis: Mosby; 1994:2370. Reprinted by permission from Mosby.)

SURGICAL TECHNIQUE　Vitrectomy is performed depending on the eye's specific condition (see Chapter 23). General comments include the following:

- Be careful before turning on the infusion (see earlier).
- The sclerotomies are not prepared or should be plugged until at least some of the SCH has been drained.
- Carefully monitor the IOP, never allowing the eye to become hypotonous.
- The PFCL "sinks" posteriorly and helps to push the remaining SCH through the drainage sclerotomy, which may be placed more anteriorly than usual.
- The peripheral retina may be displaced anteriorly and adheres to the iris; that is, it appears attached when in fact it is not. In such cases, one must either:
  ◦ start through limbal incisions and break the iridoretinal adhesions; or
  ◦ anticipate the need for a large peripheral retinectomy.

Outcomes and Prognosis

The prognosis of SCH is guarded, determined by:

- whether the initial wound closure was timely[44];
- the presence and nature of associated conditions (e.g., central choroidal apposition, vitreous or retinal incarceration, retinal detachment, APD, duration of central retinal apposition[46]); and
- the effectiveness of the secondary reconstruction.

The visual outcome is increasingly poor as the category/complexity of SCH increases.[47] Immediate retinal detachment is a poor prognostic indicator.[48]

---

[f]Most vitreoretinal surgeons consider it a fairly strong argument for intervention.

SUMMARY

Choroidal rupture in the posterior pole occurs in up to 10% of contused eyes. Poor initial visual acuity is due to a rupture underneath the fovea or to overlying subretinal/vitreous hemorrhage. Late decrease in vision is typically caused by a serosanguineous macular detachment because of CNV development. CNV may spontaneously regress or be photocoagulated or surgically removed, although the visual prognosis is guarded. Choroidal rupture, on the other hand, should not be regarded as a contraindication to surgery for other trauma-related conditions such as a macular hole.

SCH is a dreaded complication because of the potential for expulsion of intraocular contents and/or central retinal apposition. Intraoperative management includes immediate closure of the wound(s). Drainage during the primary management is rarely advocated. Postoperatively, the IOP, inflammation, and pain must be controlled. Indications for drainage/surgery include uncontrollable IOP and pain and certain posterior segment conditions (e.g., central retinal apposition, vitreous hemorrhage, vitreous/retinal incarceration, retinal detachment, retained lens fragments). The secondary reconstruction is ideally delayed for 1 to 2 weeks to allow clot liquefaction, determined by echography. The outcome is usually poor, although it varies with the complexity of the associated clinical findings. Immediate wound closure and meticulous reconstructive surgery, with drainage of the SCH if necessary, may improve the prognosis.

REFERENCES

1. USEIR, 2000.

2. Aguilar JP, Green WR. Choroidal rupture: a histopathologic study of 47 cases. *Retina*. 1984:4:269–275.

3. Postel EA, Meiler WF. Posterior segment manifestations of blunt trauma. In: Guyer DG, Yannuzi LA, Chang S, Shields JA, Green WR, eds. *Retina-Vitreous-Macula*. Vol 1, Philadelphia: WB Saunders; 1999:834–836.

4. Wyszynski RE, Grossniklaus HE, Frank KE. Indirect choroidal rupture secondary to blunt ocular trauma. A review of eight eyes. *Retina*. 1988;8:237–243.

5. Gitter KA, Slusher MM, Justice J Jr. Traumatic hemorrhagic detachment of the retinal pigment epithelium. *Arch Ophthalmol*. 1968;79:729–732.

6. Gass JDM. *Stereoscopic Atlas of Macular Disease. Diagnosis and Treatment*. 3rd ed. St. Louis: CV Mosby; 1987:170–171.

7. Kohno T, Miki T, Hayashi K. Choroidopathy after blunt trauma to the eye: a fluorescein and indocyanine green angiographic study. *Am J Ophthalmol*. 1998;126:248–260.

8. Dean Hart JC, Natsikos VE, Raistrick ER, Doran ML. Indirect choroidal tears at the posterior pole: a fluorescein angiographic and perimetric study. *Br J Ophthalmol*. 1980;64:59–67.

9. Baltatzis S, Ladas ID, Panagiotidis D, Theodossiadis GP. Multiple posttraumatic choroidal ruptures obscured by hemorrhage: imaging with indocyanine green angiography. *Retina*. 1997;17:352–354.

10. Kohno T, Miki T, Shiraki K, Kano K, Hirabayashi-Matsushita M. Indocyanine green angiographic features of choroidal rupture and choroidal vascular injury after contusion ocular injury. *Am J Ophthalmol*. 2000;129:38–46.

11. Secretan M, Sickenberg M, Zografos L, Piguet B. Morphometric characteristics of traumatic choroidal ruptures associated with neovascularization. *Retina*. 1998;18:62–66.

12. Fuller B, Gitter KA. Traumatic choroidal rupture with late serous detachment of macula. Report of successful argon laser treatment. *Arch Ophthalmol*. 1973;89:354–355.

13. Smith RE, Kelley JS, Harbin TS. Late macular complications of choroidal ruptures. *Am J Ophthalmol*. 1974;77:650–658.

14. Hilton GF. Late serosanguineous detachment of the macula after traumatic choroidal rupture. *Am J Ophthalmol*. 1975;79:997–1000.

15. Luxenburg MN. Subretinal neovascularization associated with rupture of the choroid. *Arch Ophthalmol*. 1986;104:1233.

16. Wood CM, Richardson J. Chorioretinal neovascular membranes complicating contusional eye injuries with indirect choroidal ruptures. *Br J Ophthalmol*. 1990;74:93–96.

17. Glaser BM, Campochario PA, Davis JL, Sato M. Retinal pigment epithelial cells release an inhibitor of neovascularization. *Arch Ophthalmol*. 1985;103:1870–1875.

18. Gross JG, King LP, de Juan E Jr, Powers T. Subfoveal neovascular membrane removal in patients with traumatic choroidal rupture. *Ophthalmology*. 1996;103:579–585.

19. Hawkins WR, Schepens CL. Choroidal detachment and retinal surgery. *Am J Ophthalmol*. 1966;62:813–819.

20. Last RJ, ed. *Eugene Wolff's Anatomy of the Eye and Orbit*. 6th ed. Philadelphia: WB Saunders; 1968:90–93.

21. Chu TG, Green RL. Suprachoroidal hemorrhage. *Surv Ophthalmol*. 1999;43:471–486.

22. Lakhanpal V. Experimental and clinical observations on massive SCH. *Trans Am Ophthalmol Soc*. 1989;91:545–652.

23. Beyer CF, Peyman GA, Hill JM. Expulsive choroidal hemorrhage in rabbits. A histopathologic study. *Arch Ophthalmol*. 1989;107:1648–1653.

24. Sekine Y, Takei K, Saotome T, Hommura S. Survey of risk factors for expulsive choroidal hemorrhage: case reports. Substantiation of the risk factors and their incidence. *Ophthalmologica*. 196;210:344–347.

25. Speaker MG, Guerriero PN, Met JA, Coad CT, Berger A, Marmor M. A case-control study of risk factors for intraoperative suprachoroidal expulsive hemorrhage. *Ophthalmology*. 1991;98:202–210.

26. Tabandeh H, Sullivan PM, Smahliuk P, Flynn HW, Schiffman J. Suprachoroidal hemorrhage during pars plana vitrectomy. Risk factors and outcomes. *Ophthalmology*. 1999;106:236–242.

27. Fastenberg DM, Perry HD, Donnenfeld ED, Schwartz PL, Shakin JL. Expulsive SCH with scleral buckling surgery. *Arch Ophthalmol*. 1991;109:323.

28. Williams DK, Rentiers PK. Spontaneous expulsive choroidal hemorrhage: a clinicopathologic report of 2 cases. *Arch Ophthalmol*. 1970;83:191–194.

29. Perry HD, Hsieh RL, Evans RM. Malignant melanoma of the choroid associated with spontaneous expulsive choroidal hemorrhage. *Am J Ophthalmol*. 1977;84:205–208.

30. Chorich LJ, Derick RJ, Chambers RB, et al. Hemorrhagic ocular complications associated with the use of systemic thrombolytic agents. *Ophthalmology*. 1998;105:428–431.

31. Margo CE, Bullington WD, Pautler S. Occult SCH and posterior scleral rupture. *Am J Ophthalmol*. 1988;106:358–359.

32. Reynolds MG, Haimovici R, Flynn HW, DiBernardo C, Byrne SF, Feuer W. Suprachoroidal hemorrhage. Clinical features and results of secondary surgical management. *Ophthalmology*. 1993;100:460–465.

33. Kuhn F, Morris R, Mester V, Witherspoon D. Management of intraoperative expulsive choroidal hemorrhage during anterior segment surgery. In: Stripe M, ed. *Anterior and Posterior Segment Surgery: Mutual Problems and Common Interests*. New York: Ophthalmic Communications Society; 1998:191–203.

34. Verhoff FH. Scleral puncture for expulsive SCH following sclerotomy: scleral puncture for postoperative separation of the choroid. *Ophthalmic Res.* 1915;24:55–59.

35. Gordon JA, Wulc AE, Budenz DL, Nevyas HJ. Delayed SCH mimicking acute retrobulbar hemorrhage. *Surv Ophthalmol.* 1995;40:229–231.

36. Chu TG, Cano MR, Green RL, Liggett PE, Lean JS. Massive SCH with central retinal apposition. A clinical and echographic study. *Arch Ophthalmol.* 1991;109:1575–1581.

37. Sternberg P Jr. Trauma: principles and techniques of treatment. In: Ryan SJ, ed. *Retina.* 2nd ed. St. Louis: Mosby; 1994:2369–2371.

38. Lakhanpal V, Schocket SS, Elman MJ, Nirankari VS. A new modified vitreoretinal surgical approach in the management of massive SCH. *Ophthalmology.* 1989;96:793–800.

39. Eller AW, Adams EA, Fanous MM. Anterior chamber maintainer for drainage of SCH. *Am J Ophthalmol.* 1994;118:258–259.

40. Lambrou FH Jr, Meredith TA, Kaplan HJ. Secondary management of expulsive choroidal hemorrhage. *Arch Ophthalmol.* 1987;105:1195–1198.

41. Abrams GW, Thomas MA, Williams GA, Burton TC. Management of postoperative SCH with continuous-infusion air pump. *Arch Ophthalmol.* 1986;104:1455–1458.

42. Alexandridis E. Silicone oil tamponade in the management of severe hemorrhagic detachment of the choroid and ciliary body after surgical trauma. *Ophthalmologica.* 1990;200:189–193.

43. Desai UR, Peyman GA, Chen CJ, et al. Use of perfluoroperhydrophenanthrone in the management of SCHs. *Ophthalmology.* 1992;99:1542–1547.

44. Berrocal JAR. Adhesion of the retina secondary to large choroidal detachments as a cause of failure in retinal detachment surgery. *Mod Prob Ophthalmol.* 1979;20:51–52.

45. Weinberg DV, Rosenberg LF. Retina to retina adhesions following SCH. *Br J Ophthalmol.* 1996;80:674.

46. Scott IU, Flynn HW, Schiffman J, Smiddy WE, Ehlies F. Visual acuity outcomes among patients with appositional SCH. *Ophthalmology.* 1997;104:2039–2046.

47. Wirostkko WJ, Han DP, Mieler WF, Pulido JS, Connor TB Jr, Kuhn E. Suprachoroidal hemorrhage. Outcome of surgical management according to hemorrhage severity. *Ophthalmology.* 1998;105:2271–2275.

48. Welch JC, Spaeth GL, Benson WE. Massive SCH. Follow-up and outcome of 30 cases. *Ophthalmology.* 1988;95:1202–1206.

Chapter 23

VITREOUS AND RETINA

Kah-Guan Au Eong, David Kent, and Dante J. Pieramici

The incidence of serious[a] ocular injuries shows no sign of abating. This is despite intensive efforts to heighten public awareness through robust educational campaigns and explicit warnings directed at prevention in the home, at the workplace, and during recreation (see Chapters 4 and 27). The physical, psychological, and socioeconomic suffering of individuals afflicted with severe ocular trauma can last a lifetime, and the financial implications, both personal and in terms of national productivity and health care maintenance, are incalculable.

In the last decade, refined microsurgical techniques and instrumentation, the availability of intraocular antibiotics, and a better understanding of the pathophysiology of the severely injured eye have resulted in the improvement of the visual outcome in patients with severe ocular trauma (see Chapters 8 and 24). Even in cases with a discouraging visual prognosis, the benefits in terms of good cosmetic reconstruction and repair should not be underestimated (see Chapters 25 and 31).

This chapter deals with the clinical features, pathophysiology, and management of closed and open trauma involving the two structures of the posterior segment that are most commonly injured. Trauma involving the choroid, IOFBs, and the optic nerve are discussed in Chapters 22, 24, and 37, respectively; Chapters 16 and 26 address additional issues related to the vitreous and the retina.

EPIDEMIOLOGY AND PREVENTION

Recent epidemiological data confirm the disturbing trend in the prevalence of severe ocular trauma.[1] The home has now surpassed the workplace as the most common site for serious ocular injury, testament perhaps to the huge growth of the "do-it-yourself" home enthusiast and/or a decrease in work-related injury (see Chapter 4). They also confirm that most eye injuries are preventable, occurring in people who wear no eye protection.[1–4,b]

Traumas from blunt and sharp objects are the two major causes of severe ocular injuries, and in the USEIR, the retina and vitreous are second only to the cornea as the most frequently involved ocular tissues.[1] It is no coincidence, therefore, that the posterior segment manifestations of severe ocular trauma are foremost as the cause of severe and permanent visual morbidity (Fig. 23–1).

Retinal detachment following contusion is not uncommon[5,6] and is observed primarily in males,[4,7–10] especially in the younger age groups.[1,2,8–10]

The USEIR found the following information.

Rate of retinal involvement among all serious injuries: 31%.

- Among closed globe injuries: 34%.
- Among open globe injuries: 29%.

---

[a]Defined by the USEIR as trauma resulting in permanent and significant structural and/or functional changes to the eye (see Chapter 4).

[b]The protection afforded by ordinary prescription spectacles (see Chapter 4) is of some benefit in reducing or preventing eye injury.[1,2]

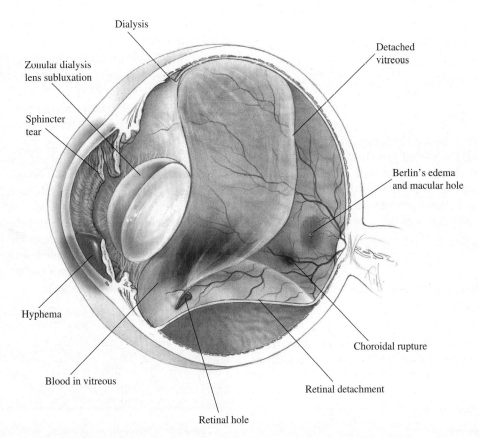

FIGURE 23–1 Various intraocular injuries involving both the anterior and posterior segments can result from trauma by blunt objects. (From Aaberg TM and Sternberg P. Blunt and penetrating ocular injuries. In: Regillo CD, Brown GC, Flynn HW, ed. *Vitreoretinal Diseases: The Essentials.* New York: Thieme; 1999:515.)

Rate of vitreous involvement among all serious injuries: 31%.

- Among closed globe injuries: 22%.
- Among open globe injuries: 40%.

Rate of vitreoretinal involvement among all serious injuries: 44%.

Age (years):

- range: 0–103;
- mean: 30;
- ≤15: 25%;
- 20 to 39: 49%;
- ≥60: 8%.

Sex: 82% *males*.

Place:

- Home: 41%;
- Place for recreation and sport: 15%;
- Industrial premises: 14%;
- Street and highway: 11%.

Cause:

- blunt object: 32%
- sharp object: 14%
- BB/pellet gun: 9%;
- gunshot: 8%;
- hammering: 7%
- MVC: 7%;
- fireworks: 6%;
- nail: 6%.

Among retinal injuries (=100%):

- hemorrhage: 35%;
  ◦ macular: 5%;
- defect: 20%;
  ◦ macular hole: 0.07%; among eyes with contusion:[c] 1.4%; among eyes with open globe injury:[d] 0.15%;

---

[c]Eyes with contusion = 100%.

[d]Eyes with open globe injury = 100%.

- retinal commotio: 9%
  - macular commotio: 4%;
- retinal detachment: 26%;
  - hemorrhagic: 7%;
  - rhegmatogenous: 8%;
  - macular: 2%.

Despite tremendous advances in therapy, the mainstay of tackling the global problem of ocular trauma (see Chapter 4) remains prevention. Time and again, it has been shown that regardless of the setting, the correct ocular protection not only prevents injuries[11–14] but also markedly reduces the severity of injury.

RETINA

Closed Globe Injury
Pathophysiology

High-speed cinematography was used to study experimentally the effects of contusion resulting from high-speed pellets.[15] The ocular damage resulting from the impact could be explained in four phases of globe deformation:

1. compression;
2. decompression;
3. overshooting;
4. oscillations.

It appears that both retinal dialysis and peripheral retinal tears occur secondary to tractional forces generated at the vitreous base as the equatorial diameter of the globe increases rapidly.[16]

> **PEARL...** The vitreous body is relatively inelastic and cannot stretch when the eye is rapidly compressed.

Retinal breaks can occur via the following mechanisms:

- *Vitreous base avulsion.* Extreme traction on the vitreous base may cause its anterior border to be ripped from either the retina or pars plana.[16] The distribution of the retinal tears in this model mirrors closely the retinal changes seen clinically.[17,18]

> **PEARL...** It is probably the site of the initial impact that determines the exact distribution of the consequent retinal abnormalities.[16]

- *Abnormal sites of vitreoretinal adhesion* (e.g., lattice degeneration).
- *Coup injury.* Local trauma at the site of scleral impact[19] induces a direct, concussive, full-thickness necrosis of the overlying retina.[20,e]
- The induction of *sudden posterior vitreous detachment*.

Evaluation

Fundamental in the evaluation of any patient presenting with ocular trauma is a comprehensive history and a careful physical examination (see Chapters 8 and 9).

The precise circumstances surrounding the injury must be thoroughly elucidated and the exact mechanism of the injury[f] must be ascertained; this helps predict whether vitreoretinal involvement must be anticipated. It is essential to establish the shape of the agent, that is, blunt versus sharp.

> **PEARL...** In cases of a projectile causing ocular trauma, the foreign body must be assumed intraocular until proved otherwise (see Chapter 24).

The importance of examining *both* eyes cannot be overemphasized.

> **PEARL...** "In the heat of moment" the physician is often preoccupied with ascertaining the full extent of damage to the eye the patient is referring to or the eye obviously involved, while the other eye may also harbor serious disease.[g]

> ▼ **PITFALL**
>
> The possibility of bilateral ocular injury should always be excluded despite a unilateral presentation.[2]

---

[e]In open globe trauma, a direct injury mechanism may also contribute; see later.

[f]For example, a patient presenting with a history of pounding metal on metal needs to be thoroughly evaluated for an IOFB; in case of injury caused by a knife, it is very unlikely that an object is retained inside the globe.

[g]Individuals presenting with trauma caused by a blunt object often have a history of repeated trauma to either eye.[2]

Corroborative sources of information should be sought and questioned even after the initial presentation.

- Regardless of how mild or severe an ocular injury first appears, a baseline visual acuity for *both* eyes should be recorded (see Chapter 9).
- The presence or absence of an APD should be documented as this provides vital prognostic information for the visual outcome (see Chapter 3).[21]
- It is imperative to comment on the integrity of each ocular structure in turn.
- Media opacities (e.g., corneal edema, hyphema, cataract, vitreous hemorrhage) can make thorough evaluation of the posterior segment extremely difficult or even impossible.

PEARL... In the absence of a clear IBO view of the ocular fundus, B-scan ultrasonography is an excellent alternative (see Chapter 9). It should be repeated periodically until the view improves or intraocular pathology requiring surgical intervention is detected.

PITFALL

The presence of an anatomically normal anterior segment, normal vision, or lack of pain should not deter the examiner from seeking the possibility of serious and sight-threatening posterior segment pathology.[10]

It must be remembered that retinal tears and detachment may develop years after the original trauma.

PEARL... All patients with a history of contusion should be followed at least until the ora serrata can be viewed for 360°.[17,18,22,23]

Clinical Conditions

***Commotio Retinae*[h]** is a relatively common consequence of contusion.

CLINICAL FEATURES First described in 1873,[24] this injury is typically caused by contusion and is characterized by transient gray-white discoloration or opacification of the outer sensory retina. The opacification may be confined to the macula or may involve extensive areas of the peripheral retina.[25]

When the posterior pole is affected, a cherry-red spot at the fovea mimicking that in acute central retinal artery occlusion may be seen. There may be associated hemorrhage (preretinal, retinal, subretinal) and choroidal rupture (Fig. 23–2).[25]

The symptoms are determined primarily by the location of the lesion, for example, its relation to the macula. The patient may have no visual complaints if only the peripheral retina is involved or severe visual impairment if extensive macular lesions are present. As the retinal opacification resolves, vision may return to normal and there may be no ophthalmoscopic findings after the resolution.

---

[h]That is, retinal contusion or Berlin's edema.

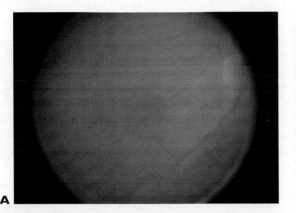 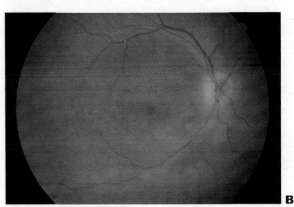

FIGURE 23–2 **(A)** Patient presents following severe contusion to eye. Examination discloses retinal whitening in the posterior pole and in the periphery consistent with commotio retinae. **(B)** Within a few days, the retinal whitening has subsided and RPE pigmentary disturbance in noted in the macula.

<table><tr><td>

PITFALL

A macular hole may rapidly develop, and, if untreated, it may permanently impair vision.
</td></tr></table>

Pigmentary disturbance may occur following commotio retinae; with resolution of the edema, it may mimic retinitis pigmentosa.[26,27]

PATHOPHYSIOLOGY   The pathophysiology of commotio retinae has been the subject of much controversy. It was originally postulated that the retinal opacification was due to extracellular edema.[24] Later experimental studies, however, identified disruption of the photoreceptor outer segments as the main histopathologic findings.[28–30] One experimental study[28] found the following.

• Disruption of photoreceptor outer segments occurred immediately after injury.
• Phagocytosis of the fragmented outer segments by RPE cells developed at 24 hours.
• Within 48 hours after the injury, RPE cells had begun to migrate among the outer segment fragments and into the outer retina. This migration reached as far as the ganglion cell and inner plexiform layers.
• The RPE became a multilayered, disorganized structure on Bruch's membrane with atrophy of the overlying photoreceptor outer segment.
• In areas of severe atrophy, the photoreceptor outer segment could not be detected at all, resulting in direct apposition of the inner segment with the RPE.
• There was *no* evidence of intracellular or extracellular retinal edema in this animal model, which appears clinically similar to patients with this condition.
  ○ No leakage of fluorescein from retinal capillaries could be demonstrated at any time after injury.

PEARL... Commotio retinae is associated not with extracellular edema but with disruption of photoreceptor outer segments.[28]

An FA study[30] found the following.

• No fluorescein leaked from the retinal vessels 30 minutes after injury, but there was progressive staining of the RPE in the posterior pole.

• Following severe ocular contusion, the RPE underlying the opacified retina undergoes significant anatomic and functional changes.
• These changes range from cellular disruption immediately after the injury to rounding up and migration of RPE cells into the outer layers of the neurosensory retina.
• Eventually, hyperplasia of the RPE occurs.

A histopathologic study[31,i] in humans found the following.

• Photoreceptor outer segment disruption and damage to the RPE.
• Only a minimal amount of albumin around retinal vessels was detected by immunohistochemistry, indicating the minimal role of the blood-retinal barrier defect in the pathogenesis of commotio retinae.

Disruption of the blood-retinal barrier at an average of 16 hours after injury was confirmed in a clinical study using FA and vitreous fluorophotometry.[32]

PEARL... There is no treatment of proven benefit for commotio retinae. Visual acuity tends to recover in the majority of cases, except in those with severe macular involvement or other associated intraocular damage.[33]

MANAGEMENT AND PROGNOSIS   In a prospective study:[33]

• 60% of patients with commotio retinae affecting the macular region had recovery of visual acuity within 2 weeks of injury;
• 40% were left with permanent macular damage and varying degrees of visual loss.[j]

Chorioretinitis Sclopetaria   is an uncommon consequence of trauma by a blunt object.

PEARL... Chorioretinitis sclopetaria is a distinct closed globe injury typically caused by transmitted shock waves from a high-velocity missile penetrating the orbit and grazing, but not perforating, the sclera.

---

[i]In an eye enucleated 24 hours after injury after clinical diagnosis of commotio retinae.

[j]Most of these eyes had other ocular injuries including choroidal rupture, cataract, and lens subluxation.

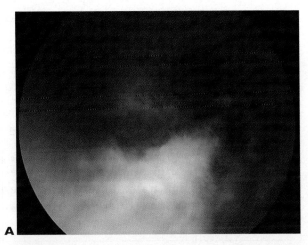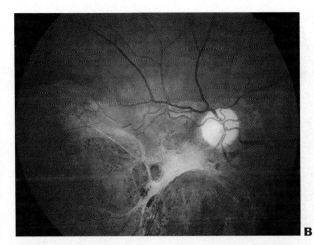

FIGURE 23–3 Chorioretinitis sclopetaria. **(A)** Inferior part of the posterior pole in a 15-year-old boy after he was shot with an air gun from a distance of 15 meters. The bullet penetrated his right lower eyelid and was lodged in the inferior part of the orbit. He noted immediate loss of vision in the right eye. IBO on the day of the injury disclosed a radially oriented chorioretinal break in the inferior part of the fundus with overlying vitreous hemorrhage and a preretinal hemorrhage over the macula. **(B)** Six weeks following the injury, note the bare sclera visible through the defect of the choroid, Bruch's membrane, and retina, with surrounding hyperpigmentation, as a result of direct injury to the inferior retina adjacent to the path of the high-velocity missile. Note the irregular pigmentary disturbances and the preretinal gliotic membrane involving the optic disk and macula as a result of indirect injury of the posterior pole. The macular lesion is not contiguous with the inferior lesion. Visual acuity is counting fingers. (From Beatty S, Smyth K, Au Eong KG, Lavin MJ. Chorioretinitis sclopetaria. *Injury.* 2000;31:55–60. Reprinted by permission from Elsevier Science.)

HISTORY AND EPIDEMIOLOGY   Although the term was first used in the German literature in 1901,[34] the earliest description of the condition was in a book on war injuries published in 1872.[35,k]

Chorioretinitis sclopetaria is relatively rare,[36] especially during peacetime; the largest published series includes only eight cases.[37] It is typically caused by gun injuries[37–39] but has been described in association with injuries from objects such as the nozzle of a high-pressure water hose,[37] metal rod,[37] and fishing line sinker.[40]

PATHOPHYSIOLOGY   There are typically two distinct areas of injury in chorioretinitis sclopetaria (Fig. 23–3).

1. The first site is the area adjacent to the path of the missile; the injury is caused directly by the concussive force of the missile.
   - Rapid deformation of the globe by a high-velocity missile or its shock waves causes a sudden increase in stress in the sclera, choroid, retina, and posterior vitreous cortex.[37]
   - These tissues rupture in areas where the induced tensile stress is greater than the tensile strength of the tissue.

   - Typically, there is full-thickness rupture of the choroid, Bruch's membrane, and retina. This is accompanied by retraction of these tissues to expose the underlying sclera.
   - The chorioretinal rupture is oriented radially if the missile has come to rest deep in the orbit.[37]
2. The second area of injury is remote from the path of the missile and typically involves the macula.
   - The injury is believed to result indirectly from transmission of shock waves through the wall of the eye (see Chapter 22).
   - When the force is severe, there may be only one large lesion involving both areas.[41]

CLINICAL FEATURES   include the following.
- Immediately following the injury, acute loss of vision.
  - Visual acuity in the range of counting fingers is not uncommon because of the severity of the force.[37,39]
- There are usually extensive retinal and choroidal hemorrhages as well as tears in these layers.
- The sclera remains intact.
- Preretinal and vitreous hemorrhages are often present.[39]
- The vitreous hemorrhage may obscure the view of the fundus, and only after the blood has cleared can the typical pigmentary disturbance and retinal scarring be seen (Fig. 23–4).

---

[k]The term "sclopetaria" may have been derived from the verb "slow," an old English variant of "sclaw"; from "claw," which means to scratch, pull, or tear[36]; or from the Latin word "sclopetum," which refers to a type of 14th century Italian handgun.[36]

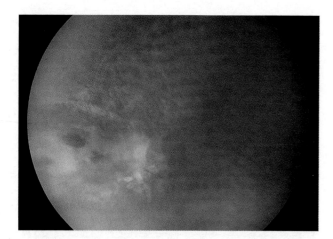

FIGURE 23–4   Within weeks of orbital missile injury an area of healing sclopetaria is present in the periphery. As the blood clears, fibrous proliferation as well as RPE proliferation and mottling are present. In some areas, bare sclera may be evident.

- The lesion heals with the development of white, fibrous scar tissue with pigment at its edges.[41,42]
- Acute retinal detachment is rare.

PEARL...   That acute retinal detachment is so uncommon in chorioretinitis sclo-petaria may be explained by the fact that the retraction of the choroid and retina as a single unit and the typically intact posterior hyaloid face prevent the access of fluid to the subretinal space.[37] In addition, patients tend to be relatively young and have formed vitreous, thus lowering the risk of retinal detachment.[37]

- In the later stages, the resultant spontaneous "retinopexy" usually does not allow a retinal detachment to occur in areas of pigmentary retinal changes.

PITFALL

Late retinal detachment has been reported in one fourth of patients in one study, due to retinal breaks at a site distant from the original chorioretinal rupture.[37]

MANAGEMENT   The clinical findings of a large retinal break with surrounding retinal edema may prompt surgical intervention for treatment of a presumed retinal detachment.

SPECIAL CONSIDERATION

Despite the lesion's striking appearance, observation, *not* surgical intervention, is the appropriate initial management for these injuries because acute retinal detachment is so rare.[37]

- Pars plana vitrectomy may be necessary for nonclearing vitreous hemorrhage, which is more common in young patients with formed vitreous gel.
- It is important for ophthalmologists to be familiar with the clinical features of this condition so that an accurate diagnosis can be promptly established and unwarranted surgical intervention avoided.[39]

PROGNOSIS   The visual prognosis of chorioretinitis sclopetaria is variable. If there is severe scarring of the macula, the visual prognosis is poor. However, cases with return of vision to 20/20 have been reported.[37]

PEARL...   The physician's primary goal with chorioretinitis sclopetaria is to make a prompt and accurate diagnosis so that unwarranted surgical intervention is avoided.[39]

Traumatic Macular Hole   is a relatively common complication of contusion, and may occur within hours of the incident.

CLINICAL FEATURES   The fovea, devoid of the inner retinal layers or blood supply, is vulnerable to full-thickness hole formation following contusion.

- Traumatic macular hole is believed to account for fewer than 10% of all macular holes.[43]
- Macular hole is most commonly caused by contusion[44–47] but has also been reported in association with accidental laser injury[48,49] and retrobulbar needle globe perforation.[50]
- A traumatic macular hole typically ranges in size from 0.2 to 0.5 disk diameter and may be oval or round.[51]
- Patients with traumatic macular holes tend to be young, and posterior vitreous detachment is typically absent in these eyes.[51,52]

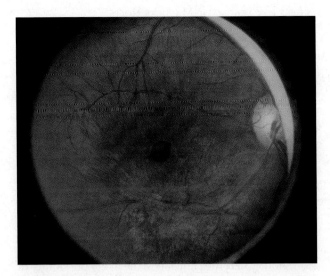

FIGURE 23–5   Traumatic macular holes often have associated macular findings that result from the contusion injury. In this patient, in addition to the large central full-thickness hole, adjacent RPE disturbances can be seen. Some epiretinal proliferation is also present.

- In one series, the traumatic macular holes were associated with other injuries including:
  - commotio retinae in 35%;
  - massive vitreous hemorrhage in 25%;
  - hyphema in 25%; chorioretinal atrophy in 25%;
  - choroidal rupture in 20%;
  - angle recession in 20%;
  - peripheral retinal tears in 10%; and
  - retinal dialysis with retinal detachment in 5% (Fig. 23–5).[51]

PATHOPHYSIOLOGY   The exact mechanism by which traumatic macular hole develops is not well understood.

Possible mechanisms mentioned earlier were contusion necrosis, subfoveal hemorrhage, and vitreous traction.[25] In one documented case the macular hole enlarged from a tiny dehiscence in the fovea after trauma.[47] Based on recent data, surface traction has been identified as a major component in the etiology of traumatic macular holes.[53] Rigidity of the ILM may play an important role (R. Morris, F. Kuhn, J. Dalma, personal communication).

Vision is usually in the range of 20/100 to 20/400 following the development of a full-thickness macular hole. Occasionally, the hole may spontaneously close,[54,*l*] with or without full recovery of the visual acuity (Fig. 23–6).

MANAGEMENT   Until recently, there was no treatment for macular hole.[6] Based on a theory regarding pathogenesis for idiopathic macular holes[55] and the success with surgery for idiopathic and traumatic holes,[47,49,50,52,53,56–61] it is now more difficult for the surgeon to justify foregoing intervention.

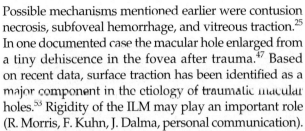

CONTROVERSY

Spontaneous closure of traumatic macular holes does occur in a few cases, especially in young patients. However, observation is a dubious initial treatment option, since most holes are not expected to close without surgical intervention and may lessen the chance of a good anatomical and functional recovery.[53,*m*]

---

*l*Glial cell proliferation may play an important role in spontaneous closure of the macular hole.

*m*See Chapter 8 for some general thoughts.

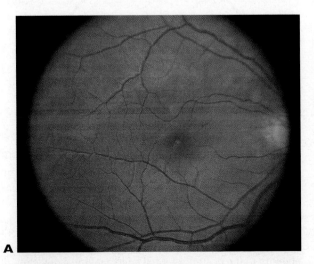

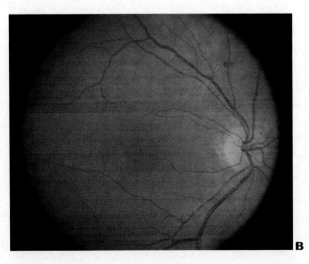

FIGURE 23–6   **(A)** Following an MVC and contusion to the eye, a small, full-thickness macular hole developed with 20/100 vision. **(B)** Over the next 4 months, there was gradual closure of the hole without surgery, and vision returned to 20/30.

Table 23–1   Literature Review of the Major Studies on Surgery for Traumatic Macular Holes

Author, Reference	Number of Eyes	Surgical Technique	Anatomical Success Rate	Functional Success Rate*	Remark
Amari[52]	16	No adjunct, no ILM removal	79% with one, 96% with two surgeries	87%	One or more surgeries
Chow[60]	15	Autologous plasmin, no ILM removal	94%	69%	
Garcia-Arumi[59]	14	Platelet concentrate, no ILM removal	93%	In all eyes with hole closure	One or more surgeries
Kuhn[53]	17	No adjunct, ILM removal	100%	94%	Single surgery

*At least two Snellen lines.

The current standard treatment includes a three-port pars plana vitrectomy, peeling of the posterior hyaloid face from the posterior pole, intravitreal gas tamponade, and postoperative face-down positioning for about up to 2 weeks. ILM removal is becoming increasingly popular.

> **PEARL...**   As with surgery for idiopathic macular holes, removal of the macular ILM appears to increase the anatomical and functional success rates in patients with traumatic macular holes.[53] It also seems from published data that early intervention has distinct advantages, possibly even more so than for an idiopathic macular hole.

PROGNOSIS   Vitreous surgery, with or without adjuvant therapy or ILM peeling, can lead to hole closure and visual improvement in most eyes. The favorable results may be due to the younger age of these patients and the shorter duration of the macular hole.[52] Table 23–1 provides an overview of the major studies.

Vitreous Base Avulsion   is rare.

CLINICAL FEATURES   Avulsion of the vitreous base per se does not cause retinal detachment and usually does not require intervention other than observation. The symptoms may be minimal.[n]

> **PEARL...**   It is the presence of avulsion, recognized as part of the vitreous base draped over the peripheral retina (the so-called bucket-handle) sign, that confirms the history of significant contusion.

The pathognomic presence of vitreous base avulsion should alert the clinician to the likely possibility of severe underlying ocular pathology (e.g., retinal dialysis, peripheral [giant] retinal tears, angle recession).

MANAGEMENT   No surgical intervention is necessary. However, close follow-up is recommended until the ora serrata and pars plana area can be adequately visualized to rule out retinal dialysis or tears of the pars plana.[62]

Retinal Dialysis   is probably more common than generally perceived.

CLINICAL FEATURES   Retinal dialysis is the most frequent traumatic retinal break.[5] It almost always occurs at the time of the injury.[16,18] It may be defined as a break or separation occurring at the anterior edge of the ora serrata and, unlike tears secondary to posterior vitreous detachment with or without a history of trauma, the vitreous remains attached to the posterior edge of the dialysis[63,64] (Fig. 23–7). This intimate

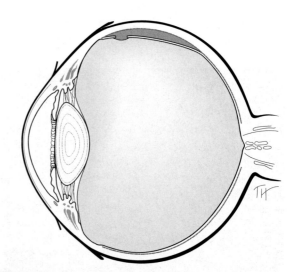

FIGURE 23–7   A retinal dialysis differs from a giant retinal tear as the vitreous spans the retinal defect and provides stability to the posterior retinal edge, making a detachment less likely. (From Tiedeman JS. Retinal tears and rhegmatogenous retinal detachments. In: Regillo CD, Brown GC, Flynn HW, ed. *Vitreoretinal Diseases: The Essentials.* New York: Thieme; 1999;476.)

[n]A vague complaint of floaters.

anatomical relationship is probably responsible for the slow progression from retinal dialysis to retinal detachment.

A retinal dialysis may be difficult to visualize initially because of the minimal separation between the retina and ora serrata. The difficulty in early detection is borne out by published reports. In one series, 41% of retinal detachments associated with retinal dialyses were first diagnosed more than 1 year following the original injury.[63]

Scleral depression may aid the diagnosis, but is rarely possible in a child.

> **PITFALL**
>
> Caution is advised at the initial evaluation with respect to scleral depression: it may cause further damage to an already compromised eye.

Retinal detachments related to dialysis are usually slow to develop,[65] giving the ophthalmologist a window of opportunity to detect and treat them, provided regular follow-up and meticulous examination of the patient are performed.

> **PITFALL**
>
> A retinal dialysis may not be visible at the initial examination and may be overlooked at subsequent examinations.[22,63,66]

It is difficult to overstate the importance of proper examination of the *entire*[o] ora serrata. In one study:[23]

- 66% of dialyses were located in the *inferotemporal* quadrant;
- 10% in the superotemporal quadrant;
- 4% in the inferonasal quadrant;
- 6% of retinal dialyses occurred in more than one quadrant.

The predilection for the inferotemporal and, to a lesser extent, superonasal quadrants has been confirmed in several reports.[16–18,22,65,67,68]

---

[o]That is, 360°.

> **PEARL...** The most common retinal dialysis location is the inferotemporal quadrant.[7,63,65,69] However, because the dialysis can occur in any quadrant, thorough evaluation of the *entire* ora serrata is necessary.

MANAGEMENT   includes the following.

- In the absence of retinal detachment, most retinal dialyses should be treated prophylactically with transscleral cryoretinopexy or, preferably, laser retinopexy.
- Early recognition of retinal dialysis is the key to avoiding more extensive intervention.

Not all retinal dialyses lead to retinal detachment. Occasionally, a dialysis will seal spontaneously due to a vigorous chorioretinal response to the insult.

> **PEARL...** If the surgeon elects not to treat a retinal dialysis, regular follow-ups are mandatory, and the patient should be counseled (see Chapters 5 and 8) with respect to this management strategy.

Peripheral Retinal Breaks   are a common source of posttraumatic retinal detachment.

CLINICAL FEATURES   The location and configuration of flap *horseshoe or "U" tears* tend to mimic those associated with a spontaneous posterior vitreous detachment. The typical appearance of the horseshoe flap or an operculum confirms an etiology secondary to vitreous traction.

The symptoms are also similar with complaints of:

- floaters;
- photopsia; and/or
- blurred vision from primary or secondary vitreous hemorrhage.

> **PEARL...** The risk of progression to retinal detachment in case of a horseshoe tear is much greater than with a retinal dialysis.

Tears from full-thickness retinal *necrosis* are usually slower to evolve and are more likely than tears from vitreous traction to be associated with periretinal hemorrhage. These tears also tend to be large, more irregular, and located at the site of direct ocular contusion.

PEARL... In most cases, contusion-related retinal tears are located inferotemporally, probably because the bony orbit affords less protection at this location and the eye is rolled upward due to Bell's phenomenon associated with the impending approach of any noxious stimulus.

- Peripheral retinal breaks without visible evidence of traction (retinal *holes*) tend to be small and round.
- *Stretch* tears supposedly occur in the setting of rapid horizontal expansion of the eye. They are usually located anterior to the equator and have a curvilinear configuration. They may progress to retinal detachment or seal spontaneously.
- *Giant* retinal tears, defined as retinal tears involving 90° or more of the circumference of the globe, are commonly associated with contusion[70,71] (Fig. 23–8).
  - Myopic males appear to be at a higher risk of developing giant retinal tears from contusive injury.[71]

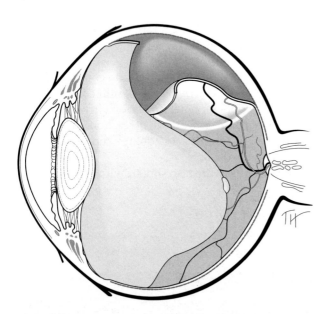

FIGURE 23–8 In a giant retinal tear the vitreous separates from the posterior edge of the retina, allowing the retinal edge to detach and roll over in some cases. (From Tiedeman JS. Retinal tears and rhegmatogenous retinal detachments. In: Regillo CD, Brown GC, Flynn HW, ed. *Vitreoretinal Diseases: The Essentials.* New York: Thieme; 1999;475.)

- Occasionally, giant tears can be seen secondary to trauma-induced full-thickness retinal necrosis.

PEARL... The presence of periretinal hemorrhage following ocular trauma should alert the clinician to the possibility of underlying retinal tears.

PATHOPHYSIOLOGY   A retinal tear secondary to contusion occurs when the transmission of an external force causes sudden and rapid distortion of the globe.

- The eye shortens anteroposteriorly and elongates equatorially.
- The relative inelasticity of the eyewall, coupled with the fact that the eye is a fluid-filled structure and therefore relatively resistant to compression, means that the globe cannot adequately stretch in response to this deformation.
- The volume of the eye remains virtually constant during/following contusion because the aqueous outflow facility cannot adjust rapidly enough to the sudden volume displacement.
- Compression of one part of the globe therefore effectively means that a corresponding volume of fluid must be displaced elsewhere within this closed system.
- This sudden violent change in shape without a corresponding change in volume generates tractional forces within the globe. This discrepancy can be extremely destructive to ocular tissues.
- All these factors conspire to make the posterior segment particularly susceptible to a contusive insult.

MANAGEMENT   In most instances, traumatic retinal tears should be treated with laser retinopexy or, less prefereably, cryoretinopexy. Holes that have undergone spontaneous closure due to chorioretinal adhesion can be observed but should be followed closely to detect possible progression to retinal detachment.

CONTROVERSY

A giant retinal tear, even in the absence of retinal detachment, may require a prophylactic scleral buckle as a reasonable alternative to retinopexy because of the associated vitreous traction and risk of PVR development.

PITFALL

The risk of progression to retinal detachment is too great in contused eyes with retinal breaks outside the fovea; therefore, prophylactic treatment should at least be considered for all of these eyes.

Traumatic Rhegmatogenous Retinal Detachment is the most common cause of permanent visual loss.

CLINICAL FEATURES   Trauma accounts for up to 12% of rhegmatogenous retinal detachments and remains the most common cause of detachments in children.[72,73]

Traumatic retinal detachment may occur secondary to:

- retinal dialysis;
- flap/horseshoe tears;
- giant retinal tears;
- full-thickness retinal necrosis; or
- stretch tears.

PEARL... With the exception of giant retinal tears as the cause, traumatic retinal detachments in general tend to progress slowly.[4,65] This is particularly true if a formed vitreous is present.

Retinal detachments secondary to peripheral retinal tears tend to progress more quickly than those due to retinal dialysis, which can sometimes take years to develop or to become symptomatic. Consequently, if considerable time elapses between injury and presentation, differentiation of this type of retinal detachment from nontraumatic types may be difficult. A search for other signs of trauma, especially if unilateral, may be particularly rewarding in unraveling the precise etiology.

The *symptoms* of traumatic rhegmatogenous retinal detachment are similar to those associated with rhegmatogenous retinal detachment in nontraumatic settings; they range from:

- floaters and
- photopsia to
- progressive visual field loss and eventual

- loss of central vision from macular involvement.

In some cases, presentation may be delayed until the retinal detachment involves the macula and causes decreased visual acuity.

PEARL... Delayed presentation typically occurs for retinal detachments following retinal dialysis, evolving over several months or even years.

In eyes with a slowly developing retinal detachment, the examination may reveal:

- progressive "high or tide water marks" beneath the detached retina;
- a retina that is thin/atrophic; and
- an appearance of the retina similar to retinoschisis.[63,65]

The presence of subretinal macrocysts is also an indicator of chronicity.[63,65] The bullous appearance characteristic of so many rhegmatogenous detachments is more likely to be seen with:

- large retinal dialyses;
- superior retinal detachment;
- avulsion of the vitreous base;
- posterior vitreous detachments; or
- persistent traction on a retinal break.

PVR can occur in any setting but is more likely to be associated with giant retinal tears.[65,74,75]

PEARL... If a thorough search of the retina fails to yield the cause of a rhegmatogenous retinal detachment in a case of contusion, then the pars plana should be evaluated as the source of hole formation.[62]

MANAGEMENT   Surgical success in the treatment of a rhegmatogenous retinal detachment secondary to contusion depends on a thorough examination and careful planning prior to surgery. Injury in the posterior segment rarely occurs in isolation. Significant involvement of the anterior ocular structures (see Chapters 14, 17, 21, and 25) may also require surgical intervention before vitreoretinal issues can be addressed.

- The aim of surgery is to reattach the retina, and, to this end, all retinal breaks must be identified and closed and all vitreous traction must be released.

- Depending on the circumstances of the causative retinal breaks, *uncomplicated* traumatic rhegmatogenous detachments can be treated with:
  - pneumatic retinopexy (if the break is superior);
  - scleral buckling; or
  - vitrectomy.

> **P**EARL... **The surgeon's preference is an additional factor in determining the surgical option.**

- Extensive tractional membranes or vitreous opacities typically require vitrectomy to achieve successful retinal reattachment.
- A retinal detachment in the presence of a *giant retinal tear* needs special consideration for a number of reasons.
  - The posterior margin of the tear, free from any vitreous attachment, tends to scroll on itself and may require careful surgical manipulation to unroll.
  - Failure to reattach the retina further increases the likelihood of PVR.[p]
  - A pars plana vitrectomy with or without a lensectomy[q] is almost always required in such cases.
  - If the posterior flap is scrolled, it can be unfolded and repositioned using PFCL (see the Appendix).
  - Correct repositioning of the posterior flap permits the application of laser retinopexy.
  - The anterior flap should be removed.

> **PITFALL**
>
> Failure to remove the anterior aspect of the flap allows it to act as a potential nidus for anterior PVR formation with eventual ciliary body detachment and ocular hypotony (see Chapter 19 and Fig. 23–9).

- Because the anterior retina receives its blood supply from posteriorly, a giant retinal tear renders the adjacent anterior retinal flap an ischemic source for the development of ocular neovascularization.

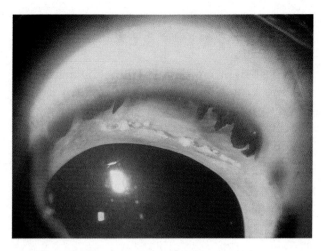

FIGURE 23–9 Hypotony following open globe injury. Because the iris and lens are absent, a fibrous epiciliary membrane can be seen with traction on the ciliary body.

- After fixation of a broad encircling band,[r] the PFCL should be removed (see the Appendix).
- Finally, the eye is filled with silicone oil for permanent postoperative tamponade (see the Appendix).

PVR is the most common reason for surgical failure. The term PVR is used clinically to describe the fibrous membranes seen either in association with rhegmatogenous retinal detachment or as a complication of its surgical management. At its simplest, it may be considered an anomalous wound-healing process.

HISTORY The term was coined in 1983,[s] emphasizing that proliferation at the cellular level is thought to be pivotal in its pathogenesis.

> **P**EARL... **A common misperception among ophthalmologists is that PVR is a new condition. In reality, it was recognized as long ago as the 1930s ("preretinal organization"). It has gained prominence in the past decades because of the emergence of the sophisticated equipment and techniques necessary to not only recognize but understand and treat it.**

---

[p]Remember, this risk is *already* high in the presence of a giant retinal tear.

[q]See Chapter 21 and the Appendix.

[r]It is increasingly common among vitreoretinal surgeons not to use a buckle in the treatment of retinal detachments due to a giant tear; slippage, a frequent cause of failure, cannot occur in the absence of a slope.

[s]By the Retina Society Terminology Committee.

The occurrence of PVR following trauma appears to be associated with the type of injury; perforating injury shows the highest incidence (see Chapter 26).[76]

PITFALL

Vision loss in posterior segment trauma occurs not only as a result of the initial insult but also because of the development of PVR. Indeed, it is PVR that is the principal cause of vision loss in these patients.[77–80] Consequently, PVR remains a formidable adversary of the vitreoretinal surgeon despite recent microsurgical advances.

CLASSIFICATION A disease with such a diverse spectrum as PVR makes a classification system necessary with respect to the disease's:

- severity;
- location; and
- extent.

Since the first attempt at grading the condition in 1978,[81] the classification of PVR has evolved to the currently accepted system published in 1991.[82] This updated version not only takes into account disease location but also includes a description of the *types of contraction* that are now accepted to be pivotal in disease progression.[t]

Such a classification of PVR is necessary so that:

- disease severity, extent, and location are universally meaningful;
- results from studies can be compared and interpreted in a uniform and standardized way;
- appropriate surgical intervention can be planned according to the available management strategies;
- surgeons are aware of the prognosis and the expected outcomes; and
- findings from clinical and biomedical research studies can be disseminated in a meaningful way to the medical community at large.

PATHOPHYSIOLOGY Histopathologically, PVR is characterized by the following findings.

- The formation and contraction of fibrocellular membranes on both retinal surfaces (i.e., epiretinal

and subretinal). RPE cells appear to be pivotal in the development of these membranes.[83] In early PVR formation, some RPE cells lose their normal adhesiveness to Bruch's membrane (Figs. 23–10 through 23–12). These free cells phenotypically assume the roles of and behave like wound fibroblasts or macrophages.[84] They travel to the surfaces of the detached neurosensory retina through one or more retinal breaks.

- A concomitant breakdown of the blood-retinal barrier resulting from retinal detachment permits the recruitment of inflammatory cells, while glial cells from adjacent retina also migrate to this evolving membrane. However, it is the fibroblast-like cells that are most abundant. Available evidence points to the RPE as the source of these cells.[85,86]

- The presence of fibroblasts is fundamental in generating the forces necessary for PVR membrane contraction by remodeling of the extracellular matrix. In this remodeling of the extracellular matrix, individual cells draw collagen toward them, akin to a sailor pulling in the sheets of a sail.[87] The process manifests itself clinically as folds within the neurosensory retina, which eventually causes a secondary tractional and/or combined tractional/rhegmatogenous retinal detachment.

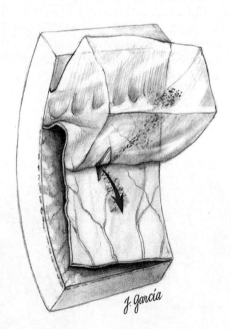

FIGURE 23–10 Retinal tear formation stimulates the release of RPE cells into the vitreous while breakdown of the blood-retinal barrier generates a cytokine-mediated recruitment of inflammatory cells. Clinically, this is characterized by the presence of pigments clumps or "tobacco dust" suspended within a hazy vitreous humor.

---

[t]The updated classification also shows how difficult it is to define the line between being accurate and simple; systems that are too complex do not gain acceptance in everday use.

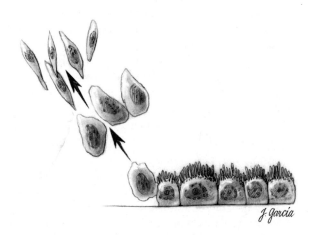

FIGURE 23-11 Liberation of RPE from Bruch's membrane triggers a redifferentiation of these cells that causes them not only to assume a wound-healing phenotype but also to behave as such with proliferative, migratory, and adhesion properties identical to those of typical wound fibroblasts.

- As with wound repair elsewhere, it is now recognized that PVR membranes are in a state of flux with membranes of different clinical durations undergoing a time-dependent buildup of extracellular material.[88] This interdependence between cells and matrix has led to the discovery of many extracellular matrix molecules in PVR membranes. These range from glycosaminoglycans such as heparin sulfate[89] to components of the clotting system such as plasminogen.[90]

SPECIAL CONSIDERATION

Breakdown of the blood-retinal barrier is an inevitable consequence of surgical repair of retinal detachment and will thus provide one of the key ingredients to the initiation or perpetuation of PVR. RPE cells can also be liberated from Bruch's membrane as a result of scleral depression or cryotherapy at the time of surgery.[75] This liberation of RPE cells coupled with iatrogenic blood-retinal barrier breakdown will further enhance the likelihood of PVR.

PITFALL

In retinal detachment associated with trauma, there is significant blood-retinal barrier breakdown and therefore these eyes are at particular risk of developing PVR.

Other potential risk factors[76,91–93] for the development of PVR following trauma include:

- poor vision at presentation;
- preexisting retinal detachment;
- complete extrusion of lens at the time of injury;
- vitreous hemorrhage;

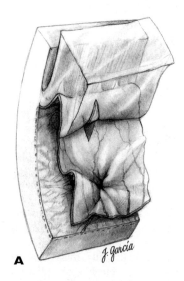

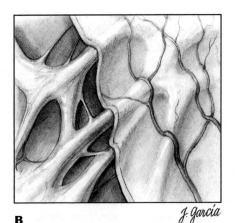

FIGURE 23-12 **(A)** Migration and adhesion of these cells cause remodeling of newly synthesized extracellular matrix in the vitreous and on the retinal surfaces, giving rise to the wrinkling, star fold, and membrane formation seen clinically. **(B)** When the membranes are subretinal, they appear as bands with draped retina overlying.

- vitreous prolapse;
- long, posteriorly located wound; and
- persistent inflammation.

The clinical spectrum of PVR in association with rhegmatogenous retinal detachment varies from mild to very severe.

- The earliest detectable change is the appearance of so-called *tobacco dust* in the vitreous.

> **PEARL...** The presence of tobacco dust is not synonymous with progression to a more severe disease.

- ○ Tobacco dust consists of clumps of RPE cells that have been liberated from Bruch's membrane and have gained access to the vitreous through one or more defects in the neurosensory retina.[94]
- ○ These cells are thought to settle on the retinal surface to initiate membrane formation.[83]
- ○ Contraction of these membranes gives rise to the familiar clinical changes.
- *Mild* PVR is characterized by the following:
  - ○ retinal surface wrinkling;
  - ○ retinal vascular tortuosity; and
  - ○ rolling of the edges of retinal breaks.
- With *more advanced* contraction, characteristic "star folds" become evident.
- *Further progression* of these star folds gives rise to localized tractional retinal detachment. Previously closed retinal breaks may reopen or new breaks may develop.
- *Eventually*, a funnel-shaped, total retinal detachment with taut vitreous ensues.

From a clinical and surgical point of view, *anterior PVR*, defined as PVR occurring at or anterior to the posterior insertion of the vitreous base, merits special attention. Its effects are potentially catastrophic not only to vision but also to the eye as a whole. Anterior PVR is the most common cause of failure to achieve retinal reattachment following vitrectomy for PVR (see Chapters 19 and 25 and the Appendix).[95,96]

Tractional membranes can grow over the:

- lens;
- IOL; and
- ciliary body, eventually leading to ciliary body detachment and intractable ocular hypotony with phthisis (see Chapter 8).[97,98]

Contraction of PVR membranes generates three types of tractional forces (Fig. 23–13).

- anteroposterior;
- circumferential; and
- perpendicular.

The process evolves over time.

- Initially, there is *proliferation of RPE and glial cells* within the vitreous base. The de novo synthesis and remodeling of collagen by these cells lead to shortening and overlap of the anterior and posterior aspects of the vitreous base.
- Further cellular proliferation can lead to the *seeding of various surfaces* (e.g., lens, IOL, ciliary body, iris), causing even greater foreshortening of the vitreous base and anteroposterior traction on the retina, recognized as circumferential retinal folds that are parallel to the equator of the globe.
- Progressive, 360° *contraction* within the vitreous base produces circumferential traction that results in radial folds within the retina.

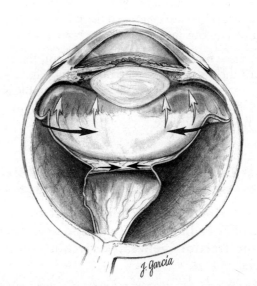

FIGURE 23–13 PVR generates three kinds of tractional forces: anteroposterior, circumferential, and perpendicular. All result from deposition and remodeling of extracellular matrix within the vitreous base by proliferating cells. Anteroposterior traction can cause foreshortening of the vitreous base that in turn pulls the retina anteriorly so that it adheres to the pars plana or even to the iris and lens (white arrows). Meanwhile, vitreous base contraction also generates circumferential traction (curved arrows), which cause radial folds within the retina. Finally, perpendicular traction pulls the retina toward the center of the vitreous cavity, causing the characteristic funnel configuration seen clinically (straight arrows).

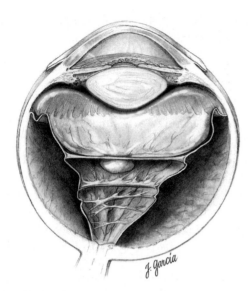

FIGURE 23–14   With continued intravitreal, epiretinal, and subretinal proliferation, a classic funnel configuration of the retinal detachment is seen clinically.

• *Perpendicular traction* usually arises from contractile forces that are generated mainly along the posterior vitreous face.

As these membranes shorten, they pull the retina toward the center of the vitreous cavity (Fig. 23–14). This process, if unchecked, will give rise to the characteristic funnel-shaped retinal detachment and opacified vitreous face.

SPECIAL CONSIDERATION

In anterior PVR, circumferential traction results in radial retinal folds and anteroposterior traction generates circumferential folds.

MANAGEMENT PRINCIPLES   The principles governing the surgical management of PVR are identical to those of conventional retinal reattachment surgery.

Identification of all retinal breaks.

• Failure to identify all retinal breaks may result in persistence or recurrent retinal detachment.
• Initially, the identification of breaks can be frustrating because extensive PVR can make adequate visualization virtually impossible. Only after release of traction following the removal of membranes will all breaks become apparent.

Release of all retinal traction (Figs. 23–15 through 23–19).

• It is necessary to eliminate both preretinal and subretinal membranes and the relief of transvitreal traction. This may require:
  ○ membrane stripping;
  ○ retinotomy; and/or
  ○ retinectomy.

PEARL...   If the price to pay for complete traction relief is the creation of a retinal lesion (e.g., a tear or even a large retinectomy), this is still the lesser of the two evils: any residual traction will eventually lead to retinal redetachment.

Retinal reattachment and long-term retinal stabilization.

• Only after relief of all traction can complete apposition of the retina to the RPE be achieved and closure of retinal breaks be performed.
• Long-term closure of breaks can be achieved with laser retinopexy or cryopexy. Laser photocoagulation is preferred because cryotherapy causes the release of viable RPE cells into the vitreous cavity and possibly greater breakdown of the blood-retinal barrier. This could potentially exacerbate the preexisting PVR, particularly when a giant retinal tear is present (see Chapter 24 and the Appendix).[75]

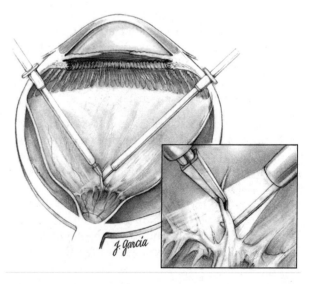

FIGURE 23–15   After removing the vitreous, further relief of traction is achieved by peeling of the membranes on the vitreous surface of the retina. Membranes can either be delaminated or segmented before removal. *Inset:* Microforceps are used to stabilize the membrane on the retina while it is peeled with a lighted pick.

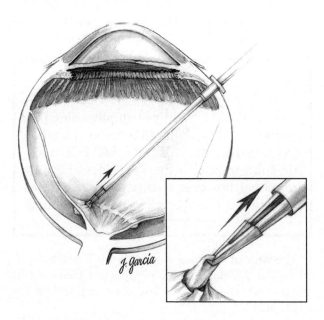

FIGURE 23–16 If traction still persists despite adequate removal of all membranes on the vitreous side of the retina, removal of subretinal membranes is performed. Access to the subretinal space can be gained through a retinotomy or retinectomy, maneuvers that allow the membranes to be grasped and removed with forceps.

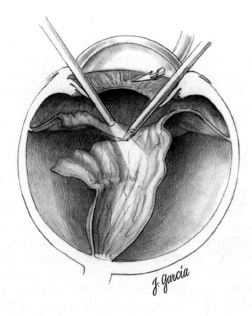

FIGURE 23–17 In severe PVR where the retina has been foreshortened, traction and therefore detachment will persist despite meticulous removal of membranes on both surfaces of the retina. Such a scenario usually requires a retinectomy. Essentially the anterior retina is incised circumferentially to relieve traction from this anterior PVR.

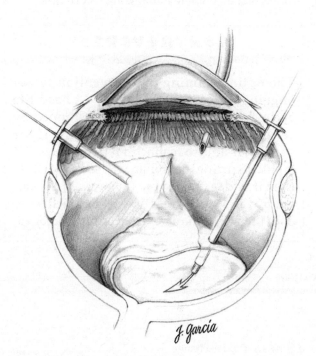

FIGURE 23–18 Following the relief of all traction, the retina can be reattached. Reapposition to the wall of the globe can be facilitated by injecting a heavy liquid, which displaces subretinal fluid, thereby permitting attachment of the neurosensory retina to the RPE.

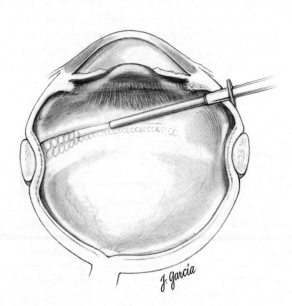

FIGURE 23–19 Enhancement of more long-term attachment between the retina and the RPE can be facilitated by the application of an endolaser to the sites of breaks and also retinectomies or retinotomies if present.

Prevention of persistent/recurrent PVR.[u]

- Despite massive strides in improving the surgical success of retinal reattachment in PVR, the surgical techniques and instrumentation currently employed do not address the ongoing fibrocellular proliferation that characterizes the condition. Essentially two processes drive PVR formation:
  1. proliferating cells with secondary contraction; and
  2. inflammation that is exacerbated at the time of surgery.
- Several agents, some of which have worked in experiments, have been tried clinically but with only limited success. These include corticosteroids,[99] fluoropyrimidines,[100] daunomycin,[101] low-molecular-weight heparin,[102] and colchicine.[103] Success with these agents has been disappointing because of either minimal effect or unacceptable side effects/toxicity within the therapeutic range.[104] Further research is required into pharmacological agents to control PVR at the cellular level and thereby prevent the need for multiple surgeries.

For ease of understanding, it is often convenient to divide the management anatomically into anterior and posterior PVR.

- The posterior[v] PVR is usually tackled first because posterior traction has to be released to allow the posterior retina to flatten. PFCL provides tremendous assistance in stabilizing the retina and thereby permitting the more anterior component to be addressed.
- Conversely, if PFCL is not used, anterior traction should be relieved prior to posterior dissection. The posterior membranes will help stabilize the posterior retina while dissection is carried out anteriorly. Posterior PVR membranes are then removed after complete anterior dissection. Tables 23–2 and 23–3

---

[u]Chapter 26 has additional information on PVR development and therapy.

[v]Defined as PVR posterior to the vitreous base.

summarize the properties and uses of PFCL (see also the Appendix).

PITFALL

Any break that could potentially come into contact with PFCL should be freed of traction first to reduce the chance of the PFCL tracking subretinally. If the PFCL does become subretinal, however, it can easily be aspirated through the retinal break (see the Appendix).

The issue of *timing* of surgery in PVR remains controversial. No data from a prospective trial exist to suggest whether early or late intervention is more appropriate.

- Advocates of an *early approach* suggest that this period offers the best opportunity for successful retinal reattachment, with the maximal chance for preservation of vision.
- On the other hand, those advocating *later surgery* hold the view that waiting permits this anomalous wound-healing process to stabilize and purport that this assists in the surgical removal of more mature membranes[105] while minimizing recurrence.

CONTROVERSY

The optimal timing of intervention for an ongoing PVR is still debated. PVR has a life cycle, which is not shortened or stopped by surgical intervention. Consequently, if the surgeon is able to reattach a retina while PVR is still occurring, the retina will soon redetach, even if under silicone oil. If, however, the surgeon waits until the PVR cycle reaches its end, the retina may be irreversibly damaged.

TABLE 23–2   PFCLs: Properties and Their Clinical Implications

Property	Implication
Low viscosity	Easy to handle
High vapor pressure	Enhances evaporation during air–fluid exchange
Stable carbon-fluorine bonds	Inert
Specific gravity > water	Sinks in water and therefore able to displace subretinal fluid anteriorly
Transparent	Optically clear and free of aberrations
High boiling point	Permits laser photocoagulation without vaporization

TABLE 23–3 USES OF PFCL

Stabilization of posterior retina allows anterior dissection of periretinal membranes

Drainage of subretinal fluid through anterior retinal breaks

Serves as a stabilizing factor during dissection ("third hand")

Unfolding of giant retinal tears

PVR is a disease spectrum that allows the surgeon to tailor the approach to each individual patient depending on disease severity and location. For example, very early stages of PVR may be managed conventionally with scleral buckling or pneumoretinopexy without resorting to pars plana vitrectomy techniques,[w] which are required for more severe disease where traction is prominent. Tables 23–4 and 23–5 summarize the essential surgical steps in the management of posterior and anterior PVR, respectively, by pars plana vitrectomy techniques.

PEARL... Failure to relieve anterior contraction despite meticulous membrane dissection is an indication for relaxing retinotomy/retinectomy.

[w]It must be mentioned that an increasing number of surgeons see vitrectomy, not scleral buckling, as the primary treatment approach to retinal detachment, even if PVR is present.

SURGICAL MANEUVERS AND ADJUNCTS commonly utilized for both posterior and anterior PVR are:

Subretinal membrane dissection

- The presence of these membranes does not have the same clinical or prognostic significance as do preretinal membranes.
- Although present in almost half of all PVR cases, only rarely do subretinal membranes prevent retinal reattachment[106] and hence merit removal.
- For this reason, the decision to proceed with their removal should be considered only after meticulous dissection of anterior and posterior preretinal membranes.

PEARL... Only after relief of all anterior traction on the retina can the surgeon fully appreciate the necessity to excise a subretinal membrane. At this point it becomes obvious whether such a membrane is preventing retinal reattachment.

- Subretinal membrane dissection requires one or more retinotomies. This permits the membrane to be grasped with special intraocular forceps and pulled out through the retinotomy. The location and size of a membrane govern the difficulty associated with removal, the number of retinotomies required, and ultimately whether a retinectomy is necessary.

TABLE 23–4 ESSENTIAL SURGICAL STEPS IN PARS PLANA VITRECTOMY FOR POSTERIOR PVR

Surgical Step	Goal/Effect
Broad and high scleral buckle	Reduces traction if anterior PVR develops postoperatively
Core pars plana vitrectomy	Allows placement of dissecting instruments within the eye
Additional removal of vitreous	Permits some relief of transvitreal traction
Separation of posterior hyaloid	Permits retina to "relax," facilitating more complete removal of vitreous. Reduces chance of epiretinal membrane
Shaving of vitreous base	Reduces scaffold for anterior proliferation
Removal of periretinal membranes posterior to equator	Identification of associated retinal breaks and relief of traction
Injection of PFCL	Flattens posterior retina
	Drains subretinal fluid through anterior breaks
	Causes countertraction on retina, stabilizes posterior retina, draws vitreous base posteriorly, allows complete anterior dissection of membranes, reduces risk of further breaks and/or vitreous or retinal incarceration
Relaxing retinotomy/retinectomy	Necessary if retina still cannot be reattached despite above measures
Subretinal membrane dissection	May be necessary if significant traction is still present
Air–fluid exchange	Drainage of subretinal fluid, flattening of retina, and application of photocoagulation to retinal breaks
Endolaser photocoagulation	Closure of breaks and prophylaxis against potential future breaks
Silicone oil or C_3F_8 injection	Long-term retinal tamponade

TABLE 23–5   ESSENTIAL SURGICAL STEPS IN PARS PLANA VITRECTOMY FOR ANTERIOR PVR

Surgical Step	Goal/Effect
Broad and high scleral buckle	Relieves transvitreal traction
Core pars plana vitrectomy	Further relief of transvitreal traction
Incision and removal of anterior and posterior hyaloid vitreous	Relief of anteroposterior contraction
Vertical relaxing incisions within vitreous base	Relief of circumferential traction
Relaxing retinotomy/retinectomy	Necessary if retina still cannot be reattached despite above measures
Subretinal membrane dissection	May be necessary if significant traction is still present
Fluid-air exchange	Drainage of subretinal fluid, flattening of retina and application of photocoagulation to retinal breaks
Endolaser photocoagulation	Closure of breaks and prophylaxis against potential future breaks
Silicone oil or C_3F_8 injection	Long-term retinal tamponade

PITFALL

Occasionally, the usually easy-to-detach subretinal membrane adheres very strongly to the retina, and forceful removal attempts will result in iatrogenic retinal tears. In these eyes, the membrane may be only partially removed or simply severed.

PEARL... Special forceps, designed for this very purpose, help in the removal of subretinal membranes. In general, it is advisable to create the retinotomy for extraction at some distance from the membrane.

Relaxing retinotomy/retinectomy. The indications for these maneuvers include:

- significant subretinal membranes; and, much more commonly,
- residual traction, typically in the presence of anterior PVR.[107]

As a general rule:

- the retinal incision should be performed as anteriorly as possible[x]; and
- the remaining anterior retina should be excised.[y]

Persistent anterior traction can lead to recurrent retinal detachment postoperatively.

PEARL... Adequate hemostasis at the edge of the incision must be achieved because bleeding is a further risk factor for PVR. This can be achieved by performing the incision between a double row of diathermy burns. Residual blood is especially dangerous if the eye is filled with silicone oil.

Subretinal fluid removal. This permits complete *intraoperative*[z] reattachment of the retina. Drainage of subretinal fluid can be achieved in a number of ways.

- Fluid–air exchange through:
  - an existing posterior break;
  - a posterior "drainage" retinotomy; or
  - an existing anterior break using a flexible-extendable silicone cannula.
- Using PFCL and draining through:
  - an existing anterior break; or
  - a retinotomy created anteriorly.

Endolaser photocoagulation

- Retinal reattachment allows the application of confluent photocoagulation burns around all retinal breaks, including the edges of retinotomy or retinectomy sites.

---

[x]To preserve as much of the retina as the situation allows and to minimize the surface of the bare RPE.

[y]Because it can act as a scaffold for PVR.

[z]One of the advantages of using vitrectomy, rather than buckling, for retinal detachment repair.

- Laser treatment can be applied in eyes filled with:
  - BSS;
  - gas;
  - silicone oil;
  - PFCL (see the Appendix).

Endolaser treatment should not be applied, however, to a retina with persistent traction as this can lead to further break- or hole formation.

PEARL... In addition to laser treatment in the areas of visible pathology, prophylactic 360° IBO or endolaser cerclage may be considered (see the Appendix).

Intraocular tamponade.[aa]

- This is necessary to allow adequate chorioretinal adhesion to form. Agents available include air, SF_6, C_3F_8, and silicone oil.
- In general, longer term tamponade is necessary in PVR surgery to achieve higher rates of retinal

reattachment and better visual outcomes.[108,109] Tables 23–6 and 23–7 summarize the advantages and disadvantages of using C_3F_8 and silicone oil, respectively.

A few additional comments.

- Following retinal reattachment, a nonexpansile 14% concentration of C_3F_8 is exchanged for air. However, if there are numerous inferior retinal breaks or an inferior retinectomy is present, an expansile concentration of 16–20% can be used.[bb]
- If the surgeon elects to use silicone oil, it is best instilled into the eye following retinal reattachment with a fluid-air exchange.
  - If PFCL has been used, a direct PFCL–silicone oil exchange can be performed.
  - If the patient is aphakic or has an AC IOL, an inferior peripheral iridotomy is performed[110] and the patient remains face down for one day to allow the AC to be filled with aqueous.
- There is general consensus among vitreoretinal surgeons that in most cases, silicone oil can (should) be removed 3 to 6 months after surgery in most eyes.

[aa]See the Appendix for further details.

[bb]Most surgeons in this situation prefer silicone oil.

TABLE 23–6 ADVANTAGES AND DISADVANTAGES OF C_3F_8 GAS AS INTERNAL TAMPONADE

Advantages	Disadvantages
Dissolves spontaneously and therefore does not require removal	Tamponade is not permanent
Can be "topped up" at the slit lamp	Requires posturing that may not be possible in elderly or children
May be superior to silicone oil in eyes undergoing vitrectomy for the first time	Restricts vision
	Cataractogenic
	Can cause keratopathy
	Prevents immediate air or high-altitude travel

TABLE 23–7 ADVANTAGES AND DISADVANTAGES OF SILICONE OIL AS INTERNAL TAMPONADE

Advantages	Disadvantages
Permanent long-term tamponade	Requires removal
After first 24 hours, posturing is usually unnecessary and therefore early mobilization is possible	Cataractogenic
Permits earlier visual rehabilitation than C_3F_8	Causes keratopathy
Permits air travel	Can cause perisilicone PVR
Lower likelihood of hypotony	Can cause postoperative elevated IOP

PEARL... The Silicone Oil Study, begun in 1985 and completed in 1990, was designed to compare the success rates between silicone oil and long-acting gases as intraocular tamponades in the treatment of PVR and the frequency of complications between silicone oil and long-acting gases. In all, this study group published a total of 11 reports.[109] The major findings of the study are summarized in Table 23–8.[108,111–119]

Prognosis and Outcome Following Surgery   Ultimately, the success of the surgical management of PVR depends on the:

- condition's severity;
- condition's location; and
- the number of procedures required to achieve anatomic success.[cc]

There are additional factors to consider.

- Before attempts were made to grade PVR and adopt a uniform classification, direct comparisons between various studies were difficult or impossible. These difficulties were further compounded as the techniques of treatment and instrumentation evolved.
- Results of conventional surgery (i.e., without vitrectomy) in severe PVR were poor, with retinal reattachment achieved in less than one third of cases.[120]

[cc]Early research results suggest that there is also a personal predilection; patients with higher levels of certain humoral factors have a higher risk of PVR development despite otherwise successful surgery (Clyde Guidry, PhD, personal communication).

TABLE 23–8   Major Findings of the Silicone Oil Study

Silicone oil was found to be superior to SF_6 for the management of severe PVR. Specifically, silicone oil–treated eyes had a higher rate of functional and anatomic success and lower rates of complication such as hypotony and keratopathy.[109]

Silicone oil and C_3F_8 were equally efficacious in achieving retinal tamponade for severe PVR with respect to both anatomic and functional success in patients who had not undergone initial vitrectomy.[108,119]

For first-time-vitrectomy cases, C_3F_8 was slightly superior to oil in achieving retinal reattachment. However, there was no significant difference with respect to visual outcome or complications.[119]

- Posterior PVR has a better outcome than anterior PVR,[118] and anatomic success with a single procedure achieves ambulatory vision around 60% of the time as opposed to around 30% in those that require multiple surgeries.[113]
- With modern vitrectomy techniques, retinal reattachment rates of 60 to 80% can be expected even in the more severe cases.[108,109]
  - However, anatomic success does not necessarily correlate with visual outcome and functional ability. Despite adequate reattachment of the posterior retina, visual outcome may be poor due to macular changes (e.g., postsurgical macular edema or persistent membranes).[121]

Open Globe Injury

Open globe ocular trauma involving the posterior segment of the eye generates a wound response similar to that of other tissues in the body. From a visual perspective, it unfortunately unleashes a devastating sequence of events, which, can ultimately lead to tractional and/or rhegmatogenous retinal detachment.

The inciting events are:

- an ocular wound leading to breakdown of the blood–retinal barrier; and
- the initiation of an inflammatory response.

Subsequent events include the following:

- liberated cytokines recruit RPE cells, fibroblasts, and glial cells that proliferate and migrate within the eye.
- collagenous extracellular matrix is produced in the vitreous and on the retinal surfaces by these cells that migrate on and within this matrix scaffold, causing it to contract.
- when the contractile forces generated by the wound overcome the normal adhesive forces between the neurosensory retina and the RPE, a tractional retinal detachment ensues.
- the detachment itself mediates further breakdown of the blood-retinal barrier and a vicious circle ensues.

Clinical and pathologic observations have been instrumental in the understanding of the pathologic events that follow severe open globe injury.[79,92,93,122] Despite proper wound closure, injuries involving the posterior segment often lead to total retinal detachment and eventually ocular hypotony. The following were found in a study[123] of eyes undergoing enucleation following penetrating ocular injury (see also Chapter 26).

- The cellular proliferation begins at the sites of penetration within the first days following injury.

- Over the course of the ensuing weeks, the intraocular proliferation progresses, leading to the formation of cyclitic, epiretinal, and retroretinal membranes.
- Proliferation also occurs along the vitreous incarcerated in the wound, resulting in condensation of the vitreous fibrils.
- Posterior vitreous separation generally occurs during the first 2 weeks of injury.

PEARL... **Posterior vitreous detachment is commonly incomplete; the surgeon must look carefully for residual vitreous on the (detached) retinal surface. The "postero/anterior (P/A) vitrectomy" technique (F. Kuhn, MD, personal communication) helps achieve this goal by first detaching the posterior vitreous, before actual vitreous removal occurs.**

- The end result of this cellular proliferation and vitreous condensation is the production of contractile forces, which lead to tractional/rhegmatogenous retinal detachment.
- Vitreous hemorrhage is (or was) invariably present in eyes with open globe injury and subsequent proliferation: it is intimately involved in the promotion of trauma-related intraocular proliferation.

The precise pathological events occurring following a traumatic wound were demonstrated experimentally.[124–128,dd] Similar to what occurs during treatment in humans, the wounds were freed of the prolapsed vitreous and closed with interrupted sutures. In eyes examined during the first week following the injury, vitreous strands were nevertheless shown to be incarcerated in the wound and attached to the nonpigmented ciliary body epithelium and to the peripheral retina. Fibroblastic invasion of the vitreous started during the first week.

PITFALL

Animal experiments confirm the clinician's experience that in eyes with scleral wound and vitreous prolapse, completely freeing the wound of the vitreous before surgical wound closure is extremely difficult.

[dd] An 8-mm incision is created through the pars plana, followed by the injection of autologous blood into the vitreous cavity. The initial penetrating injury models were developed in the rabbit and then used in the rhesus monkey to better approximate the human condition.

- Fibroblastic invasion of the vitreous started during the first week.
- By the second week of injury, a posterior vitreous detachment was present in most eyes. Blood in the vitreous cavity began to show signs of hemolysis and fibrinolysis with accumulation of macrophages. Fibrous ingrowth could be seen from the wound. Ultrastructural examination demonstrated that these proliferating cells had characteristics of both fibroblasts and smooth muscle cell myofibroblasts; the myofibroblastic cells have contractile properties that are responsible for contraction of the vitreous.
- Epiretinal membranes were present over the posterior and peripheral retina at 4 weeks following the injury.
- Contraction of transvitreal and peripheral epiretinal membranes resulted in detachment of the peripheral retina as early as 6 weeks following the injury.
- A total retinal detachment occurred with continued contraction of these membranes at 8 to 10 weeks.
- Proliferation anterior to the pars plana resulted in cyclitic membrane formation and eventual detachment of the ciliary body epithelium. The end-stage appearance of the eye was often present by 4 months with a total retinal detachment, significant folding of the retina by dense epiretinal membranes, cyclitic membrane formation with choroidal effusion, and ocular hypotony.[127]

This model confirmed that the critical events necessary to initiate and sustain the pathological events leading to retinal detachment are:

- the creation of a full-thickness scleral incision; and
- injection of autologous blood.

The model also showed that pars plana vitrectomy, with removal of the vitreous gel and blood, could interrupt/arrest the events that otherwise would result in tractional/rhegmatogenous retinal detachment.[128]

The evaluation and treatment of open globe injuries are presented elsewhere in this book (see Chapters 8, 9, 13, 14, 15, 16, and 26). For the vitreoretinal surgeon, those described earlier in this chapter for closed globe trauma apply; the only significant difference is the addition of another potential cause of retinal breaks: direct trauma (e.g., a knife penetrating into the vitreous cavity through a posterior scleral wound; a nail entering through the cornea and lodged in the retina).

VITREOUS HEMORRHAGE

Vitreous hemorrhage can occur as a result of closed and open globe injuries. Following contusion, vitreous blood may occur secondary to:

- retinal tear/dialysis;
- posterior vitreous detachment;
- sclopetaria;
- optic nerve avulsion;
- cyclodialysis;
- iris tears/dialysis;
- choroidal rupture; and/or
- eyewall wound.

Blood in the vitreous cavity highlights the need for complete posterior segment evaluation. If the blood is so dense as to make adequate visualization of the posterior segment impossible, B-scan ultrasonography is necessary.

Management

Associated with Closed Globe Injury

Vitreous blood associated with contusion is initially managed with close observation for spontaneous clearing of the blood.[ee]

- Serial ultrasound examinations are obtained when the posterior segment cannot be visualized to rule out retinal detachment.
- Retinal detachment is uncommon acutely following contusion but becomes more common weeks to months after injury if a retinal tear or dialysis is present.
- If a retinal detachment is detected during follow-up, it should be managed expeditiously. Otherwise the patient can be followed for spontaneous clearing of the hemorrhage, which usually occurs weeks to months following the injury.
- Long-standing vitreous hemorrhage not uncommonly results in ghost cell glaucoma, which usually requires vitrectomy (see Chapter 20).
- Vitreous hemorrhage may clear more slowly following trauma than in other conditions because many young patients have a formed vitreous and are phakic at the time of injury.

Indications[ff] for vitrectomy include:

- associated retinal detachment or large retinal tear;
- nonclearing hemorrhage;
- ghost cell glaucoma;
- monocular patient;
- bilateral vitreous hemorrhage; or
- associated subretinal hemorrhage.

[ee] Injuries to other tissues may force the surgeon to intervene early.

[ff] We must again emphasize (see Chapter 8) that this is basically the patient's decision: if so desired by the patient, earlier vitrectomy should be performed.

Associated with Open Globe Injury

Vitreous blood in case of an open globe injury has a more ominous natural history than that in closed globe trauma (see Fig. 23–20).

> **PEARL...** Because of its potential to incite PVR, it is generally recommended that vitreous blood be removed *prior to* the formation of significant membranes and the development of retinal detachment.[gg]

- The exact *timing* of vitrectomy following open globe injury is a matter of controversy; although most authors favor waiting for 1 to 2 weeks following the primary repair, others advocate vitrectomy at the time of wound closure (see Chapter 8 and the Appendix and Table 23–9).
- A complete vitrectomy should be performed, including removal of the posterior vitreous face as this may reduce the chance of continued epiretinal proliferation.
- A wide-angle viewing system (see Chapter 8) or scleral depression permits shaving of the vitreous base (alternatively, the endoscope may prove useful; see the Appendix).
- The use of a scleral buckle following prophylactic vitrectomy is also controversial. We generally

---

[gg] In this regard, vitrectomy is recommended early, as a prophylaxis against the development of additional posterior segment complications.

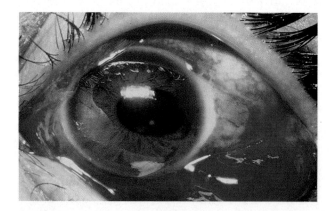

FIGURE 23–20 This patient has a ruptured globe. Blood-tinged vitreous can be seen extruding from under the medial rectus muscle. After primary wound closure and then vitrectomy 7 days following the injury to remove the vitreous blood, the proliferation cycle of events was interrupted. In cases of open globe injury with mild vitreous hemorrhage, the patient can be observed closely for the development of complications.

TABLE 23–9 ADVANTAGES OF EARLY VERSUS DELAYED VITRECTOMY IN OPEN GLOBE INJURY*

Factor	Early Vitrectomy	Delayed Vitrectomy
Less bleeding		×
Fewer procedures	×	
Posterior vitreous detachment present		×
Choroidal detachment resolved		×
Less intraocular proliferation	×	
Better surgical visualization		×

*Early vitrectomy: at the time of primary repair; delayed vitrectomy: 1 to 2 weeks following primary closure.

consider an encircling band to support the vitreous base in the following cases:

- a complete vitrectomy could not be performed,
- visualization is too poor to rule out peripheral pathology; or
- there is anterior retinal injury.

- The outcome for many of these patients is quite good as long as there is no significant retinal, optic nerve, or corneal injury.

PITFALL

Vitreous hemorrhage associated with ocular rupture has a significantly worse prognosis when compared with lacerating injury.[128]

SUMMARY

Injury to the posterior segment is a significant risk factor for irreversible visual loss. Closed globe injury leads to posterior segment lesions as a result of deformation changes of the globe; the lesions can be distant from the site of contact. Although our understanding of the pathophysiologic events that lead to posterior segment injury has greatly progressed in the last 25 years, the molecular changes that occur following contusion have not been well investigated. In open globe injury additional factors (e.g., presence of a wound, the threat of endophthalmitis, see Chapter 8) have to be taken into consideration. With advanced vitreoretinal treatment techniques available, the patient's chance of functional improvement is better today than before, although the pharmacological methods of preventing/treating PVR are still in their infancy.

Dr. K. G. Au Eong was supported by the National Medical Research Council-Singapore Totalisator Board Medical Research Fellowship, Singapore.

REFERENCES

1. May DR, Kuhn FP, Morris RE, et al. The epidemiology of serious eye injuries from the United States Eye Injury Registry. *Graefes Arch Clin Exp Ophthalmol.* 2000;238:153–157.
2. Schein OD, Hibberd PL, Shingleton BJ, et al. The spectrum and burden of ocular injury. *Ophthalmology.* 1988;95:300–305.
3. Thach AB, Ward TP, Hollifield RD, et al. Ocular injuries from paintball pellets. *Ophthalmology.* 1999;106:533–537.
4. Knorr HL, Jonas JB. Retinal detachments by squash ball accidents. *Am J Ophthalmol.* 1996;122:260–261.
5. Goffstein R, Burton TC. Differentiating traumatic from nontraumatic retinal detachment. *Ophthalmology.* 1982;89:361–368.
6. Williams DF, Mieler WF, Williams GA. Posterior segment manifestations of ocular trauma. *Retina.* 1990;10(suppl 1):S35–S44.
7. Cox MS, Schepens CL, Freeman HM. Retinal detachment due to ocular contusion. *Arch Ophthalmol.* 1966;76:678–685.
8. Moore AT, McCartney A, Cooling RJ. Ocular injuries associated with the use of airguns. *Eye.* 1987;1:422–429.
9. Winslow RL, Tasman W. Juvenile rhegmatogenous retinal detachment. *Ophthalmology.* 1978;85:607–618.
10. Filipe JA, Barros H, Castro-Correia J. Sports-related ocular injuries: a three-year follow-up study. *Ophthalmology.* 1997;104:313–318.
11. Belkin M, Treister G, Dotan S. Eye injuries and ocular protection in the Lebanon War, 1982. *Isr J Med Sci.* 1984;20:333–338.
12. Easterbrook M. Eye protection in racquet sports. *Curr Ther Sports Med.* 1990;2:365–372.
13. Pashby TJ. Eye injuries in Canadian hockey. Phase II. *Can Med Assoc J.* 1977;117:671–672, 677–678.

14. Pashby TJ, Pashby RC, Chisholm LD, et al. Eye injuries in Canadian hockey. *Can Med Assoc J.* 1975; 113:663–666, 674.

15. Delori F, Pomerantzeff O, Cox MS. Deformation of the globe under high-speed impact: its relation to contusion injuries. *Invest Ophthalmol.* 1969;8:290–301.

16. Weidenthal DT, Schepens CL. Peripheral fundus changes associated with ocular contusion. *Am J Ophthalmol.* 1966;62:465–477.

17. Assaf AA. Traumatic retinal detachment. *J Trauma.* 1985;25:1085–1089.

18. Tasman W. Peripheral retinal changes following blunt trauma. *Trans Am Ophthalmol Soc.* 1972;70:190–198.

19. Wolter RJ. The histopathology of cystoid macular edema. *Albrecht Von Graefes Arch Klin Exp Ophthalmol.* 1981;216:85–101.

20. Blight R, Dean Hart JC. Structural changes in the outer retinal layers following blunt mechanical non-perforating trauma to the globe: an experimental study. *Br J Ophthalmol.* 1977;61:573–587.

21. Joseph E, Zak R, Smith S, Best WR, Gamelli RL, Dries DL. Predictors of blinding or serious eye injury in blunt trauma. *J Trauma.* 1992;33:19–24.

22. Archer DB. Injuries of the posterior segment of the eye. Dermot Pierse lecture. *Trans Ophthalmol Soc UK.* 1985; 104:597–615.

23. Zion VM, Burton TC. Retinal dialysis. *Arch Ophthalmol.* 1980;98:1971–1974.

24. Berlin R. Zur sogenannten commotio retinae. *Klin Monatsbl Augenheilkd.* 1873;1:42–78.

25. Gass JDM. *Stereoscopic Atlas of Macular Diseases: Diagnosis and Treatment.* 4th ed. St Louis: CV Mosby; 1997.

26. Bastek JV, Foos RY, Heckenlively J. Traumatic pigmentary retinopathy. *Am J Ophthalmol.* 1981;92:621–624.

27. Cogan DG. Pseudoretinitis pigmentosa: report of two traumatic cases of recent origin. *Arch Ophthalmol.* 1969; 81:45–53.

28. Sipperley JO, Quigley HA, Gass JDM. Traumatic retinopathy in primates: the explanation of commotio retinae. *Arch Ophthalmol.* 1978;96:2267–2273.

29. Kohno T, Ishibashi T, Inomata H, Ikui H, Taniguchi Y. Experimental macular edema of commotio retinae: preliminary report. *Jpn J Ophthalmol.* 1983;27:149–156.

30. Gregor Z, Ryan SJ. Blood-retinal barrier after blunt trauma to the eye. *Graefes Arch Clin Exp Ophthalmol.* 1982;219:205–208.

31. Mansour AM, Green WR, Hogge C. Histopathology of commotio retinae. *Retina.* 1992;12:24–28.

32. Pulido JS, Blair NP. The blood-retinal barrier in Berlin's edema. *Retina.* 1987;7:233–236.

33. Eagling EM. Ocular damage after blunt trauma to the eye: its relationship to the nature of the injury. *Br J Ophthalmol.* 1974;58:126–140.

34. Goldzieher W. Beitrag zur pathologie der orbitalen Schussverletzungen. *Z Augenheilkd.* 1901;6:277–281.

35. Cohn H. *Schussverletzungen des Auges.* Breslau: Ferdinand Enke; 1872.

36. Richards RD, West CE, Meisels AA. Chorioretinitis sclopetaria. *Trans Am Ophthalmol Soc.* 1968;66:214–232.

37. Martin DF, Awh CC, McCuen BW, Jaffe GJ, Slott JH, Machemer R. Treatment and pathogenesis of traumatic chorioretinal rupture sclopetaria. *Am J Ophthalmol.* 1994;117:190–200.

38. Brown GC, Tasman WS, Benson WE. BB-gun injuries to the eye. *Ophthalmic Surg.* 1985;16:505–508.

39. Beatty S, Smyth KL, Au Eong KG, Lavin MJ. Chorioretinitis sclopetaria. *Injury.* 2000;31:55–60.

40. Katsumata S, Takahashi J, Tamai M. Chorioretinitis sclopetaria caused by fishing line sinker. *Jpn J Ophthalmol.* 1984;28:69–74.

41. Richards RD, West CE, Meisels AA. Chorioretinitis sclopetaria. *Am J Ophthalmol.* 1968;66:852–860.

42. Dubovy SR, Guyton DL, Green WR. Clinicopathologic correlation of chorioretinitis sclopetaria. *Retina.* 1997; 17:510–520.

43. Aaberg TM. Macular holes. *Surv Ophthalmol.* 1970;15: 139–162.

44. Atmaca LS, Yilmaz M. Changes in the fundus caused by blunt ocular trauma. *Ann Ophthalmol.* 1993;25:447–452.

45. Bullock JD, Ballal DR, Johnson DA, Bullock RJ. Ocular and orbital trauma from water balloon slingshots. *Ophthalmology.* 1997;104:878–887.

46. Weinstock SJ, Morin JD. Traumatic macular hole. *Can J Ophthalmol.* 1976;11:249–251.

47. Madreperla SA, Benetz BA. Formation and treatment of a traumatic macular hole. *Arch Ophthalmol.* 1997;115: 1210–1211.

48. Thach AB, Lopez PF, Snady-McCoy LC, Golub BM, Frambach DA. Accidental Nd:YAG laser injuries to the macula. *Am J Ophthalmol.* 1995;119:767–773.

49. Ciulla TA, Topping TM. Surgical treatment of a macular hole secondary to accidental laser burn. *Arch Ophthalmol.* 1997;115:929–930.

50. Sheidow TG, Gonder JR. Macular hole secondary to retrobulbar needle perforation. *Retina.* 1998;18:178–180.

51. Yanagiya N, Akiba J, Takahashi M, et al. Clinical characteristics of traumatic macular holes. *Jpn J Ophthalmol.* 1996;40:544–547.

52. Amari F, Ogino N, Matsumura M, Negi A, Yoshimura N. Vitreous surgery for traumatic macular holes. *Retina.* 1999;19:410–413.

53. Kuhn F, Morris R, Mester V, Witherspoon C. Internal limiting membrane removal for traumatic macular holes. *Ophthalmic Surg Lasers.* 2001;32:308–315.

54. Kusaka S, Fujikado T, Ikeda T, Tano Y. Spontaneous disappearance of traumatic macular holes in young patients. *Am J Ophthalmol.* 1997;123:837–839.

55. Gass JDM. Idiopathic senile macular holes: its early stages and pathogenesis. *Arch Ophthalmol.* 1988;106:629–639.

56. Kelly NE, Wendel RT. Vitreous surgery for idiopathic macular holes: results of a pilot study. *Arch Ophthalmol.* 1991;109:654–659.

57. Margherio AR, Margherio RR, Hartzer M, Trese MT, Williams GA, Ferrone PJ. Plasmin enzyme-assisted vitrectomy in traumatic pediatric macular holes. *Ophthalmology.* 1998;105:1617–1620.

58. Rubin JS, Glaser BM, Thompson JT, Sjaarda RN, Pappas SS, Murphy RP. Vitrectomy, fluid-gas exchange and

transforming growth factor-beta-2 for the treatment of traumatic macular holes. *Ophthalmology.* 1995;102: 1840–1845.

59. Garcia-Arumi J, Corcostegui B, Cavero L, Sararols L. The role of vitreoretinal surgery in the treatment of posttraumatic macular hole. *Retina.* 1997;17:372–377.

60. Chow DR, Williams GA, Trese MT, Margherio RR, Ruby AJ, Ferrone PJ. Successful closure of traumatic macular holes. *Retina.* 1999;19:405–409.

61. de Bustros S. Vitreous surgery for traumatic macular hole. *Retina.* 1996;12:451–452.

62. Alappatt JJ, Hutchins RK. Retinal detachments due to traumatic tears in the pars plana ciliaris. *Retina.* 1998; 18:506–509.

63. Ross WH. Traumatic retinal dialyses. *Arch Ophthalmol.* 1981;99:1371–1374.

64. Scott JD. Retinal dialysis. *Trans Ophthalmol Soc UK.* 1977;97:33–35.

65. Kennedy CJ, Parker CE, McAllister IL. Retinal detachment caused by retinal dialysis. *Aust N Z J Ophthalmol.* 1997;25:25–30.

66. Tasman W. Peripheral retinal changes following blunt trauma. *Mod Prob Ophthalmol.* 1974;12:446–450.

67. Hagler WS, North AW. Retinal dialyses and retinal detachment. *Arch Ophthalmol.* 1968;79:376–388.

68. Johnston PB. Traumatic retinal detachment. *Br J Ophthalmol.* 1991;75:18–21.

69. Dumas JJ. Retinal detachment following contusion of the eye. *Int Ophthalmol Clin.* 1967;7:19–38.

70. Aylward GW, Cooling RJ, Leaver PK. Trauma-induced retinal detachment associated with giant retinal tears. *Retina.* 1993;13:136–141.

71. Nacef L, Daghfous F, Chaabini M, et al. [Ocular contusions and giant retinal tears]. *J Fr Ophtalmol.* 1997;20:170–174.

72. Haimann MH, Burton TC, Brown CK. Epidemiology of retinal detachment. *Arch Ophthalmol.* 1982;100:289–292.

73. Tasman W. Retinal detachment in children. *Trans Am Ophthalmol Otolaryngol.* 1967;71:455–460.

74. Campochiaro PA, Kaden IH, Vidaurri-Leal J, Glaser BM. Cryotherapy enhances intravitreal dispersion of viable RPE cells. *Arch Ophthalmol.* 1985;103:434–436.

75. Glaser BM, Vidaurri-Leal J, Michels RG, Campochiaro PA. Cryotherapy during surgery for giant retinal tears and intravitreal dispersion of viable RPE cells. *Ophthalmology.* 1993;100:466–470.

76. Cardillo JA, Stout JT, LaBree L, et al. Post-traumatic proliferative vitreoretinopathy: the epidemiologic profile, onset, risk factors, and visual outcome. *Ophthalmology.* 1997;104:1166–1173.

77. Brinton GS, Aaberg TM, Reeser FH, Topping TM, Abrams GW. Surgical results in ocular trauma involving the posterior segment. *Am J Ophthalmol.* 1982;93: 271–278.

78. Cox MS, Freeman HM. Retinal detachment due to ocular penetration I: clinical characteristics and surgical results. *Arch Ophthalmol.* 1978;96:1354–1361.

79. Eagling EM. Perforating injuries involving the posterior segment. *Trans Ophthalmol Soc UK.* 1975;95:335–339.

80. Ryan SJ, Allen AW. Pars plana vitrectomy in ocular trauma. *Am J Ophthalmol.* 1979;88:483–491.

81. Machemer R. Pathogenesis and classification of massive periretinal proliferation. *Br J Ophthalmol.* 1978;62:737–747.

82. Machemer R, Aaberg TM, Freeman HM, Irvine AR, Lean JS, Michels RG. An updated classification of retinal detachment with proliferative vitreoretinopathy. *Am J Ophthalmol.* 1991;112:159–165.

83. Hiscott P, Sheridan C, Magee RM, et al. Matrix and the RPE in proliferative retinal disease. *Prog Retin Eye Res.* 1999;18:167–190.

84. Laqua H, Machemer R. Clinical-pathological correlation in massive periretinal proliferation. *Am J Ophthalmol.* 1975;80:913–929.

85. Hiscott PS, Grierson I, McLeod D. RPE cells in epiretinal membranes: an immunohistochemical study. *Br J Ophthalmol.* 1984;68:708–715.

86. Machemer R, van Horn D, Aaberg TM. Pigment epithelial proliferation in human retinal detachment with massive periretinal proliferation. *Am J Ophthalmol.* 1978;85:181–191.

87. Glaser BM, Cardin A, Biscoe B. Proliferative vitreoretinopathy: the mechanism of development of vitreoretinal traction. *Ophthalmology.* 1987;94:327–332.

88. Hiscott PS, Grierson I, McLeod D. Natural history of fibrocellular epiretinal membranes: a quantitative, autoradiographic, and immunohistochemical study. *Br J Ophthalmol.* 1985;69:810–823.

89. Weller M, Wiedemann P, Bresgen M, Heimann K. Vitronectin and proliferative intraocular disorders. I. A colocalisation study of the serum spreading factor, vitronectin, and fibronectin in traction membranes from patients with proliferative vitreoretinopathy. *Int Ophthalmol.* 1991;15:93–101.

90. Weller M, Wiedemann P, Bresgen M, Heimann K. Vitronectin and proliferative intraocular disorders. II. Expression of cell surface receptors for fibronectin and vitronectin in periretinal membranes. *Int Ophthalmol.* 1991;15:103–108.

91. Ehrenberg M, Thresher RJ, Machemer R. Vitreous hemorrhage nontoxic to retina as a stimulator of glial and fibrous proliferation. *Am J Ophthalmol.* 1984;97:611–626.

92. Percival SP. Late complications from posterior segment intraocular foreign bodies with particular reference to retinal detachment. *Br J Ophthalmol.* 1972;56:462–468.

93. Roper-Hall MJ. The treatment of ocular injuries. *Trans Ophthalmol Soc UK.* 1959;79:57.

94. Hamilton AM, Taylor W. Significance of pigment granules in the vitreous. *Br J Ophthalmol.* 1972;56:700–702.

95. Lewis H, Aaberg TM. Causes of failure after repeat vitreoretinal surgery for recurrent proliferative vitreoretinopathy. *Am J Ophthalmol.* 1991;111:15–19.

96. Lewis H, Aaberg TM, Abrams GW. Causes of failure after initial vitreoretinal surgery for severe proliferative vitreoretinopathy. *Am J Ophthalmol.* 1991;111:8–14.

97. Lopez PF, Grossniklaus HE, Aaberg TM, Sternberg P, Capone A, Lambert HM. Pathogenetic mechanisms in anterior proliferative vitreoretinopathy. *Am J Ophthalmol.* 1992;114:257–279.

98. Zarbin MA, Michels RG, Green WR. Dissection of epiciliary tissue to treat chronic hypotony after surgery for retinal detachment with proliferative vitreoretinopathy. *Retina.* 1991;11:208–213.

99. Tano Y, Sugita G, Abrams G, Machemer R. Inhibition of intraocular proliferations with intravitreal corticosteroids. *Am J Ophthalmol.* 1980;89:131–136.

100. Blumenkranz M, Hernandez E, Ophir A, Norton EW. 5-Fluorouracil: new applications in complicated retinal detachment for an established antimetabolite. *Ophthalmology.* 1984;91:122–130.

101. Wiedemann P, Leinung C, Hilgers RD, Heimann K. Daunomycin and silicone oil for the treatment of proliferative vitreoretinopathy. *Graefes Arch Clin Exp Ophthalmol.* 1991;229:150–152.

102. Iverson DA, Katsura H, Hartzer MK, Blumenkranz MS. Inhibition of intraocular fibrin formation following infusion of low-molecular-weight heparin during vitrectomy. *Arch Ophthalmol.* 1991;109:405–409.

103. Berman DH, Gombos GM. Proliferative vitreoretinopathy: does oral low-dose colchicine have an inhibitory effect? A controlled study in humans. *Ophthalmic Surg.* 1989;20:268–272.

104. Charteris DG. Proliferative vitreoretinopathy: pathobiology, surgical management, and adjunctive treatment. *Br J Ophthalmol.* 1995;79:953–960.

105. Michels RG. Surgery of retinal detachment with proliferative vitreoretinopathy. *Retina.* 1984;4:63–83.

106. Lewis H, Aaberg TM, Abrams GW, McDonald HR, Williams GA, Mieler WF. Subretinal membranes in proliferative vitreoretinopathy. *Ophthalmology.* 1989; 96:1403–1414.

107. Aaberg TM. Management of anterior and posterior proliferative vitreoretinopathy. XLV Edward Jackson memorial lecture. *Am J Ophthalmol.* 1988;106:519–532.

108. Vitrectomy with silicone oil or perfluoropropane gas in eyes with severe proliferative vitreoretinopathy: results of a randomized clinical trial. Silicone Study Report 2. *Arch Ophthalmol.* 1992;110:780–792.

109. Vitrectomy with silicone oil or sulfur hexafluoride gas in eyes with severe proliferative vitreoretinopathy: results of a randomized clinical trial. Silicone Study Report 1. *Arch Ophthalmol.* 1992;110:770–779.

110. Ando F. Usefulness and limit of silicone in management of complicated retinal detachment. *Jpn J Ophthalmol.* 1987;31:138–146.

111. McCuen BW, Azen SP, Stern W, et al. Vitrectomy with silicone oil or perfluoropropane gas in eyes with proliferative vitreoretinopathy. Silicone Study Report 3. *Retina.* 1993;13:279–284.

112. Barr CC, Lai MY, Lean JS, et al. Postoperative intraocular pressure abnormalities in the Silicone Study. Silicone Study Report 4. *Ophthalmology.* 1993;100:1629–1635.

113. Blumenkranz MS, Azen SP, Aaberg TM, et al. Relaxing retinotomy with silicone oil or long-acting gas in eyes with severe proliferative vitreoretinopathy. Silicone Study Report 5. The Silicone Study Group. *Am J Ophthalmol.* 1993;116:557–564.

114. Hutton WL, Azen SP, Blumenkranz M, et al. The effects of silicone oil removal. Silicone Study Report 6. *Arch Ophthalmol* 1994;112:778–785.

115. Abrams GW, Azen SP, Barr CC, et al. The incidence of corneal abnormalities in the Silicone Study. Silicone Study Report 7. *Arch Ophthalmol.* 1995;113:764–769.

116. Cox MS, Azen SP, Barr CC, et al. Macular pucker after successful surgery for proliferative vitreoretinopathy. Silicone Study Report 8. *Ophthalmology.* 1995;102:1884–1891.

117. Lean J, Azen SP, Lopez PF, Qian D, Lai MY, McCuen B. The prognostic utility of the Silicone Study Classification System. Silicone Study Report 9. Silicone Study Group. *Arch Ophthalmol.* 1996;114:286–292.

118. Diddie KR, Azen SP, Freeman HM, et al. Anterior proliferative vitreoretinopathy in the silicone study. Silicone Study Report Number 10. *Ophthalmology.* 1996;103:1092–1099.

119. Abrams GW, Azen SP, McCuen BW, Flynn HW, Lai MY, Ryan SJ. Vitrectomy with silicone oil or long-acting gas in eyes with severe proliferative vitreoretinopathy: results of additional and long-term follow-up. Silicone Study Report 11. *Arch Ophthalmol.* 1997;115:335–344.

120. Wilkinson CP, Rice TA. *Michels Retinal Detachment.* 2nd ed. St Louis: Mosby-Year Book, 1997.

121. Bonnet M. Macular changes and fluorescein angiographic findings after repair of proliferative vitreoretinopathy. *Retina.* 1994;14:404–410.

122. Johnston S. Perforating eye injuries: a five year survey. *Trans Ophthalmol Soc UK.* 1971;91:895–921.

123. Winthrop SR, Cleary PE, Minckler DS, Ryan SJ. Penetrating eye injuries: a histopathological review. *Br J Ophthalmol.* 1980;64:809–817.

124. Cleary PE, Jarus G, Ryan SJ. Experimental posterior penetrating eye injury in the rhesus monkey: vitreous-lens admixture. *Br J Ophthalmol.* 1980;64:801–808.

125. Cleary PE, Ryan SJ. Posterior perforating eye injury. Experimental animal model. *Trans Ophthalmol Soc UK.* 1978;98:34–37.

126. Cleary PE, Ryan SJ. Method of production and natural history of experimental posterior penetrating eye injury in the rhesus monkey. *Am J Ophthalmol.* 1979; 88:212–220.

127. Cleary PE, Ryan SJ. Histology of wound, vitreous, and retina in experimental posterior penetrating eye injury in the rhesus monkey. *Am J Ophthalmol.* 1979; 88:221–231.

128. Cleary PE, Ryan SJ. Vitrectomy in penetrating eye injury: results of a controlled trial of vitrectomy in an experimental posterior penetrating eye injury in the rhesus monkey. *Arch Ophthalmol.* 1981;99:287–292.

Chapter 24

INTRAOCULAR FOREIGN BODIES

Ferenc Kuhn, Viktória Mester, and Robert Morris

IOFBs are traditionally defined as intraocularly retained, unintentional projectiles, although surgeons commonly remove objects of different types from the eye (see Table 24–1). IOFBs have typically caused so much concern to both patients and health care providers (from ancient barbers to modern ophthalmologists) as to prompt urgent extraction. This urge all too commonly has taken precedence over the most important goal: vision.[1]

HISTORY

IOFB extraction dates back thousands of years[2]; the first successful magnetic IOFB removal was reported in 1624.[3] The EEM, introduced by Hirschberg in 1789, became the ultimate tool with a high success rate in extracting fresh ferrous IOFBs, even if these were invisible. The EEM also served diagnostic purposes,[4] verifying the IOFB's magnetic nature by inflicting pain on the unanesthetized patient. The introduction of vitrectomy not only improved the results considerably: it refocused the ophthalmologist's attention from IOFB removal to complex visual rehabilitation.[5]

> **PEARL...** The primary goal in managing IOFB injuries is to treat/prevent associated conditions such as endophthalmitis, retinal detachment, and late metallosis. Only occasionally is removal of the IOFB in the vitrectomy era the sole or ultimate *purpose* of the management; rather, it is the *means* to preserve vision.

TABLE 24–1 "EXPLODED" IOFB DEFINITION: CONDITIONS/MATERIALS REQUIRING CONSIDERATION OF SURGICAL REMOVAL

	Example	
Condition	Anterior Segment	Posterior Segment
External material: intentional		
Still in place but causing complications/useful no more	IOL	Drug-releasing device
Dislocated	Retinal tack[132]	Silicone oil trapped subretinally[133]
External material: unintentional	Rubber lost during Healon injection[134]	Metal fragments lost during phacoemulsification[135,136]
Surgical trauma		
Causing dislocation of (ocular) tissue	Vitreous in AC	Lens material in vitreous, cilia[137]
Surgical trauma causing extravasation	Hyphema	Subretinal hemorrhage
Traditional interpretation of an IOFB	Glass in AC	Nail in retina

Epidemiology and Prevention

Incidence[a]:

- 18–41% among open globe injuries[6–9] (USEIR: 16%).

Age (years):

- average: 29–38[8,10–13] (USEIR: 31);
- range: 3–79[8,10–12] with 66% between 21 and 40[14] (USEIR: 2–76 with 61% between 21 and 40 and only 3% being 60).

Sex: males in 92–100%[8,10–13,15,16] (USEIR: in 93%).

Place:

- work in 54–72%[8,12,13,16] (USEIR: 33%);
- home in 30%[8,16] (USEIR: 42%).

Cause:

- hammering in 60–80%[14–17] (USEIR: 53%);
- power or machine tools in 18–25%[14,17];
- weapon-related in 19% (USEIR).

IOFB injury is rare in persons wearing eye protection[10,18]; in the USEIR, only 3% of patients claimed having safety goggles on when the injury occurred.

> **P**EARL... It is the ophthalmic community's responsibility to call the public's attention to the importance of using adequate safety glasses while conducting dangerous activities such as hammering[18] and fireworks[19,20] or power tool[14,17] use (see Chapters 4 and 27).

---
[a]Typically in penetrating injuries; only exceptionally are IOFBs encountered in ruptures.

Pathophysiology

Occasionally, an IOFB has so much momentum[b] that the damage is incompatible with anatomical reconstruction (see Chapters 8 and 31). However, in the vast majority of cases the injury allows globe preservation via appropriate surgery, during which typically the following consequences must be addressed:

- entrance wound (must have occurred by definition);
- inflammation; and
- immediate and secondary
  - physical (mechanical);
  - chemical; and
  - other complications (e.g., endophthalmitis; see Table 24–2).

Entrance Wound

The IOFB must possess certain energy to perforate the eye's protective wall. The length of the entry wound is predictive of the risk of retinal damage: the shorter the wound, the less energy to be lost during penetration (see Table 24–3).

> **P**EARL... Objects entering the eye through the sclera preserve more energy than those entering through the cornea[21] and are thus more likely to exit the eye posteriorly (i.e., causing a perforating injury).

Mechanical Intraocular Damage

Little or no damage is expected if the IOFB has completely lost its kinetic energy upon entry. Typically,

---
[b]Kinetic energy delivered to the eye upon, and immediately following, entry.

Table 24–2 Selected Primary and Secondary Consequences of an IOFB Injury

Complications	Mechanical (only the most common are listed)	Chemical	Other
Immediate	Scleral/corneal wound Bleeding (e.g., hyphema vitreous/retinal/subretinal) Iris lesion/deformity Lens fragments, cataract Retinal break(s) Rhegmatogenous retinal detachment	Chalcosis	Endophthalmitis Inflammation
Secondary	Glaucoma Posterior vitreous detachment Vitreous organization EMP Retinal break(s) Rhegmatogenous/tractional retinal detachment PVR	Siderosis Chalcosis Metallosis	Inflammation Hypotony

TABLE 24–3 THE RELATIONSHIP BETWEEN WOUND LENGTH AND THE RISK OF RETINAL IMPACTION

Length of Corneal/Scleral Wound (mm)	Proportion of Eyes with Retinal Injury (%)
3	43
4–6	26
7	5

Source: F. Kuhn and R. Morris, unpublished data from the USEIR.

however, intraocular tissue injury also occurs. The primary impact may be followed by additional impaction(s) via ricocheting (see Table 24–4 and the following). Blunt IOFBs are more destructive than sharp objects.[22]

PEARL... A posterior segment IOFB has a 68% chance of causing one and a 21% chance of resulting in two or more retinal lesions.[23]

Inflammation

Breach of the eyewall, intraocular hemorrhage, and lens/vitreous admixture, among other lesions, incite an inflammatory response. Inflammation can cause synechia formation and IOP elevation and has been implicated in the development of PVR.[24]

Chemical Implications

Metallic IOFBs are rarely pure.[25] The damage an alloy inflicts is generally proportional to the content of the harmful component.[26] Toxicity is more closely related to the active surface area than to the volume of the IOFB.[27,c]

Siderosis

IOFB-related corrosion is caused by the interaction between trivalent iron ions and proteins primarily in the eye's epithelial cells. The cytotoxicity involves

enzyme liberation and lysosome breakdown, leading to cell degeneration.[28] The ferric iron, stored in siderosomes as ferritin, is thought to be toxic by generating free radicals.[29]

PITFALL

Siderosis may develop as early as a few days[30] or as late as several years[2] after injury.

Siderotic changes include the following clinical findings:

- iron deposits on the corneal endothelium;
- chronic open-angle glaucoma;
- brownish discoloration of the iris, leading to conspicuous heterochromia in people with light-colored irises[d];
- dilated, nonreactive pupil (another common first sign[32]),[e] which may also show light/near reaction dissociation and supersensitivity to weak miotics[33];
- yellow cataract with brown deposits on the anterior capsule;
- pigmentary retinal degeneration, eventually leading to attenuated vessels and visual field loss; and
- optic disk swelling/hyperemia.[34]

The clinical diagnosis is confirmed by characteristic ERG changes such as:

- increased A wave initially; and a
- progressive reduction of the B wave subsequently.

The threat of siderosis is a powerful argument to remove all fresh ferrous IOFBs. Nevertheless, siderosis is not inevitable; see Table 24–5 for various misconceptions. If there is associated IOP elevation despite removal of the foreign body, filtration surgery may be required.

---

[c]That is, the shape of the IOFB is another factor to consider when toxicity is estimated.

[d]Discovery of the difference in iris colors commonly causes people to seek medical attention.[31]

[e]Siderosis affects the parasympathetic neurons of the iris, leading to a dilated and poorly reactive pupil. The pupils react normally to diluted (0.1%) pilocarpine, but there is no response to phospholine iodide.

TABLE 24–4 THE RISKS OF POSTERIOR SEGMENT IOFBs CAUSING RETINAL LESION(S)[23]

Location of IOFB	Risk of Development of at Least One Retinal Lesion (%)	Risk of Development of Multiple Retinal Lesions (%)
Vitreous	62	8
Retinal/subretinal	76	29
Posterior segment	68	21

Table 24-5 Common Myths and Truths Regarding Siderosis

Myth	Truth
All IOFBs with iron content eventually cause siderosis	Neither electrophysiologic nor clinical signs of siderosis are inevitable[138,139]
Once siderotic changes occur, they are permanent	Timely removal of the IOFB can improve the visual acuity,[140] the visible siderotic changes,[138] and the ERG signs; even marked reduction of the ERG B wave may be reversible[141]
Intralenticular IOFBs do not cause siderosis	Siderosis has been reported to develop even if the IOFB is intralenticular[142,143] as iron eventually may "leak out" from the lens[25]; these changes can occur as early as weeks after the injury.[144] The threat of siderosis is greater when the IOFB is located in the lens periphery[40]
Encapsulated IOFBs do not cause siderosis	The fibrous tissue, forming around an intraretinal IOFB usually within 10 days after injury,[145] does not necessarily prevent iron dissolution into the inner eye, and severe loss of vision may develop[146]
The condition of the eye, once stable, remains so	Intraocular manipulations may dislodge the IOFB and lead to late siderosis development[34]

PITFALL

Rarely, siderosis is caused by objects presumed not to have a free iron content (steel, stone)[35–37] and by vitreous hemorrhage.[38]

It is best to discuss all treatment options with the patient, who must make the ultimate decision in cases of a chronic IOFB with threatening or existent siderosis (see Table 24–6 for our guidelines). If an IOFB is retained, regular follow-up of the informed patient is necessary using visual acuity, slit lamp, IBO, ERG, and diagnostic x-ray spectrometry.[39] The ERG is especially important because electrophysiologic signs of siderosis may arise earlier

Table 24-6 Management Recommendations for Ferrous IOFBs

IOFB/Eye's Condition	Location	Electrophysiologic and/or Clinical Signs of Siderosis	Recommendation
Fresh	Anywhere	−	Remove
Chronic	Anterior segment	−	Remove/retain
Chronic	Lens (no cataract)	−	Retain
Chronic	Lens (no cataract)	+	Remove
Chronic	Lens (cataract)	−	Remove/retain
Chronic	Lens (cataract)	+	Remove
Chronic	Vitreous	−	Retain/remove
Chronic	Vitreous	+	Remove
Chronic	Encapsulated in retina	−	Retain/remove
Chronic	Encapsulated in retina	+	Remove
Chronic	Subretinal	−	Retain
Chronic	Subretinal	+	Remove
Blind, painful, phthisical eye	Anywhere	+/−	Enucleate

than clinical changes.[40] If the patient is not expected to return for follow-up, IOFB removal should be recommended.

Chalcosis

PITFALL

Although uncommon, copper IOFBs cause particular concern because they can elicit a rapid, sterile, but endophthalmitis-like reaction[41] including corneal/scleral melting, hypopyon, and retinal detachment.[2,42] Untreated, this violent response may lead to loss of vision within a few hours,[2,f] eventually leading to phthisis.[43]

Once the danger of the acute reaction has passed, however, the risk of toxicosis drops dramatically and the IOFB may be tolerated for many years without complications.

Copper tends to deposit in membranes (e.g., Descemet's, lens capsules, ILM[2,44]) and causes destruction by increasing lipid peroxidation.[26] The typical clinical findings include:

- copper particles in the aqueous;
- green discoloration of the iris;
- greenish/brown-colored sunflower cataract with spokes of copper deposits radiating from a central ring;
- copper particles in the vitreous; and
- copper deposits on the retinal surface.[2]

Unlike siderosis, chronic chalcosis rarely leads to blindness, and even the associated cataract does not severely impede vision. Improvement may occur spontaneously or after surgical removal[45]; conversely, the chalcosis may intensify despite successful IOFB removal due to the intraocular retention of copper powder[2].

"Inert" Substances

Substances generally well tolerated inside the eye (e.g., gold, glass, plastic, porcelain) may on occasion cause substantial damage[40]:

---

[f]Pure copper, experimentally implanted into the rat vitreous,[27] caused irreversible retinal damage after only 2 days when the particle's surface area exceeded 1.3 mm².

- hot plastic can lead to massive foreign body reaction and eventual loss of the eye[46];
- aluminum may result in metallosis[42];
- sharp edges of glass can inflict secondary mechanical damage[47];
- lead may result in medically uncontrollable glaucoma[48];
- nucleus material left in the vitreous after cataract surgery may cause a foreign body reaction[49] (see Chapter 21).

EVALUATION

Based on a detailed history, inspection at the slit lamp and by ophthalmoscopy, and certain diagnostic tests (see later in this Chapter and Chapter 9), the ophthalmologist should (be able to) determine whether an IOFB is indeed present. The medicolegal implications are considerable; missed IOFBs constitute up to 56% of all trauma-related legal claims (see Chapter 7).[50] The following basic questions must be answered:

- Is there a foreign body?
- Is the foreign body truly in the eye (IOFB) or is it in the orbit?
- Are there multiple IOFBs?
- Exactly where inside the eye is the IOFB situated?
- What were the circumstances of the injury?
- What associated conditions are present (e.g., endophthalmitis, vitreous hemorrhage) or threaten (e.g., retinal detachment)?

PITFALL

Multiple IOFBs are especially common in young patients,[51] in cases of explosion or war trauma,[52] and in MVCs if the windshield is not laminated.[53]

History

Ask specific questions to determine the circumstances of the injury (when, where, how, by whom and what, distance, energy, material, etc.), and keep in mind that:

- most patients seek medical attention shortly after injury because of pain and/or visual complaints;

- if the history is suspicious but no IOFB is found, it is best to continue the search for an elusive IOFB[54,55];
- IOFBs may not be discovered until siderotic signs appear[33].

PITFALL

An estimated 20% of the patients do not experience pain,[53–55] and vision may remain excellent.[33] Children, observers, and passers-by are especially susceptible to being unaware of the injury, even if specifically asked,[56] and are prone to late presentation. In addition, IOFBs may be present despite a negative history[57] because the person is in denial (see Chapter 30); IOFBs as large as 13 × 1 mm have gone undetected.[56] The physician should suspect an IOFB in virtually all cases of open globe injury.[58]

External Inspection and Slit Lamp

An anterior entrance wound is commonly visible to the naked eye (use a penlight if necessary) or there may be warning signs (e.g., hemorrhage over the sclera, localized corneal edema, nonsurgical hole in the iris[g]).

PITFALL

Even in fresh cases with fairly large IOFBs, the entrance wound may be impossible to find,[56,59] especially if the wound is posterior.

Reports on wound size vary widely (1 to 17 mm[16,60]); most wounds are <5 mm. *Slit-lamp biomicroscopy* is mandatory, and a 90-diopter lens can provide additional information regarding IOFB position and composition as well as the associated intraocular damage. Gonioscopy, performed after wound closure, may also be helpful (see Table 24–7 for literature data on the distribution of the entry sites).

PEARL... Even in inside-out (i.e., rupture) or apparently closed globe injuries, or in the presence of uveal prolapse[14] or lens dislocation,[61] IOFBs can be present.

---

[g]Presence of an entry wound and an iris hole provides trajectory information.

TABLE 24–7   Locations of Entry Wounds (%; Literature Overview)

Corneal	Scleral	Limbal/ Corneoscleral	Reference (Source)
53	40	7	23
50	30	20	(USEIR, 1999)
32	45	23	11
52	34	15	12
66	17	NA	59
59	25	16	13
41	37	26	60
65	25	10	16

Ophthalmoscopy

By also showing the damage to intraocular tissues (see Table 24–8 for literature data on risk factors) and the IOFB's relationship to these tissues, information provided by direct visualization is superior to that by any other diagnostic technique.[10] Especially if located anteriorly, however, IOFBs may be missed, even in the presence of clear media.[29]

Ultrasonography

In the hands of an experienced clinician, ultrasonography is a very effective method to detect the presence and location of even nonmetallic IOFBs. It is the best indirect method to find associated tissue injuries such as choroidal and vitreous hemorrhages and retinal detachment[10,62] and to follow eyes after the primary repair.

PITFALL

False-negative results are possible on echography if the IOFB is small, wooden, or of vegetable matter, and a false-positive result may be found in the presence of gas bubbles.[10,62]

With extreme caution, ultrasonography may be performed on eyes with an open wound;[63] alternatively, it is used on the operating table once the wound is closed. The B scan tends to overestimate the size of the IOFB and should not be used for measuring purposes.[64]

For finding and localizing small, nonmetallic IOFBs in the anterior segment, ultrasound biomicroscopy is superior to CT, MRI, and contact B-scan ultrasonography.[65,66] It is limited in its ability, however, to distinguish between different materials and cannot be used if the globe has an open wound.[65]

TABLE 24-8 THE RISK OF DEVELOPING SELECTED ASSOCIATED INJURIES/CONDITIONS WITH IOFB TRAUMA (%)

Endophthalmitis	Hyphema	Cataract	Vitreous Hemorrhage	Retinal Lesion(s)	Retinal Detachment	Reference
9	3	48	45	45	9	23
3	45	38	45	15	9	12
0	NA	NA	52	16	20	13
13	30	59	37	19	15	60
0	40	25	30	NA	50	51
7	NA	33	45	NA	7	8
13	NA	47	37	26	21	16
0	NA	50	50	12	25	147

Radiology

Plain X-Ray

Although still widely used, this traditional method is slowly being replaced by CT as the primary radiological diagnostic tool. Inaccuracies have been described in numerous individual case reports and large studies.[17,31,67–73] Screening by plain x-ray has been found unnecessary.[74] Dental x-ray is more helpful by virtue of its bone-free image.

CT

With a sensitivity of 45 to 65% for IOFBs <0.06 mm^3 and of 100%[75] for IOFBs >0.06 mm^3, CT is the best indirect method for both detecting and localizing IOFBs. Appropriate software and technique allow some differentiation of IOFB composition, although CT still cannot distinguish between various types of metals.[62,76,77]

PITFALL

CT can miss plastic,[78] even metallic[79] IOFBs, especially if too wide cuts are used or the eye moves during the procedure.[67] Wood may cause problems by giving an image similar to that caused by air. Conversely, a false-positive finding can also occur (see Fig. 24–1).

Although both are able to find IOFBs as small as 0.048 mm^3,[75] *helical (spiral) CT*:

- provides an image superior to that of a conventional axial CT[80,81];
- has a shorter examination time;
- has the ability to reconstruct coronal/sagittal images without further scanning; and
- reduces motion artifacts and radiation.[82]

MRI

A powerful tool for cross-sectional and soft-tissue analyses, MRI is very sensitive in detecting IOFBs, allowing discovery even when performed for nonophthalmological indications.[83]

CONTROVERSY

The literature is rather confusing in determining whether MRI is safe in cases of ferrous IOFBs.[h] Some reports found that IOFB movement is rare,[85] whereas others have shown that movement is not only very common[86] but may occur even when the test is performed for distant body problems such as a lumbar spine herniation.[87] Furthermore, damage due to IOFB movement during MRI has not been seen by some authors[88] but reported to occur by others.[89]

PITFALL

The most important diagnostic question is whether the foreign body is intra- or extraocular. Unfortunately, the margin of error of radiological methods is greatest when the object is closest to the eyewall. Personal consultation with the radiologist *before* the test is conducted and making an effort to *personally read the test results* reduce the incidence of radiological errors.

---

[h]Shotgun pellets in the United States are not made of lead any more but of steel, making them potentially hazardous for MRI.[84]

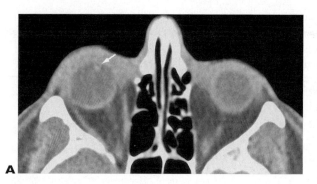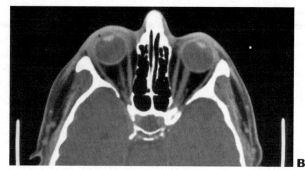

FIGURE 24–1 Even a positive CT finding is not infallible. **(A)** Preoperative CT scan; the radiologist described an IOFB 3 mm from the surface inside the right eye (his arrow is still visible on the scan). Careful investigation failed to detect the IOFB during vitrectomy. **(B)** Postoperative CT scan shows a right orbit without any foreign object.

Metal Detectors

Having been supplanted by superior diagnostic methods[90] or because they are not commercially available,[39] metal detectors are rarely used today.

Table 24–9 summarizes certain shortcomings of ultrasonography, plain x-ray, and CT; Table 24–10 shows some of the potential diagnostic traps, threatening even when different evaluation methods are combined.[10] It must be emphasized that in the vitrectomy era:

- accurate preoperative IOFB localization is less important;[55] and
- the IOFB may move from its predetermined position before or during surgery.[37]

PITFALL

If an IOFB is not found during surgery, the most likely locations are behind the iris in the vitreous cavity at 6 o'clock, subretinally, or in the angle, in which case only gonioscopy may help in discovering it.[i]

---

[i]Rarely, the path of the IOFB is posteroanterior (e.g., having entered the eye through the sclera from below or when the patient was looking up).

MANAGEMENT STRATEGY AND COUNSELING

Before designing and discussing with the patient the management plan, all data must be analyzed carefully to answer the following crucial questions:

- Is this a high-risk injury?[j] If yes, immediate intervention is advised.
- Is a retinal break and/or detachment present? The more likely that retinal damage has occurred (see Table 24–4), the more urgent the intervention. If media opacity prevents retinal visualization, use indirect clues such as:
  - wound length (see Table 24–3);
  - circumstances of the injury (the greater the kinetic energy of the object and the sharper it is, the more likely that deep penetration has occurred); and
  - wound location (i.e., corneal vs. scleral).

Additional helpful factors to consider are:

- IOFB characteristics (see Table 24–11);
- risks and types of associated intraocular tissue damage (see Table 24–8);

---

[j]For endophthalmitis development (e.g., vegetable matter, soil contamination) and IOFBs with copper content.

TABLE 24–9 THE (IN)ACCURACY OF VARIOUS DIAGNOSTIC MODALITIES IN IOFB RECOGNITION AND LOCALIZATION (%)

	Ultrasonography	X-ray	CT
Detection			
False positive	6[68]–26[69]	0[68]*	14[73] (see Fig. 24–1)
False negative	8[69]–11[68]	5[69]–60[68]	5[69]
Inaccurate localization	Anecdotal evidence	11[69]–30[17]	2[69]

*To the less careful observer, an artifact may appear as an IOFB.

TABLE 24–10   REPORTED DIAGNOSTIC TRAPS WITH IOFBs

Trap	Reference
IOFB masquerading as globe rupture	148
IOFB masquerading as idiopathic chronic iridocyclitis	57,149
IOFB masquerading as a choroidal melanoma, even as one with extrascleral extension	72,150,151,152
IOFB causing subretinal neovascularization	153
Ocular calcification masquerading as IOFB	154
Encapsulated preretinal hemorrhage masquerading as IOFB	155

TABLE 24–11   CHARACTERISTICS OF IOFBs

Variable	Findings	Reference (Source)
Number	Multiple in 8–25% of eyes	11,12,60,51
Location	58% in posterior segment	(USEIR, 2000)
	13–24% in anterior segment	8,9,17,60,97
	7–10% in lens	8,17,156
	25–48% in vitreous	8,17,60,97
	16–44% in retina	8,17,60
	52% retina and choroid	92
	0–15% subretinally	8,16,60
Size (mm)	Average: 3.5 (range: 0.5–25)	60,97
	73% > 3	97
	45% ≥ 2	13
	2 × 1 to 5 × 9	11
Material	41–89% magnetic	10,11,12,14,60
	78–100% metallic	9,10,11,12,60
	5–18% glass	8,9,60

- the surgeon's experience, expertise, and the equipment available; and
- the legal environment.

> **PITFALL** ▼
>
> A surgeon unfamiliar with the techniques of *comprehensive* globe reconstruction should *not* attempt removal of a posterior segment IOFB (see Chapter 8).

Figure 24–2 shows the management options; remember that:

- if they are fresh, even inert IOFBs are best removed (see Figs. 24–3 and 24–4, and Table 24–12);
- if IOFB removal is decided upon and the eye shows associated tissue damage, it is better to perform complex reconstruction simultaneously than as a secondary reconstructive procedure because:
  - vision is not improved just by IOFB removal;[14] and
  - the risk of endophthalmitis is reduced only if the "cultured media" (i.e., vitreous) is also promptly removed[9,23];

- in cases of posterior segment IOFBs, a decision must be made whether to perform vitrectomy:
  - the more extensive the intraocular tissue damage, the more vitrectomy is indicated to treat existing lesions and to prevent subsequent retinal detachment[91];
  - an IOFB invisible due to vitreous hemorrhage is an absolute indication.

In addition, decisions must be made regarding:

- instrumentation (see later in this Chapter);
- timing (see later in this Chapter); and
- the use of prophylactic antibiotics (see Chapter 28 and the Appendix).

General anesthesia is preferred, especially if the IOFB is in the posterior segment. If the intervention is urgent (high-risk case) and the patient ate recently, alternative methods are available (see Chapter 8).

SO has become so rare (see Chapters 8 and 29) that we feel it justified not to consider it as a major factor when the management plan is designed. The patient must nevertheless be fully informed (see Chapter 7), especially when deciding whether to retain a permanently blind eye, and careful follow-up is always advised.

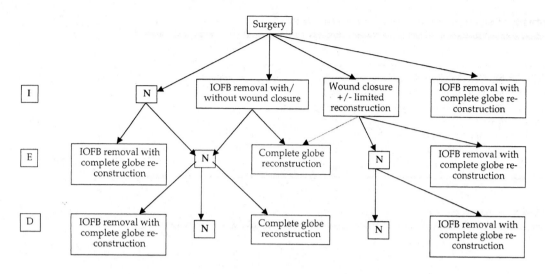

I: Immediate management; E: early management (2-7 days); D: delayed management (≥8 days); N: no surgery. To a varying degree, all of these options are practiced clinically.

FIGURE 24–2 Flowchart showing the management options in eyes with IOFB injury.

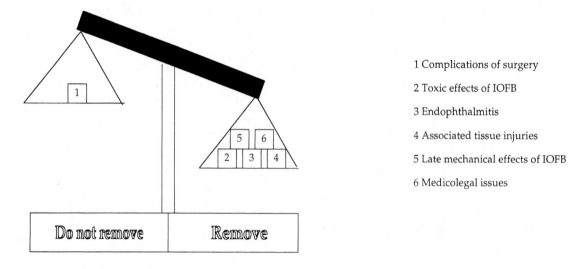

1 Complications of surgery

2 Toxic effects of IOFB

3 Endophthalmitis

4 Associated tissue injuries

5 Late mechanical effects of IOFB

6 Medicolegal issues

FIGURE 24–3 Scaling the decision whether to perform surgery to remove an *acute* IOFB.

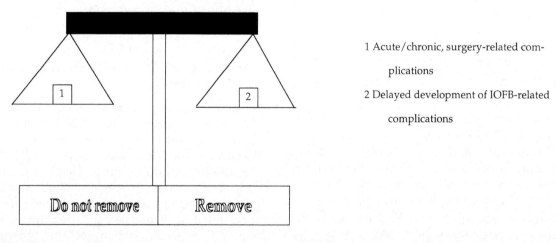

1 Acute/chronic, surgery-related complications

2 Delayed development of IOFB-related complications

FIGURE 24–4 Scaling the decision whether to remove a *chronic* IOFB, which causes no visual complaints, no signs of metallosis, and no electrophysiologic alterations.

TABLE 24–12   FRESH IOFB: REMOVAL RECOMMENDATIONS

IOFB Location	Removal?	Method*	Comment
Anterior chamber	Yes		Avoid injury to lens/endothelium
Lens	Yes/no	ICCE	
		ECCE + IOM/forceps	
		Phacoemulsification + IOM/forceps	Decision based on the extent of lens
		Vitrectomy probe + IOM/forceps	injury and patient's request
Vitreous	Yes		Look for retinal injury
Retinal	Yes		Look for additional retinal injury
Subretinal	Yes		Protect photoreceptors; use viscoelastics if necessary

*See Table 24–17 for further details.

TIMING

Literature data regarding the optimal time for intervention are conflicting. Endophthalmitis prevention is the primary goal (Table 24–13), for which as early surgery as reasonably possible is recommended for both medical and legal reasons.[k] Conversely, a recent study has confirmed earlier reports that there is no difference whether surgery is performed in the first 48 hours or later.[92] Delaying the intervention nevertheless requires vigilance (see Chapter 28) to quickly note signs of a developing infection.[l]

> **P**EARL...   The vast majority of eyes that develop endophthalmitis do so *before* the patient presents.[9,10] With time, the risk of endophthalmitis development is rapidly and dramatically reduced.

- IOFBs in the AC are usually removed at the time of primary repair.
- Intralenticular IOFBs are typically extracted in conjunction with cataract removal.
- IOFBs in the posterior segment require careful analysis of the risks and advantages (see Table 24–14).

Certain additional factors to consider (see Chapter 8 for details):

- less experienced surgeons may want to delay the intervention because:
  - the earlier the surgery is performed, the greater the danger of the development of difficult-to-control intraoperative hemorrhage;
  - spontaneous detachment[93] makes the critical step of posterior hyaloid face removal technically easier[42] while significantly improving the prognosis[94];
  - early intervention may reduce[91] the current 11%[24] incidence of PVR development;
- especially in cases of central corneal wounds, edema may initially prevent adequate visualization; intensive steroid therapy can substantially improve conditions in just a few days;
- the delay should not exceed 14 days: a few weeks will increase almost fourfold the risk of proliferation and subsequent tractional retinal detachment[93];
- no statistically significant visual/anatomical difference is seen whether vitrectomy is performed during the first or the second week after injury[8];
- spontaneous posterior hyaloid detachment may occur in a few days,[95,m] especially if vitreous hemorrhage is present.[96]

SPECIAL CONSIDERATION

Should the ophthalmologist perform emergency surgery on a patient presenting at 10 PM with a normal-risk injury or can the intervention be delayed until the morning? Take into consideration the tissue damages as well as the surgeon's expertise and experience, the staff/equipment available at night versus in the morning, the patient's general condition, and the legal environment.

---

[k]In the United States, IOFB injuries are almost always considered to be an emergency.

[l]Rarely, endophthalmitis may develop weeks or even months after the trauma if the IOFB is retained.

[m]This may not occur within the first 2 postinjury weeks as commonly as some literature reports suggest. We found that at 10 days after injury, half of the eyes still have an attached vitreous posteriorly.[23]

Table 24–13   Endophthalmitis in IOFB Injuries: A Literature Overview

Variable	Finding	Reference (Source)
Incidence	0–48%	10,60,128,157, 158,159
	5%	(USEIR, 2000)
Incidence according to IOFB location	Anterior segment: 3.9%; posterior segment: 8.8%	9
Organisms involved (literature review)	*Bacillus* species (43%); *Staphylococcus* species (31%); Gram negatives (9%); *Streptococcus* species (3%); fungi (3%)	128
(single series)	*Staphylococcus* species (27%); *Streptococcus* species (21%); *Bacillus* species (15%)	160
Culture positivity and endophthalmitis	No correlation	15
	High culture positivity rate without clinical endophthalmitis; culture should not by itself determine management decisions	60,161
Risk factors for endophthalmitis development	Primary repair after 24 hours; iv antibiotic therapy not started within 24 hours; lens injury; wound >5 mm;	162
	posterior segment involvement;	163
	timing of intervention: 3.5% if <24 hours, 13.4% if >24 hours	9
	rural setting	158
Not risk factors for endophthalmitis development	IOFB location; uveal prolapse; lens injury; whether IOFB removed completely/partially/not at all; size of IOFB	9
Effect of treatment timing	Delay in surgery not a risk factor for endophthalmitis development	13,116,164
	Endophthalmitis incidence rises if IOFB removal and reconstruction delayed >24 hours	17,165
Effect of therapy on endophthalmitis development	Endophthalmitis developing despite immediate IOFB removal[11] and intravitreal prophylactic antibiotics	
Time of endophthalmitis development	Endophthalmitis present at the time of evaluation in 91–100% of eyes	9,10
	The later the patient presents, the less likely	10
	Usually ≤36 hours after injury	128
Endophthalmitis development	No statistically significant difference whether endophthalmitis develops	16
	Outcome determined by initial damage, virulence, surgery timing	9
Retinal problems in endophthalmitis	Severe prognostic factor	95,166
Endophthalmitis prophylaxis	See Chapter 28	60

Although many surgeons still delay for a few days, without adverse effects, vitrectomy and IOFB extraction if endophthalmitis has not yet developed,[10,23,97] recently there has been a shift toward early intervention.

Management of chronic IOFBs is based on:

- whether metallosis is present (Table 24–6);
- whether mechanical damage (e.g., from an intravitreal glass particle) threatens; and

TABLE 24-14 IMMEDIATE VERSUS DELAYED INTERVENTIONS FOR POSTERIOR SEGMENT IOFB
REMOVAL AND GLOBE RECONSTRUCTION

Variable	Immediate*	Delayed†
Endophthalmitis risk	−/+	++
Corneal wound causing visibility difficulty	++	+/−
Adequate time to plan surgery/management	−/+	++
Chalcosis risk	−/+	+
Siderosis risk	−	−
Intraoperative (expulsive) hemorrhage risk	++	+
Difficulty of posterior hyaloid face removal	++	+
Retinal detachment risk	−/+	+/++
Risk of encapsulation of retinal IOFB	−	+
Threat of lawsuit	+	++

*Within 12 hours.
†Between 5 and 10 days after injury.

- the patient's desire when assessing:
  - the risks of removal versus
  - the inconvenience of regular follow-up visits.

INSTRUMENTATION

Although occasionally other tools may also be utilized (e.g., paper clips,[98] intraocular lasso,[99] intraocular cryoprobe [K. Packo, MD, Vitreous Society, Rome, Italy, August 1999], gravity,[100] cannulated extrusion needle,[101] forceps-fitted magnet[102]), there are three basic types of instruments for IOFB removal: EEMs, forceps, and IOMs (see Tables 24–15 to 24–17). EEMs may be equipped with intraocular attachments,[103] but they are bulkier and less convenient to use than IOMs.

TABLE 24-15 COMPARISON OF INSTRUMENTS COMMONLY USED FOR IOFB REMOVAL

Variable	EEM	Forceps	IOM	Comment
IOFB size critical	−	+	−	Different forceps designs may be required
IOFB shape critical	−	+	−	Different forceps designs may be required
IOFB surface critical	−	+	−	Different forceps designs may be required
IOFB composition critical	+	−	+	The higher the ferrum content, the more effective the magnet
IOFB location important in planning extraction	+	+	−	The closer the IOFB to the EEM's tip, the less risk of secondary damage; with forceps, the surgeon may be forced to use nondominant hand
May be used in hazy media	−	−	−/+	IOM may help find invisible IOFB (e.g., lying in a pool of subretinal blood or attached to posterior iris surface)
Useable for encapsulated IOFB	−	−	−	
Useable for freed IOFB	+/−	+	+	EEM can still cause secondary tissue damage
Instrument moves toward IOFB	−	+	+	Excellent visibility may be crucial with forceps and IOM
IOFB moves toward instrument	+++	−	+	IOM: movement is <2 mm
Process of contacting IOFB with instrument entirely controlled by surgeon	−−	+	++	Forceps may pose danger if sharp-edged IOFB on retina
Process of IOFB removal entirely controlled by surgeon	−	+	+++	
Dexterity required	−	+++	+	
Surgeon able to reduce secondary complications via careful planning/execution	+	+++	+++	
Loss of IOFB at extraction incision	+	++	+	

Table 24–16   Extraction of Ferrous IOFBs from the Posterior Segment: Vitrectomy or EEM?

Media Clear	IOFB Visible	IOFB Location	Vitrectomy	EEM
−	−	vitreous	+	−
−	−	retina	+	−
−	−	subretinal	+	−
+ anteriorly, mild vitreous hemorrhage	+	vitreous	+*	−
+ anteriorly, mild vitreous hemorrhage	+	retina	+	−
+ anteriorly, mild vitreous hemorrhage	+	subretinal	+	−
+	+	vitreous, single retinal impact site	+*	−
+	+	retina	+	−
+	+	subretinal	+	−
+	+	vitreous, no visible retinal injury	+*,†	+‡
+	−	retina	+	−

*IOM may be used without performing vitrectomy.
†Vitrectomy carries all the standard risks of the operation.
‡The danger of iatrogenic damage to intraocular tissues during extraction still exists. Another alternative to vitrectomy would be to use an IOM rather than the EEM.

Table 24–17   Instrument Recommendations for IOFB Extraction

IOFB Position/ Composition	Instrument	Comment
Ferrous IOFBs in AC	IOM > forceps	Viscoelastic and miosis can help protect lens if forceps used
Nonmagnetic IOFBs in AC	Forceps	Viscoelastic and miosis can help protect lens
Ferrous/nonmagnetic IOFBs in lens	IOM/forceps/cataract removal device	Cataract is not necessary to develop; therefore observation is a viable option[167] or the IOFB may be extracted without lens removal[168]
Ferrous IOFBs in posterior segment	IOM > forceps	Occasionally the EEM may be an alternative to IOM or use forceps in eyes with a small IOFB floating freely in the vitreous, preferably close to the extraction site in eyes with no more than minimal vitreous hemorrhage and only limited retinal pathology
Nonmagnetic IOFBs in the posterior segment	Forceps	Vitreoretinal pathology determines whether vitrectomy is needed

EEM

Traditionally, magnet strength and usefulness in ophthalmology were thought to be proportionally related.[″] The tips were intentionally designed to increase the pull force and the distance at which this force is efficient.[104]

The inherent problem of the EEM is that the surgeon has to view the removal process from an angle, making it difficult to align the following:

- external magnetic pole,
- surgical incision/instrument tip; and
- IOFB (Fig. 24–5).

[″]Lancaster criteria: "Unless a giant magnet can pull a small steel ball 1 mm in diameter with a force of over 50 times its weight at a distance of 20 mm, and unless a hand magnet will pull such a ball in contact with its tip with a force over 5,000 times its weight, they are not ophthalmologically effective."[2]

PITFALL

The EEM is able to exert significant pull force, yet the success rate in removing *encapsulated* IOFBs drops to as low as 59%.[105] Using an EEM to extract encapsulated IOFBs is contraindicated, however, because of the danger of iatrogenic retinal injury.

The potential for complications is determined as much by statistical luck as by surgical expertise and is significant[106]: the retinal detachment rate reached 27% in one study[105] and increased from 2% preoperatively to 24% postoperatively in another report.[14] Special-

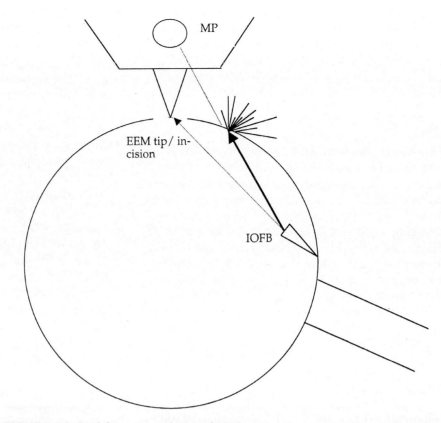

Unless the magnetic pole (MP), the instrument's tip/extraction incision, and the IOFB fall onto the same axis, the IOFB tends to fly toward the MP (solid arrow and dotted line), striking the eyewall first, rather than to the EEM's tip (dotted arrow).

FIGURE 24–5   Schematic rendering of EEM use.

ized EEM designs such as the "Innenpolmagnet"[107] have not become popular. The EEM has a tendency to overheat,[108] reducing efficiency and possibly burning the patient's skin (Fig. 24–6). The weight (up to 1 ton)[104] can cause logistical difficulties.

> **PEARL...**   Although some authors[11,60,97] found no statistically significant outcome difference whether eyes underwent EEM or vitrectomy surgery (Table 24–16), these studies did not compare eyes with similar injuries. Eyes with no or only minimal associated injuries are typically selected for EEM IOFB removal; vitrectomy is employed in eyes with extensive damage. In a study in which the eyes in the two groups had comparable damage, statistically significantly better anatomical° and functional results were found in eyes managed by vitrectomy/IOM than by EEM.[23]

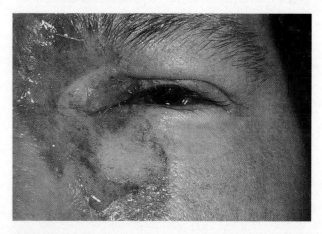

FIGURE 24–6   Patient has severe skin burn due to inappropriate EEM use.

Forceps

Intraocular forceps allow controlled maneuvers but may require considerable dexterity to grasp the IOFB (e.g., lifting up sharp objects from the retinal surface) or to adjust its position (e.g., aligning the IOFB's longest axis with that of the instrument). Use of additional tools such as PFCL[109] provides limited help (see Chapter 21 and the Appendix).

°Determined by the rate of nucleation, evisceration, phthisis, or irreparable PVR.

Either the forceps is designed in such a fashion that it "engulfs" the IOFB (e.g., spoon or Wilson forceps) or its jaws must be serrated.[p] Because IOFBs come in different sizes, shapes, and surface textures, surgeons should have several types of forceps at their disposal.[110–112]

IOM

These permanent magnets allow controlled IOFB removal with no need for special dexterity. Free-flying of the IOFB, inherently considerable with EEMs, is ≤ 2 mm. Most IOMs gradually lose power with time[108] and have a limited pull force, commonly requiring concurrent forceps use.[13,59] At least one IOM design,[q] however, has no such drawbacks and is ideal for ferrous IOFBs of any size, shape, weight, surface texture, and location.[113] Such IOMs allow removal of objects from the orbit as well (see Chapter 36).

Vitrectomy and the IOM appear to be superior to forceps/IOM use.[23,97] See Table 24–17 for details of instrumentation.

MANAGEMENT

A summary of our recommendations may be found in Table 24–18; Figure 24–7 shows the surgical details of IOFB removal. Additional issues to consider:

- Both the removed specimen (e.g., vitreous) and the IOFB should be *cultured*, even if culture positivity is not synonymous with endophthalmitis development (and it may yield false-positive results, see Chapter 28).[60]

- Never rely on visual experience when estimating the *size* of the IOFB and thus the required length of the extraction incision.[r] Because of the effect of the vitrectomy lens, the precorneal fluid, the cornea, the crystalline lens, and the vitreous substitute (e.g., air), the virtual and true IOFB sizes may differ considerably[114] (see Fig. 24–8).

- With appropriate protection of the corneal endothelium, extremely large IOFBs may be extracted via a *limbal* route.[115]

- To avoid iatrogenic retinal complications, *encapsulated IOFBs* must be completely freed before removal is attempted.[116,117] Use sharp instruments (MVR blade, needle, scissors) to adequately open the commonly strong capsule.

- *Intraretinal IOFBs* are associated with a 29[116] to 36%[118] incidence of EMP formation, even if the posterior hyaloid is carefully removed; the postoperative retinal detachment rate may reach 79%[118] with 50% of eyes developing PVR.

- *Subretinal IOFBs*, commonly hidden by blood, can be removed through an adjacently prepared retinotomy or through a peripheral (existing) retinal break[101,119]; viscoelastics may be used for photoreceptor protection.

- *Prophylactic retinopexy* should be considered for fresh retinal breaks.
  - If the vitreous has been completely removed from around a small posterior break (see Fig. 24–9), however, retinopexy is probably not necessary, especially as it may increase surface proliferation.[120]
  - Because cryopexy may stimulate cellular proliferation,[121] laser is preferred.
  - Pigmentation around the break does not necessarily imply that the lesion is sealed.
  - Older impact lesions do not require treatment.
  - The location of the break must also be considered: the more anterior a lesion, the more retinopexy is desired.

> **PEARL...** The retinopexy scar requires time to reach meaningful strength,[122] advocating deferral of surgery for several days after laser treatment[23,59] and even more following cryopexy.[59,122]

- *Prophylactic scleral buckling* may be considered to reduce the development of traction around the vitreous base. It has been found useful in some studies for open globe injuries,[95] especially if peripheral vitrectomy cannot be performed satisfactorily and the threat of PVR is significant (e.g., severe vitre-

---

[p] Even though it decreases the actual area of contact if the IOFB is rigid, serration is required to account for IOFBs of irregular shape and/or surface to provide sufficient traction.

[q] Available from Geuder GmbH, Heidelberg, Germany (catalogue number: 31900).

[r] A "good surgeon" is defined not by how small an extraction is created but by the low rate of complications associated with surgical management.

ous hemorrhage and/or retinal lesions are present)[13] or the volume of the IOFB exceeds 4 mm³.[59] However, an adverse effect of prophylactic scleral buckling has also been reported.[123]

> **PEARL... By helping to achieve complete vitreous removal in the base area, the endoscope may play a major role in the future in the prevention of anterior PVR development, thereby reducing the need for (prophylactic) buckling (see the Appendix).**

- Treatment of existing/intraoperatively developing retinal detachment does not differ from that performed in the absence of an IOFB (see Chapter 23).

ALTERNATIVE TREATMENT METHODS

No vitrectomy: trans-pars plana EEM/forceps/IOM removal may be performed if a visible IOFB is floating freely in the vitreous cavity (Table 24–16). This approach is not recommended if the IOFB is large or there is substantial associated damage to the posterior segment.

Scleral cutdown for IOFBs encapsulated anterior to the equator spares the surgeon of having to open the capsule internally.[59] However, very accurate localization of the IOFB is required, and vitrectomy may still be necessary for vitreous incarceration in the wound. This method is used with decreasing frequency: in one study, it was employed in 7% of eyes, as opposed to a 74% vitrectomy and a 15% EEM rate.[60] In other large studies, scleral cutdown was not[8,16,23,97] or rarely[92] utilized.

Endoscopic IOFB removal has been reported if corneal opacity prevented adequate visualization of the posterior segment.[124] In such cases, however, the TKP[125] (see Chapter 25) allows comprehensive reconstruction of the posterior segment as well as creation of a clear visual axis anteriorly.

LATE COMPLICATIONS

These may be due to:

- the composition of the IOFB (e.g., chalcosis, siderosis);

- the initial trauma caused by the IOFB (e.g., cataract, retinal impact site);
- subsequent scarring (e.g., PVR, choroidal neovascularization); or
- the surgical interventions themselves either as an:
  ○ expected consequence (e.g., postvitrectomy EMP development) or as an
  ○ iatrogenic trauma (e.g., peripheral retinal tear, macular phototoxicity[126]).

The management of these complications does not differ from that of complications occurring without IOFB involvement and is discussed elsewhere in this book.

SPECIAL ISSUE

Objects entering the eye only partially represent a unique management dilemma; nails and fishhooks are common examples (see Fig. 24–10 and Chapter 14).

> **PITFALL**
>
> In most cases, the attending physician should *not* remove the IOFB before referral; for instance, improperly extracted fishhooks can cause great damage.[127] If it is feared that additional trauma will be inflicted during transportation (e.g., a child cannot be adequately sedated/immobilized and may push/pull on a nail), extremely careful removal of the IOFB may be attempted, but the risks of ECH and additional intraocular damage are significant.

ANTIBIOTIC USE[s]

Prophylactic treatment:

- topical use always recommended;
- iv or oral use generally recommended, although they do not appear to reduce the endophthalmitis rate: 6.8% with, 7.2% without[9];
- intravitreal use should be considered[128] in high-risk cases[60,t];

---

[s]For dosage, see Chapter 28 and the Appendix.

[t]We recommend it.

TABLE 24–18 IOFB Injuries: Surgical Recommendations in Various Clinical Situations

Case Description	Surgical Steps	Comment
AC IOFB without lens involvement	Inspect wound in its entirety	Use conjunctival dissection if necessary
	Clean and close still open original wound if not self-sealing unless IOFB can be extracted through wound without further traumatizing eye	
	Introduce viscoelastics to maintain chamber depth/protect endothelium and lens	
	If necessary, make new incision at a convenient location	Preferably 90°–180° away from the IOFB's current position to ensure ample maneuvering room
	Extract IOFB	Use IOM/forceps as appropriate
	Restore iris diaphragm if and as necessary	
	Remove viscoelastics	
	Close extraction incision	
AC IOFB with lens involvement/ intralenticular IOFB	Same as above plus:	
	Determine whether cataract present/inevitable (a capsular tear ≤2 mm usually heals, larger ones lead to cataract[142]);	
	If the answers are "no": leave lens intact	
	If the answers are "yes": remove IOFB	Using IOM/forceps/cataract removal device as appropriate
		Suction cutter preferred to scissors
	Perform anterior vitrectomy	Anterior lensectomy or phacoemulsification /ECCE
	Remove lens	
	Consider IOL implantation when determined that no (serious) posterior segment injury is present	
Posterior segment IOFB	Inspect wound in its entirety	Use conjunctival dissection if necessary
	Clean and close still open original wound if not self-sealing unless IOFB can be extracted through wound without further traumatizing eye[147]	
	Prepare three pars plana incisions for vitrectomy unless IOFB can be removed through a pars plana incision without the need for vitreous surgery	
	Detach posterior hyaloid face	To reduce EMP incidence
	Complete vitrectomy	

Action	Notes
Locate IOFB and determine its size by comparing it with optic disk or an intraocular instrument	Optic disk in emmetropic eyes: 1.5 mm horizontally and 1.85 mm vertically[169]; fiberoptic light: 0.9 mm in diameter; always use the cross section, not just one dimension of IOFB; remember that the original wound is almost always smaller than the longest dimension of the IOFB due to tissue elasticity and stretching upon entry[170]
Free IOFB from remaining vitreous strands and/or capsule	
Prepare scleral incision at pars plana, usually extending an existing one	Consider a "T" or "L" shape incision if too long a linear incision would be required; incise choroid using MVR blade; as the choroidal wound is always shorter than the scleral one because the choroid is very elastic, extend incision using (Vanras) scissors
Make contact with IOFB using IOM/forceps	
Remove fiberoptic light once IOFB elevated into midvitreous	
Use toothed forceps to open scleral wound	
Slowly remove IOFB	Loss of IOFB at the incision occurs either because wound is too small or because extraction is too rapid
Place suture in scleral wound to restore it to vitrectomy length	
Search for retinal lesions	Using scleral indentation and the IBO if needed, especially posterior to pars plana wounds
Consider treatment of exiting lesions	Laser or cryopexy
Consider prophylactic treatment	Because of the threat of late retinal detachment from iatrogenic peripheral breaks, IBO/endolaser cerclage may be considered[171]; deliver 800–1200 spots from the ora serrata to the equator, sparing the horizontal meridians
Consider vitreous tamponade	Air; gas (SF_6, C_3F_8, etc.); silicone oil
Close pars plana incisions	

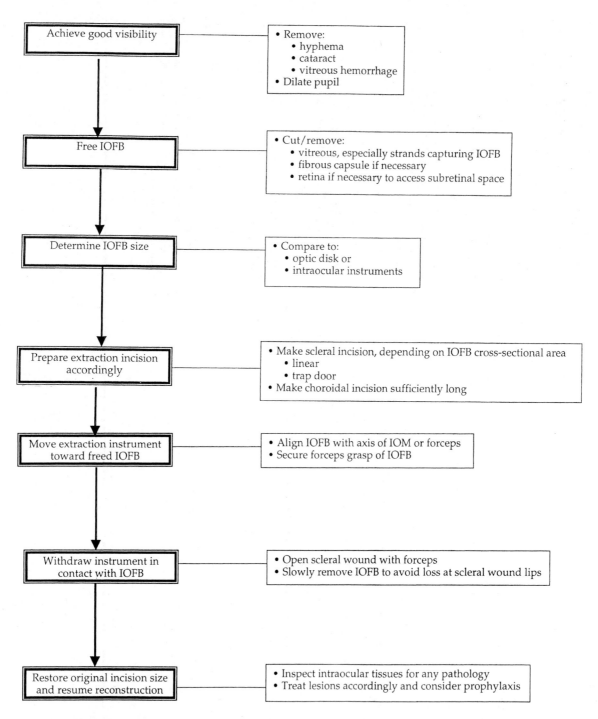

FIGURE 24–7 Important surgical steps in IOFB removal from the posterior segment.

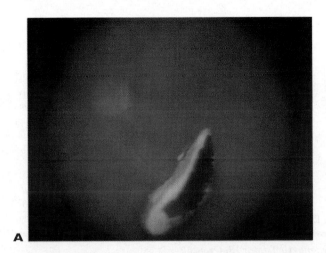
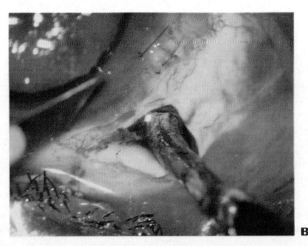

FIGURE 24–8   The misleading appearance of IOFB size. **(A)** Inside the eye. **(B)** Even though the IOFB is only partially delivered, it is obviously larger than suggested by the intraocular image (A and B: identical magnification).

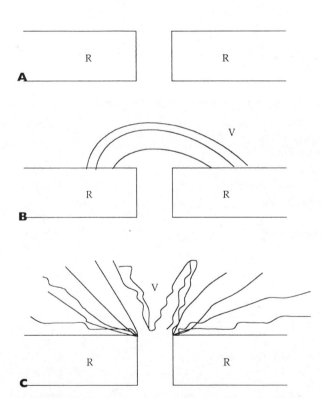

FIGURE 24–9   The vitreous and the need for retinopexy in case of a small, posterior retinal break caused by IOFB impact. **(A)** Complete vitreous removal, no traction; retinopexy is probably not necessary. **(B)** The vitreous has been trimmed around the break but a "plug" still covers the break; retinopexy is probably not necessary. **(C)** Vitreous traction remains; retinopexy is highly recommended (R, retina; V, vitreous).

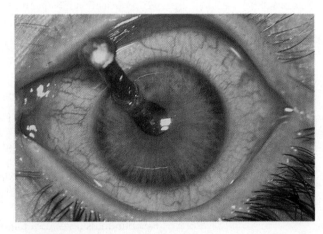

FIGURE 24–10   Nail penetrating the cornea with a substantial portion remaining external, representing a management dilemma: should you "pull the plug"? (See the text for details).

- signs of toxic retinopathy (hemorrhagic Roth's spots) remote from areas of mechanical trauma may coincide with bacterial presence before clinical signs of endophthalmitis develop.

Endophthalmitis treatment:

- topical use always recommended;
- iv or oral use always recommended;
- intravitreal use always recommended.

Prognosis and Outcome

It has been reported that open globe injuries with an IOFB have a better outcome than those without,[129] although the opposite has also been found.[59] The prognosis is nonetheless better today than even in the recent past; most eyes escape enucleation and achieve good vision. The improvement is due, among other factors, to technological advances such as vitrectomy and the IOM,[5,108] a better understanding of the pathophysiology,[91,93,96,130] and an evolving management philosophy[131]. The most important factor responsible for poor outcome is not retinal detachment but the initial tissue damage[42] such as a macular impact site.[u]

A large number of variables appear in published reports and the data are conflicting; it is therefore impossible to cite an overall prognostic figure. Tables 24–19 and 24–20 provide an overview of the prognosis and outcome.

---

[u]In the USEIR, 8% of injuries involved the macula.

Table 24–19 Prognostic Factors in Eyes with IOFBs: A Literature Review

Variable	Prognostic Factor [Reference]: Yes	No
Mechanism of injury	Poor outcome with firearm/BB injury[12,172]	[16]
Type of injury	65% blindness if rupture, 21% blindness if penetrating[8]	
Size of IOFB	42% enucleation if >15 mm, 1% if <1 mm[17] 1 mm increase of largest IOFB diameter increases RR of poor outcome by a 1.21[12] factor	[10]
	Better prognosis if IOFB: smaller[8,76], cross section <5 × 2 mm²[164], length <3 mm[97]	
	85% good vision if <2 mm, 15% if >10 mm[173]	
Shape of IOFB	Worse prognosis if blunt[12,172]	[16]
Material of IOFB	Worse prognosis if nonmetallic,[11] glass[174]	
Location of IOFB	Enucleation rate: higher if in posterior segment[14]	[16]
	74% if IOFB in vitreous/retina/choroid[17]	
	Worse prognosis if in posterior segment[76]	
Location of wound	70% blindness if posterior, 20% blindness if anterior[8]	[16]
	Corneoscleral: prognostic factor for poor outcome[12]	[7]
Size of wound	≥4 mm: predictive of ≤5/200 outcome[16]	
Uveal/vitreous prolapse	[12]	[7]
	64% blindness if yes, 19% blindness if no[8]	
Initial mechanical damage	[42]	
	Hyphema[12]	
	Lens injury[11]	
	Vitreous hemorrhage[147]	
	Retinal detachment rate: 42% if present, 5% if not[105]	
	Risk factor for postoperative PVR[24]	
	Macular impact site[23]	
	Retinal impact site inside vascular arcades[11]	[16, 97]
	Retinal detachment[10]	[16, 97]
	Optic nerve head involvement[11]	
APD	[10]	
Endophthalmitis	[175]	[16]
Initial visual acuity	46% blindness if <20/400, 7% blindness if ≥20/400	[11]
	≤5/200 for poor outcome, ≥20/40 for good outcome[16]	
Type of intervention	≥20/60 outcome: 72% with vitrectomy, 27% with EEM[23]	[11]*
	Blindness if posterior segment involved: 56% with vitrectomy, 82% without[8]	[16]*
Number of interventions	≤2 operations: predictive of ≥20/40 outcome[16]	
Late complications	Secondary cataract[10]	
	Retinal detachment[10]	

*Selection bias: severity of initial injuries was different in the two groups.

TABLE 24–20   THE OUTCOME IN EYES WITH IOFBs: A LITERATURE REVIEW

Variable	Finding [Reference]
Enucleation rate	Depends on surgical technique: 0% with vitrectomy, 7% with EEM[23]
	6%,[176] 7%,[15] 9%,[17,18] 11%,[8] 20% (per 5-year intervals: 30%, 23%, 17%, 14%[14]), 29%[1]
	Depends on IOFB size: 13% if <16 mm^3; 28% if >16 mm^3[14]
	Depends on IOFB location: 1.7% if in AC; 19% if in vitreous; 16% if in lens; 20% if in retina[14]
Visual improvement	47%,[11] 58%[13]
	Depends on surgical technique: 68% with vitrectomy, 23% with EEM[23]
Visual deterioration	11%,[11] 15%,[13] 18%[147]
	Depends on surgical technique: 15% with vitrectomy, 53% with EEM[23]
	Not expected over long-term follow-up[14]
Final vision NLP	8%,[97] 12%,[8] 20%,[14] 33%[177]
	Depends on surgical technique: 9% with vitrectomy, 33% with EEM[23]
Final vision <20/400	28%[8]
Final vision <20/200	20%,[10] 22%,[97] 29%,[11] 30%,[8] 42%,[14] 49%,[147] 76%[18]
	Depends on surgical technique: 21% with vitrectomy, 50% with EEM[23]
Final vision ≥ 20/40	26%,[177] 50%,[157] 51%,[10] 62%,[13] 60%,[16] 68%,[97] 71%[92]
	Depends on surgical technique: 68% with vitrectomy, 20% with EEM[23]
Retinal detachment rate	Depends on IOFB position: 25% if in vitreous, 28% if intraretinal/choroid, 2% if elsewhere[17]
	If EEM route anterior: 50%, if pars plana: 21%; if direct posterior: 19%[17]
	23% after successful EEM[105]

CONTROVERSIES

It is not surprising that a topic as important and complex as the management of eyes with IOFBs has generated so many controversies (see Table 24–21).

SUMMARY

The most important tasks in treating patients with fresh IOFBs are the following:

- determine whether an IOFB is indeed present;
- determine whether the injury is high risk, requiring immediate intervention;
- determine what associated injuries are present;
- discuss the eye's condition and the management options with the patient;
- perform surgery as appropriate: in most cases, either:
  - close the wound, remove the IOFB and repair all tissue injuries, take a specimen(s) for culturing, and start antibiotics therapy; or
  - take a specimen for culturing, close the wound, and start antibiotic therapy; remove the IOFB and repair all tissue injuries during a secondary procedure in a few days.

THE NONOPHTHALMOLOGIST'S ROLE

PEARL...   The nonophthalmologist should presume that *all* open globe injuries involve an IOFB. Shield the eye, give *systemic* medication for pain/anxiety/nausea as needed, and refer the patient urgently to the nearest capable ophthalmologic institution. Personal discussion with the ophthalmologist is highly advised. Unless it is a high-risk injury and/or a long delay in transportation is expected, there is no need to start antibiotic therapy, but tetanus prophylaxis may be given (see Chapter 8 and the Appendix).

Table 24-21 Controversies in the Management of Eyes with IOFBs

Variable	Opinion	Counter Opinion	Resolution
Preoperative IOFB localization	Critical for optimal planning	Not important in vitrectomy era	Critical to know if foreign body intraocular; accurate intraocular location less important
Use of prophylactic *intravitreal* antibiotics	Always	Never	Only in high risk cases: it would be unnecessary in approximately 90% of eyes, and possibly increase the risk of bacterial resistance to the most potent antibiotics
Eyes should undergo immediate IOFB removal and reconstruction	Always	Delay of a few days beneficial	High risk eyes or those with endophthalmitis should have immediate surgery; otherwise a delay of up to two weeks may be acceptable
Vitrectomy necessary for all posterior segment IOFBs	Yes	No	Consider risks versus benefits of vitrectomy
Use of EEM	Yes	No	Only if minimal damage associated with small and visible IOFB free in vitreous, preferably close to extraction site; IOM or forceps gives more control
Fate of lens if IOFB intralenticular	Remove	Retain	Depends on individual situation
Removal of posterior hyaloid face	Always	Not necessary	Unless removal very risky (young patient with strong vitreous adhesion to retina), removal preferred; if impossible, circumcise it
Retinopexy for all retinal lesions	Always	Not necessary	Fresh retinal lesions, especially if posterior hyaloid could not completely be removed, probably better be treated; laser preferred to cryopexy
Improvement of prognosis by vitreous surgery	Yes	No	The more difficult the case, the more likely that vitreous surgery offers anatomically and functionally better prognosis over other methods
Primary implantation of IOLs	Yes	No	Individual preference, but presence of IOL makes secondary reconstruction (e.g., for PVR) more difficult

REFERENCES

1. Niiranen M. Perforating eye injuries. *Acta Ophthalmol Suppl.* 1978;135:1 87.

2. Duke-Elder S. *System of Ophthalmology.* London: Henry Kimpton; 1972:451–649.

3. Straub W. The ophthalmology of Fabricius Hildanus in the 17th century. *Doc Ophthalmol.* 1990;74:21–29.

4. Hildebrand H. Sixty-six magnet operations with successful extraction of particles of iron from the inferior of the eye in fifty-three cases. *Arch Ophthalmol.* 1996;114:762–763.

5. Kuhn F, Morris R, Witherspoon CD. Magnetische intraokulare Fremdkörper im hinteren Augenaschnitt. *Ophthalmologe.* 1993;90:539–548.

6. Shock JP, Adams D. Long-term visual acuity results after penetrating and perforating injuries. *Am J Ophthalmol.* 1985;100:714–718.

7. de Juan E, Sternberg P Jr, Michels R. Penetrating ocular injuries. *Ophthalmology.* 1983;90:1318–1322.

8. Punnonen E, Laatikainen L. Prognosis of perforating eye injuries with intraocular foreign bodies. *Acta Ophthalmol.* 1989;66:483–491.

9. Thompson JT, Parver LM, Enger CL, Mieler WF, Liggett PE. Infectious endophthalmitis after penetrating injuries with retained intraocular foreign bodies. *Ophthalmology.* 1993;100:1468–1474.

10. Souza DS, Howcroft M. Management of posterior segment intraocular foreign bodies: 14 years' experience. *Can J Ophthalmol.* 1999;34:23–29.

11. Pavlovic S, Schmidt KG, Tomic Z, Dzinic M. Management of intra-ocular foreign bodies impacting or embedded in the retina. *Aust N J Ophthalmol.* 1998;26:241–246.

12. Chiquet C, Zech J, Denis P, Adeleine P, Trepsat C. Intraocular foreign bodies. Factors influencing final visual outcome. *Acta Ophthalmol Scand.* 1999;77:321–325.

13. Camacho H, Mejia LF. Extraction of intraocular foreign bodies by pars plana vitrectomy. *Ophthalmologica.* 1991;202:173–179.

14. Roper-Hall MJ. Review of 555 cases of intra-ocular foreign bodies with special reference to prognosis. *Br J Ophthalmol.* 1954;38:65–99.

15. Behrens-Baumann W, Praetorius G. Intraocular foreign bodies. *Ophthalmologica.* 1989;198:84–88.

16. Williams DF, Mieler WF, Abrams GW, Lewis H. Results and prognostic factors in penetrating ocular injuries with retained intraocular foreign bodies. *Ophthalmology.* 1988;95:911–916.

17. Percival SPB. A decade of intraocular foreign bodies. *Br J Ophthalmol.* 1972;56:454–461.

18. Owen P, Keightley SJ, Elkington AR. The hazards of hammers. *Injury.* 1987;18:61–62.

19. Kuhn F, Morris R, Witherspoon C, et al. Serious fireworks-related eye injuries. *Ophthalmic Epidemiol.* 2000;7:139–148.

20. Wilson R. Ocular fireworks injuries and blindness an analysis of 154 cases and a three-state survey comparing the effectiveness of model law regulation. *Ophthalmology.* 1902;09:291–297.

21. Brown I. Nature of injury. *Int Ophthalmol Clin.* 1968;8:147–152.

22. Potts A, Distler JA. Shape factor in the penetration of intraocular foreign bodies. *Am J Ophthalmol.* 1985;100:183–187.

23. Mester V, Kuhn F. Ferrous intraocular foreign bodies retained in the posterior segment: management options and results. *Int Ophthalmol.* 2000;22:355–362.

24. Cardillo J, Stout J, LaBree L, et al. Posttraumatic proliferative vitreoretinopathy. The epidemiologic profile, onset, risk factors, and visual outcome. *Ophthalmology.* 1997;104:1166–1173.

25. Virata SR, Kylstra JA, Peiffer RL. The ocular effects of intralenticular iron foreign bodies in rabbits. *Ophthalmic Surg.* 1995;26:142–144.

26. McGahan M, Bito L, Myers B. The pathophysiology of the ocular microenvironment. II. Copper-induced ocular inflammation and hypotony. *Exp Eye Res.* 1986;42:595–605.

27. Schmidt JGH, Mansfield-Nies R, Nies C. On the recovery of the electroretinogram after removal of intravitreal copper particles. *Doc Ophthalmol.* 1987;65:135–142.

28. Tawara A. Transformation and cytotoxicity of iron in siderosis bulbi. *Invest Ophthalmol Vis Sci.* 1986;27:226–236.

29. Hope-Ross M, Mahon GJ, Johnston PB. Ocular siderosis. *Eye.* 1993;7:419–425.

30. Davidson M. Siderosis bulbi. *Am J Ophthalmol.* 1933;16:331–335.

31. Barr CC, Vine AK, Martonyi CL. Unexplained heterochromia. Intraocular foreign body demonstrated by computed tomography. *Surv Ophthalmol.* 1984;28:409–411.

32. Monterio MLR, Coppeto JR, Milani JAA. Iron mydriasis. *J Clin Neuroophthalmol.* 1993;13:254–257.

33. Weiss MJ, Hofeldt AJ, Behrens M, Fisher K. Ocular siderosis. Diagnosis and management. *Retina.* 1997;17:105–108.

34. Yamaguchi K, Tamai M. Siderosis bulbi induced by intraocular lens implantation. *Ophthalmologica.* 1989;198:113–115.

35. Macken PL, Boyd SR, Feldman F, Heathcote JG, Steiner M, Billson FA. Intralenticular foreign bodies: case reports and surgical review. *Ophthalmic Surg.* 1995;26:250–252.

36. Schocket SS. Siderosis from a retained intraocular stone. *Retina.* 1981;1:201–207.

37. Steel DHW, Rosseinsky DR, James CR. Acute retinal toxicity caused by the bimetallic electrochemical action of a galvanized steel intraocular foreign body. *Retina.* 1998;18:77–79.

38. Cibis P, Yamashita T, Rodriguez F. Clinical aspects of ocular siderosis and hemosiderosis. *Arch Ophthalmol.* 1959;62:46–53.

39. Neumann R, Belkin M, Loenthal E, Gorodetsky R. A long-term follow-up of metallic intraocular foreign bodies, employing diagnostic X-ray spectrometry. *Arch Ophthalmol.* 1992;110:1269–1272.

40. Knave B. Electroretinography in eyes with retained intraocular metallic foreign bodies: a clinical study. *Acta Ophthalmol.* 1969;S100:1–63.

41. Micovic V, Milenkovic S, Opric M. Acute aseptic panophthalmitis caused by a copper foreign body. *Fortschr Ophthalmol.* 1990;87:362–363.

42. Cooling RJ, McLeod D, Blach RK, Leaver PK. Closed microsurgery in the management of intraocular foreign bodies. *Trans Ophthalmol Soc UK.* 1981;101:181–183.

43. Rao NA, Tso MOM, Rosenthal R. Chalcosis in the human eye: a clinicopathologic study. *Arch Ophthalmol.* 1976;94:1379–1384.

44. Barry D. Effect of retained intraocular foreign bodies. *Int Ophthalmol Clin.* 1968;56:454–461.

45. Dayan M, Gottrell D, Mitchell K. Reversible retinal toxicity associated with retained intravitreal copper foreign body in the absence of intraocular inflammation. *Acta Ophthalmol.* 1999;77:597–598.

46. Rohrbach JM, Schlote T, Kriegerowski M, Klier R. Massive foreign body reaction after intraocular penetration of hot, liquid plastic. *Klin Monatsbl Augenheilkd.* 1997;210:65–67.

47. Saar I, Raniel J, Neumann E. Recurrent corneal oedema following late migration of intraocular glass. *Br J Ophthalmol.* 1991;75:188–189.

48. Katz LJ, Maus M, Eagle RC. Secondary glaucoma in a case of a lead foreign body in the angle. *Ophthalmic Surg.* 1994;25:482–484.

49. Wolter JR. Foreign body reaction to firm nuclear lens substance. *Ophthalmic Surg.* 1983;14:135–138.

50. Bettman JW. Seven hundred medicolegal cases in ophthalmology. *Ophthalmology.* 1990;97:1379–1384.

51. Williams DF, Mieler WF, Abrams GW. Intraocular foreign bodies in young people. *Retina.* 1990;10:S45–S49.

52. Heimann K, Lemmen KD. Perforating eye injuries with multiple intraocular foreign bodies following military maneuver accidents. *Klin Monatsbl Augenheilkd.* 1986;188:221–224.

53. Kuhn F, Collins P, Morris R, et al. Epidemiology of motor vehicle crash-related serious eye injuries. *Accid Anal Prev.* 1994;26:385–390.

54. Irvine AR. Old and new techniques in the management of intraocular foreign bodies. *Ann Ophthalmol.* 1981;12:41–47.

55. Kuhn F, Halda T, Witherspoon CD, Morris R, Mester V. Intraocular foreign bodies: myths and truths. *Eur J Ophthalmol.* 1996;6:464–471.

56. Arora R, Gupta A, Mazumdar S, Gupta A. A retained intraretinal foreign body. *Ophthalmic Surg Lasers.* 1996;27:885–887.

57. Alexandrakis G, Balachander R, Chaudhry NA, Filatov V. An intraocular foreign body masquerading as idiopathic chronic iridocyclitis. *Ophthalmic Surg Lasers.* 1998;29:336–337.

58. Hamanak N, Ikeda T, Inokuchi N, Shirai S, Uchihori Y. A case of intraocular foreign body due to graphite pencil lead complicated by endophthalmitis. *Ophthalmic Surg Lasers.* 1999;30:229–231.

59. Ahmadieh H, Sajjadi H, Azarmina M, Soheilian M, Baharivand N. Surgical management of intraretinal foreign bodies. *Retina.* 1994;14:397–403.

60. Mieler WF, Ellis MK, Williams DF, Han DP. Retained intraocular foreign bodies and endophthalmitis. *Ophthalmology.* 1990;97:1532–1538.

61. Yuen HY, Kew J, Metreweli C. Case quiz. Lens dislocation due to foreign body. *Australas Radiol.* 1998;42:395–396.

62. McNicholas MMJ, Brophy DP, Power WJ, Griffin JF. Ocular trauma: evaluation with US. *Radiology.* 1995;195:423–427.

63. Rubsamen PE, Cousins SW, Winward KE, Byrne SF. Diagnostic ultrasound and pars plana vitrectomy in penetrating ocular trauma. *Ophthalmology.* 1994;101:809–814.

64. Cascone G, Filippello M, Ferri R, Sicmone G, Zagami A. B-scan echographic measurement of endobulbar foreign bodies. *Ophthalmologica.* 1994;208:192–194.

65. Barash D, Goldenberg-Cohen N, Tzadok D, Lifshitz T, Yassur Y, Weinberger D. Ultrasound biomicroscopic detection of anterior ocular segment foreign body after trauma. *Am J Ophthalmol.* 1998;126:197–202.

66. Laroche D, Ishikawa H, Greenfield D, Liebmann JM, Ritch R. Ultrasound biomicroscopic localization and evaluation of intraocular foreign bodies. *Acta Ophthalmol.* 1998;76:491–495.

67. Barnes E, Griffiths M, Elliott A. Intraocular foreign body missed by computed tomography. *BMJ.* 1993;306:1542.

68. Bryden FM, Pyott AA, Bailey M, McGhee CNJ. Real time ultrasound in the assessment of intraocular foreign bodies. *Eye.* 1990;4:727–731.

69. Lindahl S. Computed tomography of intraorbital foreign bodies. *Acta Radiol.* 1987;28:235–240.

70. McElvanney AM, Fielder AR. Intraocular foreign body missed by radiography. *BMJ.* 1993;306:1060–1061.

71. Newman DK. Eyelid foreign body mimics an intraocular foreign body on plain orbital radiography. *Am J Emerg Med.* 1999;17:283–284.

72. Park SS, Theodossiadis PG, Gragoudas ES. Intrascleral foreign body simulating extrascleral extension of uveal melanoma. *Arch Ophthalmol.* 1994;112:1620–1621.

73. Spierer A, Tadmor R, Treister G, Blumenthal M, Belkin M. Diagnosis and localization of intraocular foreign bodies by computed tomography. *Ophthalmic Surg.* 1985;16:571–575.

74. Bray LC, Griffiths PG. The value of plain radiography in suspected intraocular foreign body. *Eye.* 1991;5:751–754.

75. Chacko JG, Figueroa RE, Johnson MH, Marcus DM, Brooks SE. Detection and localization of steel intraocular foreign bodies using computed tomography. *Ophthalmology*. 1997;104:319–323.

76. Hadden OB, Wilson JL. The management of intraocular foreign bodies. *Aust N Z J Ophthalmol*. 1990;18:343–351.

77. Zinreich SJ, Miller NR, Aguayo JB, Quinn C, Hadfield R, Rosenbaum AE. Computed tomographic three-dimensional localization and compositional evaluation of intraocular and orbital foreign bodies. *Arch Ophthalmol*. 1986;104:1477–1482.

78. Duker JS, Fischer DH. Occult plastic intraocular foreign body. *Ophthalmic Surg*. 1989;20:169–170.

79. Wu JT, Lam DS, Fan DS, Lam WW, Tham CC. Intravitreal phaco chopper fragment missed by computed tomography. *Br J Ophthalmol*. 1998;82:460–461.

80. Lakits A, Steiner E, Scholda C, Kontrus M. Evaluation of intraocular foreign bodies by spiral computed tomography and multiplanar reconstruction. *Ophthalmology*. 1998;105:307–312.

81. Prokesch R, Lakits A, Scholda C, Bankier A, Ba-Ssalamah A, Imhof H. Spiral CT and conventional CT in the preoperative imaging of intraocular metal foreign bodies. *Radiologe*. 1998;38:667–673.

82. Lakits A, Prokesch R, Scholda C, Bankier A, Weninger F, Imhof H. Multiplanar imaging in the preoperative assessment of metallic intraocular foreign bodies. *Ophthalmology*. 1998;105:1679–1685.

83. Wheatcroft S, Benjamin L. Magnetic resonance imaging and the dangers of orbital foreign bodies. *Br J Ophthalmol*. 1996;80:1116.

84. Taylor W. MRI for metallic foreign bodies? *Ophthalmology*. 2000;107:410.

85. Williams S, Char DH, Dillon WP, Lincoff N, Moseley M. Ferrous intraocular foreign bodies and magnetic resonance imaging. *Am J Ophthalmol*. 1988;105:398–401.

86. Lagouros PA, Langer BG, Peyman G, Mafee MF, Spigos DG, Grisolano J. Magnetic resonance imaging and intraocular foreign bodies. *Arch Ophthalmol*. 1987;105:551–553.

87. Kremmer S, Schiefer U, Wilhelm H, Zrenner E. Mobilization of intraocular foreign bodies by magnetic resonance tomography. *Klin Monatsbl Augenheilkd*. 1996;208:201–202.

88. Williamson TH, Smith FW, Forrester JV. Magnetic resonance imaging of intraocular foreign bodies. *Br J Ophthalmol*. 1989;73:555–558.

89. Ta C, Bowman R. Hyphema caused by a metallic intraocular foreign body during magnetic resonance imaging. *Am J Ophthalmol*. 2000;129:533–534.

90. Roper-Hall MJ. An intra-ocular foreign body locator. *Trans Ophthalmol Soc UK*. 1957;77:239–250.

91. Ryan SJ. Traction retinal detachment. XLIX Edward Jackson Memorial Lecture. *Am J Ophthalmol*. 1993;115:1–20.

92. Greven C, Engelbrecht N, Slusher M, Nagy S. Intraocular foreign bodies. Management, prognostic factors, and visual outcomes. *Ophthalmology*. 2000;107:608–612.

93. Cleary PE, Ryan SJ. Vitrectomy in penetrating eye injury. *Arch Ophthalmol*. 1981;99:287–292.

94. Alfaro D, Tran V, Runyan T, Chong L, Liggett P. Vitrectomy for perforating eye injuries for shotgun pellets. *Am J Ophthalmol*. 1992;114:81–85.

95. Brinton G, Topping T, Hyndiuk R, et al. Posttraumatic endophthalmitis. *Arch Ophthalmol*. 1984;102:547–550.

96. Cleary PE, Ryan SJ. Histology of wound, vitreous, and retina in experimental posterior penetrating eye injury in the rhesus monkey. *Am J Ophthalmol*. 1979;88:221–231.

97. Chiquet C, Zech J, Gain P, Adeleine P, Trepsat C. Visual outcome and prognostic factors after magnetic extraction of posterior segment foreign bodies in 40 cases. *Br J Ophthalmol*. 1998;82:801–806.

98. Walker TD. A radio translucent intraorbital foreign body. *Aust N Z J Ophthalmol*. 1989;17:199–200.

99. Erakgun T, Ates H, Akkin C, Kaskaloglu M. A simple "lasso" for intraocular foreign bodies. *Ophthalmic Surg Lasers*. 1999;30:63–66.

100. Ferencz J, Harel O, Assia E. Utilizing gravity in the removal of a large intraocular foreign body. *Ophthalmic Surg Lasers*. 1997;28:508–509.

101. Joondeph BC, Flynn HW. Management of subretinal foreign bodies with a cannulated extrusion needle. *Am J Ophthalmol*. 1990;110:250–253.

102. Mansour A. New attachment for the ocular magnet. *Ann Ophthalmol*. 1988;20:239.

103. May DR, Noll FG, Munoz R. A 20-gauge intraocular electromagnetic tip for simplified intraocular foreign-body extraction. *Arch Ophthalmol*. 1989;107:281–282.

104. Bronson NR. Practical characteristics of ophthalmic magnets. *Arch Ophthalmol*. 1968;79:22–27.

105. Percival SPB. Late complications from posterior segment intraocular foreign bodies. *Br J Ophthalmol1*. 1972;56:462–468.

106. Amalong R. Retinal detachment after manipulation of magnetic foreign body. *Am J Ophthalmol*. 1970;70:10–13.

107. Heimann K. Chirurgie der Fremdkoerperverletzungen. In: *Augenärtzliche Operationen*. Berlin: Springer–Verlag; 1989:641.

108. Parel JM. Progress in foreign body extractors. In: *Basic and Advanced Vitreous Surgery*. Padova: Liviana Press; 1986:321–328.

109. Ruddat MS, Johnson MW. The use of perfluorocarbon liquid in the removal of radiopaque intraocular glass. *Arch Ophthalmol*. 1995;113:1568–1569.

110. Wilson DL. A new intraocular foreign body retriever. *Ophthalmic Surg*. 1975;6:64.

111. Hickingbotham D, Parel J-M, Machemer R. Diamond-coated all purpose foreign body forceps. *Am J Ophthalmol*. 1981;91:267–268.

112. Hutton WL. Vitreous foreign body forceps. *Am J Ophthalmol*. 1977;83:430–431.

113. Kuhn F, Heimann K. Ein neuer Dauermagnet zur Entfernung intraokularer ferromagnetischer Fremdkoerper. *Klin Monatsbl Augenheilkd*. 1991;198:301–303.

114. Kuhn F, Morris R, Witherspoon CD. Intraocular foreign body (posterior segment). In: *Masters Techniques in Ophthalmic Surgery*. Baltimore: Williams–Wilkins; 1995:1201.

115. Hanscom TA, Landers MB. Limbal extraction of posterior segment foreign bodies. *Am J Ophthalmol*. 1979; 88:777–778.

116. Kuhn F, Kovacs B. Management of postequatorial magnetic intraretinal foreign bodies. *Int Ophthalmol*. 1989;13:321–325.

117. Heimann K, Paulmann H, Tavakolian U. The intraocular foreign body. *Int Ophthalmol*. 1983;6:235–242.

118. Slusher MM, Sarin LK, Federman JL. Management of intraretinal foreign bodies. *Ophthalmology*. 1982;89: 369–373.

119. Kuhn F. Management of subretinal foreign bodies. *Vitreoretinal Surg Technol*. 1989;6:1.

120. Ambler J, Meyers S. Management of intraretinal metallic foreign bodies without retinopexy in the absence of retinal detachment. *Ophthalmology*. 1991; 98:391–394.

121. Campochiaro PA, Gaskin HC, Vinores SA. Retinal cryopexy stimulates traction retinal detachment in the presence of an ocular wound. *Arch Ophthalmol*. 1987; 105:1567–1570.

122. Kita M, Negi A, Kawano S, Honda Y. Photothermal, cryogenic, and diathermic effects on retinal adhesive force in vivo. *Retina*. 1991;11:441.

123. Hermsen V. Vitrectomy in severe ocular trauma. *Ophthalmologica*. 1984;189:86–92.

124. Norris JL, Cleasby GW. Intraocular foreign body removal by endoscopy. *Ann Ophthalmol*. 1982;14: 371–372.

125. Kuhn F, Witherspoon CD, Morris R. Endoscopic surgery vs. temporary keratoprosthesis vitrectomy. *Arch Ophthalmol*. 1991;109:768.

126. Kingham JD. Photic maculopathy in young males with intraocular foreign body. *Mil Med*. 1991;156: 44–47.

127. Aiello L, Iwamoto M, Guyer D. Penetrating ocular fish-hook injuries. Surgical management and long-term visual outcome. *Ophthalmology*. 1992;99:862–866.

128. Seal DV. Criteria for intravitreal antibiotics during surgical removal of intraocular foreign bodies. *Eye*. 1992;6:465–468.

129. Hutton WL, Fuller DG. Factors influencing final visual results in severely injured eyes. *Am J Ophthalmol*. 1984;97:715–722.

130. Cleary PE, Ryan SJ. Method of production and natural history of experimental posterior penetrating eye injury in the rhesus monkey. *Am J Ophthalmol*. 1979; 88:212–220.

131. Morris R, Kuhn F, Witherspoon CD. Management of the recently injured eye with no light perception vision. In: *Vitrectomy in the Management of the Injured Globe*. Philadelphia: Lippincott Raven; 1998:113–125.

132. Lewis H, Aaberg TM, Packo KH, Richmond PP, Blumenkranz MS, Blankenship GW. Intrusion of retinal tacks. *Am J Ophthalmol*. 1987;103:672–680.

133. Honda Y, Ueno S, Miura M, Yamaguchi H. Silicone oil particles trapped in the subretinal space: complications after substitution of the vitreous. *Ophthalmologica*. 1986;192:1–5.

134. Salminen L. Intraocular foreign body from a Healon syringe. *Am J Ophthalmol*. 1987;104:427–428.

135. Martinez-Toldos JJ, Elvira JC, Hueso JR, et al. Metallic fragment deposits during phacoemulsification. *J Cataract Refract Surg*. 1998;24:1256–1260.

136. Tyagi AK, Kheterpal S, Callear AB, Kirkby GR, Price NJ. Simultaneous posterior chamber intraocular lens implant combined with vitreoretinal surgery for intraocular foreign body injuries. *Eye*. 1998;12:230–233.

137. Gottlieb F, Finestone J, Ackerman JL. Intravitreal cilia and retinal detachment. *Ann Ophthalmol*. 1982;14: 541–544.

138. Peyman G, Raichand M, Goldberg MF, Brown S. Vitrectomy in the management of intraocular foreign bodies and their complications. *Br J Ophthalmol*. 1980; 64:476–482.

139. Wolter RJ. The lens as a barrier against foreign body reaction. *Ophthalmic Surg*. 1981;12:42–45.

140. Sneed SR, Weingeist TA. Management of siderosis bulbi due to retained iron-containing intraocular foreign body. *Ophthalmology*. 1990;97:375–379.

141. Kuhn F, Witherspoon CD, Morris R, Skalka H. Improvement of siderotic ERG. *Eur J Ophthalmol*. 1992;2:44–45.

142. Keeney AH. Intralenticular foreign bodies. *Arch Ophthalmol*. 1971;86:499–501.

143. Klemen UM, Freyer H. Siderosis lentis et bulbi durch ein intralentales Rostpartikel. *Klin Monatsbl Augenheilkd*. 1978;172:258–261.

144. O'Duffy D, Salmon JF. Siderosis bulbi resulting from an intralenticular foreign body. *Am J Ophthalmol*. 1999;127:218–219.

145. De Bustros S. Posterior segment intraocular foreign bodies. In: *Eye Trauma*. St. Louis: Mosby Year Book; 1991:232.

146. Sneed SR. Ocular siderosis. *Arch Ophthalmol*. 1988; 106:997.

147. Coleman DJ, Lucas BC, Rondeau MJ, Chang S. Management of intraocular foreign bodies. *Ophthalmology*. 1987;94:1647–1653.

148. Lins M, Kopietz L. Foreign body masquerading as a ruptured globe. *Ophthalmic Surg*. 1985;16:586–588.

149. Kamath MG, Nayak IV, Satish KR. Case report: intraocular foreign body in the angle masquerading as uveitis. *Indian J Ophthalmol*. 1991;39:138–139.

150. Cunliffe I, Singh A, Mody C, Innes J, Rennie I. Retained intraocular foreign body simulating choroidal melanoma: a report of two cases. *Ger J Ophthalmol*. 1993;2:416–418.

151. Lebowitz HA, Couch JM, Thompson JT, Shields JA. Occult foreign body simulating a choroidal melanoma with extrascleral extension. *Retina*. 1988;8:141-144.

152. Khouri AS. Civilian eye injuries in warfare. *Surv Ophthalmol*. 1998;42:390–391.

153. Trimble SN, Schatz H. Subretinal neovascularization following metallic intraocular foreign-body trauma. *Arch Ophthalmol*. 1986;104:515–519.

154. Mora J, Gross K, Murray N, Chisholm B. A diagnostic dilemma: one foreign body or two? *Arch Ophthalmol*. 1993;111:1171–1172.

155. Barnard TA, Weidenthal DT. Intraocular mass simulating a retained foreign body. *Am J Ophthalmol*. 1998;126:149–150.

156. Roper-Hall MJ. Treatment of ocular injuries. *Trans Ophthalmol Soc UK*. 1959;79:57–69.

157. Tomic Z, Pavlovic S, Latinovic S. Surgical treatment of penetrating ocular injuries with retained intraocular foreign bodies. *Eur J Ophthalmol*. 1996;6:322–326.

158. Boldt H, Pulido J, Blodi C, et al. Rural endophthalmitis. *Ophthalmology*. 1989;101:332–341.

159. Kazokoglu H, Saatci O. Intraocular foreign bodies: results of 27 cases. *Ann Ophthalmol*. 1990;22:373–376.

160. Alfaro D, Roth D, Liggett P. Posttraumatic endophthalmitis: causative organisms, treatment, and prevention. *Retina*. 1994;14:206–211.

161. Rubsamen PE, Cousins S, Martinez JA. Impact of cultures on management decisions following surgical repair of penetrating ocular trauma. *Ophthalmic Surg Lasers*. 1997;28:43–49.

162. Schmidseder E, Mino de Kaspar H, Klauss V, Kampik A. Post-traumatic endophthalmitis after penetrating eye injuries. Risk factors, microbiological diagnosis and functional outcome. *Ophthalmologe*. 1998;95:153–157.

163. Duch-Samper AM, Menezo JL, Hurtado-Sarrio M. Endophthalmitis following penetrating eye injuries. *Acta Ophthalmol Scand*. 1997;75:104–106.

164. Karel I, Diblik P. Management of posterior segment foreign bodies and long-term results. *Eur J Ophthalmol*. 1995;5:113–118.

165. Jonas JB, Budde WM. Early versus late removal of retained intraocular foreign bodies. *Retina*. 1999;19:193–197.

166. Nelsen PT, Marcus DA, Bovino JA. Retinal detachment following endophthalmitis. *Ophthalmology*. 1985;92:1012–1017.

167. Foss AJE, Forbes JE, Morgan J. An intralenticular foreign body and a clear lens. *Br J Ophthalmol*. 1993;77:828.

168. Pieramici D, Capone AJ, Rubsamen PE, Roseman RL. Lens preservation after intraocular foreign body injuries. *Ophthalmology*. 1996;103:1563–1567.

169. Lempert P. Optic disc size. *Ophthalmology*. 1996;103:348–349.

170. Eisner G. *Eye Surgery*. Berlin: Springer–Verlag; 1990:56.

171. Morris R, Kuhn F, Mester, V. Prophylactic scleral buckle for prevention of retinal detachment following vitrectomy for macular hole. *Br J Ophthalmol* 2000;84:673.

172. Sternberg P Jr, de Juan E, Michels RG. Penetrating ocular injuries in young patients. *Retina*. 1984;4:5–8.

173. Neubauer H. Intraocular foreign bodies. *Trans Ophthalmol Soc UK*. 1975;95:496–501.

174. Gopal L, Banker AS, Deb N, et al. Management of glass intraocular foreign bodies. *Retina*. 1998;18:213–220.

175. Affeldt J, Flynn H, Forster R, et al. Microbial endophthalmitis resulting from ocular trauma. *Ophthalmology*. 1987;94:407–413.

176. Khan MD, Kundi N, Mohammed Z, Nazeer AF. A 6 1/2-years survey of intraocular and intraorbital foreign bodies in North-west Frontier Province, Pakistan. *Br J Ophthalmol*. 1987;71:716–719.

177. Elder MJ. Penetrating eye injuries in children of the West Bank and Gaza Strip. *Eye*. 1993;7:429–432.

Chapter 25

SEVERE COMBINED ANTERIOR AND POSTERIOR SEGMENT TRAUMA

C. Douglas Witherspoon, Robert Morris, Robert Phillips,
Ferenc Kuhn, Suzanne Nelson, and Robert Witherspoon

In dealing with the more severe eye injuries, it becomes less valuable to separate their classification and treatment artificially based on anatomical designations. Not surprisingly, the most serious injuries often involve both the anterior and posterior segments of the eye, crosscutting not only anatomical designations but also traditional ophthalmological disciplines (see Fig. 25–1). Corneal opacities/edema, hyphema, traumatic cataract, and choroidal and vitreous hemorrhages frequently obstruct visualization of the retina and may prevent safe and timely posterior segment reconstruction before the onset of severe scarring. Unfortunately, many of these severely injured eyes are still enucleated, without giving the surgeon a chance to visualize the postequatorial retina and the optic disk and thus accurately assess the viability of these vital tissues.

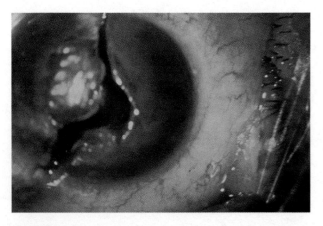

FIGURE 25–1 Open globe injury typical of trauma requiring TKP vitrectomy.

HISTORY

In 1981 the first TKP model (Landers-Foulks[a]) was introduced[1] (see Table 25–1). This PMMA device permits pars plana vitrectomy for complete and timely treatment of severe posterior segment injuries in eyes with corneal opacification. A soft silicone rubber TKP model (Eckardt) was designed in 1987; this allowed a better view of the peripheral retina and, by having a shorter cylinder, was suitable for use even in phakic eyes.[2,b]

Since its original description, the Landers TKP has undergone a number of modifications, and it is now available with wide-field optics, a short cylinder, and a broad flange (see Fig. 25–2A and B).

> **PEARL...** Both types of TKP are valuable as optical devices for exploration and reconstruction of the posterior segment of the globe in the presence of an opaque cornea. The results published in earlier series are encouraging.[3–5]

---

[a] The original model was later modified by Landers.

[b] A soft silicone rubber flange allows customized suture placement as sutures are placed directly through the silicone flange at any site without the restricton of preplaced suture holes. It is helpful when corneal lacerations cross the recipient bed trephination.

TABLE 25–1   COMPARISON OF TKP DEVICES

Property	Landers*	Eckardt
Material	PMMA	Silicone rubber
Multiple use	Yes	Yes, but limited
Variable suture fixation	No	Yes
Wide-field optics available	Yes	Yes
Useful for phakic and pseudophakic eyes	Yes (short-cylinder version)	Yes
Useful with miotic pupil	Yes (standard cylinder version)	No; must use iris retractors
Available size (cylinder diameter in mm)	7.2, 8.2	7
Manufacturer	Wöhlk Contactlinsen, Kiel, Germany	Ocular Instruments, Bellevue, WA

*The wide-field, short cylinder model

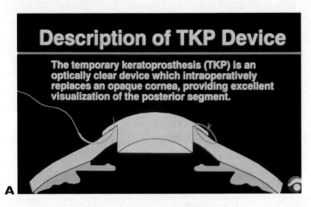 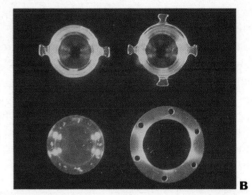

FIGURE 25–2   **(A)** TKP, schematic. **(B)** TKP models, clockwise from upper left: two-strut Landers-Foulks; four-strut Landers-Foulks; Eckardt; Landers wide-field.

CLINICAL RATIONALE FOR TKP USE

In very severely injured eyes, it is common for the surgeon to advise enucleation, instead of a direct inspection of the retina and optic disk. If, however, the retina and optic disk appear to be viable to the experienced trauma specialist, major intraocular reconstruction may be justified—provided the patients are adequately counseled regarding the relative risks and benefits and they desire the procedure (see Chapters 5, 7, and 8).

PEARL... The availability of even ambulatory vision as a "spare" to the better eye is of significant value to most patients.

PEARL... The TKP allows direct visual inspection of the postequatorial retina and optic disk by an experienced eye trauma surgeon so that a decision can be made whether to proceed with intraocular reconstructive efforts or, if appropriate, enucleation (see Chapter 8).

Alternatives to the TKP include:

- delayed surgery;
- inadequate surgery due to poor visualization;
- sequential surgery;
- no surgery; or
- endoscopic surgery.

None of these options allows *timely, direct* inspection and globe reconstruction utilizing all capabilities of modern vitreoretinal surgery while simultaneously restoring corneal transparency.

SURGICAL TECHNIQUE

In most cases, TKP vitrectomy is jointly performed by an *anterior-* and a *posterior segment surgical team.* The surgeons alternate responsibilities during the operation, each team adding its unique expertise to the procedure. In this way, the constellation of problems associated with severe combined anterior and posterior segment injuries can be addressed optimally while minimizing the potential complications associated with such a complex procedure.

We prefer *general anesthesia* as TKP vitrectomies tend to be lengthy and often unpredictable. There are, however, no absolute contraindications to local anesthesia if the surgeons feel that its benefits outweigh the potential complications or if the patient's condition so requires (see Chapter 8).

Establishing the Surgical Field

The Posterior Segment Team

Typically, the vitreoretinal surgeon starts the procedure by opening the surgical field and preparing the eye for the intraocular reconstruction.

- A 360-degree conjunctival incision is made 2 to 3 mm posterior to the limbus to avoid disturbing the perilimbal stem cell population.
- The four rectus muscles are isolated on sutures to allow:
  - control of the globe;
  - inspection of the external quadrants of the globe (if the primary repair was performed elsewhere, this may be the first time that the surgeon has the opportunity to visualize the extent and quality of the initial repair); and, if desired,
  - scleral buckling later in the procedure.
- Primary wound repairs or surgical incisions are reinforced if found not to be watertight.
- The sclera is also inspected for any evidence of wounds that might have been missed at the time of primary repair; if present, these wounds are revised as necessary.
- Unless there is significant uncertainty regarding the anterior anatomical relationships, the infusion cannula is usually placed at this time.

> **PEARL...** The infusion is not turned on until the cannula can actually be confirmed to be free within the vitreous cavity. Often this is not possible until *after* the TKP is actually placed.

- We generally initiate the intraocular segment of the surgery with an IOP of 25 mm Hg, set by a GFLI system.[c] The GFLI has the following advantages:
  - allows accurate setting of the IOP[d];

- has a simple mechanism to change the IOP as operative conditions demand;
- the IOP change can be rapid if the need arises;
- allows fast changes between fluid and gas environments as required throughout the operation; and
- has a digital IOP display, clearly visible to all operating room personnel even in the dark.

> **PEARL...** The authors use and recommend the GFLI for *all* vitrectomies.

- The cannula is typically placed in the inferotemporal quadrant, through the pars plana at 3.5 mm posterior to the limbus. Either a 4- or a 6-mm cannula can be used, similarly to standard vitrectomy cases. Typically, a special silicone oil infusion cannula set is chosen.
  - Silicone oil cannula infusion sets differ from standard infusion sets; they have thicker walls, are less compliant than standard infusion tubing, and have a tubing that is firmly bonded to the cannula to reduce the risk of tubing disconnections or "blowouts."

> **PEARL...** Silicone oil cannula infusion sets are inexpensive and their use is preferable to suture-tying the tubing to the cannula in an attempt to prevent disconnection.[e]

- At this time, the posterior segment surgery team inspects the globe a last time prior to the placement of the TKP. The degree of corneal opacity is reassessed in cases where there is still some doubt about the possibility of performing a safe, effective, and complete posterior segment reconstructive procedure through the damaged cornea.
- Vitrectomy may be attempted with the option of converting to a TKP vitrectomy procedure if necessary.

---

[c]Consisting of tubing set connecting an air pump to the air pocket in the infusion bottle via a spiked tubing.

[d]Crucial to control sudden intraoperativa bleeding (see Chapter 22).

[e]Should the tubing become disconnected from the cannula, it is usually necessary to replace the cannula and its attached tubing completely with a new one. The reduced friction caused by silicone coating of the connecting surfaces makes it nearly impossible to maintain cannula attachment once tubing disconnection occurs.

PEARL... The wide-angle viewing system is very helpful in cases of modest corneal opacity (see Chapter 8).

PITFALL

With a "standby" TKP procedure, often some time passes before corneal failure occurs during vitrectomy. A posterior segment surgeon may be reluctant to call for the corneal surgery team if the latter has been waiting[f] for some time. This may cause the posterior segment surgeon to try to complete the procedure with an inadequate view or unnecessarily lengthen the duration of the surgery. As a result, compromise becomes more likely, and a gap may rapidly develop between what could be done with the optimal view through the TKP and what can actually be accomplished under suboptimal operating conditions.

The Anterior Segment Team

The anterior segment surgeon takes over at this point.

- The initial step is to remove the damaged central cornea with a vacuum trephine.
  - Vacuum trephines allow a stable platform on an often irregular surface. Higher than normal vacuums may be required.
  - The size and placement of the trephination and the type of TKP to be used depend on multiple factors specific to each case and are best determined by a consensus between the participating surgeons at the time of the operation.
  - The authors have extensive experience with both the Landers(-Foulks) and the Eckardt style of TKPs. In recent years, we have preferred the modified Landers wide-field lens with the short cylinder. The short-cylinder model works well in pseudophakic as well as aphakic patients. This version is easy to insert, provides a very clear image, and is reusable.[g]

PEARL... A good starting point for the novice TKP trauma surgeon is the 7.2-mm modified Landers wide-field prosthesis with a short cylinder and a broad flange.

- The standard cylinder TKP is valuable for maintaining an adequate pupillary opening during surgery when miosis is present or iris/ciliary body damage causes obstruction of the central visual axis; most of these eyes have iris damage or loss.
- As an alternative, iris retractors can be used with the short-cylinder design.[h]
- The 7.2-mm wide-angle prosthesis is placed in a 7.25- or 7.5-mm[i] recipient bed.
  - The use of a trephine that is 0.25 mm larger than the diameter of the TKP cylinder allows for easier placement and does not dilate the recipient opening.
  - Rarely, it is necessary in some severely damaged corneas to create the bed using a "freehand" technique; this, however, should be avoided if possible because of the superior results obtained using a vacuum trephine. Regardless of the technique used, every attempt is made to maintain as normal anatomical relationships as possible (see Chapter 14 and the Appendix).
- The cornea may be marked with a tissue dye prior to trephination to document the tissue relationships so that proper alignment can be established later in the procedure when corneal transplantation is performed.

PEARL... At all times during the reconstructive procedure, it is impossible to predict the postoperative vision potential, and it would be imprudent to place arbitrary restrictions during the surgery based on pessimistic assumptions.

- It is quite common for the pars plana region to be severely disrupted and scarred in eyes selected for TKP vitrectomy. Often, safe insertion of the pars plana infusion cannula or even the TKP itself may require limited, open-sky anterior segment

---

[f]Perhaps after normal working hours or during a busy day's schedule.

[g]Being made of hard polymer rather than silicone rubber.

[h]In eyes without sufficiently wide pupil, the standard cylinder TKP is preferred.

[i]This sizing is preferred and suggested by the authors.

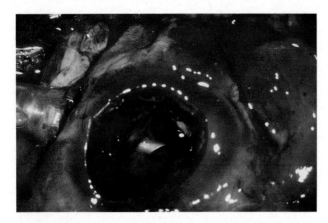

FIGURE 25-3 Open sky view, prior to TKP placement. Almost clear tissue is seen around the cannula prior to cleaning and turning the infusion on.

reconstruction initially, including removal of a cataractous and/or ruptured lens and limited open sky vitrectomy (Fig. 25–3).

- IOLs are removed only if absolutely necessary, although they are rarely present in these eyes. Their removal is not required for placement of the TKP itself if the short-cylinder model is used.

PEARL... Open-sky procedures should be limited to those absolutely necessary so as to limit the exposure to ECH in the absence of a closed, pressurized system. The blood pressure must be closely monitored and all other precautions taken; see Chapter 22.

- More major open-sky procedures are occasionally justified, particularly when extensive ciliary body or retroiridal scar tissue dissection is required (for phthisis prophylaxis, see Fig. 26–3) and peripheral visualization through the TKP is not adequate; in such cases, the endoscope may prove extremely helpful (see Chapter 19 and the Appendix).

PEARL... The endoscope holds the promise of becoming an important tool in conjunction with TKP surgery during major intraocular reconstructive operations following severe combined anterior and posterior segment trauma. It is, however, *not* recommended to use the endoscope as a substitute for TKP vitrectomy.

PEARL... Iris reconstruction is best avoided until the later stages of the surgery to allow unrestricted access to the ciliary body and the posterior segment structures during the procedure.

- As much of the iris diaphragm should be preserved as possible (see Chapters 16 and 18). This is extremely important for maintaining the silicone oil within the vitreous cavity, away from the graft endothelium to help maintain graft clarity (see the Appendix).
- If a cyclodialysis cleft has been identified, it is generally repaired at this time.

PEARL... It is best to repair cyclodialysis clefts *prior to* opening the infusion line during pressurized surgery so that fluid is not diverted into the suprachoroidal space.

All efforts up to this point in the operation have been directed at establishing an adequate surgical field. The surgical field is complete once the infusion cannula is positively identified to be free within the vitreous cavity and the eye is pressurized with the TKP in place.[j]

Vitrectomy

The Posterior Segment Team

The posterior segment surgeon continues the operation.

Once the conditions listed above are established, an exploratory vitrectomy is performed. The goal of this procedure is to allow a direct and clear view of the postequatorial retina and optic disk to determine their viability.[k] Once these critical structures have been inspected, a decision is made whether to proceed with complete intraocular reconstruction.

---

[j]The suturing of the TKP is determined by its type. A braided suture (e.g., 7/0 vicryl) is preferred to a monofilament suture that tends to break with scleral depression.

[k]It is often difficult to expose these structures adequately as the retina is frequently tightly sandwiched between dense subretinal and vitreous blood.

PEARL... Once the postequatorial retina and the optic disk are clearly visualized, it is usually possible for an experienced trauma surgeon to determine whether these structures are viable (i.e., reconstruction is possible for the purpose of achieving functional improvement) or irreparably damaged (i.e., functional reconstruction is not possible).

PITFALL

The surgeon must also take into consideration the condition of the ciliary body, which is commonly the cause of the procedure's failure (see Chapter 19 and the Appendix).

If reconstruction is decided upon, initially a small core "working area" is created in the central anterior vitreous cavity, using a vitrectomy probe (Fig. 25–4).

- The most difficult part of the procedure is *the identification of the retina and the establishment of the proper surgical plane among the monotonous, amorphous layers of blood, vitreous, scar, and debris.*
  - The retina is often pale and sandwiched between layers of blood. Blood vessels may be normal, poorly perfused, or not perfused at all.
  - Streaks of blood may mimic blood vessels, and, when lying on flat, partially organized layers of vitreous and debris, the appearance may strongly resemble the retina.[l]
  - To further complicate matters, there are usually many such layers, usually densely packed together and intimately adherent to the retina, making it extremely difficult to identify and separate the retina.
- A useful surgical tactic is to choose one quadrant to begin the search for the retinal surgical plane. All other factors being equal, the starting quadrant should:
  - be located superiorly to avoid an inferior break, if one is created inadvertently;
  - be located where a retinotomy is likely to be needed during the reconstruction;
  - contain the least posterior segment damage;
  - be as far away from posterior scleral wound(s) as possible;
  - have an attached retina[m]; and
  - be free of choroidal detachment.
- Once a quadrant is chosen, the layers (as thin as possible), are shaved away one by one, gradually moving more posteriorly within this quadrant.
- Sometimes, after breaking through a detached vitreous face, retrovitreal blood must be evacuated, and eventually the retina is reached.
- The dissection is then very carefully expanded laterally to confirm that the retina has indeed been identified.
- When the plane of the retina has been found, the dissection is expanded from this starting point, gradually exposing more of the retina and eventually the optic disk as well.

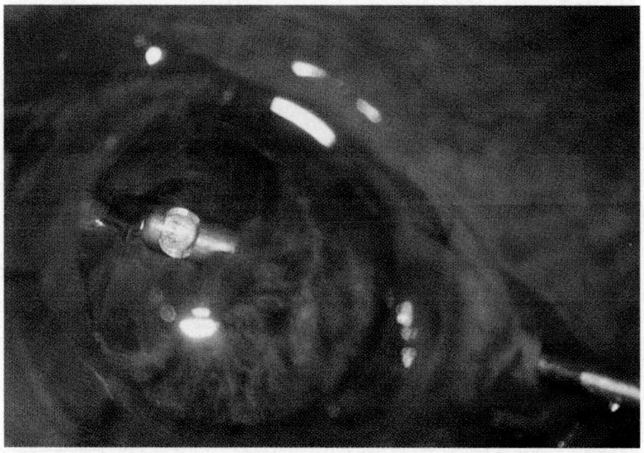

FIGURE 25–4 Vitrectomy, initial stage through perfectly clear TKP view.

SPECIAL CONSIDERATION

It is generally more productive to work from the less damaged quadrants toward the more severely injured quadrants and from the midperiphery toward the central retina. The more identifiable retina that can be found, the easier it is to follow and remain in the proper surgical plane. In this way, there is less chance of creating inadvertent retinal breaks.

[l]In other words, what may appear as vitreous is in reality retina or vice versa.

[m]Or at least less detachment than other quadrants.

- After identification of the retina and expansion of the surgical plane, the posterior segment reconstruction can proceed much more rapidly. Particular attention is paid to achieving a complete anterior vitreous removal and removal of all scar tissues, including those over the ciliary body.
- Retinotomy and/or retinectomy may be used where irreducible traction is encountered. Retinal tacks, intraocular air or other gas mixtures, silicone oil, PFCLs, indirect or endolaser photocoagulation, and scleral buckling are used as needed (see Chapter 23 and the Appendix for certain details; more can be found in vitreoretinal textbooks).
- The working sclerotomies are closed, but the infusion cannula remains in place for later adjustment of the IOP, gas, or silicone oil levels following corneal transplantation.

Anterior Segment Surgery

The Anterior Segment Team
After completion of the intraocular reconstruction by the vitreoretinal specialist, the anterior segment surgeon removes the TKP and performs any iris reconstruction necessary to restore the normal anatomy of the iris diaphragm as much as possible.

- If the iris is completely destroyed, an artificial iris device maybe sutured into place (see Chapter 18).
- If the iris is relatively intact following reconstruction and liquid silicone oil is used, an inferior, peripheral iridectomy is created to accommodate the altered aqueous humor dynamics created by silicone oil placement (see the Appendix). This should be basal and large. Meticulous hemostasis should be maintained during the creation of the iridectomy because of the tendency of fibrin formation to lead to closure of the iridectomy in the early postoperative period.

IOL implantation is rarely performed at this stage, mainly because of the severity of the injuries and the complexity of the reconstructive surgery. An AC IOL may be used, but more commonly a PC IOL is sutured into the ciliary sulcus.[n] In eyes in which lensectomy has been performed earlier in the procedure or at the time of primary repair, a PC IOL may be placed in the ciliary sulcus if sufficient capsular support is preserved (see Chapter 21).

PEARL... We prefer to perform lensectomy with preservation of *both* the anterior and posterior capsules, allowing placement of the IOL in either the capsular bag or the ciliary sulcus.

After the TKP is removed, the PK procedure is completed by placing an 8.0-mm donor graft in the recipient bed (provided a 7.25 or 7.5 vacuum trephine has been used).

PEARL... A graft slightly larger than the trephine's diameter helps to compensate for stretching of the recipient bed that may take place during the procedure; this is especially true if any dilation of the recipient bed from the TKP has occurred. A larger graft also helps to counteract the corneal flattening (see the Appendix) often seen in postoperative TKP patients with smaller donor grafts.[o]

Suturing of the graft requires special considerations.

- In eyes with complicated corneal lacerations, we prefer to use interrupted corneal graft sutures *combined with* a running suture. This allows greater flexibility in closure and postoperative adjustment, particularly where the corneal laceration crosses the graft-host junction.
- Solely interrupted sutures are preferred if there is concern that a running suture might pull through lacerated tissue.

PEARL... Rarely, in cases with very complicated corneal lacerations and especially where tissue maceration is present, the recipient cornea must be retrephined or a new recipient bed created freehand outside the original TKP bed. A large donor graft is then used to replace the entire defect. Additional suturing of the recipient lacerations may be needed. Intraoperative keratometry may be used for cylinder control but cannot be used for silicone oil due to distorted mires.

---

[n]Scarring over the pars plana must be taken into account when suturing a lens into the sulcus.

[o]Grafts are normally flat in the early postoperative period but become more convex with time.

Final Closure

The Posterior Segment Team

Final closure is performed by the posterior segment surgeon. The main focus is the adjustment of the silicone oil level and the IOP. In most cases, the ideal closure would leave the silicone oil level essentially flat at the pupillary level, with silicone oil completely filling the vitreous cavity and aqueous completely filling the AC. Adjustments in the silicone oil level, however, must be made to compensate for anticipated changes in postoperative volume (e.g., choroidal edema, true [hemorrhagic] choroidal detachment).

PITFALL

During lengthy keratoplasty, aqueous may reaccumulate posterior to the silicone oil, giving rise to inadequate postoperative fill of the vitreous cavity. If this is suspected, the posterior segment surgeon may search for and remove all aqueous after keratoplasty, before final closure.

After closing the sclerotomies, the conjunctiva is sutured. Every effort is made to leave the conjunctiva smooth; it may even cover portions of the corneal graft.

CASE SERIES

An analysis of a case series of 127 eyes of 127 consecutive patients, in whom we performed exploration by TKP vitrectomy for severe combined anterior and posterior segment trauma using the techniques just described, showed the following results.

- Most of these patients previously underwent surgery for repair of corneal and/or scleral lacerations/ruptures as part of a primary stabilizing operation.
- The TKP vitrectomy was performed an average of 20 days following the primary repair.
- After we directly inspected the postequatorial retina and the optic disk and they appeared nonviable, the eye was usually enucleated, although in rare cases anatomic reconstruction followed, in accordance with the patient's strong desire and following counseling regarding the potential disadvantages including the risk of SO (see Chapters 5, 8, and 29).
- Confirmation of a viable optic nerve head and postequatorial retina was followed by posterior segment reconstruction by TKP vitrectomy.
- 20 eyes were enucleated without further attempts at intraocular reconstruction (Fig. 25–5).

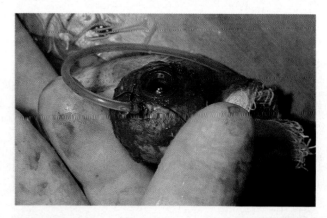

FIGURE 25–5 Enucleation. After end-stage retinal damage is confirmed, the eye is removed with TKP and infusion in place.

- 107 eyes underwent attempted intraocular reconstruction by TKP vitrectomy.
  - The median follow-up time was 464 days (range, 6–3035 days).
  - *Preoperatively*: The best corrected visual acuity was 2/200–20/400 in 6%, hand motion to light perception in 21%, light perception in 55%, and NLP in 19%. The retina was detached in 94%.
  - *Postoperatively*[p]: 38% of eyes were unstable; 24% of these were secondarily enucleated or eviscerated. 62% of eyes were stable, with an IOP of ≥8 mm Hg *and* an attached retina (Fig. 25–6).
  - 30% of eyes were NLP at the final follow-up, as opposed to 27% preoperatively. Of eyes undergoing TKP vitrectomy with NLP initial vision, 40% improved to at least light perception vision, with 10% of eyes reaching 20/40 to 20/100.

SUMMARY

The TKP provides an excellent view to allow performing timely reconstructive surgery on eyes with severe combined anterior and posterior segment trauma. The functional and anatomical results of this complicated surgery are very promising; chronic hypotony is now the most common late postoperative complication. Additional research is needed into the cause and treatment of ciliary body dysfunction; the endoscope may be helpful in advancing this field further.

Severely traumatized eyes deserve surgical exploration with direct visualization of the posterior retina and optic disk by an experienced eye trauma surgeon before nonreversible triage decisions are made. Fig. 25–7 shows the general thought process the surgeon uses when approaching patients with so severe eye trauma.

---

[p] After at least 6 months follow-up.

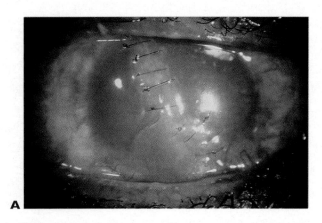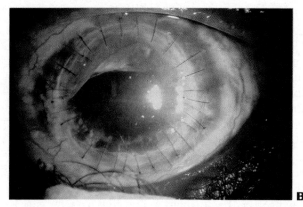

FIGURE 25–6   **(A)** Preoperative view prior to TKP vitrectomy, showing poor visualization through damaged cornea. **(B)** Postoperative view after TKP vitrectomy and PK.

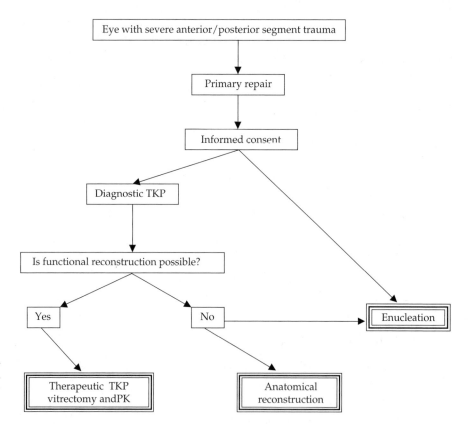

FIGURE 25–7   Flowchart showing the strategic thinking in managing eyes with severe anterior/posterior segment trauma.

REFERENCES

1. Landers MBI, Foulks GN, Landers DM, Hickingbotham D, Hamilton RC. Temporary keratoprosthesis for use during pars plana vitrectomy. *Am J Ophthalmol.* 1981;91:615–619.

2. Eckardt C. A new temporary keratoprosthesis for pars plana vitrectomy. *Retina.* 1987;191:243.

3. Garcia-Valenzuela E, Blair NP, Shapiro MJ, et al. Outcome of vitreoretinal surgery and penetrating keratoplasty using temporary keratoprosthesis. *Retina.* 1999;19:424–429.

4. Beckhuis W, Zivojnovic R. Use of temporary keratoprosthesis in the management of severe ocular trauma with retinal detachment and proliferative vitreoretinopathy. *Dev Ophthalmol.* 1989;18:86–89.

5. Witherspoon CD, Kuhn F, Morris R, Collins W P, Phillips R. Anterior and posterior segment trauma. In: Roy H, ed. *Master Techniques in Ophthalmic Surgery.* Baltimore: Williams & Wilkins; 1995:538–547.

Chapter 26

MANAGEMENT OF EYES WITH PERFORATING INJURY

Stephen G. Schwartz and William F. Mieler

The Ocular Trauma Classification Group classified perforating ocular injuries as *type D*, typically involving *zone III* (see Chapters 1 and 2). These injuries are usually[1-11] associated with a worse outcome[a] than contusions, IOFBs and penetrating trauma, and they can occasionally be as serious as ruptures. This chapter describes the unique aspects of treating eyes with injuries involving both entrance and exit wounds.

EPIDEMIOLOGY

- The *incidence* of perforating injuries varies widely and is reported between 7% and 31%, depending on study criteria and terminology.[1-5,7,12]
  - Among all injured eyes undergoing vitreoretinal surgery, the incidence decreases to 4–10%.[2,3,7]
  - If limited to injuries caused by high-speed projectiles, (e.g., industrial nail guns,[13] BB guns,[14,15] and shotguns,[6,10,16,17]), the incidence rises to 50–92%.
  - The rate is 0.075% among retrobulbar injections.[18]
  - Missiles are the cause in three fourths of eyes.[19,20]

The following is the epidemiological information found by the USEIR.

Rate of perforating injury among all serious injuries: 3%.

Rate of perforating injury among open globe injuries: 5%.
Age (years):
- range: 2–77;
- average: 24.

Sex: 87% *male.*
Place of injury:
- home: 40%;
- industrial premises: 18%;
- recreation and sport: 15%;
- street and highway: 9%;
- public building: 4%.

Source of injury:
- gunshot: 38%;
- various sharp objects: 18%;
- BB/pellet gun: 17%;
- hammering on metal: 9%;
- various blunt objects: 4%;
- MVC: 3%;
- explosion: 2%.

Rate of corneo/scleral perforations[b]: 53%.

Rate of sclero/scleral perforations: 47%.

---

[a] Perforating injury is one of the prognostic factors identified by, and used in, the OTS (see Chapter 3).

[b] Among those where this information was provided.

PATHOPHYSIOLOGY AND PROGNOSIS

The typical perforating injury is caused by:

- a high-speed projectile or missile (e.g., BB or shotgun pellet); or, less commonly,
- a sharp object (e.g., blade, nail, broken glass).

Most projectiles are blunt; some,[19] but not all,[3] studies report a worse prognosis associated with projectile injuries (see Table 26–1 for the muzzle velocities of projectiles causing perforating trauma).

> **P**EARL... Blunt objects (e.g., BB or shotgun pellet) require higher velocity (i.e., kinetic energy[34]) to enter (rupture/perforate) the globe. The energy is absorbed by the eye, causing significant damage (see Chapters 1 and 3).

A sharp object is able to perforate the eye at a much lower velocity, often causing less severe coincidental damage[18,20,21] unless resulting in retinal detachment, submacular hemorrhage, direct macular or optic nerve injury, or *multiple* posterior exit wounds ("sewing machine injury"[22]).

Nails fired from an industrial nail gun[c] are sharp projectiles.[d] There are limited data regarding their prognosis.[13]

The damage occurring at the time of a perforating injury is compounded by scarring (i.e., consequences of the eye's own healing response; see Chapter 8),[23–26] which is frequently far more deleterious to the eye than the initial trauma.

Contracting membranes may be present as early as 6 hours after injury.[26] Several factors, including blood[28–30,e] and lens injury,[31,32] may contribute to the development of tractional retinal detachment.

Fibrosis, the first step in PVR, begins at the scleral wound(s). The amount of new collagen increases most dramatically between 14 and 30 days, especially in the presence of autologous blood.[33,34] The tract connecting the entry and exit wounds becomes a scaffold for fibroblast proliferation as early as 4 days after injury,[35] leading to anteroposterior traction.[36]

TABLE 26-1   VELOCITIES OF PROJECTILES DOCUMENTED TO CAUSE OCULAR PERFORATING INJURIES*

Projectile	Muzzle Velocity (m/sec)
Shotgun pellet[16]	243
BB (pump-action rifle)[71]	213
Nail (industrial nail gun)[13]	125
BB (spring-loaded rifle)[16]	91

*The velocity of a projectile is highest immediately upon being fired (muzzle velocity) and is progressively slowed by air resistance. As a reference, the estimated velocity of a BB necessary to perforate an eye consistently is 73 m/sec for the rabbit, 103 m/sec for the human, and 113 m/sec for the dog.[27] (It should be noted, however, that there is significant individual variability in these measurements, as BBs from a spring-loaded rifle [muzzle velocity 91 m/sec] have been documented to cause perforating injuries.[16]) Generally, shotgun pellets cause more severe damage than BBs because of their higher velocities. However, newer pump-action BB rifles achieve muzzle velocities approaching those of shotguns, and devastating injuries may ensue (e.g., perforating the cornea, lens, vitreous, and optic disk and coming to rest in the substance of the optic nerve 2 mm posterior to the lamina cribrosa[71]). A shotgun pellet may also fragment upon striking the anterior surface of the eye, resulting in multiple exit wounds.[56,57]

> **P**EARL... The two most important factors in PVR development appear to be vitreous hemorrhage and vitreous incarceration in the wound[37]; injury to the lens, vitreous, and/or ciliary epithelium appears to accelerate this process[26].

Traumatic vitreopathy[f] may make visualization more difficult; the developing partial posterior vitreous separation accentuates the anteroposterior traction between the exit wound and the vitreous base.[39]

> **PITFALL**
>
> In the previtrectomy era, the majority of eyes with perforating trauma eventually lost light perception, became phthisical, or required enucleation, typically because of irreparable retinal detachment and hypotony.[9,16,40,41]

---

[c] Muzzle velocity: 100–150 m/sec.

[d] In comparison: a BB traveling at 101 m/sec completely traverses the eye in 0.5 msec.[27]

[e] For example, purified fibronectin or platelet-derived growth factor.

---

[f] Collapsed, disorganized vitreous collagen, which combines with hemorrhage to form a matrix interconnecting the wound(s) with the cortical vitreous.[38]

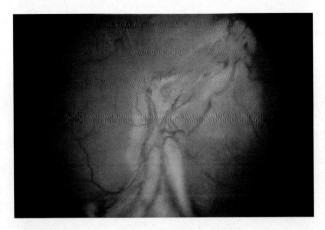

FIGURE 26–1   Dart injury with a posterior exit wound along the inferior vascular arcade. The patient had minimal vitreous hemorrhage, allowing direct visualization of the extent of posterior segment damage. Vision was hand motions due to development of a retinal detachment with PVR. Vitrectomy was performed with retinectomy of the incarcerated tissue, laser photocoagulation, and placement of silicone oil. Final vision was 5/200.

SURGICAL TREATMENT

Vitrectomy

Timely vitrectomy[1,9,26,35,39,42–51] serves many purposes, including:

- removal of:
  - clotted hyphema;
  - injured lens;
  - vitreous hemorrhage; and
  - IOFBs; as well as

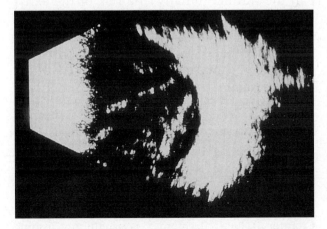

FIGURE 26–3   B-scan echogram documenting marked disruption of the posterior sclera with overlying choroidal and retinal detachment. This patient sustained a shotgun injury, with the large pellet coming to rest in the orbit. Dense vitreous hemorrhage and cataract formation precluded direct visualization of the posterior segment. Surgical repair was successful in reestablishing anatomic integrity including an attached retina, though vision was eventually lost because of hypotony and phthisis.

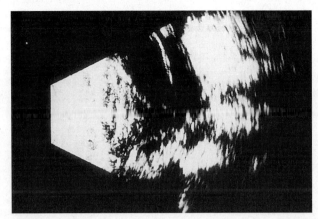

FIGURE 26–2   B-scan echogram suggesting a subtle defect in the posterior sclera as a result of an assault with an ice pick. The area of abnormality is marked by the presence of retinal and vitreous incarceration into the scleral wound. Presence of an exit wound was confirmed at the time of vitrectomy, and the incarcerated tissue was removed.

- treatment of all treatable lesions (see Figs. 26–1 through 26–4) in the posterior segment.

> **PEARL...** Vitrectomy improves the prognosis for perforating eye injuries when compared with the natural history.[52]

A meta-analysis of published reports[1,5,11,13,15,17,19,21,22,53–58] on eyes undergoing *vitrectomy* for *perforating*

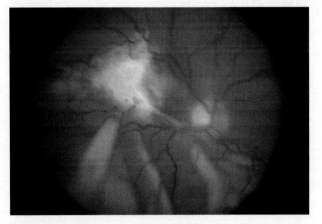

FIGURE 26–4   Color photograph of a posterior exit wound just superotemporal to the macula. One month after vitrectomy, reproliferation and recurrent inferior retinal detachment are seen. The patient underwent repeat vitreous surgery, and the final vision is 2/200.

Table 26–2 Meta-analysis of Eyes with Vitrectomy for Perforating Ocular Injuries

Study	Anatomic Success*	Visual Success†
Hutton[1]	2/5 (40%)	2/5 (40%)
Hanscom and Krieger[53]	3/3 (100%)	3/3 (100%)
Sternberg et al.[5]	NA	5/14 (36%)
Ramsay et al.[54]	11/18 (58%)	10/18 (53%)
Brown et al.[15]	2/9 (22%)	0/9 (0%)
Vatne and Syrdalen[55]	25/41 (61%)	23/41 (56%)
Roden et al.[17]	4/5 (80%)	8/14 (57%)
Morris et al.[10]	11/14 (64%)	8/14 (57%)
Schneider et al.[21]	4/7 (57%)	4/7 (57%)
Ford and Barr[56]	3/3 (100%)	3/3 (100%)
Martin et al.[19]	41/51 (80%)	32/51 (63%)
Grizzard et al.[22]	9/12 (75%)	8/12 (67%)
Alfaro et al.[57]	14/22 (50%)	11/22 (50%)
Lee and Sternberg[13]	1/2 (50%)	1/2 (50%)
Pulido et al.[58]	6/6 (100%)	5/6 (83%)
Total	136/198 (69%)	123/221 (56%)

*Typically defined as restoration of ocular integrity, combined with retinal attachment.
†Defined as postoperative visual acuity of 5/200 or better.

trauma (excluded were series not satisfying both criteria[2,3,4,6,7,11,52]) showed anatomical[8] success in 69% and a visual acuity of ≥5/200 in 56% of eyes. See Tables 26–2 and 26–3 for risk factors for a poor outcome.

Timing

The timing of vitrectomy for perforating ocular trauma remains controversial. Some authors[3] found no significant difference in the outcome; others recommended early surgery[33,49,59,60] There are three alternatives:

1. early (2 days);
2. delayed (7–14 days); or
3. late (after 30 days).

---

[8] Restoration of ocular integrity and an attached retina.

Table 26–3 Factors Associated with a Poor Visual Outcome in Perforating Injuries

Injuries due to projectiles (particularly shotgun pellets)
Preoperative visual acuity of <5/200
Dense preoperative vitreous hemorrhage
Preoperative retinal detachment
Direct injury to the macula or optic nerve
Multiple exit wounds
Absence of spontaneous posterior vitreous separation prior to vitrectomy
Inability to relieve all vitreous adhesions from the exit wound

▼ **PITFALL**

Early vitrectomy (i.e., within 2 days after injury) is rather difficult because of the lack of posterior hyaloid separation and the increased risk of severe intraoperative bleeding (see Chapter 8). Visibility may also be compromised if the cornea was involved in the trauma. Finally, the risk of the exit wound's reopening remains a serious threat: retinal incarceration and loss may be the consequence, especially if the IOP must be elevated intraoperatively because of a severe hemorrhage (see Chapter 22 and the Appendix).

Delayed vitrectomy eliminates the difficulties seen with too early surgery,[7,19,39,55,58] especially if adequate anti-inflammatory treatment was administered (see Chapter 8). Late vitrectomy[53] is usually not recommended/practiced today.

Management of the Posterior Exit Wound

Typically, the posterior hyaloid eventually separates posteriorly, except at the exit wound,[58] where it remains tightly adherent.

PITFALL

Surgical closure of a large and/or posterior exit wound can potentially prevent incarceration of the vitreous/retina,[39] but the risks of the procedure usually outweigh its benefit[60] (see Chapter 16).

Delayed vitrectomy allows spontaneous closure of the exit wound by fibrous tissue. This, however, may be the very source of PVR; an individual decision must be made regarding treatment, although pulling this "tissue plug" must be avoided to prevent hemorrhage.[19] Chapter 16 describes the management of retinal incarceration.

Prophylactic Scleral Buckle

The value of prophylactic scleral buckle remains controversial: some authors[9,3,7] find it beneficial because of the theoretically reduced risk of retinal detachment, but others[55] disagree. It remains an individual decision, but a few facts are important to remember.

- Subsequent *rhegmatogenous* retinal detachment is often not directly related to the site of the posterior exit wound[h] but develops secondary to a new retinal break in the vitreous base region within two clock hours of the wound.[60]
- To counter subsequent *traction* at the vitreous base, as complete as possible vitrectomy may be just as effective as a prophylactic buckle, avoiding the associated morbidity.

Two devices offer considerable help in achieving total removal of the peripheral vitreous:

1. a wide-angle viewing system (see Chapter 8); and
2. an endoscope (see the Appendix).

Special Issue: Needle Perforation

Retinal breaks should be treated in the standard fashion with demarcating laser photocoagulation (or, less preferably, cryopexy). If significant subretinal hemorrhage is present, adhesive therapy may not be necessary,[22] but the submacular blood should be evacuated early to prevent permanent photoreceptor damage. Actual rhegmatogenous retinal detachment should be repaired using standard techniques (see Chapter 23).

Adjunctive Therapy

Because vitrectomy itself may induce membrane formation,[61] researchers try to find alternative/complementary treatments.

- *Systemic corticosteroids*[33] have demonstrated no efficacy.
- *Intravitreal corticosteroids* have shown an effect in some,[62] but not all,[63] studies.
- *Beta-aminopropionitrile,[i]* used topically and systemically in experimental work,[35] resulted in improvement at 2 weeks after injury—but this difference disappeared at 5 weeks.[64]
- *Systemic and intravitreal penicillamine*[65] reduced the intravitreal proliferation compared to control eyes.
- *Intravitreal and periocular 5-fluorouracil* not only has shown limited efficacy[66] but also may be toxic to both the cornea and the photoreceptors.[67]
- *Combined use of intravitreal 5-fluorouracil and beta-aminopropionitrile* has successfully reduced the strength of vitreous membranes.[68]
- *Hematoporphyrin derivative, activated by laser photoradiation*, has demonstrated some efficacy experimentally.[69,70]
- *Brachytherapy with cobalt 60* has shown a possible protective effect experimentally.[31]

In summary, pharmacological prophylaxis/treatment of PVR, although an ideal approach in principle, is currently not available for the clinician.

SUMMARY

Perforating ocular injuries represent an unusual but particularly severe form of open globe trauma. They are often caused by high-speed projectiles, which induce significant incidental damage. Surgical repair must not only address the initial damage but also try to prevent PVR development. Meta-analysis of the existing literature indicates a 69% anatomical and a 56% visual success rate with vitrectomy techniques. Technical advances in vitreous surgery may further improve these results. Adjunctive treatment with pharmacotherapy may play a prominent role in the future.

---

[h] It is usually difficult to place a buckle over the exit wound and also involves potentially high morbidity.

[i] An inihibitor of collagen cross-linking.

References

1. Hutton WL. Symposium: pars plana vitrectomy: the role of vitrectomy in penetrating ocular injuries. *Trans Am Acad Ophthalmol Otol.* 1976;81:OP-414–OP-419.

2. Appiah AP. The nature, causes, and visual outcome of ocular trauma requiring posterior segment surgery at a county hospital. *Ann Ophthalmol.* 1991;23:430–433.

3. Ahmadieh H, Soheilian M, Sajjadi H, Azarmina M, Abrishami M. Vitrectomy in ocular trauma: factors influencing final visual outcome. *Retina.* 1993;13:107–113.

4. Shock JP, Adams D. Long-term visual acuity results after penetrating and perforating ocular injuries. *Am J Ophthalmol.* 1985;100:714–718.

5. Sternberg P Jr, de Juan E Jr, Michels RG. Penetrating ocular injuries in young patients: Initial injuries and visual results. *Retina.* 1984;4:5–8.

6. Hill JC, Peart DA. The visual outcome of ocular bird-shot injuries. *S Afr Med J.* 1986;70:807–809.

7. Hermsen V. Vitrectomy in severe ocular trauma. *Ophthalmologica.* 1984;189:86–92.

8. De Juan E Jr, Sternberg P Jr, Michels RG. Penetrating ocular injuries: types of injuries and visual results. *Ophthalmology.* 1983;90:1318–1322.

9. Hutton WL, Fuller DG. Factors influencing final visual results in severely injured eyes. *Am J Ophthalmol.* 1984;97:715–722.

10. Morris RE, Witherspoon CD, Feist RM, Byrne JB, Ottemiller DE. Bilateral ocular shotgun injury. *Am J Ophthalmol.* 1987;103:695–700.

11. Hay A, Flynn HW Jr, Hoffman JI, Rivera AH. Needle penetration of the globe during retrobulbar and peribulbar injections. *Ophthalmology.* 1991;98:1017–1024.

12. Adhikary HP, Taylor P, Fitzmaurice DJ. Prognosis of perforating eye injury. *Br J Ophthalmol.* 1976;60:737–739.

13. Lee BL, Sternberg P Jr. Ocular nail gun injuries. *Ophthalmology.* 1996;103:1453–1457.

14. Sternberg P Jr, de Juan E Jr, Green WR, Hirst LW, Sommer A. Ocular BB injuries. *Ophthalmology.* 1984;91:1269–1277.

15. Brown GC, Tasman WS, Benson WE. BB-gun injuries to the eye. *Ophthalmic Surg.* 1985;16:505–508.

16. Drummond J, Kielar RA. Perforating ocular shotgun injuries: relationship of ocular findings to pellet ballistics. *South Med J.* 1976;69:1066–1068.

17. Roden D, Cleary P, Eustace P. A five-year survey of ocular shotgun injuries in Ireland. *Br J Ophthalmol.* 1987;71:449–453.

18. Ramsay RC, Knobloch WH. Ocular perforation following retrobulbar anesthesia for retinal detachment surgery. *Am J Ophthalmol.* 1978;86:61–64.

19. Martin DF, Meredith TA, Topping TM, Sternberg P Jr, Kaplan HJ. Perforating (through-and-though) injuries of the globe. Surgical results with vitrectomy. *Arch Ophthalmol.* 1991;109:951–956.

20. Seelenfreund MH, Freilich DB. Retinal injuries associated with cataract surgery. *Am J Ophthalmol.* 1980;89:654–658.

21. Schneider ME, Milstein DE, Oyakawa RT, Ober RR, Campo R. Ocular perforation from a retrobulbar injection. *Am J Ophthalmol.* 1988;106:35–40.

22. Grizzard WS, Kirk NM, Pavan PR, Antworth MV, Hammer ME, Roseman RL. Perforating ocular injuries caused by anesthesia personnel. *Ophthalmology.* 1991;98:1011–1016.

23. Newsome DA, Rodrigues MM, Machemer R. Human massive periretinal proliferation: in vitro characteristics of cellular components. *Arch Ophthalmol.* 1981;99:873–880.

24. Kampik A, Kenyon KR, Michels RG, Green WR, de la Cruz ZC. Epiretinal and vitreous membranes: comparative study of 56 cases. *Arch Ophthalmol.* 1981;99:1445–1454.

25. Grierson I, Rahi AHS. Structural basis of contraction in vitreal fibrous membranes. *Br J Ophthalmol.* 1981;65:737–749.

26. Coles WH, Haik GM. Vitrectomy in intraocular trauma: its rationale an its indications and limitations. *Arch Ophthalmol.* 1972;87:621–628.

27. Tillett CW, Rose HW, Herget C. High-speed photographic study of perforating ocular injury by the BB. *Am J Ophthalmol.* 1962;54:675–678.

28. Cleary PE, Ryan SJ. Posterior perforating eye injury: experimental animal model. *Trans Ophthalmol Soc UK.* 1978;98:34–37.

29. Cleary PE, Ryan SJ. Histology of wound, vitreous, and retina in experimental posterior penetrating eye injury in the rhesus monkey. *Am J Ophthalmol.* 1979;88:221–231.

30. Yeo JH, Sadeghi J, Campochiaro PA, Green WR, Glaser BM. Intravitreous fibronectin and platelet-derived growth factor: new model for traction retinal detachment. *Arch Ophthalmol.* 1986;104:417–421.

31. Chakravarthy U, Maguire CJF, Archer DB. Experimental posterior perforating ocular injury: a controlled study of the gross effects of localized gamma irradiation. *Br J Ophthalmol.* 1986;70:561–569.

32. Cleary PE, Jarus G, Ryan SJ. Experimental posterior penetrating eye injury in the rhesus monkey: vitreous-lens admixture. *Br J Ophthalmol.* 1980;64:801–808.

33. Pilkerton AR, Rao NA, Marak GE, Woodward SC. Experimental vitreous fibroplasia following perforating ocular injuries. *Arch Ophthalmol.* 1979;97:1707–1709.

34. Ussmann JH, Lazarides E, Ryan SJ. Traction retinal detachment: a cell-mediated event. *Arch Ophthalmol.* 1981;99:869–872.

35. Topping TM, Abrams GW, Machemer R. Experimental double-perforating injury of the posterior segment in rabbit eyes: the natural history of intraocular proliferation. *Arch Ophthalmol.* 1979;97:735–742.

36. Winthrop SR, Cleary PE, Minckler DS, Ryan SJ. Penetrating eye injuries: a histopathological review. *Br J Ophthalmol.* 1980;64:809–817.

37. Eagling EM. Perforating injuries involving the posterior segment. *Trans Ophthalmol Soc UK.* 1975;95:335–339.

38. Coleman DJ. Symposium: pars plana vitrectomy: the role of vitrectomy in traumatic vitreopathy. *Trans Am Acad Ophthalmol Otol.* 1976;81:OP-406–OP-413.

39. Michels RG. Vitrectomy methods in penetrating ocular trauma. *Ophthalmology.* 1980;87:629–645.

40. Kreshon MJ. Eye injuries due to BB-guns. *Am J Ophthalmol.* 1964;58:858–861.

41. Bowen DI, Magauran DM. Ocular injuries caused by airgun pellets: an analysis of 105 cases. *Br Med J.* 1973;1:333–337.

42. Cleary PE, Ryan SJ. Vitrectomy in penetrating eye injury: results of a controlled trial of vitrectomy in an experimental posterior penetrating eye injury in the rhesus monkey. *Arch Ophthalmol.* 1981;99:287–292.

43. Gregor Z, Ryan SJ. Complete and core vitrectomies in the treatment of experimental posterior penetrating eye injury in the rhesus monkey. I. Clinical features. *Arch Ophthalmol.* 1983;101:441–445.

44. Gregor Z, Ryan SJ. Complete and core vitrectomies in the treatment of experimental posterior penetrating eye injury in the rhesus monkey. II. Histologic features. *Arch Ophthalmol.* 1983;101:446–450.

45. Faulborn J, Atkinson A, Olivier D. Primary vitrectomy as a preventive surgical procedure in the treatment of severely injured eyes. *Br J Ophthalmol.* 1977;61:202–208.

46. Michels RG. Early surgical management of penetrating ocular injuries involving the posterior segment. *South Med J.* 1976;69:1175–1177.

47. Conway BP, Michels RG. Vitrectomy techniques in the management of selected penetrating ocular injuries. *Ophthalmology.* 1978;85:560–583.

48. Brinton GS, Aaberg TM, Reeser FH, Topping TM, Abrams GW. Surgical results in ocular trauma involving the posterior segment. *Am J Ophthalmol.* 1982;93:271–278.

49. Ryan SJ, Allen AW. Pars plana vitrectomy in ocular trauma. *Am J Ophthalmol.* 1979;88:483–491.

50. Meredith TA, Gordon PA. Pars plana vitrectomy for severe penetrating injury with posterior segment involvement. *Am J Ophthalmol.* 1987;103:549–554.

51. Abrams GW, Topping TM, Machemer R. Vitrectomy for injury: the effect on intraocular proliferation following perforation of the posterior segment of the rabbit eye. *Arch Ophthalmol.* 1979;97:743–748.

52. de Juan E Jr, Sternberg P Jr, Michels RG, Auer C. Evaluation of vitrectomy in penetrating ocular trauma: a case-control study. *Arch Ophthalmol.* 1984;102:1160–1163.

53. Hanscom T, Krieger AE. Late vitrectomy in double perforating ocular injuries. *Ophthalmic Surg.* 1979;10:78–80.

54. Ramsay RC, Cantrill HL, Knobloch WH. Vitrectomy for double penetrating ocular injuries. *Am J Ophthalmol.* 1985;100:586–589.

55. Vatne HO, Syrdalen P. Vitrectomy in double perforating eye injuries. *Acta Ophthalmol.* 1985;63:552–556.

56. Ford JG, Barr CC. Penetrating pellet fragmentation: a complication of ocular shotgun injury. *Arch Ophthalmol.* 1990;108:48–50.

57. Alfaro DV, Tran VT, Runyan T, Chong LP, Ryan SJ, Liggett PE. Vitrectomy for perforating eye injuries from shotgun pellets. *Am J Ophthalmol.* 1992;114:81–85.

58. Pulido JS, Gupta S, Folk JC, Ossoinig KC. Perforating BB gun injuries of the globe. *Ophthalmic Surg Lasers.* 1997;28:625–632.

59. Coleman DJ. Early vitrectomy in the management of the severely traumatized eye. *Am J Ophthalmol.* 1982;93:543–551.

60. Cooling RJ. Immediate management of posterior perforating trauma. *Trans Ophthalmol Soc UK.* 1982;102:223–224.

61. Stern WH, Fisher SK, Anderson DH, et al. Epiretinal membrane formation after vitrectomy. *Am J Ophthalmol.* 1982;93:757–772.

62. Tano Y, Sugita G, Abrams G, Machemer R. Inhibition of intraocular proliferations with intravitreal corticosteroids. *Am J Ophthalmol.* 1980;89:131–136.

63. Weiss JF, Belkin M. Glucocorticosteroid inhibition of intraocular proliferation [letter]. *Am J Ophthalmol.* 1982;92:133.

64. Moorhead LC. Effects of beta-aminopropionitrile after posterior penetrating injury in the rabbit. *Am J Ophthalmol.* 1983;95:97–109.

65. Weiss JF, Belkin M. The effect of penicillamine on post-traumatic vitreous proliferation. *Am J Ophthalmol.* 1981;92:625–627.

66. Blumenkranz M, Hernandez E, Ophir A, Norton EWD. 5-Fluorouracil: new applications in complicated retinal detachment for an established antimetabolite. *Ophthalmology.* 1984;91:122–130.

67. Stern WH, Guerin CJ, Erickson PA, Lewis GP, Anderson DH, Fisher SK. Ocular toxicity of fluorouracil after vitrectomy. *Am J Ophthalmol.* 1983;96:43–51.

68. Moorhead LC, Sepahban S, Armeniades CD. Evaluation of drug treatments for proliferative vitreoretinopathy using vitreous microtensiometry. *Ann Ophthalmol.* 1991;23:349–355.

69. Folk JC, Assouline J, Tse D, Blodi C, Cutkomp J. Hematoporphyrin photoradiation of rabbit dermal fibroblasts [ARVO abstract]. *Invest Ophthalmol Vis Sci.* 1984;25:271.

70. Thomas EL, Chong L. Prevention of transvitreal band and traction retinal detachment formation by the use of hematoporphyrin derivative and photoradiation therapy [ARVO abstract]. *Invest Ophthalmol Vis Sci.* 1984;25:271.

71. Dinkel TA, Ward TP, Frey DM, Hollifield RD. Dissection along the optic nerve axis by a BB. *Arch Ophthalmol.* 1997;115:673–675.

Chapter 27

INJURY TO THE POSTSURGICAL EYE

Paul F. Vinger

 Eye injuries are common and expensive (see Chapter 4),[1–4] making it essential for society to determine whether and how common surgical procedures affect the globe's resistance to trauma. A few of the most obvious questions include the following.

- How much force does it take to penetrate or rupture the eye?
- Is the postsurgical eye more prone to serious injury? If so, how much?
- What is the velocity difference between paintballs causing contusion versus rupture?
- When is it appropriate for a patient to resume full activity after ocular surgery?

▼ PITFALL

A new drug's safety must be clearly proved before it becomes available, but no such requirements exist for new types of ocular surgeries or to reveal their potential for complications, which surgeons have a natural bias to underreport.

The true incidence of postsurgical trauma–related complications is thus difficult to determine. Injuries remain a largely neglected public health problem.[5]

THE MECHANISM OF EYE INJURIES

Expansion of the eyeball perpendicular to the direction of impact is the cause of many closed globe injuries (e.g., angle recession, iridodialysis, lens subluxation, choroidal rupture; see Chapters 17, 20, 21, and 23).

- The damage is more severe as the impact force increases and the time to maximum force decreases.
- Because the energy is transmitted throughout the globe, the tissue damage may occur distant from the impact site.

When the globe is penetrated/perforated/ruptured, the eyewall's tensile strength is exceeded by a combination of local strain, shock waves, increased IOP, and acute cavitation of dissolved intraocular gas.

Because ruptures have the worst prognosis (see Chapter 3),[6–9] the major concern is *whether eyes sustain rupture, rather than contusion, because a prior surgery weakened the eyewall*. Table 27–1 summarizes the energy various objects require to cause an open globe injury in the unoperated eye. Less energy is required to penetrate or rupture the eye with high-speed, small, hard missiles (BB) than with low-speed, softer, larger missiles (squash ball).

PEARL... **The external factors that determine an eye's injury include maximum force, time to maximum force, area of contact, and properties of the impacting object.**

TABLE 27–1   OPEN GLOBE INJURY*[10] CORRELATION AMONG IOP, OBJECT HARDNESS, SIZE, AND KINETIC ENERGY[10–22]

	Diameter/Weight	Human Eye	Monkey Eye	Pig Eye
Elevated IOP[11–14]	NA	67 psi (3500 mm Hg)		76 psi (4000 mm Hg)
Sharp object[15]	NA	Energy required to penetrate globe varies with sharpness, but it is usually low		
BB[16,17]	4.5 mm/0.35 g	236 ft/s (161 mph), 0.91 J		
Metal rod[18]	12.5 mm/303 g		12.2 ft/s (8.3 mph), 2.1 J	
Paintball[19]	17.5 mm/3.55 g			290 ft/s (198 mph),13.9 J
Golf ball[†]	43 mm/45.4 g			86 ft/s (59 mph), 15.6 J
Squash ball[20,21]	41 mm/24.7 g			150 ft/s (102 mph), 25.8 J
Baseball[22,‡]	73.8 mm/143.9 g	81 ft/s (55 mph), 43.5 J		

*Penetration and rupture of individual eyes vary.

[†]P.F. Vinger, unpublished data.

[‡]Standard major league baseball: peak force 3768 N; onset rate 3486 N/ms. Note that when a soft baseball (146.5 g) with a similar cover and diameter was used to strike the other eye of the cadaver, the eye did not rupture at 110 ft/s (75 mph). While the energy delivered by the soft baseball (82.33 J) was greater than that delivered by the standard baseball, the peak force (3208 N) and the onset rate (3486 N/ms) of the soft baseball were less than the peak force and onset rate for the harder major league baseball.

Theoretical Considerations[a]

Energy transmitted to the eye via impact depends on the mass and velocity of the object.[23] The entire spectrum of eye trauma can be produced by varying the impact force and the onset rate. For instance, when changing the speed of a 0.345 g BB:[17]

- at 13 m/s, the energy is less than the 0.03 J required to cause contusion;
- at 62.3 m/s, retinal tears occur at the vitreous base;
- at 72.0 m/s, the globe is penetrated;
- at 124 m/s, even bone is penetrated.[16,17]

Test devices[24] and mathematical models[25] have been devised for documenting the eye injury potential of various products. The force onset rate needed to produce clinically detectable contusion is ~750 N/ms. Certain toy dart guns propelling suction cups exceed this level[26] (see Fig. 27–1). Certain protective eyewears[27] prevent/reduce injury by decreasing the force onset rate and the peak force by spreading the total force over time.

---

[a]Mass is measured in kg; force is measured in newton (N), which is analogous to the pound; 1 kg mass weighs 9.8 (~2.2 pounds); a force of 1 N over a distance of 1 m uses 1 J—if done in 1 s, 1 watt of power is required; the onset rate is measured in newton per millisecond (N/ms).

SPECIAL CONSIDERATION

Injury as related to force onset rate applies only to total forces in a limited range, which is yet undetermined. Even with an onset rate below 750 N/ms, the slowly applied force of a bulldozer would cause significant injury.

Structural Anatomy of the Eyewall

The eyewall is a union of two thin-walled (~0.5 mm) spheres (radii: 8 mm and 12 mm) with centers 5 mm apart.[28] At the junction of the optic nerve sheath, which may be represented by a cylinder (radius: 2 mm), the scleral sphere is perforated by multiple openings (lamina cribrosa,[29] Fig. 27–2). However, the eyewall is not of uniform thickness,[30] is significantly thinner in myopia,[31] and loses elasticity with age.[32] The intact eyewall tends to rupture where its structural strength is weakest:

- at the limbus where the radius of curvature changes;
- near the equator behind exertion of the extraocular muscles where the sclera is thinnest; and
- at the lamina cribrosa where the sclera is perforated.[33]

How does a surgical incision influence the force necessary to open the eyewall?

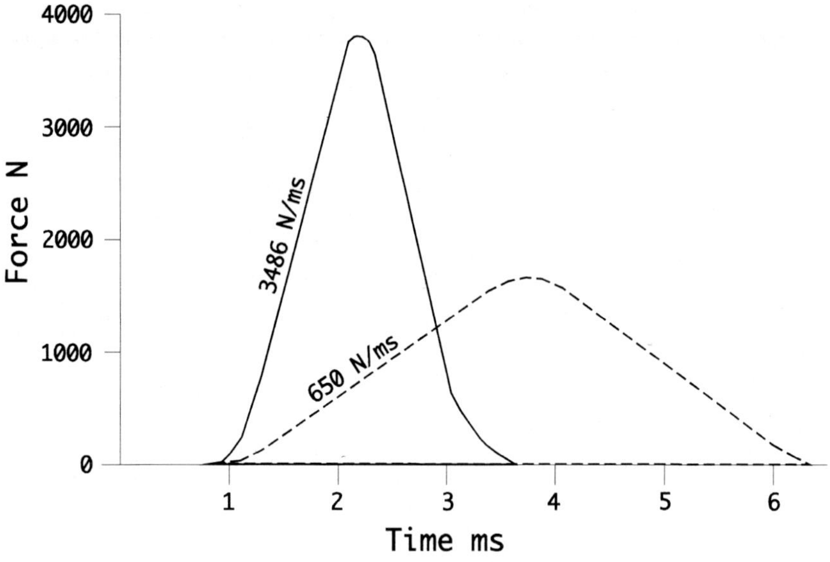

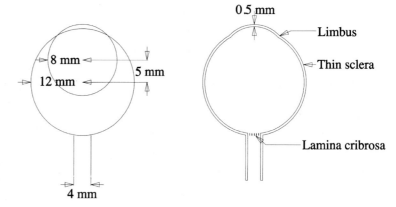

FIGURE 27–1 The same total force (area beneath the curves) with different onset rates and durations. (Solid curve) Major league baseball ruptures a human cadaver eye in an artificial orbit; peak force of 3768 N, onset rate of 3486 N/ms.[22] (Dotted curve) Force spreads over time and has a peak onset rate below the 750 N/ms required to cause contusion.

FIGURE 27–2 An unoperated eyewall ruptures at the limbus, equatorial sclera, and lamina cribrosa.

THE EFFECTS OF COMMON SURGICAL INCISIONS

PITFALL

The wound is most susceptible to rupture during the healing process. Full healing in the cornea requires 2 to 3 months, but the wound still develops only half of the original tensile strength.[34,35] It would take an ideal glue for surgical incisions not to weaken the globe's structural resistance.

When the healing process is complete but the wound is not as strong as the surrounding normal tissue, the stress concentration caused by the incisional notch must be considered.[36] For example, the presence of an epithelial plug creates stress concentration at the RK incision site, a risk factor for rupture.

The required force is hard to predict and may depend on factors such as the size of the plug and the strength of the wound collagen.[37]

It is the combination of stress concentration and a diminished tensile strength that causes eyes to rupture at the site of surgical incision—*provided the incision site has less tensile strength than the limbus, the equatorial sclera, or the lamina cribrosa* (see Fig. 27–3).

PEARL... Not all incisions are prone to rupture; for example, even though a tapering 1-mm paracentesis incision has some weakening effect locally, this eye is still more likely to rupture at the limbus or equatorial sclera.

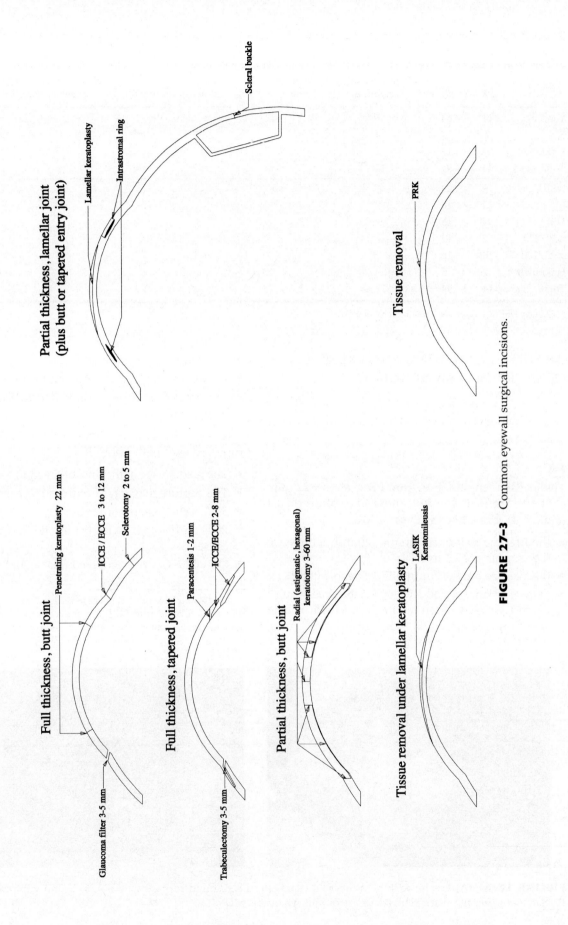

Full thickness, butt joint

Penetrating keratoplasty 22 mm

ICCE / ECCE 3 to 12 mm

Sclerotomy 2 to 5 mm

Glaucoma filter 3-5 mm

Full thickness, tapered joint

Paracentesis 1-2 mm

ICCE/ECCE 2-8 mm

Trabeculectomy 3-5 mm

Partial thickness, butt joint

Radial (astigmatic, hexagonal) keratotomy 3-60 mm

Tissue removal under lamellar keratoplasty

LASIK
Keratomileusis

Partial thickness, lamellar joint (plus butt or tapered entry joint)

Lamellar keratoplasty

Intrastromal ring

Scleral buckle

Tissue removal

PRK

FIGURE 27–3 Common eyewall surgical incisions.

283

TABLE 27–2 INJURED EYE RUPTURED AT THE SURGICAL INCISION AND THE BEST CORRECTED POSTOPERATIVE VISUAL ACUITY*

	PK	Cataract	Prior Eyewall Laceration	Trabeculect-omy	RK	Strabismus	IOFB	Retinal Detachment	Surgery Not Specified	Total
Yes	44	64	6	2	1				15	132
No		27	4			2	1	1		35
Unknown		3	2		1					6
Total	44	94	12	2	2	2	1	1	15	173
NLP	9	29	1			1	1		4	45
LP	9	16	7	1	1			1	5	40
HM	9	15	2	1					2	29
<20/200	5	12								17
≥20/200	10	16	2		1	1			4	34
Unknown	2	6								8
Total	44	94	12	2	2	2	1	1	15	173

*173 eyes; USEIR December 1988–September 1999.

TRAUMA FOLLOWING DIFFERENT TYPES OF INTRAOCULAR SURGERY

Of 4798 eyes with open globe injury in the USEIR,[38] 3.6% of eyes were reported to have had prior surgery (Table 27–2).

PK

The incision length for a 7-mm PK graft is ~22 mm, prone to rupture due to trauma by a blunt object (Fig. 27–4). Of patients with prior PK:

- the lifetime risk of traumatic wound dehiscence (i.e., rupture) is 2.5 to 5.7%[39–41];
- the average time of rupture is 3.4 years after PK;
- there is no time period after which the eye is "safe": PK incisions have been reported to dehisce as long after the procedure as 13,[42] 25,[43] and even 75[38] years;

- the trauma may be trivial[b];
- sutures do not help in retaining the graft[42]; and
- the prognosis is poor: only 28.6 to 33% of eyes recover ≥20/200 vision.[40,49]

The following information is from the USEIR on ruptured eyes with prior PK.

- The median age at the time of the injury is 45 years.
- The rupture may have occurred 75 years after PK.
- 59% of the patients are male.
- Falls and assaults with fist are the most common causes.
- Only 21% of eyes recovered final ≥20/200 vision.

---

[b] For example, accidental pokes in the eye,[44] digital massage for glaucoma 6 years after PK,[45] use of suction cup device (force: 1.86–1.96 N) for contact lens removal,[46,47] and sports.[48]

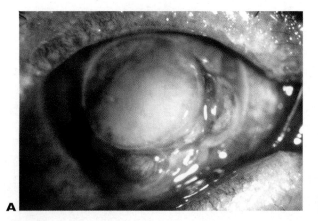
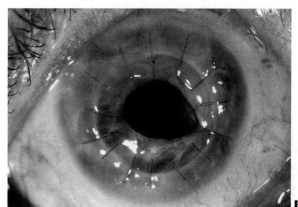

FIGURE 27–4   (A) Eye hit with blunt object 4 years after PK. Wound rupture with iris, lens, and vitreous prolapse. (B) Same eye after reconstruction. (Courtesy of Kathryn Colby, MD)

Cataract

- Rupture of ICCE and ECCE wounds (Fig. 27–5) often occurs long after surgery.
- The visual outcome is commonly poor.
- Frequent causes include falls and even minor trauma (e.g., a dog's paw).[52–55]
- The lifetime risk of rupture is 1.4% with large-incision operations.[56]
- Phacoemulsification scleral pocket wounds 7.5 mm in length may also dehisce.[57–58,c]

[c] Although subjected to internal/external pressure, a 5.1-mm-long no-stitch flap incision has greater wound integrity than a 7.0-mm-long sutured incision.[59]

- PC IOLs are more resistant to minor ocular trauma[d] than AC or iris-fixated IOLs (see Chapter 21).[55]
- Improperly constructed small-incision clear corneal wounds may fail after even trivial trauma[61]; the length of the posterior lip is important.[62]

CONTROVERSY

Clear corneal incisions 3.0 or 3.5 mm wide and at least 2.0 mm long have less tendency to rupture than shorter incisions and are comparable to similarly constructed scleral tunnel incisions.[63] Conversely, square corneoscleral incisions with a 1.5-mm internal corneal lip have been found to offer greater stability and safety than the conventional rectangular clear corneal incision (3.2 × 2.0 mm).[64]

- Incisions with an internal corneal lip, which creates a self-sealing valve, provide a more pressure-resistant wound.[65,66]

[d] Even PC IOLs require relatively little energy (0.68 J) to extrude.[60] Unincised eyes, when struck with a 12.5-mm-diameter metal rod, require 2.08 J to rupture.[18]

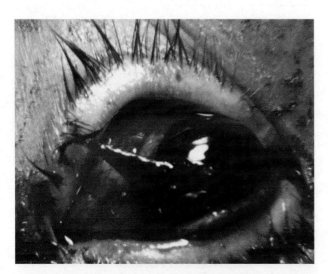

FIGURE 27–5 ICCE incision (no IOL implanted), rupturing 2 weeks postoperatively from a fall. Choroidal hemorrhage.

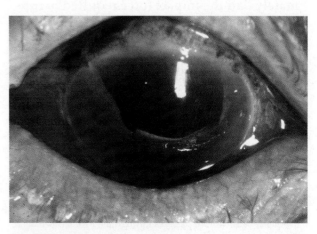

FIGURE 27–6 Fall causing a 4-mm phaco wound to rupture. (Courtesy of Roberto Pineda, MD)

- Manipulation of the entry wound during surgery may create a situation in which a longer incision is stronger than a shorter one.[e]

> **PEARL...** Self-sealing small sutureless cataract incisions, if properly constructed, provide a strong, pressure-resistant wound, which is unaffected even by scleral buckling.[68]

Analysis of the USEIR data shows that:

- 68% of eyes, rupturing after cataract surgery, do so at the surgical wound;
- the dehiscence may occur a long time after surgery:
  - 20% in 9 months to 15 years and only 16% in less than 5 weeks;
- the median age at the time of injury is 77 years;
- women slightly outnumber men (56% vs. 44%);
- the most common etiology is falling (54%);
- wearing eyeglasses does not appear to offer good protection;
- the IOL is extruded in 80% of eyes; and
- the prognosis is poor: less than 19% of eyes recover ≥20/200 vision.

Refractive Surgery

Incisional (radial, hexagonal, astigmatic) Keratotomy

This operation increases the susceptibility of the globe to rupture[69,70] because of the following.

- The presence of epithelium in the wound.[71-75]
- The irregular scar tissue[76] never regains the strength of the uncut corneal fibrils.[77,f]

> **SPECIAL CONSIDERATION**
>
> Standard RK incisions rupture at approximately half the impact force required to rupture unoperated eyes.[78-81]

- The total incision length is >30 mm in an 8-incision and >60 mm in a 16-incision RK.
- The incisions cut through 80 to 95% of the 0.5-mm corneal thickness.[83,84]
- The incisions often cut to or through the limbus.

[e]4.0-mm self-sealing incisions with a Prodigy inserter rupture at a pressure similar to that of a sutured limbal incision, both at one fourth the pressure of a 5.2-mm self-sealing incision. Suturing the self-sealing incisions does not significantly change the rupturing pressure.[67]

[f]Squash balls rupture pig eyes through the RK incisions at significantly lower speeds than unoperated eyes (typically rupturing at the limbus or sclera).[20] BBs, shot at velocities causing only hyphema in unoperated cat eyes, ruptured the globe along the RK incision lines in 31% of eyes that underwent RK 8 weeks earlier.[82]

> **PITFALL**
>
> RK and hexagonal keratotomy wounds not only require less energy (even the force of a clear corneal incision for cataract has been sufficient to dehisce an 8-month RK incision) than unoperated corneas to rupture but also remain susceptible for many years (Fig. 27–7).[85-100,g] The site of rupture also differs (see Table 27–3). Reducing the incision length appears to reduce the risk of corneal rupture, but as the IOP is increased, even eyes with "mini" RK eventually rupture.[102,103]

> **PITFALL**
>
> It is impossible to perform a keratotomy incision still effective for refractive purposes but short enough to prevent rupture at energy levels lower than those in unoperated eyes. Consequently, all patients considering such surgery should be counseled about blunt object–related risks of open globe injury, even if the risk is not absolute.[104,105] The concept that the rupture of an RK incision "saves vision"[106] is consistent neither with the poor clinical results nor with experimental data (Fig. 27–8), which demonstrate the explosive loss of ocular contents upon squash ball impact.

[g]The post-RK risk limits employment opportunities such as enlistment in the U.S. Armed Forces.[101]

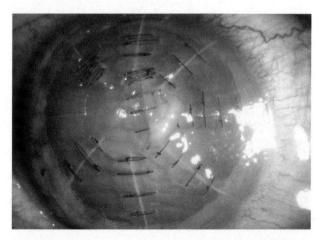

FIGURE 27–7 Two years postoperatively an air bag deployment ruptured seven of eight RK incisions, involving unincised clear central cornea. (Courtesy of Marc Goldberg, MD)

TABLE 27–3   THE IMPACT REQUIRED TO RUPTURE PIG CORNEAS SUBJECTED TO BLUNT FORCE*

Prior Surgery	Force (N)	Location of Rupture	% of the Total
None (control eye)	746.3	Limbus	100
Standard RK	246.2	Surgical incision	33
"Mini" RK, 3.5-mm incisions	351.3	Surgical incision	47
"Mini" RK, 2.0-mm incisions	514.2	Surgical incision	69

*See the text for more details.

PRK, ALK, PTK, and LASIK

Following such surgery, the energy required to rupture the eye is not significantly different from that for normal eyes.[20,21,107] PRK does not weaken the cornea after degrees of ablation up to 42 D; if ruptures occur, they are at the limbus or behind the extraocular muscle insertions.[108,h] In human experiments, the energy required to rupture normal eyes versus eyes after

----

[h] Of control pig eyes that were subjected to lateral compression, 90% ruptured at the sclera and one at the optic nerve; RK eyes ruptured at the corneal incisions; PRK eyes ruptured at the sclera; after PTK, the corneal rupture occured when the ablations were at least 40% in depth.[109]

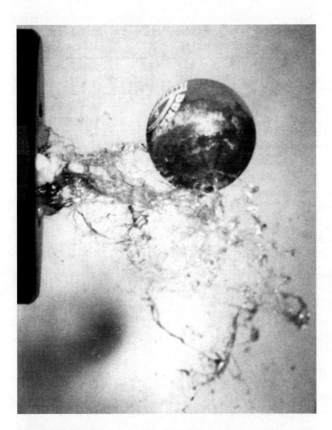

FIGURE 27–8 Pig eye with eight-incision, 95% depth, standard RK. Soft squash ball (129.5 mph) results in wound dehiscence (involves clear cornea and sclera) and explosive tissue loss.

ALK/PRK/LASIK was not significantly different,[110] but the latter tended to rupture near the flap edge or the limbus.

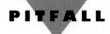

PITFALL

Flap dehiscence by trauma after LASIK is a long-term concern.[111,112]

Intrastromal Corneal Ring

Stromal healing following implantation seems satisfactory,[113] but no information is available regarding the effects of trauma on these eyes.

Glaucoma

A filter or a trabeculectomy is a butt joint from which tissue was removed. Eyes that have had glaucoma surgery are more prone to rupture through the incision.[114]

Procedures Associated with Scleral Buckling

The consequences depend on the type of procedure.

- *Transscleral diathermy:* The scleral weakening is significant.[115]
- *Transscleral cryopexy/diode photocoagulation:* No significant scleral weakening occurs.[116]

Vitrectomy

No significant weakening occurs if the cornea and limbus are not involved.

PREVENTION

Prophylaxis of an eye injury is especially important in eyes that have undergone (open globe) surgery.

- Eye protection is not necessarily offered by streetwear/sunglasses, although the type and severity of the injury may be affected.
- It is the obligation of the surgeon to advise the patient of the need for long-term use of protective eyewear[51] that prevents the external force from striking the eye.

- Wound dehiscence has not been reported from strain (lifting, working out, sports) or from indirect trauma (e.g., head injury, sudden deceleration in MVC).
- People with conditions that weaken the structure of the globe should *not*:
  - deactivate their air bags[117–120]; or
  - be discouraged from work or sports.[i]
- For patients with average risk, the advice in Table 27–4 (should be supplied with all eyeglass prescriptions) is adequate.
- To protect eyes at risk (Table 27–5), it is necessary to have a polycarbonate lens that does not shatter[121] (Fig. 27–9).[122]
- For patients with high risk, the frame should meet the industrial standard specifications (ANSI Z87) or preferably the more rigid requirements of the sports standard (ASTM F803).[123,124]

PEARL... It is essential for the ophthalmologist to discuss the need for appropriate protective eyewear with *every patient undergoing operation*, even if this is "only" refractive surgery.[125]

---

[i]They should, however, be given warning/advice regarding the increased risk, the need for prevention in the desired activity, and a specific prescription for protective eyewear (see Chapter 7).[125]

TABLE 27–4   Safety Recommendations*

Unless there is a specific reason for another lens material, prescribe *polycarbonate* lenses, especially for children, functionally one-eyed people, and active adults. These lenses absorb UV and are coated for scratch resistance; therefore, no further UV- or scratch-resistant coating is suggested.

For sports that have the potential for eye contact with a ball or racket, 3-mm-thick polycarbonate lenses in a frame that passes ASTM F803 are recommended. The frame must be certified by the PECC for the specific sport or the manufacturer must supply a test report from an accredited and unrelated testing laboratory, certifying that the eyewear passes ASTM F803 for the intended sport. ASTM F803 covers the racquet sports, women's lacrosse and field hockey, baseball, and basketball. For other sports, protectors should meet or exceed ASTM F803 standard specifications for squash.

For sports with high impact (e.g., ice hockey, batter/base runner in youth baseball), a face shield mounted on a helmet designed for the sport is required. Paintball protectors must conform to the requirements of ASTM F1776.

Working people exposed to flying chips or using power tools should have protectors meeting ANSI Z87.1. Goggles are safest. Only polycarbonate lenses should be used.

Many workplace activities, (e.g., chain saw use) require, in addition to safety glasses, a helmet with a face shield designed for the activity.

*See Chapter 7.

TABLE 27–5   Risk of Trauma-Related Globe Rupture in Eyes with Prior Surgery

High	PK
	Large incision, butt joint ICCE, ECCE
	Standard RK with incisions to limbus
	Hexagonal keratotomy
Moderately high	Large-incision tapered joint ICCE, ECCE
	Trabeculectomy or other filtration surgery
	Prior repair of corneal and/or scleral laceration
Moderate	Small-incision butt joint ECCE
	"Mini" RK
	Astigmatic keratotomy
Moderately low	Small tapered incision ECCE
	Scleral buckle with diathermy
No more than in eyes with no prior surgery	Paracentesis
	Scleral buckle with cryopexy or laser
	Strabismus surgery
	Lamellar keratoplasty/pterygium
	LASIK*
	PRK
	Keratomileusis*

*Late traumatic dehiscence of corneal flap remains a potential future problem.

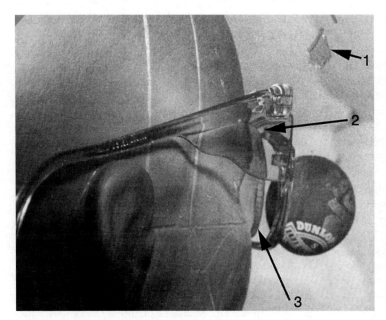

FIGURE 27–9   This industrial safety frame conforms to ANSI Z87, which is *not satisfactory for sports* and fails with a 90 mph squash ball: (1) sharp shards break off; (2) frame breaks; (3) polycarbonate lens (no shattering) strikes the eye (glass or allyl resin plastic, permitted under ANSI Z87, lenses would have shattered).

SUMMARY

Severe blunt force has the potential to lead to contusion rupture. In cases of rupture, the eye tends to open at its weakest point. In eyes that have undergone surgery, the weakest point is usually at the site of the surgical incision, even many years following the surgery. Examination of a severely injured eye must include focused evaluation of the previous incision to rule out a full-thickness eyewall defect. The increased risk of open globe injury resulting from incisional surgery needs to be discussed with the patient preoperatively and appropriate precautions taken postoperatively.

[The author wishes to thank Don Moodie, John Crocker, and Clause DesRochers for engineering assistance]

REFERENCES

1. Katz J, Tielsch JM. Lifetime prevalence of ocular injuries from the Baltimore Eye Survey. *Arch Ophthalmol.* 1993;111:1564–1568.

2. Feist RM, Farber MD. Ocular trauma epidemiology. *Arch Ophthalmol.* 1989;107:503–504.

3. Schein OD, Hibberd PL, Shingleton BJ, et al. The spectrum and burden of ocular injury. *Ophthalmology.* 1988; 95:300–305.

4. Jeffers J. An ongoing tragedy: pediatric sports-related eye injuries. *Semin Ophthalmol.* 1990;5:216–223.

5. Parver LM. Eye trauma: the neglected disorder. *Arch Ophthalmol.* 1986;104:1452–1453.

6. Hahn HJA. Perforating wounds of the eye. *J R Nav Med Serv.* 1976;62:73–81.

7. Gilbert CM, Soong HK, Hirst LW. A two-year prospective study of penetrating ocular trauma at the Wilmer Ophthalmological Institute. *Ann Ophthalmol.* 1987;19: 104–106.

8. Groessl S, Nanda SK, Mieler WF. Assault-related penetrating ocular injury. *Am J Ophthalmol.* 1993;116: 26–33.

9. Cherry PMH. Rupture of the globe. *Arch Ophthalmol.* 1972;88:498–507.

10. Kuhn F, Morris R, Witherspoon CD, Heimann K, Jeffers JB, Treister G. A standardized classification of ocular trauma. *Ophthalmology.* 1996;103:240–243.

11. Burnstein Y, Klapper D, Hersh PS. Experimental globe rupture after excimer laser photorefractive keratectomy. *Arch Ophthalmol.* 1995;113:1056–1059.

12. Bullock JD, Warwar RE, Green WR. Ocular explosions from periocular anesthetic injections: a clinical, histopathologic, experimental, and biophysical study. *Ophthalmology.* 1999;106:2341–2352.

13. Bullock JD, Warwar RE, Green WR. Ocular explosion during cataract surgery: a clinical, histopathological, experimental, and biophysical study. *Trans Am Ophthalmol Soc.* 1998;96:243–276.

14. Magnante DO, Bullock JD, Green WR. Ocular explosion after peribulbar anesthesia: case report and experimental study. *Ophthalmology.* 1997;104:608–615.

15. Vinger PF. The eye and sports medicine. In: Duane TD, Jaeger EA, eds. *Clinical Ophthalmology.* Vol 5. Philadelphia: JB Lippincott; 1985:chap 45.

16. Delori F, Pomerantzeff O, Cox MS. Deformation of the globe under high speed impact: its relation to contusion injuries. *Invest Ophthalmol*. 1969;8:290–301.

17. Preston JD. Review of standard consumer safety specification for non-powder guns (ANSI/ASTM F589-78) and non-powder gun projectiles and propellants (ANSI/ASTM F590-78). Mechanical and Textile Division, Engineering Sciences, CPSC, Washington, February 8, 1980.

18. Green RP, Peters DR, Shore JW, Fanton JW, Davis H. Force necessary to fracture the orbital floor. *Ophthalmol Plast Reconstr Surg*. 1990;6:211–217.

19. Vinger PF, Sparks JJ, Mussack KR, Dondero J, Jeffers JB. A program to prevent eye injuries in paintball. *Sports Vision*. 1997;3:33–40.

20. Umlas JW, Galler El, Vinger PF, Wu HK. Ocular integrity after quantitated trauma in radial keratotomy eyes. Presented at Association for Research in Vision and Ophthalmology, May 16, 1995, Ft. Lauderdale, FL. Abstracts in *Invest Ophthalmol Vis Sci*. 1995;36(4):S583.

21. Galler El, Umlas JW, Vinger PF, Wu HK. Ocular integrity after quantitated trauma following photorefractive keratectomy and automated lamellar keratectomy. Presented at Association for Research in Vision and Ophthalmology, May 16, 1995, Ft. Lauderdale, FL. Abstracts in *Invest Ophthalmol Vis Sci*. 1995; 36(4):S580.

22. Vinger PF, Duma SM, Crandall J. Baseball hardness as a risk factor in eye injuries. *Arch Ophthalmol*. 1999;117:354–358.

23. Bloomfield LA. *How Things Work: The Physics of Everyday Life*. New York: John Wiley & Sons; 1997.

24. Berger RE, Huckeba JA. Impact on human eyes by propelled objects. Report to Consumer Product Safety Commission NBSIR 80-2037, Bethesda, MD, 1980.

25. Berger RE. A model for evaluating the ocular contusion injury potential of propelled objects. *J Bioeng*. 1978;2:345–358.

26. Berger RE. System for assessing eye injury potential of propelled objects. *J Res Natl Bur Stand*. 1979;84:9–19.

27. Crocker J, DesRochers C, Delbridge G, Vinger P. Optimization of lens edge design for safety eyewear using experimentally validated finite element (FE) impact analysis. 7th International Conference on Product Safety Research, October 1, 1999, Bethesda, MD.

28. Duke-Elder S, Wybar KC. The anatomy of the visual system. *System of Ophthalmology*. Vol 2. St. Louis: CV Mosby, 1961.

29. Jonas JB, Mardin CY, Schlotzer-Schrehardt U, Naumann GO. Morphometry of the human lamina cribrosa surface. *Invest Ophthalmol Vis Sci*. 1991;32:401–405.

30. Olsen TW, Aaberg SY, Geroski DH, Edelhauser HF. Human sclera: thickness and surface area. *Am J Ophthalmol*. 1998;125:237–241.

31. Funata M, Tokoro T. Scleral change in experimentally myopic monkeys. *Graefes* Arch Clin Exp Ophthalmol. 1990;228:174–179.

32. Friberg TR, Lace JW. A comparison of the elastic properties of human choroid and sclera. *Exp Eye Res*. 1988; 47:429–436.

33. Duke-Elder S, MacFaul PA. Injuries: Part 1. Mechanical injuries. *System of Ophthalmology*. Vol 14. St. Louis: CV Mosby; 1972.

34. Gasset AR, Dohlman CH. The tensile strength of corneal wounds. *Arch Ophthalmol*. 1968;79:595–602.

35. Masuda K. Tensile strength of corneoscleral wounds repaired with absorbable sutures. *Ophthalmic Surg*. 1981;12:110–114.

36. Pilkey WD. Peterson's Stress Concentration Factors. New York: John Wiley & Sons; 1997:65–66.

37. Bryant MR, Szerenyi K, Schmotzer H, McDonnell PJ. Corneal tensile strength in fully healed radial keratotomy wounds. *Invest Ophthalmol Vis Sci*. 1994;35:3022–3031.

38. United States Eye Injury Registry, PO Box 5556, Birmingham, AL 35255.

39. Tseng SH, Lin SC, Chen FK. Traumatic wound dehiscence after penetrating keratoplasty: clinical features and outcome in 21 cases. *Cornea*. 1999;18:553–558.

40. Sambursky DL, Maadel K, Cuite C, Sambursky RP, Sperber LTD. Wound dehiscence following penetrating keratoplasty. Scientific Poster, American Academy of Ophthalmology, Chicago, 1993.

41. Bowman RJ, Yorston D, Aitchison TC, McIntyre B, Kirkness CM. Traumatic wound rupture after penetrating keratoplasty in Africa. *Br J Ophthalmol*. 1999;83:530–534.

42. Farley MK, Pettit TH. Traumatic wound dehiscence after penetrating keratoplasty. *Am J Ophthalmol*. 1987;104:44–49.

43. Rohrbach JM, Weidle EG, Steuhl KP, Meilinger S, Pleyer U. Traumatic wound dehiscence after penetrating keratoplasty. *Acta Ophthalmol Scand*. 1996;74:501–505.

44. Agrawal V, Wagh M, Krishnamachary M, Rao GN, Gupta S. Traumatic wound dehiscence after penetrating keratoplasty. *Cornea*. 1995;14:601–603.

45. MacRae SM, Van Buskirk EM. Late wound dehiscence after penetrating keratoplasty in association with digital massage. *Am J Ophthalmol*. 1986;102:391–392.

46. Yu DD, Kletzky DH, Lempo MA. Corneal-graft dehiscence secondary to suction-cup device use for contact lens removal. *Arch Ophthalmol*. 1992;110:1050–1051.

47. Ingraham HJ, Perry HD, Epstein AB, et al. Suction cup/contact lens complications following penetrating keratoplasty. *CLAO J*. 1998;24:59–62.

48. Rehany U, Rumelt S. Ocular trauma following penetrating keratoplasty: incidence, outcome, and postoperative recommendations. *Arch Ophthalmol*. 1998;116:1282–1286.

49. Raber IM, Arentsen JJ, Laibson PR. Traumatic wound dehiscence after penetrating keratoplasty. *Arch Ophthalmol*. 1980;98:1407–1409.

50. Zagelbaum BM, Starkey C, Hersh PS, Donnenfeld ED, Perry HD, Jeffers JB. The National Basketball Association eye injury study. *Arch Ophthalmol*. 1995;113:749–752.

51. Swan KC, Meyer SL, Squires E. Late wound separation after cataract extraction. *Ophthalmology*. 1978;85:991–1003.

52. Johns KJ, Sheils P, Parrish CM, Elliott JH, O'Day DM. Traumatic wound dehiscence in pseudophakia. *Am J Ophthalmol.* 1989;108:535–539.

53. Liggett PE, Mani N, Green RE, Cano M, Ryan SJ, Lean JS. Management of traumatic rupture of the globe in aphakic patients. *Retina.* 1990;10(suppl 1):59–64.

54. Kass MA, Lahav M, Albert DM. Traumatic rupture of healed cataract wounds. *Am J Ophthalmol.* 1976;81:722–724.

55. Assia EI, Blotnick CA, Powers TP, Legler UF, Apple DJ. Clinicopathologic study of ocular trauma in eyes with intraocular lenses. *Am J Ophthalmol.* 1994;117:30–36.

56. Lambrou FH, Kozarsky A. Wound dehiscence following cataract surgery. *Ophthalmic Surg.* 1987;18:738–740.

57. Stevens JD, Claoue CM, Steele AD. Postoperative blunt trauma to 7.5 mm scleral pocket wounds. *J Cataract Refract Surg.* 1994;20:344–345.

58. Pham DT, Anders N, Wollensak J. Wound rupture 1 year after cataract operation with 7 mm scleral tunnel incision (no-stitch technique). *Klin Monatsbl Augenheilkd.* 1996;208:124–126.

59. Heier JS, Walton WT, Enzenauer RW, Rice W, Tuman D. Wound strength comparison of a 5.1-millimeter no-stitch with a 7.0-millimeter sutured incision in human cadaver globes. *Ophthalmic Surg.* 1994;25:685–687.

60. Magargal LE, Shakin E, Bolling JP, Robb-Doyle E. Traumatic extrusion of posterior chamber lenses: clinical and experimental correlations. *J Cataract Refract Surg.* 1986;12:670–673.

61. Hurvitz LM. Late clear corneal wound failure after trivial trauma. *J Cataract Refract Surg.* 1999;25:283–284.

62. Frieling E, Steinert RF. Intrinsic stability of 'self-sealing' unsutured cataract wounds. *Arch Ophthalmol.* 1993;111:381–383.

63. Mackool RJ, Russell RS. Strength of clear corneal incisions in cadaver eyes. *J Cataract Refract Surg.* 1996;22:721–725.

64. Ernest PH, Lavery KT, Kiessling LA. Relative strength of scleral corneal and clear corneal incisions constructed in cadaver eyes. *J Cataract Refract Surg.* 1994;20:626–629.

65. Ernest PH, Kiessling LA, Lavery KT. Relative strength of cataract incisions in cadaver eyes. *J Cataract Refract Surg.* 1991;17(suppl):668–671.

66. Berger RR, Van Coller B. The "lock-and-valve" incision: truce in the "suture wars." *Ophthalmic Surg.* 1993;24:689–691.

67. Kondrot EC. Rupturing pressure in cadaver eyes with three types of cataract incisions. *J Cataract Refract Surg.* 1991;17(suppl):745–748.

68. Wyszynski RE, Khosrof S, Shands P, Kalski RS, Bruner WE. Effect of scleral buckling on unsutured cataract wound strength. *Ophthalmic Surg Lasers.* 1996;27:787–789.

69. Vinger PF, Mieler WF, Oestreicher JH, Easterbrook M. Ruptured globes following radial and hexagonal keratotomy surgery. *Arch Ophthalmol.* 1996;114:129–134.

70. Rashid ER, Waring GO. Complications of refractive keratotomy. In: Waring GO, ed. *Refractive Keratotomy for Myopia and Astigmatism.* St. Lewis: Mosby; 1992:863–936.

71. Deg JK, Binder PS. Wound healing after astigmatic keratotomy in human eyes. *Ophthalmology.* 1987;94:1290–1298.

72. Ingraham HJ, Guber D, Green R. Radial keratotomy. Clinicopathologic case report. *Arch Ophthalmol.* 1985;103:683–688.

73. Waring GO, Steinberg EB, Wilson LA. Slit-lamp appearance of corneal wound healing after radial keratotomy. *Am J Ophthalmol.* 1985;100:218–224.

74. Yamaguchi T, Tamaki K, Kaufman HE, Katz J, Shaw EL. Histologic study of a pair of human corneas after anterior radial keratotomy. *Am J Ophthalmol.* 1985;100:281–292.

75. Binder PS, Nayak SK, Deg JK, Zavala EY, Sugar J. An ultrastructural and histochemical study of long-term wound healing after radial keratotomy. *Am J Ophthalmol.* 1987;103:432–440.

76. Melles GRJ, Binder PS, Anderson JA. Variation in healing throughout the depth of long-term, unsutured, corneal wounds in human autopsy specimens and monkeys. *Arch Ophthalmol.* 1994;112:100–109.

77. Lindquist TD. Complications of corneal refractive surgery. *Int Ophthalmol Clin.* 1992;32:97–114.

78. Larson BC, Kremer FB, Eller AW, Bernadino VB. Quantitated trauma following radial keratotomy in rabbits. *Ophthalmology.* 1983;90:660–667.

79. Luttrull JK, Jester JV, Smith RE. The effect of radial keratotomy on ocular integrity in an animal model. *Arch Ophthalmol.* 1982;100:319–320.

80. Campos M, Lee M, McDonnell PJ. Ocular integrity after refractive surgery: effects of photorefractive keratectomy, phototherapeutic keratectomy, and radial keratotomy. *Ophthalmic Surg.* 1992;23:598–602.

81. Rylander HG, Welch AJ, Fremming B. The effect of radial keratotomy in the rupture strength of pig eyes. *Ophthalmic Surg.* 1983;14:744–749.

82. McKnight SJ, Fitz J, Gianqiacomo J. Corneal rupture following radial keratotomy in cats subject to BB gun injury. *Ophthalmic Surg.* 1988;19:165–167.

83. Thornton SP, Gardner SK, Waring GO. Surgical instruments used in refractive keratotomy. In: Waring GO, ed. *Refractive Keratotomy for Myopia and Astigmatism.* St. Louis: Mosby; 1992:407–489.

84. Waring GO. Atlas of surgical techniques of radial keratotomy. In: Waring GO, ed. *Refractive Keratotomy for Myopia and Astigmatism.* St. Louis: Mosby; 1992:507–639.

85. Binder PS, Waring GO, Arrowsmith PN, Wang C. Histopathology of traumatic corneal rupture after radial keratotomy. *Arch Ophthalmol.* 1988;106:1584–1590.

86. Glasgow BJ, Brown HH, Aizuss DH, Mondino BJ, Foos RY. Traumatic dehiscence of incisions seven years after radial keratotomy. *Am J Ophthalmol.* 1988;106:703–707.

87. Reichel MB, Busin M, Koch F, Sekundo W. Traumatic wound dehiscence and corneal rupture 3 1/2 years after radial keratotomy. *Klin Monatsbl Augenheilkd.* 1995;206:266–267.

88. Panda A, Sharma N, Kumar A. Ruptured globe 10 years after radial keratotomy. *J Refract Surg.* 1999;15:64–65.

89. Simmons KB, Linsalata RP. Ruptured globe following blunt trauma after radial keratotomy: a case report. *Ophthalmology.* 1987;94(suppl):148.

90. McDonnell PJ, Lean JS, Schanzlin DJ. Globe rupture from blunt trauma after hexagonal keratotomy. *Am J Ophthalmol.* 1987;103:241–242.

91. Zhaboyedov GD, Bondavera GS. Traumatic rupture of the eyeball after radial keratotomy. *Vestn Oftalmol.* 1990;106:64–65.

92. Pearlstein ES, Agapitos PJ, Cantrill HL, Holland EJ, Williams P, Lindstrom RL. Ruptured globe after radial keratotomy. *Am J Ophthalmol.* 1988;106:755–756.

93. McDermott ML, Wilkinson WS, Tukel DB, Madion MP, Cowden JW, Puklin JE. Corneoscleral rupture ten years after radial keratotomy. *Am J Ophthalmol.* 1990; 110:575–577.

94. Forstot SL, DaMiano RE. Trauma after radial keratotomy. *Ophthalmology.* 1988;95:833–835.

95. Nolan BT. Perforation by a foreign body through a pre-existing radial keratotomy wound. *Mil Med.* 1991; 156:151–154.

96. Bloom HR, Sands J, Schneider D. Corneal rupture from blunt trauma 22 months after radial keratotomy. *Refract Corneal Surg.* 1990;6:197–199.

97. Girard LJ, Rodrizuez J, Nono N, Wesson M. Delayed wound healing after radial keratotomy. *Am J Ophthalmol.* 1985;99:484–486.

98. Deg JK, Zavala EY, Binder PS. Delayed wound healing after radial keratotomy. *Ophthalmology.* 1985;92:734–740.

99. Budak K, Friedman NJ, Koch DD. Dehiscence of a radial keratotomy incision during clear corneal cataract surgery. *J Cataract Refract Surg.* 1998;24:278–280.

100. Basuk WL, Zisman M, Waring GO, et al. Complications of hexagonal keratotomy. *Am J Ophthalmol.* 1994;117:37–49.

101. Enzenauer RW, Wolter A, Cornell FM, Tucker S. Radial keratotomy in the soldier-aviator. *Mil Med.* 1993;158:521–528.

102. Pinheiro MN Jr, Bryant MR, Tayyanipour R, Nassaralla BA, Wee WR, McDonnell PJ. Corneal integrity after refractive surgery. Effects of radial keratotomy and mini-radial keratotomy. *Ophthalmology.* 1995;102: 297–301.

103. Steinemann TL, Baltz TC, Lam BL, Soulsby M, Walls RC, Brown HH. Mini radial keratotomy reduces ocular integrity. Axial compression in a postmortem porcine eye model. *Ophthalmology.* 1998;105:1739–1744.

104. Casebeer JC, Shapiro DR, Phillips S. Severe ocular trauma without corneal rupture after radial keratotomy: case reports. *J Refract Corneal Surg.* 1994;10:31–33.

105. John ME Jr, Schmitt TE. Traumatic hyphema after radial keratotomy. *Ann Ophthalmol.* 1983;15:930–932.

106. Marmer RJ. RK saves vision. *Ocular Surg News.* February 1 1994:3.

107. Schmitt-Bernard CF, Villain M, Beaufrere L, Arnaud B. Trauma after radial keratotomy and photorefractive keratectomy. *J Cataract Refract Surg.* 1997;23:803–804.

108. Burnstein Y, Klapper D, Hersh PS. Experimental globe rupture after excimer laser photorefractive kera-tectomy. *Arch Ophthalmol.* 1995;113:1056–1059.

109. Campos M, Lee M, McDonnell PJ. Ocular integrity after refractive surgery: effects of photorefractive keratectomy, phototherapeutic keratectomy, and radial keratotomy. *Ophthalmic Surg.* 1992;23:598–602.

110. Peacock LW, Slade SG, Martiz J, Chuang A, Yee RW. Ocular integrity after refractive procedures. *Ophthalmology.* 1997;104:1079–1083.

111. Leung AT, Rao SK, Lam DS. Traumatic partial unfolding of laser in situ keratomileusis flap with severe epithelial ingrowth. *J Cataract Refract Surg.* 2000;26:135–139.

112. Chaudhry NA, Smiddy WE. Displacement of corneal cap during vitrectomy in a post-LASIK eye. *Retina.* 1998;18:554–555.

113. Quantock AJ, Kincaid MC, Schanzlin DJ. Stromal healing following explantation of an ICR (intrastromal corneal ring) from a nonfunctional human eye. *Arch Ophthalmol.* 1995;113:208–209.

114. Zeiter JH, Shin DH. Traumatic rupture of the globe after glaucoma surgery. *Am J Ophthalmol.* 1990;109:732–733.

115. Schwartz A, Rathbun E. Scleral strength impairment and recovery after diathermy. *Arch Ophthalmol.* 1975; 93:1173–1177.

116. Han DP, Nash RW, Blair JR, O'Brien WJ, Medina RR. Comparison of scleral tensile strength after transscleral retinal cryopexy, diathermy, and diode laser photocoagulation. *Arch Ophthalmol.* 1995;113:1195–1199.

117. Tsuda Y, Wakiyama H, Amemiya T. Ocular injury caused by an air bag for a driver wearing eyeglasses. *Jpn J Ophthalmol.* 1999;43:239–240.

118. Ghafouri A, Burgess SK, Hrdlicka ZK, Zagelbaum BM. Air bag-related ocular trauma. *Am J Emerg Med.* 1997;15:389–392.

119. Manche EE, Goldberg RA, Mondino BJ. Air bag-related ocular injuries. *Ophthalmic Surg Lasers.* 1997; 28:246–250.

120. Kuhn F, Morris R, Witherspoon CD. Eye injury and the air bag. *Curr Opin Ophthalmol.* 1995;6:38–44.

121. Vinger PF, Parver L, Alfaro DV, Woods T, Abrams BS. Shatter resistance of spectacle lenses. *JAMA.* 1997;277:142–144.

122. Vinger PF, Woods BA. Prescription safety eyewear: impact studies of lens and frame failure. Proceedings American Society of Safety Engineers, 1999 ASSE Professional Development Conference and Exposition. Des Plaines, IL, 1999:445–463.

123. Vinger PF. Eye safety testing and standards. *Ophthalmol Clin North Am.* 1999;12:345–358.

124. Vinger PF. Injury prevention: where do we go from here? *J Am Optom Assoc.* 1999;70:87–98.

125. Kuhn F, Johnston WT, Mester V, Török M, Berta A. Informed consent and radial keratotomy. *Ann Ophthalmol.* 2000;32:331–332.

Chapter 28

ENDOPHTHALMITIS

Nauman A. Chaudhry and Harry W. Flynn, Jr.

 Endophthalmitis is an uncommon but devastating consequence of open globe injury.[1] The relatively poor visual prognosis of traumatic endophtalmitis is due to:

- the higher frequency of organisms that are more virulent than those in postoperative cases;
- the associated trauma;
- the frequent delay in diagnosis; and
- the frequent delay in the initiation of treatment.[2–13]

Traumatic endophthalmitis therefore presents difficult diagnostic and management issues distinct from endophthalmitis occurring in other settings.

EPIDEMIOLOGY

The incidence of endophthalmitis after open globe injury is 5 to 14%;[1,9,12,13] In the USEIR, the incidence is 2.6%.

Traumatic endophthalmitis constitutes approximately 10 to 30% of all infectious endophthalmitis[a,4–8,12] cases. It is more common in males (85%).[10] In the USEIR, the rate is 2.8% among males and 1.4% among females.

Risk factors for the development of traumatic endophthalmitis include:

- >24 hours of delay in primary wound closure;
- presence of an IOFB (6.9–13%, independent of IOFB type)[14];

---

[a]Postoperative, endogenous, traumatic, and filtering bleb-associated.

- rural setting:
  - soil contamination is believed to result in a higher rate of endophthalmitis (30%) for open globe injuries occurring in a rural versus a non-rural setting[11]; and
- rupture of the lens capsule.[13]

CLINICAL DIAGNOSIS

The symptoms and signs are similar to those in other categories of endophthalmitis, but the diagnosis is often delayed due to masquerading signs that usually accompany severe ocular trauma. Early symptoms may include:

- photophobia;
- pain out of proportion to the clinical findings;
- visual loss worse than media opacities might suggest;
- hypopyon (Fig. 28–1);
- vitritis; and
- retinal periphlebitis.[15]

Other, less specific signs include:

- lid edema;
- conjunctival erythema and edema;
- corneal edema;
- fibrinous membrane formation on the iris, lens, or the IOL; and
- loss of the red reflex or progressively worsening view of the posterior pole.

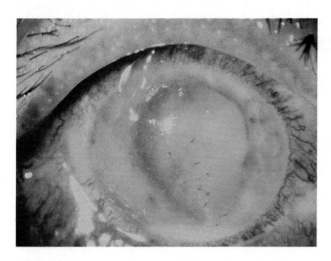

FIGURE 28–1 One day after repair of a corneal laceration, this patient developed increasing pain and hypopyon. Vitrectomy specimen revealed *Streptococcus faecalis*.

Fungal infection is more common in the following injuries:

• IOFB, especially if it is vegetable matter (e.g., thorn, wood); or
• soil contamination.

Characteristic signs of intraocular fungal infection include:

• slowly progressive inflammation after initial trauma repair;
• white "snowball-like" opacities or "string-of-pearls" configuration in the vitreous;
• chronic vitritis; and
• persistent white infiltrates around the primary wound side.[16]

> **P**EARL... Retinal periphlebitis is an early sign of endophthalmitis. However, it is often not recognized because of the common presence of media opacities.

MICROBIOLOGY

The microbiology of traumatic endophthalmitis is significantly different from that in other categories. Infections with more than one organism are common (up to 48%).[10,14] The organism is often virulent.

Gram-positive bacteria (usually cocci such as *Streptococcus* and *Staphylococcus* species) are the predomi-

nant isolates in both the adult and pediatric age groups.[8,10–12] There is a high incidence of *Bacillus* species. These infections are notable for their:

• rapid (<24 hours) onset;
• high risk of progression to panophthalmitis; and
• rate of poor visual outcome.

Endophthalmitis caused by *Bacillus* species is characterized by:

• severe pain;
• hypopyon;
• chemosis; and
• rapidly progressive proptosis and lid edema.

Additional information regarding *Bacillus* endophthalmitis includes the following.

• The characteristic ring-shaped corneal infiltrate is a late sign.
• Although rare in postoperative cases, it is rather common (up to 46% after open globe trauma) in the United States,[11] representing the second most common group after *Staphylococcus* species in IOFB injuries.[14]
• Although it was previously considered to have a uniformly poor visual prognosis, early recognition and prompt treatment of infection caused by *Bacillus* species (Fig. 28–2) may occasionally result in good visual outcome.[17,18]

Culturing for Microbiologic Analysis

The first question is: *in which cases should a sample be taken?*

> **P**EARL... When traumatic endophthalmitis is suspected, one should attempt to culture intraocular contents in all cases.

CONTROVERSY
⬅➡

Following an open globe injury, the ophthalmologist may consider routinely culturing all cases, but such an approach will yield a fair number of false-positive results and probably adds little to the clinical care of the patient (see Chapter 24).

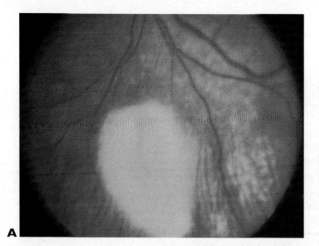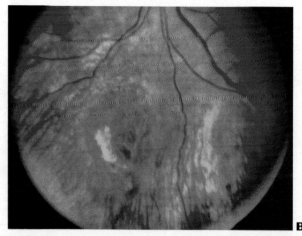

FIGURE 28–2 **(A)** An intraretinal IOFB with surrounding exudates. Infection was suspected and intravitreal vancomycin was injected during pars plana vitrectomy. The IOFB was cultured and grew *Bacillus cereus*. **(B)** The patient did not develop endophthalmitis; visual acuity eventually improved to 20/30.

The second question is: *where should the sample be taken from?*

- We do not routinely culture the wound or conjunctiva: the high risk of contamination makes a positive culture difficult to interpret.
- We do culture the wound if there is a specific indication of infection present.

In reported series of traumatic endophthalmitis, vitreous specimens have a higher rate of positive culture than aqueous samples.[19,20] The extent of vitrectomy performed to obtain samples depends on the visibility of the posterior segment and the surgeon's experience (see the Appendix for more details).

The third question is: *which culture media should be used?* Commonly used plates for bacterial and fungal cultures are:

- blood agar; and
- chocolate agar.

With a larger intraocular specimen, smears can be sent for:

- Gram, Giemsa, and fungal stains;
- Sabouraud's media (fungi);
- thioglycollate broth (all-purpose holding media); and
- anaerobic blood culture bottle.

Because the initial surgery is often performed in "off-hours," the standard culture media may not be immediately available (see also the Appendix).

PEARL... After hours or on the weekends, when the microbiology personnel may not be available to process the vitreous specimen, the vitreous aspirate can be directly injected into blood culture bottles. The culture yield of this technique appears to be comparable to that of conventional methods[21,22] (see also the Appendix).

Fungal cultures are indicated in cases in which initial bacterial cultures were negative or when fungal infection is strongly suspected.

PREVENTION: PROPHYLACTIC ANTIBIOTICS

Systemic antibiotics, although not confirmed in a randomized prospective study, may reduce the incidence of endophthalmitis in eyes with open globe injury. The selected antibiotic should:

- provide coverage against the most common pathogens known to cause traumatic endophthalmitis (i.e., *Bacillus* species and gram-positive organisms); and
- have adequate intraocular penetration after systemic administration.

The ideal antibiotic regimen remains controversial; Table 28–1 shows one protocol for prophylaxis of traumatic endophthalmitis.

Table 28–1 Prophylaxis of Traumatic Endophthalmitis

Systemic antibiotic therapy*	Vancomycin hydrochloride, 1 g iv every 12 h
	Ceftazidime, 1 g iv every 12 h
Subconjunctival antibiotic and corticosteroid therapy	Vancomycin hydrochloride, 25 mg
	Ceftazidime, 100 mg
	Dexamethasone, 12 mg
Topical therapy (started on the first postoperative day)	Antibiotic (physician's choice, commercially available antibiotic in nonfortified concentration)
	Topical cycloplegics and corticosteroids
	Optional: fortified antibiotic drops may be substituted in high-risk injuries with suspicion of infection

*Intravitreal antibiotic and corticosteroid therapy generally reserved for selected injuries with high risk of infection or when considering outpatient management of open globe injury.

- Although a first-generation cephalosporin may provide coverage for gram-positive organisms,[23] intravenous *vancomycin* is an excellent choice because it:
  - is effective against *Bacillus*, *Streptococcus*, and *Staphylococcus* species; and
  - has good intravitreal penetration.[24–27]
- Intravenous *ampicillin*/sulbactam[b] is an alternative systemic antibiotic with good intraocular penetration and generally good gram-positive coverage with variable coverage of *Bacillus* species.
- Intravenous *ceftazidime* provides good gram-negative coverage[28,29] but is less effective than vancomycin in the coverage of *Bacillus* species. Ceftazidime has a good safety profile[30] and good intravitreal penetration.[31,32]
- Oral *ciprofloxacin* has good intravitreal penetration.[33]

Systemic *aminoglycosides* are considered to have suboptimal intravitreal penetration.[34,35]

CONTROVERSY

⬅ ➡

The ideal antibiotic regimen for the prophylaxis of traumatic endophthalmitis remains controversial. The selected antibiotic should have adequate intraocular penetration after systemic administration and provide coverage against the most common causative organisms.

---

[b]Unasyn; Pfizer, New York, NY.

In addition to systemic antibiotics the following routes of administration may be considered.

- *Subconjunctival and topical* antibiotics are generally used and a postoperative cycloplegic such as scopolamine 0.25% is added.
- *Intravitreal* injection of antibiotics and dexamethasone in cases suspected to be at high risk for infection[36] (see Table 28–2) can also be considered during the initial repair.

Antifungal prophylaxis for open globe repairs is generally not recommended in the absence of clinical and microbiologic evidence for fungal infection.[16]

Alternative (Outpatient) Approach to Prophylaxis

Intravenous antibiotics often require hospitalization for administration, and many physicians admit patients with open globe injuries to the inpatient unit for 48 to 120 hours. This treatment can be expensive and disruptive to the patients' life and may be unnecessary. Alternatively, given the relatively high rates of infection following open globe injuries, most physicians would consider it to be "standard care" for these patients to receive some form of antibiotic prophylaxis.

Given the poor penetration into the posterior segment of most topical, subconjunctival, and orally administered antibiotics, these routes are probably not adequate for prophylaxis. As an alternative, one can consider intravitreal antibiotic administration at the time of wound repair. Intravitreal ceftazidime (2 mg/0.1 mL) and vancomycin (1 mg/0.1 mL) carry very low risk of intraocular toxicity and can be safely administered after the eye has been closed. In the setting of open globe injury, one should confirm ophthalmoscopically or with intraoperative ultrasound

TABLE 28–2 TREATMENT OF TRAUMATIC ENDOPHTHALMITIS

Systemic antibiotic therapy	Vancomycin hydrochloride, 1 g iv every 12 h Ceftazidime, 1 g iv every 12 h
Intravitreal antibiotic and corticosteroid therapy	Vancomycin hydrochloride, 1 mg/0.1 mL Ceftazidime, 2 mg/0.1 mL *Dexamethasone, 0.4 mg/0.1 mL
Subconjunctival antibiotic and corticosteroid therapy	Vancomycin hydrochloride, 25 mg Ceftazidime, 100 mg Dexamethasone, 12 mg
Topical therapy (started on first postoperative day)	Vancomycin hydrochloride, 50 mg/mL every hour Ceftazidime, 50 mg/mL every hour or gentamicin sulfate, 14 mg/mL every hour Topical cycloplegics and corticosteroids

*Controversial.

that large choroidal detachments or retinal detachment is not present, which might complicate the pars plana injection of these antibiotics (see the Appendix).

SPECIAL CONSIDERATION

In selected cases of open globe injury suspected to be at high risk for developing endophthalmitis or to allow outpatient management of the open globe injury, intravitreal injection of antibiotics can be considered immediately following the primary repair.

CONTROVERSY

Routine administration of prophylactic antibiotics into the vitreous is not universally accepted; it may theoretically increase the rate/speed of development of drug resistance.

TREATMENT

Bacterial Infection

Vitrectomy[c]

Early vitrectomy is recommended in most cases of clinically suspected traumatic endophthalmitis. The progression of traumatic endophthalmitis can be very

rapid because of the more virulent organisms and the often large infectious inoculum in the eye.

Vitrectomy is theoretically beneficial by:

- debulking inflammatory debris and toxins;
- removing the scaffold for tractional preretinal membranes; and
- allowing better distribution of intraocular antibiotics.

PITFALL

The results of the EVS are probably not applicable to cases of traumatic endophthalmitis as the organisms, the age of the patient, and the mechanism of inoculation are different.

CONTROVERSY

Recently, there have been successful reports of using silicone oil at the completion of vitrectomy, reducing the postoperative complications without causing recurrence of the infection or concentrating the infecting organisms in the vicinity of the inferior retina. The eyes are irrigated with a solution containing antibiotics during vitrectomy, but no antibiotics are left/injected in the vitreous once the silicone oil has been implanted.

[c]May be combined with TKP (see Chapter 25).

Performing a more complete vitrectomy (as opposed to the traditional core vitrectomy), consistent with safe *intraoperative visualization* (*proportional* pars plana vitrectomy[d]), may increase the success rate in restoring/salvaging macular function.[37]

Antibiotics

Intravitreal, periocular, topical, and *systemic antibiotics* are recommended. The current treatment of clinically diagnosed traumatic endophthalmitis is outlined in Table 28–2 (see also the Appendix regarding intravitreal antibiotics). As an alternative to ceftazidime, amikacin or gentamicin can be considered in the subconjunctival regimen. Fortified topical antibiotics are started on the first postoperative day. In eyes with early endophthalmitis with clinical improvement and susceptible organisms, the regimen may be switched to an oral systemic agent.[33,38] Animal studies of *Bacillus cereus* traumatic endophthalmitis have suggested that intravitreal imipenem may be as effective as vancomycin in these infections.[39]

Corticosteroids

Even if somewhat controversial,[40] adjunctive intravitreal corticosteroids (dexamethasone, 0.4 mg in 0.1 mL) have been successfully used in traumatic endophthalmitis.[41] Subconjunctival dexamethasone (12 to 24 mg) is also routinely given at the time of vitrectomy. Topical steroid drops (prednisone acetate 1%) are started on the first postoperative day.

Fungal Infection

To avoid the potential posterior segment toxicity of intravitreal amphotericin B,[42] it is generally reserved for secondary treatment based on the clinical history, initial clinical signs, or documented fungal cultures. Traumatic fungal endophthalmitis may be caused by yeasts (e.g., *Candida* species) or by filamentous fungi (e.g., *Aspergillus* species), which are usually sensitive to intravitreal amphotericin B (0.005 mg in 0.1 mL).

Intravenous amphotericin B may cause significant systemic side effects. Its use generally requires prolonged hospitalization, renal function monitoring, and the use of antipyretics and fluid replacement for spiking fevers, nausea, and vomiting with dehydration.

> **PEARL...** Systemic antifungal therapy is best selected and administered in consultation with an internist (e.g., oral fluconazole vs. intravenous amphotericin B).

Occasionally, fungal endophthalmitis is caused by an organism resistant to amphotericin B (e.g., *Paecilomyces lilacinious*[16]), requiring alternative intravitreal and systemic agents.

Intravitreal,[41,43] subconjunctival, and topical corticosteroids can also be considered in traumatic fungal endophthalmitis.

SPECIAL ISSUES

Persistent Endophthalmitis after Initial Treatment

Most cases of traumatic endophthalmitis are successfully managed with vitrectomy and intravitreal antibiotics. However, in the presence of persistent/worsening inflammation with a particularly virulent organism (e.g., *Bacillus* species), repeated vitrectomy and intravitreal injections can be considered.

- In one study of culture-proven endophthalmitis of various types, a second vitreous culture and antibiotic injection was needed in 52% of eyes,[44] performed 3–8 days after the initial treatment; 29% of eyes were still culture positive. Eyes in which the initial antimicrobial therapy failed to eradicate a bacterial infection had a worse outcome than those that were culture negative on repeated sampling.

- In the EVS,[45] 7.5% of patients underwent reinjection of intravitreal antibiotics within 7 days of initial treatment because of persistent or worsening inflammation/infection. These patients, along with others who had additional procedures within 7 days of the initial treatment, demonstrated substantially worse visual outcomes compared with patients who required no additional procedures.

> **SPECIAL CONSIDERATION**
>
> In cases of persistent post-traumatic endophthalmitis, repeated intravitreal antibiotic injection can be safely performed 48 to 72 hours after the initial treatment, although[e] it may enhance the risk of retinal toxicity.[46–50]

Concurrent Retinal Detachment

Concurrent presence of retinal detachment and endophthalmitis poses a management challenge in eyes with open globe injury. Improvements in early diagnosis and treatment of endophthalmitis, along with advances in vitreoretinal surgical techniques, have nevertheless

---

[d] A term coined by Robert Morris, MD

[e] Especially in patients who receive intravitreal aminoglycosides.

made it possible to achieve a favorable outcome in some cases.[51,52] Potential approaches include the following.

- The retinal detachment is repaired by pars plana vitrectomy, possible scleral buckling, fluid–air exchange, and endolaser. The air can then be exchanged for a long-acting gas such as C_3F_8. After the vitreous cavity is 50% refilled with BSS, the desired intravitreal antibiotics are injected.
- Use of antibiotics in the irrigating fluid or use of a 50% dosage into the partially gas-filled eye.
- Silicone oil use (see earlier).

The visual prognosis is often correlated with the virulence of the causative organism.[50]

- In cases requiring a more complete gas fill (inferior retinal breaks), the surgeon can inject the intravitreal antibiotics prior to the fluid–air exchange and allow adequate time (10 minutes) for the diffusion

of the antibiotics throughout the vitreous cavity. This will reduce the chance of overconcentrating the antibiotics when only a small amount of fluid is left in the cavity.

SUMMARY

Endophthalmitis associated with open globe injuries presents a formidable clinical challenge in both diagnosis and management. Early recognition of clinical signs and prompt initiation of treatment will improve the otherwise poor visual prognosis. Even in eyes with high-risk features, such as infection with *Bacillus* species or concurrent retinal detachment, successful anatomic and useful visual acuity outcomes can be achieved. Vitrectomy should be considered in all, and performed in the vast majority of, eyes; intravitreal antibiotics (and probably corticosteroids) must also be used.

REFERENCES

1. Reynolds DS, Flynn HW, Jr. Endophthalmitis after penetrating ocular trauma. *Curr Opin Ophthalmol.* 1997; 8:32–38.
2. Thompson WS, Rubsamen PE, Flynn HW Jr, Schiffman J, Cousins SW. Endophthalmitis following penetrating trauma: risk factors and visual outcome. *Ophthalmology.* 1995;102:1696–1701.
3. William DF, Mieler WF, Abrams GW, Lewis H. Results and prognostic factors in penetrating ocular injuries with retained intraocular foreign bodies. *Ophthalmology.* 1988;95:911–916.
4. Peyman GA, Carrol CP, Raichand M. Prevention and management of traumatic endophthalmitis. *Ophthalmology.* 1980;87:320–324.
5. Parish CM, O'Day DM. Traumatic endophthalmitis. *Int Ophthalmol Clin.* 1987;27:112–119.
6. Nobe JR, Gomez DS, Liggett PE, Smith RE, Jrobin JB. Traumatic and postoperative endophthalmitis: a comparison of visual outcomes. *Br J Ophthalmol.* 1987;71:614–617.
7. Vahey JB, Flynn HW Jr. Results in the management of *Bacillus* endophthalmitis. *Ophthalmic Surg.* 1991;22:681–686.
8. Verbraeken H, Rysselaere M. Traumatic endophthalmitis. *Eur J Ophthalmol.* 1994;4:1–5.
9. Barr CC. Prognosis factors in cornea scleral lacerations. *Arch Ophthalmol.* 1983;101:919–924.
10. Alfaro VD, Roth D, Liggett PE. Traumatic endophthalmitis: causative organisms, treatment and prevention. *Retina.* 1994;14:206–211.
11. Boldt HC, Pulido JS, Blodi CF, Folk JC, Weingeist TA. Rural endophthalmitis. *Ophthalmology.* 1989;96:1722–1726.
12. Brinton GS, Topping TM, Hyndiuk RA, Aaberg TM, Reeser FH, Abrams GW. Traumatic endophthalmitis. *Arch Ophthalmol.* 1984;102:547–550.

13. Affeldt JC, Flynn HW Jr, Forest RK, Mandelbaum S, Clarckson JG, Jarras GD. Microbial endophthalmitis resulting from ocular trauma. *Ophthalmology.* 1987;94:404–413.
14. Thompson JT, Parver LM, Enger C, Mieler WF, Liggett PE, for the National Eye Trauma Study (NETS). Infectious endophthalmitis after penetrating injuries with retained intraocular foreign bodies. *Ophthalmology.* 1993;100:1468–1474.
15. Packer AJ, Weingeist TA, Abrams GW. Retinal periphlebitis as an early sign of bacterial endophthalmitis. *Am J Ophthalmol.* 1983;96:66–71.
16. Pflugfelder SC, Flynn HW Jr, Zwickey TA, et al. Exogenous fungal endophthalmitis. *Ophthalmology.* 1988;95: 19–30.
17. Foster RE, Martinez JA, Murray TG, Rubsamen PE, Flynn HW Jr, Forster RK. Useful visual outcomes after treatment of *Bacillus cereus* endophthalmitis. *Ophthalmology.* 1996;103:390–397.
18. Barletta JP, Small KW. Successful visual recovery in delayed onset *Bacillus cereus* endophthalmitis. *Ophthalmic Surg Lasers.* 1996;27:70–73.
19. Donahue SP, Kowalski RP, Jewart BH, Frieberg TR. Vitreous cultures in suspected endophthalmitis—biopsy or vitrectomy? *Ophthalmology.* 1993;100:452–455.
20. Forster RK, Abbot RL, Gelender H: Management of infectious endophthalmitis. *Ophthalmology.* 1980;87:313–319.
21. Joondeph BC, Flynn HW Jr, Miller DA, Joondeph HC. A new culture method for infectious endophthalmitis. *Arch Ophthalmol.* 1989;107:1334–1337.
22. Scott A, Flynn HW Jr, Joondeph BC, Joondeph HC, Miller DA. Use of blood culture bottles for harvesting intraocular samples for infectious endophthalmitis. Manuscript in preparation.

23. Nossov PC, Alfaro DV, Michaud ME, Winter LW, Lauglin RM, Moss ST. Intravenous cefazolin in penetrating eye injuries swine model. *Retina*. 1996;16:246–249.

24. Kervick GN, Flynn HW Jr, Alfonso E, Miller D. Antibiotic therapy for *Bacillus* species infections. *Am J Ophthalmol*. 1990;110:683–687.

25. Meredith DA, Aguilar HE, Shaarawy A. Kincaid M, Dick J, Niesman MR. Vancomycin levels in the vitreous cavity after intravenous administration. *Am J Ophthalmol*. 1995;119:774–778.

26. Davis JL, Koidou-Tsiligianni A, Pflugfelder SC, Miller D, Flynn HW Jr, Forster RK. Coagulase-negative staphylococci endophthalmitis: increase in antimicrobial resistance. *Ophthalmology*. 1988;95:1404–1410.

27. Flynn HW Jr, Pulido JS, Pflugfelder SC, et al. Endophthalmitis therapy: changing antibiotic sensitivity patterns and current therapeutic recommendations. *Arch Ophthalmol*. 1991;109:175–176.

28. Irvine D, Flynn HW Jr, Miller D, Pflugfelder S. Endophthalmitis caused by gram-negative organisms. *Arch Ophthalmol*. 1992;110:1450–1454.

29. Donahue SP, Kowalski RP, Eller AW, DeVaro JM, Jewart BH. Empiric treatment of endophthalmitis; Are aminoglycosides necessary? *Arch Ophthalmol*. 1994;112:45–47.

30. Campochiaro PA, Green WR. Toxicity of intravitreal ceftazidime in primate retina. *Arch Ophthalmol*. 1992;110:1625–1629.

31. Aguilar HE, Meredith TA, Shaarawy A, Kincaid M, Dick J. Vitreous cavity penetration of ceftazidime after intravenous administration. *Retina*. 1995;15:154–159.

32. Walstad RA, Bilka S, Thurmann-Neilsen E, Halvorsen TB. The penetration of ceftazidime into the inflamed rabbit eye. *Scand J Infect Dis*. 1987;19:131–135.

33. Karen G, Ahalel A, Bartov E, et al. The intravitreal penetration of orally administered Ciprofloxacin in humans. *Invest Ophthalmol Vis Sci*. 1991;32:2388–2392.

34. Rubenstein E, Goldfarb J, Keren G, Blumenthal M, Triester G. The penetration of gentamicin into the vitreous humor. *Invest Ophthalmol Vis Sci*. 1983;24:637–639.

35. El-massry A, Meredith TA, Aguilar HE, et al. Aminoglycoside levels in the rabbit vitreal cavity after intravenous administration. *Am J Ophthalmol*. 1996;122:684–689.

36. Seal DV, Kirkness CM. Criteria for intravitreal antibiotics during surgical removal of intraocular foreign bodies. *Eye*. 1992;6:465–468.

37. Morris R, Witherspoon CD, Kuhn F, Byrne J. Endophthalmitis. In: Roy H, ed. *Master Techniques in Ophthalmic Surgery*. Baltimore: Williams & Wilkins; 1995:560–572.

38. Alfaro DV, Hudson SJ, Rafanan MM, Moss ST, Levy SP. The effect of trauma on the ocular penetration of intravenous ciprofloxacin. *Am J Ophthalmol*. 1996;122:678–683.

39. Alfaro DV, Hudson SJ, Steele JJ, et al. Experimental post-traumatic *Bacillus cereus* endophthalmitis in a swine model. Efficacy of intravitreal ciprofloxacin, vancomycin and imipenem. *Retina*. 1996;16:317–323.

40. Kwak HW, D'Amico D. Evaluation of retinal toxicity and pharmacokinetics of dexamethasone as an intra-vitreal injection. *Arch Ophthalmol*. 1992;110:259–266.

41. Schulman JA, Peyman GA. Intravitreal corticosteroids as an adjunct to the treatment of bacterial and fungal endophthalmitis. *Retina*. 1992;12:336–340.

42. Axelrod AJ, Peyman GA. Apparent toxicity of intravitreal injection of amphotericin B. *Am J Ophthalmol*. 1973;76:578–583.

43. Coats ML, Peyman GA. Intravitreal corticosteroids in the treatment of exogenous fungal endophthalmitis. *Retina*. 1992;12:46–51.

44. Shaarawy A, Grand MG, Meredith TA, Ibanez HE. Persistent endophthalmitis after intravitreal antimicrobial therapy. *Ophthalmology*. 1995;102:382–387.

45. Doft BH, Kelsey SF, Wisniewski SR. Additional procedures after the initial vitrectomy or tap-biopsy in the Endophthalmitis Vitrectomy Study. *Ophthalmology*. 1998;105:707–716.

46. McDonald HR, Schatz H, Allen AW, et al. Retinal toxicity secondary to intraocular gentamicin injection. *Ophthalmology*. 1986;93:871–872.

47. Pflugfelder SC, Hernandez E, Fiesler SJ, Alvarez J, Pfugfelder ME, Forster RK. Intravitreal vancomycin retinal toxicity, clearance and interaction with gentamicin. *Arch Ophthalmol*. 1987;105:831.

48. Gardner SK. Intravitreal antibiotics vancomycin with aminoglycosides toxicity of multiple injections *Ocul Ther Rep*. 1989;2:33–36.

49. Campochiaro PA, Conway BP. Aminoglycoside toxicity: a survey of retinal specialists. Implication for ocular use. *Arch Ophthalmol*. 1991;109:946–950.

50. Jay WM, Fishman P, Aziz M, Snockley RK. Intravitreal ceftazidime in a rabbit model: dose and time-dependent toxicity and pharmacokinetic analysis. *J Ocul Pharmacol*. 1987;3:257–260.

51. Mieler WF, Glazer LC, Bennett M, Han DP. Favorable outcome of traumatic endophthalmitis with associated retinal breaks or detachment. *Can J Ophthalmol*. 1992;27:346–352.

52. Foster RE, Rubsamen PE, Joondeph BC, Flynn HW Jr, Smiddy WS. Concurrent endophthalmitis and retinal detachment. *Ophthalmology*. 1994;101:490–498.

Chapter 29

SYMPATHETIC OPHTHALMIA

Robert A. Mittra

 SO is a rare, bilateral, diffuse granulomatous uveitis that presents insidiously after open globe injury or surgery. The injured eye is known as the *exciting* eye and the fellow eye, developing inflammation weeks to years later, as the *sympathizing* eye. Injury to one eye leading to damage in the other has been known since Hippocrates[1] but was first well-described and termed SO only in the mid-1800s.[2] Prior to steroid therapy, SO often led to a progressive, severe decline in vision.[3]

EPIDEMIOLOGY AND PREVENTION

SO is rare, but the true incidence is unknown because of a lack of pathologic proof, the difficulty in studying sufficiently large cases series,[1] and the fact that most data are from the older literature, in which SO was often confused with other forms of uveitis.[4] The incidence is:

- ~2/1000 following open globe injury;
- ~1/10,000 following routine ocular surgery[5];
- decreasing with improved surgical technique[6,7]:
  ○ no SO in the Korean and Vietnam wars[8];
- equal between the sexes[a];
- equal between the races, although
  ○ higher pigmentation may increase inflammation and epithelioid cells[9];
- higher among the elderly[b];
- increasing with severe injuries;
- increasing with multiple ocular surgeries.

---

[a] Two thirds males in one study.[1]

[b] Higher rate of ocular surgery.

PEARL... Although SO may occur after closed eye surgery, it is most common with severe open globe injury/uveal prolapse. After the primary surgery, patients should be counseled about the possibility of SO and prophylactic enucleation (see Chapter 8).

CLINICAL PRESENTATION AND EVALUATION

Table 29–1 lists conditions in which SO has been reported.

- It has been seen as early as 5 days[1] and as late as 60 years[32,33] following trauma/surgery.[c]

---

[c] See Chapter 31, Figure 31-5

TABLE 29–1 TYPES OF SURGERY OR INJURY REPRESENTING A RISK FACTOR FOR SO DEVELOPMENT

Any type of open globe injury[1-4]
Perforated corneal ulcer[10]
Any type of intraocular sugery[11-21]
External beam radiation[21]
Cyclocryotherapy[22-24]
Laser cyclophotocoagulation[25]
Radiation for choroidal melanoma[21,26]
Contact/noncontact Nd:YAG cyclophotocoagulation[27-31]

- Approximately, two thirds of cases occur between 2 weeks and 3 months after injury[3] and 90% are diagnosed within the first year.[4]
- Once SO develops, it can remain active for up to 30 years.[34]

Complaints in the fellow eye include:

- slight pain;
- sensitivity to light;
- accommodation problems; and
- mildly decreased visual acuity.

> **PEARL...** Fellow eye complaints in patients with a history of trauma/surgery and bilateral panuveitis should always be taken seriously and require an urgent examination.

Early *signs* of SO[d] include:

- bilateral uveitis with AC cells/flare and a moderate to dense posterior vitritis[35];
- ciliary injection;
- mutton-fat keratic precipitate on the corneal endothelium;
- thickened iris;
- iris nodules;
- synechiae;
- vitritis;
- optic nerve head swelling; and
- retinal edema, occasionally with serous retinal detachment and perivasculitis.[35]

In cases with prolonged inflammation, posterior synechiae and yellow nodules at the RPE (Dalen-Fuchs nodules) develop in the periphery. The diagnosis is more difficult when:

- the uveitis in the sympathizing eye is mild and nongranulomatous;
- the injured eye has been enucleated; or
- the patient is taking systemic anti-inflammatory medication.

Table 29–2 shows the conditions that have to be taken into consideration when the diagnosis is made.

FA shows multiple, deep pinpoint areas of hyperfluorescence in the early arteriovenous phase, developing into larger areas of diffuse hyperfluorescence in later phases. The FA is nearly identical to that seen in VKH. The Dalen-Fuchs nodules display early

TABLE 29–2   THE DIFFERENTIAL DIAGNOSIS OF SO

VKH syndrome*
Phacoanaphylactic endophthalmitis
Sarcoidosis
Chronic idiopathic uveitis
Infectious granulomatous uveitis[37,38]

*Dysacusis, poliosis, vitiligo, alopecia, and lymphocytosis in the cerebrospinal fluid are common in VKH but rare in SO[36]; the diagnosis of SO, although usually made on the basis of clinical features alone, may be facilitated by the use of serum sialic acid and β_2-microglobulin levels in dificult cases.[39,40]

> **PITFALL**
>
> Dalen-Fuchs nodules are present in less than 40% of eyes.

hypo- or hyperfluorescence, followed by late leakage and staining.[4,41,42]

ICG acutely shows early hypocyanescence (which then subsides) and persistent hypocyanescence later.[43]

The long-term sequelae are highly variable:

- cataract (common);
- secondary (common);
- retinal and optic atrophy; and
- choroidal neovascularization[e] (rare and may resolve spontaneously or with anti-inflammatory medication.

PATHOLOGIC FEATURES

Classic SO manifests as a diffuse, granulomatous choroidal inflammation with cellular[f] infiltration (Fig. 29–1).[47] The original theory that SO is nonnecrotizing and spares the retina and choriocapillaris[48] has been challenged.[48,49] One pathologic review found retinal detachment in 58% and intraretinal inflammation in 42%[3]; another report showed focal choriocapillaris obliteration in 40%.[48]

> **PEARL...** It appears that the retina, choriocapillaris, and optic nerve are initially spared but become involved late in the disease.

---

[d] Purely anterior or posterior forms are rare.

[e] Presumably develops from breaks in Bruch's membrane.[44–46]

[f] Lymphocytes, epithelioid cells, eosinophils, and rarely plasma cells and polymorphonuclear leukocytes.

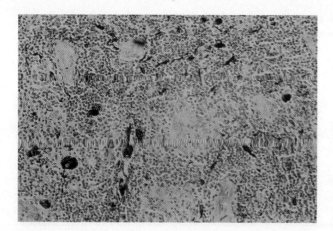

FIGURE 29–1 Histologic section of choroid showing granulomatous inflammation with lymphocytes, epithelioid cells, and giant cells. (Courtesy of Z. Nicholas Zakov, MD, Retina Associates of Cleveland.)

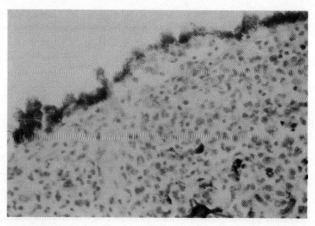

FIGURE 29–2 Dalen-Fuchs nodule showing partial attenuation of RPE. (Courtesy of Z. Nicholas Zakov, MD, Retina Associates of Cleveland.)

The Dalen-Fuchs nodules[47,50] are small collections of "epithelioid" cells and lymphocytes covered by an intact dome of RPE in the peripheral retina (Fig. 29–2), varying from focal RPE hyperplasia to disorganized nodules with degenerated RPE.[51] Originally thought to consist of transformed RPE cells,[52,53] the nodules contain T lymphocytes of the helper/inducer or cytotoxic/suppressor type.[54–61]

PATHOPHYSIOLOGY

The etiology of SO remains unknown. Most authors believe it to be an autoimmune delayed-type hypersensitivity to infectious antigens or uveal/RPE/retinal tissue, or a combination of the two.[57,62] The role of uveal melanin or "s" antigen[63] could not be confirmed.[64] Bacterial/viral particles entering the eye,[65] genetic factors,[g] and an unknown environmental factor have also been suggested.

SPECIAL CONSIDERATION

SO probably involves autoimmunity to an ocular antigen,[68,69] which gains access to the periocular lymphatics after open globe injury or surgery.

MANAGEMENT AND COMPLICATIONS

SO used to have an unrelenting course with poor visual outcome.

- Steroids decrease the severity of the inflammation and improve the vision of both eyes.[3,70] Topical, periocular, and systemic therapy (1–1.5 mg/kg/day) must be started at the first sign of the disease.[71]
- Tapering should be slow; low-dose therapy (10–25 mg/day) is commonly needed for months.[h]

SPECIAL CONSIDERATION

Those who do not respond sufficiently to high-dose steroids; develop serious side effects (e.g., glaucoma, cataract,[72] hypertension, diabetes, osteoporosis, aseptic bone necrosis, vertebral collapse); or have multiple recurrences, require immunosuppressive therapy.[73–80] *Chlorambucil, cyclosporine, azathioprine, FK506,* and *cyclophosphamide* have been used successfully but also have serious side effects.[73–80] Because recurrences are common, patients need to be followed indefinitely; a rheumatologist or other appropriate specialists should be consulted.

Enucleation of the exciting eye is controversial (Table 29–3), as is prophylactic enucleation after severe injury (see Chapter 8): removal of the injured eye within 2 weeks does not necessarily prevent SO,[85] and SO may not develop despite forgoing enucleation.[7]

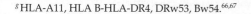

[g] HLA-A11, HLA B-HLA-DR4, DRw53, Bw54.[66,67]

[h] Purified protein derivative test for tuberculosis and a screening test for syphilis (RPR or VDRL and FTA-ABS or MHA-TP) should be obtained.

Table 29-3   Controversies Regarding the Management of SO

Variable	Opinion	Counteropinion	Resolution
Enucleation of exciting eye after SO development*	Removal before 2 weeks is beneficial for vision	Removal does not improve the prognosis and removes a potentially seeing eye	Consider enucleating eyes with light perception or worse vision and a poor prognosis
Enucleation of injured eye for SO prophylaxis	SO almost never develops if badly injured eyes are enucleated within 2 weeks	SO is extremely rare and can be effectively treated in most cases	Even if vision is NLP consider complete anatomical reconstruction and discuss with patient/family whether to retain or remove eye (see also Chapters 5 and 8)

*Can be counterproductive because this eye may eventually obtain better vision than the sympathizing eye[81]; others showed that enucleating the exciting eye within 2 weeks of SO development improves the visual outcome.[3,70,82–84]

Prognosis

The more severe the inflammation, the worse the ocular complications and visual outcome. Prompt, high-dose steroid therapy with immunosuppressive medication as needed, however, can result in vision $\geq 20/40$ in the sympathizing eye in 50% of the cases.[80]

Summary

SO is an extremely rare event following open globe injury. It has long been a much feared complication, which has led some to suggest enucleation, rather than reconstruction (evisceration), for many severely injured eyes. Given SO's apparent infrequency and its favorable response to steroid treatment when it does occur, physicians are more likely today to salvage severely injured eyes and less likely to suggest enucleation.

References

1. Albert DM, Diaz-Rohena R. A historical review of sympathetic ophthalmia and its epidemiology. *Surv Ophthalmol.* 1989;34:1–14.
2. Mackenzie W. *A Practical Treatise on the Diseases of the Eye.* 3rd ed. London: Longmans; 1840:523–534.
3. Lubin JR, Albert DM, Weinstein M. Sixty-five years of sympathetic ophthalmia. *Ophthalmology.* 1980;87:109–121.
4. Power WJ, Foster CS. Update on sympathetic ophthalmia. *Int Ophthalmol Clin.* 1995;35:127–137.
5. Liddy BSL, Stuart J. Sympathetic ophthalmia in Canada. *Can J Ophthalmol.* 1972;7:157.
6. Punnonen E. Pathological findings in eyes enucleated because of perforating injury. *Acta Ophthalmol.* 1990;68:265–269.
7. Brackup AB, Carter KD, Nerad JA, et al. Long-term follow-up of severely injured eyes following globe rupture. *Ophthalmic Plast Reconstr Surg.* 1991;7:194–197.
8. Wong TY, Seet B, Ang C. Eye injuries in twentieth century warfare: a historical perspective. *Surv Ophthalmol.* 1997;41:433–459.
9. Marak GE, Ikui H. Pigmentation associated histopathological variations in sympathetic ophthalmia. *Br J Ophthalmol.* 1980;64:220–222.
10. Dada T, Kumar A, Sharma N. Sympathetic ophthalmia associated with antecedent adherent leucoma—a rare association. *Acta Ophthalmol Scand.* 1998;76:380–381.
11. Lyons C, Tuft S, Lightman S. Sympathetic ophthalmia from inadvertent ocular perforation during conventional retinal detachment surgery. *Br J Ophthalmol.* 1997;81:612.
12. Croxatto JO, Galentine P, Cupples, et al. Sympathetic ophthalmia after pars plana vitrectomy-lensectomy for endogenous bacterial endophthalmitis. *Am J Ophthalmol.* 1981;91:342–346.
13. Gass JDM. Sympathetic ophthalmia following vitrectomy. *Am J Ophthalmol.* 1982;93:552–558.
14. Wang WJ. Clinical and histopathological report of sympathetic ophthalmia after retinal detachment surgery. *Br J Ophthalmol.* 1983;67:150–152.
15. Laroche L, Pavlakis C, Saraux H, et al. Ocular findings following intravitreal silicone injection. *Arch Ophthalmol.* 1983;101:1422–1425.

16. Tamai M, Obara J, Mizuno K, et al. Sympathetic ophthalmia: induced by vitrectomy not by trauma. *Jpn J Ophthalmol.* 1984;28:75–79.

17. Maisel JM, Vorwerk PA. Sympathetic uveitis after giant tear repair. *Retina.* 1989;9:122–126.

18. Wilson-Holt N, Hing S, Taylor DSI. Bilateral blinding uveitis in a child after secondary intraocular lens implantation for unilateral congenital cataract. *J Pediatr Ophthalmol Strabismus.* 1991;28:116–118.

19. Lakhanpal V, Dogra MR, Jacobson MS. Sympathetic ophthalmia associated with anterior chamber intraocular lens implantation. *Ann Ophthalmol.* 1991;23:139–143.

20. Stern WH. Complications of vitrectomy. *Int Ophthalmol Clin.* 1992;32:205–212.

21. Fries PD, Char DH, Crawford JB, et al. Sympathetic ophthalmia complicating helium ion irradiation of a choroidal melanoma. *Arch Ophthalmol.* 1987;105:1561–1564.

22. Sabates R. Choroiditis compatible with the histopathologic diagnosis of sympathetic ophthalmia following cyclocryotherapy of neovascular glaucoma. *Ophthalmic Surg.* 1988;19:176–182.

23. Biswas J, Fogia R. Sympathetic ophthalmia following cyclocryotherapy with histopathologic correlation. *Ophthalmic Surg Lasers.* 1996;27:1035–1038.

24. Harrison TJ. Sympathetic ophthalmia after cyclocryotherapy of neovascular glaucoma without ocular penetration. *Ophthalmic Surg.* 1993;24:44–46.

25. Bechrakis NE, Muller-Stolzenburg NW, Helbig H, et al. Sympathetic ophthalmia following laser cyclocoagulation. *Arch Ophthalmol.* 1994;112:80–84.

26. Margo CE, Pautler SE. Granulomatous uveitis after treatment of a choroidal melanoma with proton-beam irradiation. *Retina.* 1990;10:140–143.

27. Edward DP, Brown SVL, Higginbotham E, et al. Sympathetic ophthalmia following neodymium:YAG cyclotherapy. *Ophthalmic Surg.* 1989;20:544–546.

28. Minckler DS. Does Nd:YAG cyclotherapy cause sympathetic ophthalmia? *Ophthalmic Surg.* 1989;20:543.

29. Lam S, Tessler HH, Lam BL, et al. High incidence of sympathetic ophthalmia after contact and noncontact neodymium:YAG cyclotherapy. *Ophthalmology.* 1992;99:1818–1822.

30. Singh G. Sympathetic ophthalmia after Nd:YAG cyclotherapy [letter]. *Ophthalmology.* 1993;100:798–799.

31. Brown SVL, Higginbotham E, Tessler H. Sympathetic ophthalmia following Nd:YAG cyclotherapy [letter]. *Ophthalmic Surg.* 1990;21:736–737.

32. Drews RC. Delayed onset of sympathetic ophthalmia. *Ophthalmic Surg.* 1994;25:62–63.

33. Towler HMA, Lightman S. Sympathetic ophthalmia. *Int Ophthalmol Clin.* 1995;35:31–42.

34. Kinyoun JL, Bensinger RE, Chuang EL. Thirty-year history of sympathetic ophthalmia. *Ophthalmology.* 1983;90:59–65.

35. Goto H, Rao NA. Sympathetic ophthalmia and Vogt-Koyanagi-Harada syndrome. *Int Ophthalmol Clin.* 1990;30:279–285.

36. Dreyer WB, Zegarra H, Zakov ZN, et al. Sympathetic ophthalmia. *Am J Ophthalmol.* 1981;92:816–823.

37. Chan C. Relationship between sympathetic ophthalmia, phacoanaphylactic endophthalmitis, and Vogt-Koyanagi-Harada disease. *Ophthalmology.* 1988;95:619–624.

38. Chan C, Mochizuki M. Sympathetic ophthalmia: an autoimmune ocular inflammatory disease. *Springer Semin Immunopathol.* 1999;21:125–134.

39. Lamba PA, Pandey PK, Sarin GS, et al. Serum sialic acid levels in patients with sympathetic ophthalmitis. *Acta Ophthalmol.* 1993;71:833–835.

40. Sen DK, Sarin GS, Mathur MD. Serum beta-2 microglobulin level in sympathetic ophthalmitis. *Acta Ophthalmol.* 1990;68:200–204.

41. Allinson RW, Le TD, Kramer TR, et al. Fluorescein angiographic appearance of Dalen-Fuchs nodules in sympathetic ophthalmia. *Ann Ophthalmol.* 1993;25:152–156.

42. Sharp DC, Bell RA, Patterson E, et al. Sympathetic ophthalmia: histopathologic and fluorescein angiographic correlation. *Arch Ophthalmol.* 1984;102:232–235.

43. Bernasconi O, Auer C, Zografos L, et al. Indocyanine green angiographic findings in sympathetic ophthalmia. *Graefes Arch Clin Exp Ophthalmol.* 1998;236:635–638.

44. Chew EY, Crawford J. Sympathetic ophthalmia and choroidal neovascularization. *Arch Ophthalmol.* 1988;106:1507–1508.

45. Carney MD, Tessler HH, Peyman GA, et al. Sympathetic ophthalmia and subretinal neovascularization. *Ann Ophthalmol.* 1990;22:184–186.

46. Kilmartin DJ, Forrester JV, Dick AD. Cyclosporine-induced resolution of choroidal neovascularization associated with sympathetic ophthalmia. *Arch Ophthalmol.* 1998;116:249–250.

47. Fuchs E. Uber sympathisierende Entzundung (nebst Bemekungen) uber serose trumatishe iritis. *Arch Ophthalmol.* 1905;61:365–458.

48. Croxatto JO, Rao NA, McLean IW, et al. Atypical histopathological features in sympathetic ophthalmia. *Int Ophthalmol.* 1981;4:129–135.

49. Kuo PK, Lubin JR, Ni C, et al. Sympathetic ophthalmia: a comparison of the histopathological features from a Chinese and American series. *Int Ophthalmol Clin.* 1982;22:125–139.

50. Dalen A. Zur kenntnis der sogenannten Choroiditis sympathica. *Mitt Augenklin Carolin Med Chir Inst Stockh Jena.* 1904;6:1–21.

51. Reynard M, Riffenburgh RS, Minckler DS. Morphological variation of Dalen-Fuchs nodules in sympathetic ophthalmia. *Br J Ophthalmol.* 1985;69:197–201.

52. Ishikawa T, Ikui H. The fine structure of the Dalen-Fuchs nodule in sympathetic ophthalmia. *Jpn J Ophthalmol.* 1972;16:254–265.

53. Font RL, Fine BS, Messmer E, et al. Light and electron microscopic study of Dalen-Fuchs nodules in sympathetic ophthalmia. *Ophthalmology.* 1982;89:66–75.

54. Muller-Hermelink HK, Kraus-Mackiw E, Daus W. Early stage of human sympathetic ophthalmia: histologic and immunopathologic findings. *Arch Ophthalmol.* 1984;102:1353–1357.

55. Jakobiec FA, Marboe CC, Knowles DM II, et al. Human sympathetic ophthalmia; an analysis of the inflammatory infiltrate by hybridoma–monoclonal antibodies, immunochemistry, and correlative electron microscopy. *Ophthalmology.* 1983;90:76–95.

56. Chan C, Benezra D, Rodrigues MM, et al. Immunohistochemistry and electron microscopy of choroidal infiltrates and Dalen-Fuchs nodules in sympathetic ophthalmia. *Ophthalmology.* 1985;92:580–590.

57. Chan C, BenEzra D, Hsu S, et al. Granulomas in sympathetic ophthalmia and sarcoidosis. *Arch Ophthalmol.* 1985;103:198–202.

58. Rao NA, Xu S, Font RL. Sympathetic ophthalmia: an immunohistochemical study of epithelioid and giant cells. *Ophthalmology.* 1985;92:1660–1662.

59. Chan C, Nussenblatt RB, Fujikawa LS, et al. Sympathetic ophthalmia: immunopathological findings. *Ophthalmology.* 1986;93:690–695.

60. Kaplan HJ, Waldrep JC, Chan WC, et al. Human sympathetic ophthalmia: immunologic analysis of the vitreous and uvea. *Arch Ophthalmol.* 1986;104:240–244.

61. Lightman S, Chan C. Immune mechanisms in choroidoretinal inflammation in man. *Eye.* 1990;4:345–353.

62. Rao NA, Wong VG. Aetiology of sympathetic ophthalmitis. *Trans Ophthalmol Soc UK.* 1981;101:357–360.

63. Chan C, Palestine AG, Nussenblatt RB, et al. Anti-retinal auto-antibodies in Vogt-Koyanagi-Harada syndrome, Behçet's disease and sympathetic ophthalmia. *Ophthalmology.* 1985;92:1025–1028.

64. Hirose S, Kuwabara T, Nussenblatt RB, et al. Uveitis induced in primates by interphotoreceptor retinoid-binding protein. *Arch Ophthalmol.* 1986;104:1698–1702.

65. Ramadan A, Nussenblatt RB. Visual prognosis and sympathetic ophthalmia. *Curr Opin Ophthalmol.* 1996;7:39–45.

66. Reynard M, Shulman IA, Azen SP, et al. Histocompatibility antigens in sympathetic ophthalmia. *Am J Ophthalmol.* 1983;95:216–221.

67. Azen SP, Marak GE, Minckler DS, et al. Histocompatibility antigens in sympathetic ophthalmia [letter]. *Am J Ophthalmol.* 1984;98:117–119.

68. Davis JL, Mittal KK, Freidlin V, et al. HLA associations and ancestry in Vogt-Koyanagi-Harada disease and sympathetic ophthalmia. *Ophthalmology.* 1990;97:1137–1142.

69. Shindo Y, Ohno S, Usui M, et al. Immunogenetic study of sympathetic ophthalmia. *Tissue Antigens.* 1997;49:111–115.

70. Reynard M, Riffenburgh RS, Maes EF. Effect of corticosteroid treatment and enucleation on the visual prognosis of sympathetic ophthalmia. *Am J Ophthalmol.* 1983;96:290–294.

71. Hebestreit H, Huppertz H, Sold JE, et al. Steroid-pulse therapy may suppress inflammation in severe sympathetic ophthalmia. *J Pediatr Ophthalmol Strabismus.* 1997;34:124–126.

72. Reynard M, Minckler DS. Cataract extraction in the sympathizing eye. *Arch Ophthalmol.* 1983;101:1701–1703.

73. Jennings T, Tessler HH. Twenty cases of sympathetic ophthalmia. *Br J Ophthalmol.* 1989;73:140–145.

74. Tessler HH, Jennings T. High-dose short-term chlorambucil for intractable sympathetic ophthalmia and Behçet's disease. *Br J Ophthalmol.* 1990;74:353–357.

75. Leznoff A, Shea M, Binkley KE, et al. Cyclosporine in the treatment of nonmicrobial inflammatory ophthalmic disease. *Can J Ophthalmol.* 1992;27:302–306.

76. Hakin KN, Pearson RV, Lightman SL. Sympathetic ophthalmia: visual results with modern immunosuppressive therapy. *Eye.* 1992;6:453–455.

77. Leznoff A. Cyclosporine in the treatment of nonmicrobial inflammatory ophthalmic disease [letter]. *Can J Ophthalmol.* 1993;28:90.

78. Ishioka M, Ohno S, Nakamura S. FK506 treatment of noninfectious uveitis. *Am J Ophthalmol.* 1994;118:723–729.

79. Yang C, Liu J. Chlorambucil therapy in sympathetic ophthalmia. *Am J Ophthalmol.* 1995;119:482–488.

80. Chan C, Roberge FG, Whitcup SM, et al. 32 cases of sympathetic ophthalmia. *Arch Ophthalmol.* 1995;113:597–600.

81. Marak GE. Sympathetic ophthalmia [letter]. *Ophthalmology.* 1982;89:1291.

82. Tarr KH, Billson FA. Sympathetic ophthalmia: a reevaluation of management. *Trans Ophthalmol Soc N Z.* 1982;34:70–73.

83. Kraus-Mackiw E. Prevention of sympathetic ophthalmia. *Int Ophthalmol.* 1990;14:391–394.

84. Sheppard JD. Sympathetic ophthalmia. *Semin Ophthalmol.* 1994;9:177–184.

85. Bellan L. Sympathetic ophthalmia: a case report and review of the need for prophylactic enucleation. *Can J Ophthalmol.* 1999;34:95–98.

Chapter 30

UNIQUE ASPECTS OF TRAUMA IN CHILDREN

Ronald P. Danis, Daniel Neely, and David A. Plager

 Caring for children with ocular trauma involves several unique aspects such as:

- the possibility of prenatal injuries (e.g., ocular penetration by an amniocentesis needle[1]);
- predisposition to certain types of trauma (e.g., fireworks or toys related);
- diagnostic challenges due to limitations experienced during history taking and examination (see Chapter 9);
- the developing visual system and the potential for amblyopia;
- an orbit that is immature (cosmesis following enucleation or evisceration; see Chapter 31);
- the potential of eyes healing differently than adults' eyes, affecting surgical decision making; and
- the sensitivity in families and society toward suffering children, extending far beyond physical pain and disability.[2]

EPIDEMIOLOGY AND PREVENTION

The reported proportion of ocular injuries occurring in children varies according to study design,[a] population, and cultural and economic influences on admission rates. Based on data in the United States:

- children are involved in 16 to 34%[3–6] of trauma-related hospitalizations;

---
[a] Definition and age range.

- the estimated inpatient hospitalization incidence rate is 15/100,000/year[7];
- 21% of visits for ophthalmic trauma emergency care are by those under 15[8];
- 24% of all serious ocular injuries occur in those under 15 (USEIR).

The rates are similar, even higher, in some studies from other countries:

- 38% in a 12-year review of eye trauma admissions in Belfast[9];
- 47% in Israel[10];
- 47% in South India[11];
- 35% in Helsinki[12];
- 25% in Melbourne.[13]

Virtually all studies of pediatric ocular trauma show a male preponderance, which increases with age. Male/female ratios in the USEIR in 1998:

- 0–5 years: 1.9:1;
- 6–10 years: 3.4:1;
- 11–15 years: 5.1:1.

Forty-two percent of open globe injuries in patients younger than 15 years were found to have a poor prognosis.[14] The *places* and *sources* vary (Figs. 30–1 and 30–2).

- *Sports and recreation, sticks, and toys.* These represent a major etiology worldwide,[4,7,10,15–18] and the injuries are almost always preventable with adult supervision. Use of proper eye/facial protectors can reduce the rate of sports injuries. In the United States,

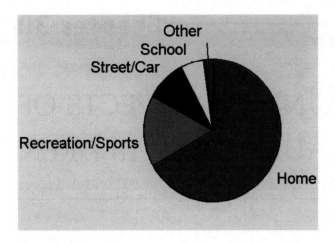

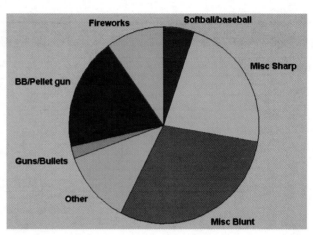

FIGURE 30-1 Place of injury for patients <15 years of age (USEIR). In 2364 reports listing the place of injury for this age group, 67% of injuries occurred in the home.

FIGURE 30-2 Source of injury for patients <15 years of age (USEIR). In 2212 reports listing the source of injury for this age group, large proportions of injuries were due to BB/pellet guns (18%), fireworks (10%), and softball/baseball (5%).

baseball is a major cause of serious ocular[19-21] and dental/facial trauma.[22,23] Mandating softer baseballs and faceguards for batters is very effective[24-26]; facial protectors in youth league hockey in Canada and the United States resulted in a 50% annual reduction in blind eyes.[27,28] Noncompliance with regulations remains responsible for continued ocular injuries.[29] Parents and children must be educated about eye protection for sports; the protectors have been standardized (ASTM)[29] and, after tests by independent laboratories,[30] certified for the consumer.

> **PEARL...** It is crucial to educate parents of monocular children, regardless of age, gender, or refractive error, about the use of safety eyewear during sports.[31]

- *Nonpowder firearms, such as paintball guns, BB guns, pellet air guns, toys that fire projectiles, and some exotic projectile-firing devices* (Figs. 30-3A–D, and 30-4A, and B). Of 32,000 such injuries in the United States each year, about 8% involve the eye with 60% of these patients being children.[32,33] Representing 5% (USEIR) to 7%[34,35] of all serious ocular injuries where air gun use is relatively unrestricted, the consequences are often dire.[34] A war game involving shooting gelatin-coated paint capsules with up to 90 m/s speed at the opponent, paintballing is increasingly popular in North America[36] and Europe. Eye injuries almost always occur when the victim is not wearing facial protection in an unsupervised environment.[37,38]

- *Fireworks.* In the EIRA, fireworks are responsible for 4.4% of all injuries and 80% of these are caused by bottle rockets.[39] Legislative action appears to be an effective means of controlling injuries from fireworks.[39,40] States that prohibit consumer fireworks sales have a much lower incidence of ocular injury from this source compared with states with less regulation.[41] U.S. and South African data have demonstrated an increased number of fireworks-related ocular injuries occurring after a legislative repeal of a ban on consumer fireworks sales.[42,43]

EVALUATION

The history of even serious pediatric ocular injury can be dubious because:

- the child's account is often vague owing to poor insight into the situation or deceptive in an effort to avoid punishment; and that

- usually there is no (available) adult eyewitness. The ophthalmologist should maintain a high index of suspicion for trauma that is less obvious (e.g., occult open globe injury or penetrating orbital injury; see Figs. 30–3 and 30–4 and Chapters 9, 10, and 15). Recognizing the presence and extent of tissue damage must be weighed against exacerbating the situation if the child is combative or there is severe lid hemorrhage (see Chapter 8). A careful consideration of the risks is necessary in deciding whether to immobilize the child forcibly (assistants, blankets, papoose board; see Fig. 30–5) and pry open the lids versus using diagnostic sedation/general anesthesia (Table 30–1).

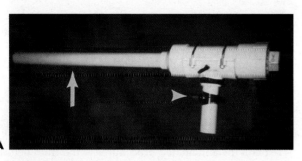

A

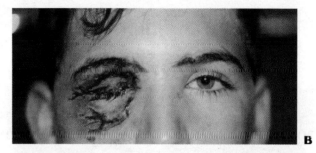

B

FIGURE 30–3A   Severe orbital and globe trauma can be caused by a homemade bazooka-like device ("potato gun"): a pipe with a large bore to accommodate a small potato as the projectile (arrow) and an attached camp stove igniter (arrowhead) that ignites the flammable explosive agent (in this case, hair spray).

FIGURE 30–3B   A 14-year-old male with severe orbital injury from accidental discharge of the device.

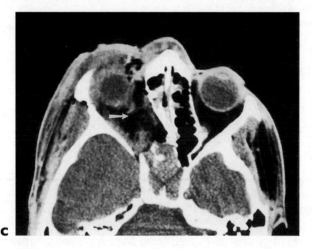

C

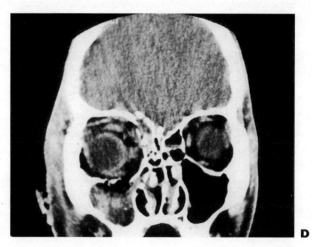

D

FIGURE 30–3   (C and D) CT scans demonstrate fracture of all walls of the orbit, optic nerve avulsion (arrow), and diffuse infiltration of the orbit with organic debris (potato).

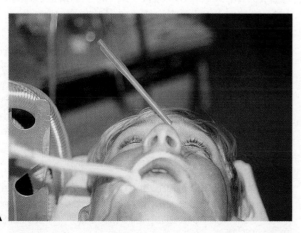

A

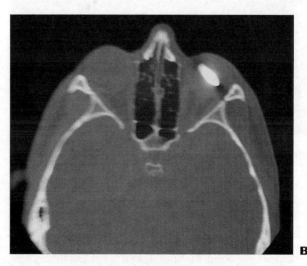

B

FIGURE 30–4   (A and B) Perforating wound due to a toy arrow fired from a crossbow. (Photograph courtesy of Rick Burgett, MD.)

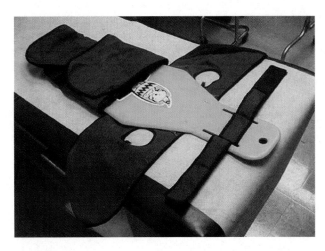

FIGURE 30–5 A papoose board is often available in emergency rooms and can be very helpful in the examination and treatment of uncooperative toddlers.

> **PEARL...** Children are especially prone to the oculocardiac reflex (Fig. 30–6), and any young patient presenting with bradycardia, nausea, somnolence, and/or syncope should be suspected of having such a reaction.

The differential diagnosis in case of a vomiting child with facial trauma includes:

- intracranial injury;

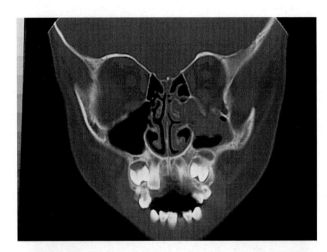

FIGURE 30–6 A 9-year-old boy hit by a pitched baseball. Coronal CT image demonstrates a left orbital floor trap-door fracture with entrapment of tissue around the inferior rectus and fluid in the left maxillary sinus. Sustained nausea and vomiting followed the injury, which prompted repeated visits to the ER and neurosurgical admission. When vomiting had not subsided 24 hours after admission, oculocardiac reflex was suspected; the orbit was explored and the fracture repaired. Nausea and vomiting resolved immediately after surgery. (Photograph courtesy of Rick Burgett, MD.)

TABLE 30–1   OPTIONS FOR EXAMINING A CHILD*

Wake child
   Have the child sit with a parent
   Give the child a token gift, such as a colorful sticker, prior to examination
   Approach in a nonthreatening manner; forced cooperation almost never works
   Talk directly to the child in a calm, soft voice
   Explain the anticipated procedures to the child before acting
   Assure the child that you will not hurt him or her
   Remove white lab coats because some children are intimidated by them
   Crying children are more likely to open their eyes if the room is darkened; this may allow you to assess chamber depth and media clarity
   Keep the ophthalmoscope's light intensity to a minimum
Sedation
   Oral dose of chloral hydrate[44] 80–100 mg/kg for the first 20 kg of body weight, supplemented as necessary with a one-time dose of 40 mg/kg; the child must be <6 years or >20 kg body weight and NPO for 4 hours; pulse oximetry and blood pressure should be monitored throughout
General anesthesia
   Brief mask anesthesia for short procedures such as superficial foreign bodies
   Intubation if longer procedure such as suturing open wounds is expected

*See also Chapter 9.

- increased IOP (e.g., from hyphema; see Chapters 17 and 20);
- uveal injury (see Chapter 16);
- extraocular muscle entrapment (see Chapter 36); and
- retrobulbar hemorrhage (see Chapter 12).

INJURIES WITH SPECIAL IMPLICATIONS

Intraocular Hemorrhages in the Neonate and Infant and Shaken/Battered Baby Syndrome

Intraretinal hemorrhages occur in ≤30% of cases of cesarean births and may take up to 2 weeks to resorb. Periretinal hemorrhages are especially important among infants <2 years of age as they are the most susceptible to injury by shaking.

The ocular (and/or intracranial) findings in the shaken/battered baby syndrome (see Chapters 10 and 33) may occur in the absence of obvious external injury and include:

- intraretinal and subhyaloid/submembranous hemorrhages (hemorrhagic macular cyst[b]), usually most dense at the posterior pole[45] (see Figs. 30–7 to 30–9);

---

[b] A term coined by Ferenc Kuhn, MD.

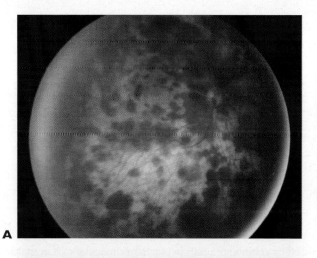

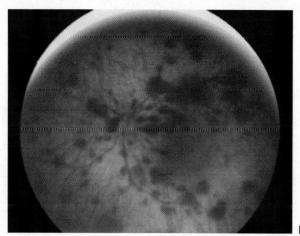

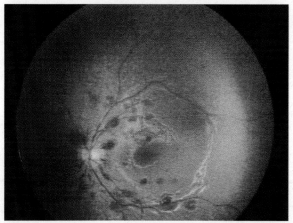

FIGURE 30–7   (A–C) The spectrum of intraretinal hemorrhages in shaken baby syndrome.

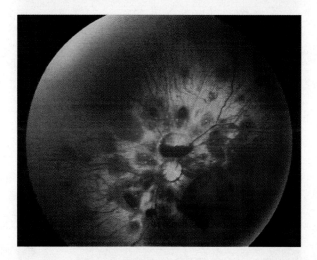

FIGURE 30–8   Large boat-shaped preretinal hemorrhages in shaken baby syndrome.

PEARL... Although typically bilateral, nonaccidental retinal hemorrhages may be asymmetric or even unilateral.[46]

• subretinal hemorrhage;
• vitreous hemorrhage (called Terson's syndrome if related to intracranial bleeding; may be associ-

ated with significant retinal and visual cortical pathology[47]);
• retinoschisis;
• retinal detachment;
• circular perimacular folds (Fig. 30–9)[48–51]; and
• optic nerve hemorrhage.

Despite surgical removal of the vitreous hemorrhage, vision commonly remains severely impaired

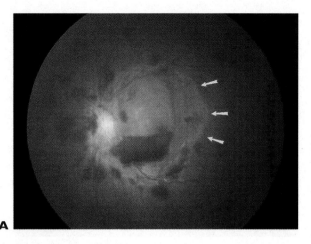 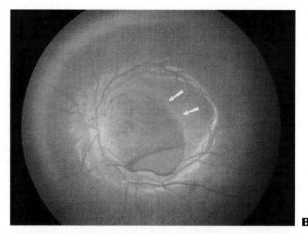

FIGURE 30–9 (**A** and **B**) Temporal macular fold (arrows) caused by submembranous hemorrhagic macular cyst in shaken baby syndrome.

because of cerebral dysfunction[52] or macular damage. Peripheral retinoschisis has been associated with high mortality.[49]

The *pathomechanism* of intraocular hemorrhages in shaken baby syndrome is controversial. Major external trauma may result in relatively minor ocular consequences.[c] Compression of the chest may raise the intracranial venous pressures and produce Purtscher's retinopathy (see Fig. 30–10 and Chapter 33).[53] Shearing produced by multiple sequences of acceleration and deceleration when an infant is shaken[54,55] disrupts both intracranial and intraocular vessels, and a vitreous gel

that is adherent to the infantile retina may explain not only the hemorrhages but also the formation of retinal detachment or retinoschisis.[51]

> **PEARL...** Since an estimated 40% of eyes show clinically visible pathology,[45] the ophthalmologist plays a pivotal role in the identification of child abuse (see Table 30–2).

Falling from a bed is insufficient to produce retinal hemorrhages; being "clumsy" does not account for orbital and lid ecchymoses. It is the eye care professional's moral and legal responsibility to report the incident for further investigation (see Chapter 7).

---

[c]We have found massive head and chest injuries but only a few intraretinal hemorrhages in children falling from as high as eight stories.

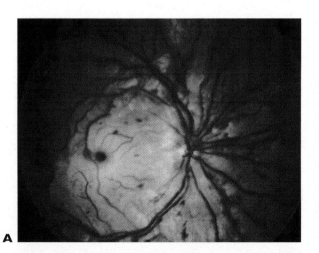 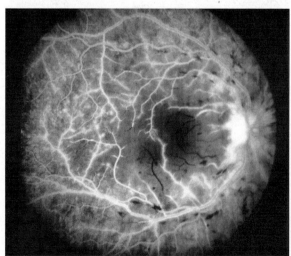

FIGURE 30–10 Purtscher-type retinopathy with no apparent head trauma in an 8-year-old male thrown from an all-terrain vehicle. (**A**) Color fundus photograph (**B**) FA.

TABLE 30–2   OCULAR MANIFESTATIONS IN THE SHAKEN/BATTERED CHILD SYNDROME*

Retinal, subhyaloid, and vitreous hemorrhages
Orbital and lid ecchymoses
Retinal detachment or dialysis
Chorioretinal atrophy
Cataract
Subluxated lens
Papilledema
Subconjunctival hemorrhage
Sixth nerve palsy
Corneal opacity and nystagmus
Optic atrophy

*Arranged in decreasing order of frequency.
Adapted from Harley R. Ocular manifestations of child abuse. *J Pediatr Ophthalmol Strabismus*. 1980;17:5–13. Reprinted by permission from Slack Incorporated.

SPECIAL CONSIDERATION

Photograph retinal hemorrhages in infants during the first 24 hours of detection for critical evidence in a child abuse investigation.

The *differential diagnosis* of retinal hemorrhages includes:

• transient bleeding (present in >11% of deliveries in the first 72 hours[56]);
• leukemia;
• subacute bacterial endocarditis;
• anemia;
• sickle cell disease;
• collagen-vascular disease;
• diabetic retinopathy (rare); and, possibly,
• cardiopulmonary resuscitation[58].[d]

Penetrating Orbital Trauma

Such injuries may be difficult to diagnose if there is no history and the wound is small. The threshold for obtaining CT, MRI, or ultrasound is higher in children because of the need for deep sedation or general anesthesia.

CT is generally the initial choice for its superior imaging of bone and blood, the safety margin with metallic foreign bodies (see Chapters 9 and 24), and the rapid scan time. MRI is slightly superior in the identification of wooden foreign bodies,[59,60] but both CT and MRI can easily miss small organic objects (Fig. 30–11).

---

[d] The data are inconclusive unless head injury, CNS disease, or sepsis is also present.[57]

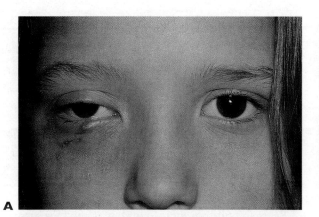
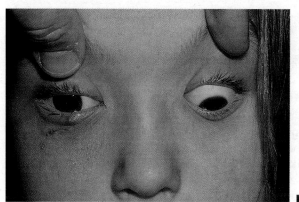
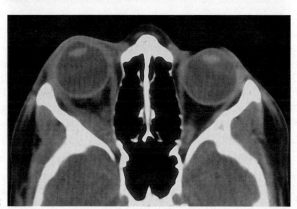
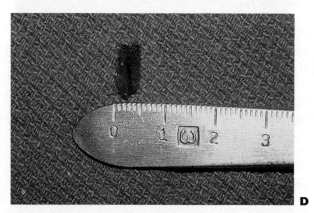

FIGURE 30–11   Occult orbital foreign body not revealed by CT. (**A** and **B**) The 7-year-old girl presented with pain, mild proptosis, and restricted motility of the right globe. (**C**) The orbital CT was read as rhabdomyosarcoma. (**D**) A lateral orbitotomy yielded a large wooden foreign body in the orbit. Subsequent history revealed that the child was struck by a sibling with a broken wooden handle from a toilet plunger. (Photographs and case report courtesy of Rick Burgett, MD.)

Metallic Foreign Bodies in the Orbit

Metallic foreign bodies with a low lead content (e.g., BB and air gun pellets, bullet fragments), may be left behind (see Chapter 36) in the orbit.[61] Objects located in the orbital apex are best observed for fear of complications (e.g., optic neuropathy, neurogenic ophthalmoplegia, ptosis). Factors favoring removal include:

- large size;
- persistent ocular motility problems; and
- anterior location.

Orbital infections may be extremely serious: prior to the era of antibiotics, one quarter of patients with orbital cellulitis died and one quarter became blind.

PEARL... An orbital abscess in the absence of orbital cellulitis may be caused by a foreign body. Surgical drainage and broad-spectrum antibiotics are required.

Nonpenetrating Orbital Trauma

Nonpenetrating orbital trauma may present differently in children,[62] whose facial bones are more elastic than those in adults; orbital roof fractures are more likely to be associated with neurocranial injuries.[63] Such fractures become more likely with facial growth and with increased sinus pneumatization: the orbital floor and the medial wall become thinner.[64]

TON

This does not seem to be different in children. The VEP is a useful diagnostic tool.[67] See Chapter 37 for details.

Loss of the Eye and Orbital Growth

The effect of anophthalmia on retarding growth of the pediatric orbit has been well documented,[68,69] but symmetric orbital growth is still possible after enucleation when using the largest possible orbital implant.[70–72]

Adnexal Injuries

Soft tissues heal rapidly in children. The primary repair should therefore be performed expeditiously.

PEARL... Skin sutures must be removed early to prevent suture scarring ("railroad tracks"). In anticipation of the difficulty in suture removal, subcuticular nonabsorbing (nylon or Prolene) pullout sutures or fine, fast-absorbing gut/mild chromic is recommended, and reinforcement with sterile adhesive strips before and after suture removal is useful.

Scars in children tend to widen as the face grows, and hypertrophic scarring is more common. The possibility of future scar revisions should be explained to the parents at the time of primary repair.

Canalicular lacerations are an easily overlooked complication of lid trauma, common in children with avulsion-type injuries involving lateral displacement of the lower lid, such as in dog bites (see Chapter 35).[73] Prompt primary repair of the canaliculus with stenting over a silicone tube is much more likely to be successful than late repair, which may require use of a Jones tube.

Persistent ptosis and post-traumatic motility disturbances due to extraocular muscle trauma threaten with the development of amblyopia.[74] Injury (generally intracranial) is the most common cause of acquired oculomotor palsy.[75,76]

Hyphema

Involving 38% of patients, it is the most frequent type of ocular trauma in the pediatric group, and ≤11% eyes may require surgery to remove the blood (USEIR). No relationship between age and rate of rebleeding, however, can be established.

Cataract and Visual Rehabilitation

The management of injured children is unsuccessful unless the *amblyopia* therapy is effective. Children ≤8 years old are at risk, with the susceptibility decreasing with increasing age. Optical rehabilitation of young children must be instituted as soon as safely possible. Principles of management include:

- prompt clearing of the visual axis;
- minimizing astigmatism during wound repair (see Chapter 14 and the Appendix);
- early removal of corneal sutures;
- rapid employment of optical correction; and
- patch occlusion of the fellow eye on a part-time basis: 50–90% of waking hours in the early postoperative period, increased to 100% later until the visual acuity reaches its plateau.[e] At this point, if the compliance has been good and the level of obtained vision remains stable, the time of daily occlusion may be gradually decreased to a maintenance level. This minimum requirement is found by trial and error and is continued until the patient is no longer of an amblyogenic age.

Over 5% of all serious eye injuries in the USEIR database are pediatric cataracts, and 40% of these are vulnerable to amblyopia. The need for surgery usually indicates a poor prognosis because of the typically severe nature of the injury and secondary amblyopia.[77,78] Surgical interventions must aim at the following goals:

- wound toilette and closure;
- removal of the cataract; and
- restoration of the lost eye's refractive power.

> **PEARL...** Corneal wounds in children heal much more rapidly than in adults; sutures are typically removed as early as 4–6 weeks postoperatively.

Amblyopia[79] is just one of the special considerations; even in children beyond the amblyogenic period,

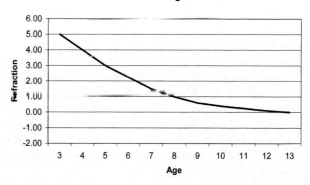

Suggested postoperative refractive goal according to age

FIGURE 30–12   The relationship between targeted postoperative refraction and the age of the patient with traumatic cataract: accounting for the anticipated myopic shift with age.

the secondary *myopic shift* must be accounted for, especially if an IOL is implanted (Fig. 30–12). Our surgical technique for a child's eye with a traumatic cataract may be employed in a primary or secondary fashion.

- Reposit/excise the prolapsed uveal tissue if present (see Chapter 16).
- Close the wound:
  - cornea: 10-0 nylon if >3–4 mm; absorbable 10-0 suture (Vicryl) otherwise;
  - sclera: 9-0 nylon.
- Decide whether to proceed with or defer lens removal (see Chapter 21); remember that lens swelling with resulting inflammation and secondary glaucoma can rapidly develop if the lens capsule is disrupted. If secondary removal is elected, intense topical steroid therapy (prednisolone every 1–4 hours) and cycloplegia (atropine 1% 2–3 times daily) are required (see Chapter 8).
- Determine the site of surgical incision:
  - scleral tunnel dissection is difficult (less rigid sclera); recommended mostly if a larger wound is needed (e.g., for placement of a sulcus-fixated IOL);
  - small clear corneal incision just anterior to the termination of the limbal vessels is preferred.
- A smaller than normal anterior capsulectomy should be performed. This is because the anterior capsule is relatively elastic and a positive vitreous pressure may be present, resulting in a distinct tendency for peripheral extension of the capsular opening.
  - The surgeon must continually direct the rhexis toward the center rather than leading it around in a circle.

---

[e]If occlusion (reverse) amblyopia occurs, patching should be discontinued until the nontraumatized eye has recovered.

○ An alternative technique is to use the vitrectomy probe, placing its port over the anterior capsule centrally, and taking multiple small bites (typical settings: 250/minute cut rate, ≤ 250 mm Hg aspiration); use a separate AC infusion.

• For nucleus/cortex removal, automated or manual aspiration is sufficient; *phacoemulsification is contraindicated*. The vitrectomy probe must be used to deal with the frequently prolapsed vitreous (see Chapter 21). Careful attention should be directed to remove all peripheral cortical material to avoid its subsequent hydration with visual and inflammatory complications.

• The integrity of the posterior capsule must be inspected.

○ If no IOL is placed, a primary posterior capsulectomy for fear of subsequent opacification should be performed (see Chapter 21), using the vitrectomy probe and followed by limited anterior vitrectomy. The capsular opening should be left small enough to permit later placement of an IOL in the bag if desired.

○ If an IOL is placed, the capsulectomy and vitrectomy should be performed through a pars plana incision after IOL insertion.

○ If the capsule is clear and the patient is expected to cooperate at the YAG laser later, however, the posterior capsule may be left intact.

SPECIAL CONSIDERATION

The pars plana is located anteriorly in young children; enter closer to the limbus than in an adult eye.

• Decide whether to proceed with or defer IOL placement. Although primary IOL placement has definite advantages,[80] it also has certain risks (see Chapter 21).

IOL implantation is very common and has a major role[81] in the optical rehabilitation of children with traumatic cataract.[f]

Children ≥9 years old are treated as adults when selecting the type and power of IOL, with the exception of a slight myopic shift.

• The difficulty of IOL power selection grows with decreasing age of the patient: the anticipated

myopic shift increases and the variability of individual responses increases.[82,83] Options include:

○ targeting emmetropia with later IOL exchange or refractive surgery;

○ "piggybacking" two IOLs with later explantation of one; or

○ anticipating the myopic shift and selecting an IOL that will approximate emmetropia in later childhood; spectacle correction is expected. Because these patients will usually require glasses for protection and carry a bifocal, we prefer this third option (Fig. 30–12). Unlike adults, children readily accept higher spectacle-corrected anisometropia despite the induced aniseikonia.

• In regard to the material and type of the IOL, no conclusive study indicates that PMMA is better than acrylic in children.

PITFALL

Rigid or foldable lenses may be employed, but silicone IOLs should be avoided because of the risk of late retinal complications requiring silicone oil use.

• The IOL can be placed in the bag, in the ciliary sulcus, or on top of the anterior capsule that has been thoroughly polished. If the capsular support is inadequate, sulcus-fixated IOLs may be used,[84] although there may be potential long-term complications (e.g., suture erosion or breakage). Our preferred method is a foldable acrylic lens placed within the bag using a small clear cornea incision.

PEARL... AC IOLs are not recommended for children.

Relatively common *alternative techniques* for restoring the eye's refractive power include:
• contact lens; and to a much lesser extent,
• epikeratophakia.

Posterior Segment Trauma

Children's lack of cooperation with postoperative positioning influences the surgeon's decisions during retinal detachment repair. Fortunately, silicone oil, requiring minimal positioning and no immobility, appears as effective in children as in adults.[85,86] Both

[f]For patients under 18 years, the FDA approves none of the currently available lenses. This fact should be disclosed to the family when obtaining informed operative consent.

silicone oil and long-acting gases, however, can lead to a high incidence of cataract formation in phakic eyes.[87]

Although PVR's higher incidence and more aggressive course in the pediatric eye is commonly asserted,[85,86] it does not seem to be supported in the literature.[14,88] Nevertheless, post-traumatic retinal detachment due to PVR is the primary cause of poor visual outcome among all pediatric age groups.[14,88]

The vitreoretinal surgeon faces increased difficulty in separating the nondetached posterior hyaloid in the pediatric eye. Nonetheless, vitreous removal must be completed as compatible with safety because leaving behind the posterior hyaloid increases the risk of PVR by providing a scaffold for proliferation at the vitreoretinal interface (see Chapters 23 and 24).[89] Enzymatic assistance in pediatric vitrectomy[90] may have a future role, although this has not been evaluated in the injured eye.

The predictors of poor outcome appear to be the same as those for adults with posterior segment injury.[14,77,88]

SUMMARY

Ocular injury, which occurs frequently in children, is an important cause of monocular blindness. As a result of the patient's age, inability to cooperate with examination, and the potential for the development of amblyopia, children presenting with eye injuries are evaluated and treated rather differently from adults. The physician should also remember that in cases of pediatric eye injury, the most concerned or anxious individuals are frequently the parents and one must not overlook their potential feelings of guilt.

REFERENCES

1. Admoni MM, BenEzra D. Ocular trauma following amniocentesis as the cause of leukocoria. *J Pediatr Ophthalmol Strabismus.* 1998;25:196–197.
2. Steiner GC, Peterson LW. Severe emotional response to eye trauma in a child: awareness and intervention [letter]. *Arch Ophthalmol.* 1992;110:753–754.
3. Schein O, Hibberd P, Shingleton B, et al. The spectrum and burden of ocular injury. *Ophthalmology.* 1988;95:300–305.
4. Grin T, Nelson L, Jeffers JB. Eye injuries in childhood. *Pediatrics.* 1987;80:13–17.
5. Zagelbaum B, Tostanoski JR, Kerner DJ, Hersh P. Urban eye trauma. A one-year prospective study. *Ophthalmology.* 1993;100:851–856.
6. Klopfer J, Tielsch JM, Vitale S, See LC, Canner JK. Ocular trauma in the United States: eye injuries resulting in hospitalization, 1984 through 1987. *Arch Ophthalmol.* 1992;110:838–842.
7. Strahlamn E, Elman M, Daub E, Baker S. Causes of pediatric eye injuries; a population-based study. *Arch Ophthalmol.* 1990;108:603–608.
8. Nash EA, Margo CE. Patterns of emergency department visits for disorders of the eye and ocular adnexa. *Arch Ophthalmol.* 1998;116:1222–1226.
9. Canavan YM, O'Flaherty MJ, Archer DB, Elwood JH. A 10-year survey of eye injuries in Northern Ireland, 1967–76. *Br J Ophthalmol.* 1980;64:618–625.
10. Rapoport I, Romem M, Kinek M, et al. Eye injuries in children in Israel. A nationwide collaborative study. *Arch Ophthalmol.* 1990;108:376–379.
11. Gothwal VK, Adolph S, Jalali S, Naduvilath TJ. Demography and prognostic factors of ocular injuries in South India. *Aust N Z J Ophthalmol.* 1999;27:318–325.
12. Niiranen M, Raivio I. Eye injuries in children. *Br J Ophthalmol.* 1981;65:436–438.
13. Fong LP. Eye injuries in Victoria, Australia. *Med J Aust.* 1995;162:64–68.
14. Sternberg P Jr, de Juan E Jr, Michels RG. Penetrating ocular injuries in young patients. Initial injuries and visual results. *Retina.* 1984;4:5–8.
15. Nelson L, Wilson T, Jeffers J. Eye injuries in childhood: demography, etiology, and prevention. *Pediatrics.* 1989;84:438–441.
16. MacEwen CJ, Baines PS, Desai P. Eye injuries in children: the current picture. *Br J Ophthalmol.* 1999;83:933–936.
17. DeRespinis PA, Caputo AR, Fiore PM, Wagner RS. A survey of severe eye injuries in children. *Am J Dis Child.* 1989;143:711–716.
18. Umeh RE, Umeh OC. Causes and visual outcome of childhood eye injuries in Nigeria. *Eye.* 1997;11:489–495.
19. Kuhn F, Witherspoon C, Morris R. Baseball-related eye injuries. In: Andrews J, Zarins B, Wilk K, eds. *Injuries in Baseball.* Philadelphia: Lippincott-Raven; 1998:395–400.
20. Rutherford G, Kennedy J, Mcghee L. *Hazard Analysis: Baseball and Softball Related Injuries to Children 5–14 Years of Age.* Washington, DC: US Consumer Product Safety Commission; 1984.
21. Schein OD, Hibberd PL, Shingleton BJ, et al. The spectrum and burden of ocular injury. *Ophthalmology.* 1988;95:300–305.
22. CPSC. *Overview of Sports-Related Injuries to Persons 5–14 Years of Age.* Washington, DC: US Consumer Products Safety Commision; 1981.
23. Tanaka N, Hayashi S, Amagasa T, Kohama G. Maxillofacial fractures sustained during sports. *J Oral Maxillofac Surg.* 1996;54:715–719.
24. Vinger PF, Duma SM, Crandall J. Baseball hardness as a risk factor for eye injuries. *Arch Ophthalmol.* 1999;117:354–358.

25. Kyle S. *Youth Baseball Protective Equipment Project Final Report*. Washington, DC: US Consumer Products Safety Commission; 1996.

26. Danis R, Hu K, Bell M. Baseball face guards are acceptable and reduce oculofacial injury in receptive youth league players. *Inj Prev*. 2000;6:232–234.

27. Vinger PF. Ocular sports injuries. Principles of protection. *Int Ophthalmol Clin*. 1981;21:149–161.

28. Pashby TJ. Ocular injuries in hockey. *Int Ophthalmol Clin*. 1988;28:228–231.

29. Napier SM, Baker RS, Sanford DG, Easterbrook M. Eye injuries in athletics and recreation. *Surv Ophthalmol*. 1996;41:229–244.

30. Vinger PF. Injury prevention: where do we go from here? *J Am Optom Assoc*. 1999;70:87–98.

31. Drack A, Kutschke PJ, Stair S, Scott WE. Compliance with safety glasses wear in monocular children. *J Ophthalmic Nurs Technol*. 1994;13(2):77–82.

32. Scribano PV, Nance M, Reilly P, Sing RF, Selbst SM. *Pediatric* nonpowder firearm injuries: outcomes in an urban pediatric setting. Pediatrics. 1997;100:E5.

33. Schein O, Enger C, Tielsch J. The context and consequences of ocular injuries from air guns. *Am J Ophthalmol*. 1994;117:501–506.

34. LaRoche GR, McIntyre L, Schertzer RM. Epidemiology of severe eye injuries in childhood. *Ophthalmology*. 1988;95:1603–1607.

35. Marshall DH, Brownstein S, Addison DJ, Mackenzie SG, Jordan DR, Clarke WN. Air guns: the main cause of enucleation secondary to trauma in children and young adults in the greater Ottawa area in 1974–93. *Can J Ophthalmol*. 1995;30:187–192.

36. Kitchens JW, Danis RP. Increasing paintball related eye trauma reported to a state eye injury registry. *Inj Prev*. 1999;5:301–302.

37. Thach AB, Ward TP, Hollifield RD, et al. Ocular injuries from paintball pellets. *Ophthalmology*. 1999;106:533–537.

38. Fineman MS, Fischer DH, Jeffers JB, Buerger DG, Repke C. Changing trends in paintball sport-related ocular injuries. *Arch Ophthalmol*. 2000;118:60–64.

39. Kuhn F, Morris R, Witherspoon CD, et al. Serious fireworks-related eye injuries. *Ophthalmic Epidemiol.*, 2000; 7:139–148.

40. Kuhn F, Mester V, Witherspoon CD, Morris R. Epidemiology and socioeconomic impact of eye injuries. In: Alfaro V, Liggett P, eds. *Vitrectomy in the Management of the Injured Globe*. Philadelphia: Lippincott Raven; 1998: 17–24.

41. Wilson RS. Ocular fireworks injuries and blindness. An analysis of 154 cases and a three-state survey comparing the effectiveness of model law regulation. Ophthalmology. 1982;89:291–297.

42. McFarland LV, Harris JR, Kobayashi JM, Dicker RC. Risk factors for fireworks-related injury in Washington State. *JAMA*. 1984;251:3251–3254.

43. Levitz LM, Miller JK, Uwe M, Drusedau H. Ocular injuries caused by fireworks. *JAAPOS*. 1999;3:317–318.

44. Fox BE, O'Brien CO, Kangas KJ, Murphree AL, Wright KW. Use of high dose chloral hydrate for ophthalmic exams in children: a retrospective review of 302 cases. *J Pediatr Ophthalmol Strabismus*. 1990;27:242–244.

45. Jensen A, Smith R, Olson M. Ocular clues to child abuse. *J Pediatr Ophthalmol Strabismus*. 1971;8:270–272.

46. Paviglianiti JC, Donahue SP. Unilateral retinal hemorrhages and ipsilateral intracranial bleeds in nonaccidental trauma. *JAAPOS*. 1999;3:383–384.

47. Terson A. De l'hémmorraghie dans le corps vitre au cours de l'hémorrhagie cérébrale. *Clin Ophthalmol*. 1900;6:309–312.

48. Lambert SR, Johnson TE, Hoyt CS. Optic nerve sheath and retinal hemorrhages associated with the shaken baby syndrome. *Arch Ophthalmol*. 1986;104:1509–1512.

49. Mills M. Funduscopic lesions associated with mortality in shaken baby syndrome. *J AAPOS*. 1998;2:67–71.

50. Massicotte SJ, Folberg R, Torczynski E, Gilliland MGF, Luckenbach MW. Vitreoretinal traction and perimacular retinal folds in the eyes of deliberately traumatized children. *Surv Ophthalmol*. 1991;98:1124–1127.

51. Greenwald MJ, Weiss A, Oesterle CS, Friendly DS. Traumatic retinoschisis in battered babies. Ophthalmology. 1986;93:618–625.

52. Matthews GP, Das A. Dense vitreous hemorrhages predict poor visual and neurological prognosis in infants with shaken baby syndrome. *J Pediatr Ophthalmol Strabismus*. 1996;33:260–265.

53. Purtscher O. Angiopathia retinae traumatica, Lymphorrhagien des Augengrundes. *Graefes Arch Ophthalmol*. 1912;82:347.

54. Ober R. Hemorrhagic retinopathy in infancy: a clinicopathologic report. *J Pediatr Ophthalmol Strabismus*. 1980; 17:17–20.

55. Caffey J. The whiplash shaken infant syndrome: manual shaking by the extremities with whiplash-induced intracranial and intraocular bleedings, linked with residual permanent brain damage and mental retardation. *Pediatrics*. 1974;54:396–403.

56. Jain IS, Singh YP, Grupta SL, Gupta A. Ocular hazards during birth. *J Pediatr Ophthalmol Strabismus*. 1980;17: 14–16.

57. Gilliland MG, Luckenbach MW. Are retinal hemorrhages found after resuscitation attempts? A study of the eyes of 169 children. *Am J Forensic Med Pathol*. 1993; 14:187–192.

58. Goetting MG, Sowa B. Retinal hemorrhage after cardiopulmonary resuscitation in children: an etiologic reevaluation. *Pediatrics*. 1990;85:585–588.

59. Nasr AM, Haik BG, Fleming JC, Al-Hussain HM, Karcioglu ZA. Penetrating orbital injury with organic foreign bodies. *Ophthalmology*. 1999;106:523–532.

60. Specht CS, Varga JH, Jalali MM, Edelstein JP. Orbitocranial wooden foreign body diagnosed by magnetic resonance imaging. Dry wood can be isodense with air and orbital fat by computed tomography. *Surv Ophthalmol*. 1992;36:341–344.

61. Finkelstein M, Legmann A, Rubin PA. Projectile metallic foreign bodies in the orbit: a retrospective study of epidemiologic factors, management, and outcomes. *Ophthalmology*. 1997;104:96–103.

62. Hopper KD, Sherman JL, Boal DK, Eggli KD. CT and MR imaging of the pediatric orbit. *Radiographics*. 1992; 12:485–503.

63. Greenwald MJ, Boston D, Pensler JM, Radkowski MA. Orbital roof fractures in childhood. *Ophthalmology*. 1989;96:491–496; discussion 96–97.

64. Koltai PJ, Amjad I, Meyer D, Feustel PJ. Orbital fractures in children. *Arch Otolaryngol Head Neck Surg*. 1995;121:1375–1379.

65. Sires BS, Stanley RB Jr, Levine LM. Oculocardiac reflex caused by orbital floor trapdoor fracture: an indication for urgent repair [letter]. *Arch Ophthalmol*. 1998;116: 955–956.

66. Macdonald D, Schneider K, Della Rocca R, Brazzo B. Childhood disorders of the orbit and adnexa. In: Nesi F, Lisman R, Levine M, eds. *Smith's Ophthalmic Plastic and Reconstructive Surgery*. 2nd ed. St. Louis: Mosby; 1998:835–847.

67. Mahapatra A. Optic nerve injury in children. A prospective study of 35 patients. *J Neurosurg Sci*. 1992; 36:79–84.

68. Apt L, Isenberg S. Changes in orbital dimensions following enucleation. *Arch Ophthalmol*. 1973;90:393–395.

69. Osborne D, Hadden OB, Deeming LW. Orbital growth after childhood enucleation. *Am J Ophthalmol*. 1974;77: 756–759.

70. Fountain TR, Goldberger S, Murphree AL. Orbital development after enucleation in early childhood. *Ophthalmol Plast Reconstr Surg*. 1999;15:32–36.

71. Reedy BK, Pan F, Kim WS, Bartlett SP. The direct effect of intraorbital pressure on orbital growth in the anophthalmic piglet. *Plast Reconstr Surg*. 1999;104:713–718.

72. Heinz GW, Nunery WR, Cepela MA. The effect of maturation on the ability to stimulate orbital growth using tissue expanders in the anophthalmic cat orbit. *Ophthalmol Plast Reconstr Surg*. 1997;13:115–128.

73. Slonim CB. Dog bite–induced canalicular lacerations: a review of 17 cases. *Ophthalmol Plast Reconstr Surg*. 1996; 12:218–222.

74. Lyon DB, Newman SA. Evidence of direct damage to extraocular muscles as a cause of diplopia following orbital trauma. *Ophthalmol Plast Reconstr Surg*. 1989;5: 81–91.

75. Schumacher-Feero LA, Yoo KW, Solari FM, Biglan AW. Third cranial nerve palsy in children. *Am J Ophthalmol*. 1999;128:216–221.

76. Holmes JM, Mutyala S, Maus TL, Grill R, Hodge DO, Gray DT. Pediatric third, fourth, and sixth nerve palsies: a population-based study. *Am J Ophthalmol*. 1999;127:388–392.

77. Alfaro DV, Chaudhry NA, Walonker AF, Runyan T, Saito Y, Liggett PE. Penetrating eye injuries in young children. *Retina*. 1994;14:201–205.

78. Baxter RJ, Hodgkins PR, Calder I, Morrell AJ, Vardy S, Elkington AR. Visual outcome of childhood anterior perforating eye injuries: prognostic indicators. *Eye*. 1994;8:349–352.

79. Keech R, Kutschke PJ. Upper age limit for the development of amblyopia. *J Pediatr Ophthalmol Strabismus*. 1995;32:89–93.

80. Anwar M, Bleik J, von Noorden G, El-Maghraby. Posterior chamber lens implantation for primary repair of corneal lacerations and traumatic cataracts in children. *J Pediatr Ophthalmol Strabismus*. 1994;31:157–161.

81. Gupta AK, Grover AK, Gurha N. Traumatic cataract surgery with intraocular lens implantation in children. *J Pediatr Ophthalmol Strabismus*. 1992;29:73–78.

82. Plager D, Kipfer H, Sprunger D, Sondhi N, Neely D. Refractive change in pediatric pseudophakia: six-year follow-up. Paper presented at: AAPOS Annual Meeting; April 2000; San Diego, CA.

83. McClatchey SK, Dahan E, Maselli E, et al. A comparison of the rate of refractive growth in pediatric aphakic and pseudophakic eyes. *Ophthalmology*. 2000;107: 118–122.

84. Buckely E. Scleral fixated (sutured) posterior chamber intraocular lens implantation in children. *J AAPOS*. 1999;3:289–294.

85. Moisseiev J, Vidne O, Treister G. Vitrectomy and silicone oil injection in pediatric patients. *Retina*. 1998;18: 221–227.

86. Scott IU, Flynn HW Jr, Azen SP, Lai MY, Schwartz S, Trese MT. Silicone oil in the repair of pediatric complex retinal detachments: a prospective, observational, multicenter study. *Ophthalmology*. 1999;106:1399–1407; discussion 407–408.

87. Blodi BA, Paluska SA. Cataract after vitrectomy in young patients. *Ophthalmology*. 1997;104:1092–1095.

88. Cardillo JA, Stout JT, LaBree L, et al. Post-traumatic proliferative vitreoretinopathy. The epidemiologic profile, onset, risk factors, and visual outcome. *Ophthalmology*. 1997;104:1166–1173.

89. Miller B, Patterson R, Ryan SJ. Retinal wound healing; cellular activity at the vitreoretinal interface. *Arch Ophthalmol*. 1986;104:281–285.

90. Margherio AR, Margherio RR, Hartzer M, Trese MT, Williams GA, Ferrone PJ. Plasmin enzyme-assisted vitrectomy in traumatic pediatric macular holes. *Ophthalmology*. 1998;105:1617–1620.

91. Harley R. Ocular manifestations of child abuse. *J Pediatr Ophthalmol Strabismus*. 1980;17:5–13.

Chapter 31

EVISCERATION AND ENUCLEATION

Michael A. Callahan

Following severe injury, several scenarios are possible:

- the eye may be impossible to reconstruct anatomically (A);
- SO may develop (B);
- the eye with no hope of functioning may have a higher than usual risk of developing SO (C);
- unbearable chronic pain may develop in a blind eye and other methods to alleviate it may prove unsuccessful or are not recommended (D);
- the eye may become phthisical and cosmetically unacceptable (E).

In case of "A," primary enucleation or evisceration is the only reasonable option; in case of "B" (see Chapter 29), it is controversial whether any, and if so which, of the potential procedures discussed in this chapter should be performed; in cases of "C" through "E," the ophthalmologist must thoroughly discuss all surgical and nonsurgical management options with the patient (see Chapters 5, 7, and 8).

DECISION MAKING[a]

Treatment options for painful, blind, and cosmetically unappealing eyes include:

- retrobulbar alcohol injection;
- cyclocryopexy (these two measures usually:
  - ruin the motility of a subsequently implanted prosthesis;

_____
[a] See also Chapter 36.

- create moderate to severe ptosis;
- create sulcus retraction secondary to fat atrophy; and
- have an effect that is temporary and unpredictable);
- evisceration; and
- enucleation.

If it is decided that the eye is best removed (see Chapter 8), the selection between evisceration and enucleation is primarily determined by:

- the expertise of the operating physician;
- the implant materials available; and
- the fear of SO development.

Extensive counseling is always required (see later in this chapter and Chapters 5 and 7).

> **PEARL...** The ophthalmologist should always explain that the patient will be fitted with a prosthesis 6 to 8 weeks postoperatively and that a patch may be needed in the interim.

SO AS A FACTOR IN DETERMINING THE MANAGEMENT

The fear of the fellow eye's involvement (see Chapter 29) and subsequent contralateral blindness are the main reason why some ophthalmologists are reluctant to recommend evisceration. The causal relationship between evisceration and SO has been debated since the 19th century. The conclusion of a literature review[1] of 1628 cases in 1963 argued against the role of evisceration as the cause of SO and recommended that evisceration, rather than enucleation, be offered to patients, unless:

- chronic inflammation is present; or
- malignancy cannot be excluded and pathologic examination is required.

It appears that this recommendation has been upheld,[b] especially because in a series of 105 cases of SO,[3] no eye was found to have undergone evisceration.[c] Furthermore, in cases of severe orbital and ocular trauma, particularly when there are a large posterior scleral rupture and extrusion of intraocular contents into the orbit, the only way to be certain that the threat of SO has been eliminated would be to remove all potential antigens. In this setting, one can reasonably argue that enucleation offers no theoretical benefit over evisceration.

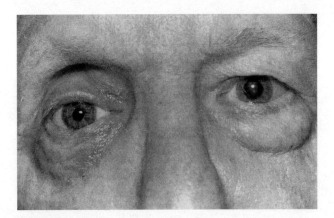

FIGURE 31-1 A 73-year-old patient showing classical signs of anophthalmic socket syndrome including hollowing of supratarsal sulcus, downward angulation of lateral canthus, and laxity of right lower lid. This patient had a quasi-integrated buried implant but nevertheless poor motility. The manifestations of the anophthalmic syndrome as depicted here are to be avoided.

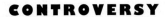

CONTROVERSY

$\longleftrightarrow$

With the increasing threat of litigation, one cannot avoid the question: is it indeed safe to recommend evisceration rather than enucleation?[1-5]

EVISCERATION

Because the sclera is retained and the extraocular muscle attachments are preserved, evisceration is usually considered to result in:

- superior motility;
- less implant migration;
- less severe manifestation of the anophthalmic socket syndrome; and
- a more physiologic solution for the orbit's long-term health (Fig. 31–1).

In addition, most ocularists until recently preferred fitting eviscerated sockets compared with enucleated sockets. Patients are also more gratified with the overall cosmetic results and motility after evisceration than after enucleation (Figs. 31–2 through 31–4).

Indications

Local and systemic factors alike may require the eye to be eviscerated rather than enucleated:

- posterior scleral rupture without hope of visual rehabilitation[d]; and
- debilitated patient too sick for general anesthesia and enucleation.

Surgical Technique

Evisceration without Keratectomy

See Figure 31–7A–C.

- Make a limbal periotomy or conjunctival incision 8 to 9 mm from the limbus over the superior 100 degrees of the globe and expose the superior rectus muscle insertion.
- Weave a double-armed suture of 6-0 Vicryl through the superior rectus insertion and "whip-lock" it on each end.
- Divide the superior rectus fascial attachments, detach the superior rectus, and tag the suture with a serrefine on a "mosquito" hemostat.
- Perform a "scratch-down" sclerotomy posterior, temporal, and nasal to the superior rectus insertion over the superior 100 degrees, but do not penetrate the choroid.
- Insert a cyclodialysis spatula to separate the potential space between the adherent anterior uveal attachments and the scleral spur. Once the correct plane is entered, avoid piercing the vitreous cavity by making small initial sweeps with the spatula hugging the sclera.

---

[b] Despite pathophysiological evidence[2] that SO *can* develop following evisceration.

[c] The author has seen one patient who, following evisceration, developed pathologically proven SO and, in spite of intensive treatment with steroids and cyclosporin A, progressed to bilateral blindness (Figs. 31–5 and 31–6).

---

[d] Evisceration preferably performed within 5 days after injury.

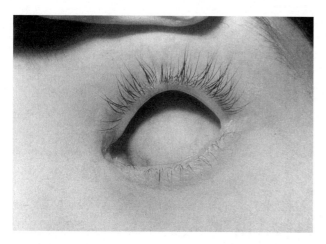

FIGURE 31–2   This 4-year-old patient suffered posterior scleral laceration and optic nerve avulsion and underwent primary evisceration with a 18-mm hydroxyapatite implant. Three months postoperatively, a beautiful socket is seen with deep fornices and almost no manifestations of the anophthalmic syndrome.

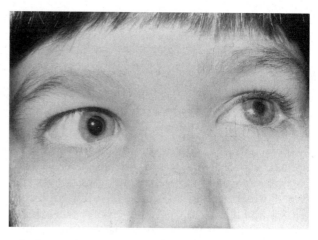

FIGURE 31–3   Same patient as shown in Figure 31–2. Eviscerated socket even without pegs has a good range of motility but not saccadic eye movement (left gaze).

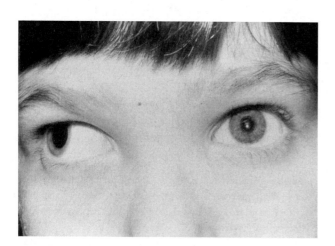

FIGURE 31–4   Same patient as in Figures 31–2 and 31–3, showing right gaze with fair motility of the eviscerated left socket without motility peg.

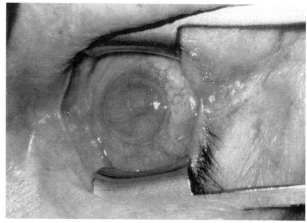

FIGURE 31–5   Pre-enucleation photograph of the *right* eye of the 69-year-old patient who underwent unsuccessful retinal detachment repair due to advanced PVR. Subsequently, nuclear sclerosis developed in her *left* eye; 4 years after cataract surgery and 12 years after unsuccessful retinal detachment repair in the *right* eye, she developed severe uveitis. The enucleated specimen demonstrated sympathetic uveitis. Despite treatment with topical periocular injections of steroids as well as oral steroids and treatment for 3 years with cyclosporine, the visual acuity in the *left* eye deteriorated from 20/20 to NLP and the eye is now phthisical. (The picture was reversed during processing from a color slide to a black and white print.)

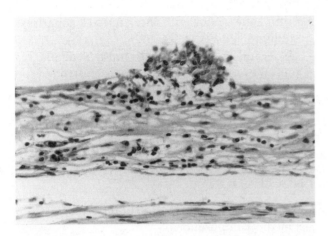

FIGURE 31–6   Pathologic specimen taken from the enucleated *right* eye of patient in Figure 31–5. Photomicrograph demonstrates Dalen-Fuchs nodule.

PEARL...   **The choroid is more easily fragmented posteriorly than at the iris root.**

- Make larger sweeps in all directions as more choroid is separated until the dissection has covered a full 360 degrees from the sclerotomy. These maneuvers are easier if the globe is normotensive. In open globes or chronically-inflamed eyes, dissection is more difficult and bleeding can be profuse. In such eyes and even with the most deliberate and meticulous initial technique, small pieces of the uvea will most likely remain attached to the sclera; these must be retrieved later.

- Once the cyclodialysis spatula has initiated the dissection, extend the scleral incision and insert a small evisceration spoon to separate the remaining uveal attachments from the sclera. Fixation of a hypotonus globe with forceps by an assistant is helpful. Keep the blade of the spoon angled firmly against the sclera during scraping. Most of the posterior dissection with the evisceration spoon is done by "feel" because the surgical field is bloody and the sclera "floppy."

- When the uvea is completely dissected, the specimen should be delivered in toto, i.e., including choroid, retina, vitreous, and lens (if present). Positioning the large evisceration spoon around the back of the specimen and scooping it out from behind "in one fell swoop" facilitates this maneuver. The profuse bleeding that usually occurs from the severed central retinal artery may be controlled via:
  - application of direct finger pressure over the optic nerve for 5 minutes;
  - cauterizing the optic nerve ab interno with bipolar cautery; or
  - Bovie cautery suction if necessary for visualization; alternatively, insert a hemostat through the sclerotomy and clamp the area of the optic disk directly. The clamp may be either left in place for 3 to 5 minutes or immediately electrocoagulated with a Bovie cautery.

- Once the field is bloodless, remove any retained uveal fragments with gauze "peanuts" tightly clamped to hemostats.

- Scrape off the corneal endothelium with absolute alcohol or iodine on a cotton-tipped applicator.

- Irrigate the scleral cavity with hydrogen peroxide, removing uveal cells and intracellular debris.

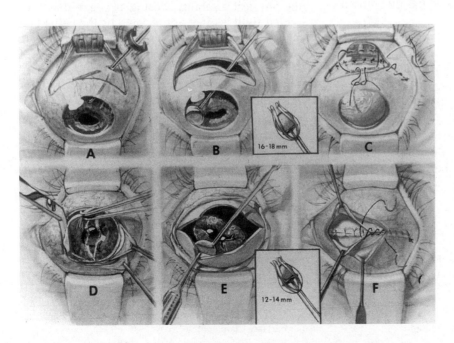

FIGURE 31–7   Technique of evisceration. **(A–C)** *Without* keratectomy. **(D–F)** *With* keratectomy. (From Callahan MA, Callahan A. Removal of eye. In: *Ophthalmic Plastic and Orbital Surgery*. Birmingham: Aesculapius Publishing Company. 1979, 43. Reprinted by permission from the Aesculapius Publishing Company, Birmingham, Alabama.)

- Irrigate the scleral cavity with an antibiotic solution (e.g., bacitracin).
- Close the sclera and conjunctiva with multiple interrupted sutures of 4-0 Vicryl.
- Reattach the superior rectus to its original insertion anterior to the scleral incision with 6-0 Vicryl.
- Suture the conjunctiva to the limbus with 6-0 chromic gut.

Evisceration with Keratectomy

See Figure 31–7D–F.[e]

- Perform a 360-degree limbal peritomy of the conjunctiva and Tenon's capsule, and remove the cornea with corneoscleral scissors. This is facilitated if the assistant fixates the globe by:
  - directly grasping the sclera or
  - using bridle sutures to hold the superior and inferior rectus muscles.
- Separate the conjunctiva from Tenon's capsule for a distance of 8 to 10 mm.[f]
- After removing the cornea, core out the attachments of the uvea to the sclera with the cyclodialysis spatula and evisceration spoon. As described previously, use initial small spoon sweeps, progressing to larger ones shearing the uvea off the sclera, ideally in a single piece.
- After the specimen is delivered, stop the bleeding as described previously.
- Inspect the inside of the sclera for any uveal remnants. Scrape them off with an evisceration spoon, curette, or gauze stretched tightly over your finger, or use peanuts.
- Excise small triangles at the edge of the sclera at 3 and 9 o'clock, converting the defect into more of an ellipse, so the sclera may be coated tightly without dog ears (inset).
- Insert an 18-mm hydroxyapatite "baseball" implant.
  - Alternatively, a 20-mm hydroxyapatite implant may be inserted by making two to four transscleral posterior relaxing incisions 3 mm in length with a Bard-Parker No. 15 blade or Colorado straight needle[g] between the muscle insertions to allow the sclera to "bow" posteriorly. (A 360-degree ab interno posterior sclerectomy around the optic nerve to detach it can be combined with the above.)
- Once the implant is inserted, irrigate the cavity with an antibiotic solution.

- Suture the sclera with interrupted or mattress sutures of 4-0 Vicryl.
- Undermine Tenon's capsule and the conjunctiva until they approximate without excessive tension and close them in two separate layers.
  - We prefer interrupted sutures of 4-0 Vicryl for Tenon's capsule and interrupted sutures of 6-0 chromic gut for the conjunctiva.

ENUCLEATION[h]

Removal of the eye has important psychological, not just medical, implications.[6]

> **PEARL...** With the introduction of hydroxyapatite orbital implants[7], evisceration does not necessarily give a cosmetic result superior to that with enucleation.

Indications

Indications include the following:

- traumatized globe having undergone multiple surgeries with large extraocular implants (scleral buckle), extraocular fibrosis, and poor ocular motility);
- a pathological diagnosis is necessary; or
- an intraocular neoplasm[i] is present or cannot be ruled out by other diagnostic techniques.

Psychological Implications[j]

Although enucleation is a straightforward procedure, its effect on the patient's and family's psyche must never be ignored: this impact may be worse than that of the physical disability. Losing an organ that once provided sight is often appreciated by the patient by an impending sense of fear, sadness, and dread (see "The Patient's Perspective"). It is the responsibility of both the operating physician and the staff (see Chapters 5 and 7) to highlight the positive aspects:

- superior cosmesis:
  - no more attention-grabbing shrunken and/or red eye;
  - a prosthetic eye that is movable;
- superior comfort:
  - pain relief;
  - no need for medications and close follow-ups;

---

[e]This technique is indicated when the cornea and sclera have been severely lacerated or the cornea has spontaneously perforated due to a necrotic ulcer.

[f]This facilitates later closure of the layers separately.

[g]Colorado Biomedical, Inc., Evergreen, Colorado.

[h]See also Chapter 36.

[i]Such a problem is uncommon in the context of a traumatized eye.

[j]Although to a lesser extent, evisceration has similar psychological implications, requiring adequate attention on the medical team's part (see Chapter 5).

- eliminated or at least significantly reduced fear for the fellow eye (i.e., SO); and
- the ability of patient to finally "get on with life" and put the encounter behind.

Surgical Technique

See Figures 31–8 through 31–23.

PITFALL

Because enucleation of the wrong eye has terrible implications for both patient and ophthalmologist, the surgeon must take specific steps to ensure that this does not happen.

- Preoperative preparations:
  - mark in advance the eye to be removed;
  - shield the fellow eye;
  - reconfirm that the correct eye has been marked by (1) asking the patient, (2) checking the patient's wristband, (3) rechecking the consent and the chart, and (4) reexamining the eye at the time of the surgery.
- After the induction of general anesthesia, administer a retrobulbar injection of 5 to 6 mL of 1% lidocaine with epinephrine (1:100,000) before the skin is prepped and draped; this will allow vasoconstricture to occur.
- Balloon the conjunctiva with the injection described previously.
- Perform a 360-degree periotomy of Tenon's capsule and the conjunctiva, precisely at the limbus. Preserve as much of these valuable tissues as possible.

- Using blunt-tipped scissors, gently spread them in progressively larger sweeps in order to dissect Tenon's capsule from the globe between the insertions of the rectus muscles in all four quadrants to expose the insertions.
- Weave a double-armed suture of 5-0 or 6-0 Vicryl through each of the muscle's insertion, whip-locking it on each edge so that it is "tagged" securely.
- Hook and detach each muscle, just as carefully as if it were a strabismus procedure. Clamp the sutures to the drape to avoid entanglement.

PITFALL

Excessive dissection, manipulation, or traction on the superior rectus may damage the levator, resulting in ptosis.

- To gain traction on the globe, take multiple bites through at least two muscle stumps 180 degrees apart with 4-0 silk sutures wedged onto a typical "CV" needle.
- Expose and transect the superior oblique muscle by grasping the superior rectus muscle's stump with forceps (e.g., locking Castroviejo), then turn the eye down and out; retract Tenon's capsule superiorly with a Desmarres retractor, and look for the whitish tendon that courses from medial to lateral just posterior and inferior to the superior rectus muscle insertion. This broad, fibrous, shiny tendon blends in with the sclera and is best found by sweeping the sclera with a small Stevens tenotomy hook. Lift it off the globe, and then snip it with scissors.

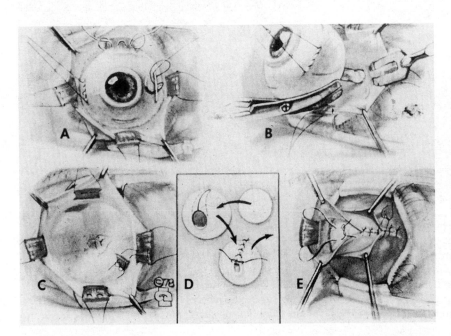

FIGURE 31–8 (A–E) Technique of enucleation with scleral-covered "baseball" implant. See the text for details. (From Callahan ME, Callahan A. Removal of eye. In: *Ophthalmic Plastic and Orbital Surgery*. Birmingham: Aesculapius Publishing Company. 1979, 46. Reprinted by permission from the Aesculapius Publishing Company, Birmingham, Alabama.)

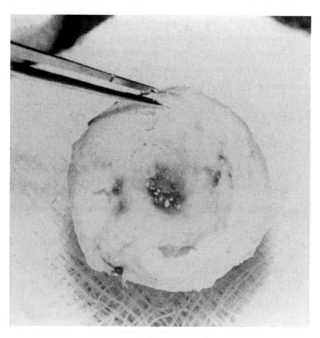

FIGURE 31-9 Preserved sclera wrapped on 18-mm hydroxyapatite sphere. Four windows have been cut anterior to equator, 90 degrees apart. Small drill holes have been placed through the scleral windows, made with an 18-gauge needle by "finger drilling" a distance within the sphere of about 1 mm to encourage vascularization. The open portion of the sphere faces posteriorly and the anterior portion of the preserved sclera faces anteriorly to help prevent extrusion.

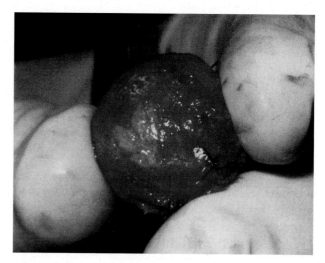

FIGURE 31-10 Posterior auricular muscle complex graft wrapped around a 20-mm hydroxyapatite sphere, an ideal implant for enucleation. Windows in the auricular muscle are cut 90 degrees apart, just anterior to the equator as shown in Figure 31–9.

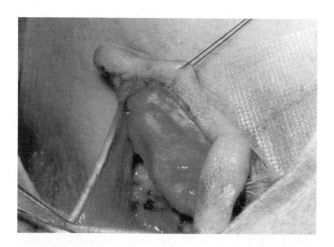

FIGURE 31-11 Intraoperative photograph showing acquisition of auricular muscle complex graft. The ear pinna has been pulled anteriorly with 4-0 silk traction sutures while the skin is retracted with forceps. The auricular muscle complex graft is very thin and adherent to the perichondrium, from which it must be delicately dissected. Surgical tape has been used to drape the patient's hair from the surgical field.

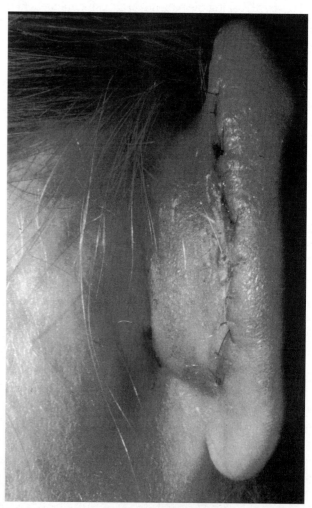

FIGURE 31-12 After harvesting of the auricular muscle complex graft, the incision is sutured with interrupted 6-0 nylon. Minimal anesthesia persists for 3 months.

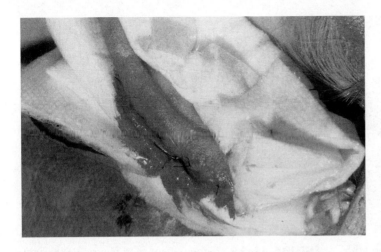

FIGURE 31–13   Telfa splitting of ear performed by placing double-armed 4-0 silk sutures or 3-0 Prolene in mattress fashion through the full thickness of the ear, sandwiching the pinna to prevent cartilaginous hematoma and necrosis.

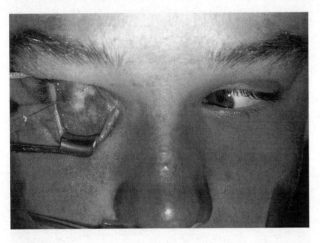

FIGURE 31–14   Critical step in the pegging process in which a pilot hole has been drilled and the patient is asked to look right. Note excursion of 25-gauge needle.

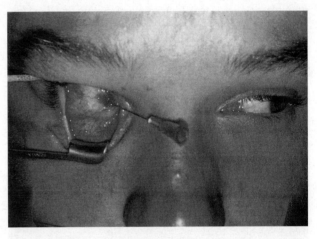

FIGURE 31–15   Same patient as shown in Figure 31–14. Note excursion of 25-gauge needle used to drill pilot hole with patient in left gaze.

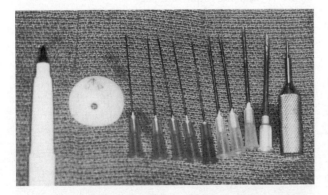

FIGURE 31–16   Instrumentation needed for metal peg system as currently used. Left to right: Skin scribe is used to mark the hole in wax template after it is inserted into the patient's socket. A 25-gauge needle is used to make a perpendicular, properly placed pilot hole within the hydroxyapatite implant. Once the excursions of the 25-gauge needle are deemed satisfactory, the pilot hole is sequentially enlarged with needles of increasing size as shown. The customized screwdriver on the right is used to insert the threaded metal peg holder.

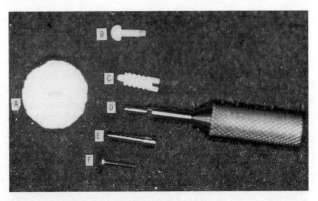

FIGURE 31–17   **(A)** Drilled hydroxyapatite implant as shown with **(C)** "old" plastic threaded peg holder. **(B)** Round-headed peg that is usually inserted by the ocularist upon prosthetic modification. The new metal peg system is shown with **(D)** screwdriver, **(E)** threaded peg holder, and **(F)** temporary flat-headed peg.

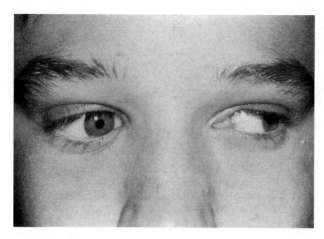

FIGURE 31–18 Patient undergoing enucleation with auricular muscle complex graft and, 12 months later, pegging with plastic peg system. Note range of motion on left gaze.

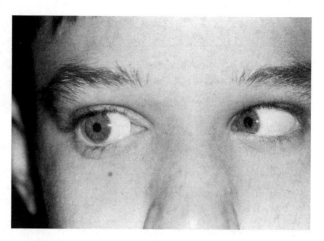

FIGURE 31–19 Same patient as in Figure 31–18; right gaze. Enucleation with 18- to 20-mm hydroxyapatite sphere, wrapped in auricular muscle complex graft and then later pegged, gives excellent motility and saccadic eye movements.

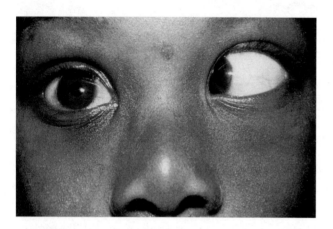

FIGURE 31–20 Enucleation of right eye with "baseball" implant and no motility peg. Enophthalmos is minimal, but motility is negligible.

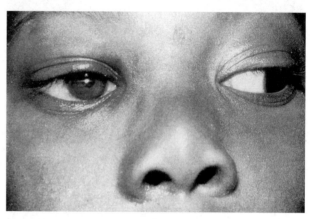

FIGURE 31–21 Same patient as shown in Figure 31–20 with somewhat better motility in left gaze, but significantly inferior to the motility when compared with the patient in Figure 31–18 (enucleation and peg).

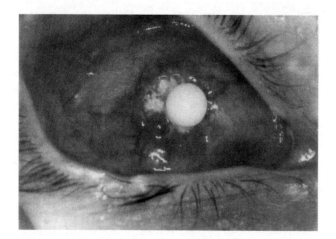

FIGURE 31–22 Plastic peg showing granulation tissue and some conjunctival erosion in an eviscerated socket.

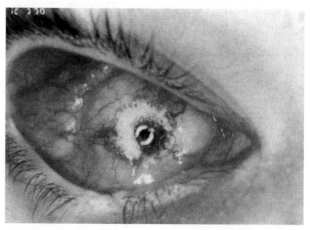

FIGURE 31–23 Replacement of plastic peg from eviscerated socket with metal peg showing less granulation tissue, and filling of hydroxyapatite pores with vascularized tissue. (Same patient as seen in Fig. 31–22.)

- Find the inferior oblique by instructing the assistant to turn the globe up and in with traction on the lateral and inferior rectus muscles' insertions while simultaneously retracting the conjunctiva and Tenon's capsule inferiorly with a Desmarres retractor.
- Hook the fleshy inferior oblique muscle first with a Stevens tenotomy hook in the posteroinferior temporal quadrant by sweeping away from the sclera with the hook's tip pointing perpendicularly away from the globe. Bluntly dissect it out with a second Stevens hook "hand over hand"; cut the muscle between two hemostats and cauterize the two ends to minimize bleeding.
- With all six extraocular muscles detached from the globe, the assistant must firmly proptose the globe by traction on the 4-0 silk sutures passed through the lateral and medial rectus insertions. This exposes the optic nerve with its posterior Tenon's capsule attachments.
- Pull the eye anteromedially and retract the orbital tissues posterolaterally, and clamp the optic nerve 4 to 5 mm behind the globe from the temporal side with a hemostat under direct visualization. Keep the hemostat for 3 to 5 minutes, then cut the nerve through the middle of the hemostat's crimp.[k] Control bleeding by direct pressure for 5 to 10 minutes with neurosurgical swab tape soaked in Neo-Synephrine. Cauterize bleeders as necessary with a bipolar cautery.
- After the globe is removed, inspect the inside of Tenon's capsule in its entirety.
- Place the 6-0 chromic gut sutures through the posterior rent in Tenon's capsule but only if it is large. Tamponade the cavity with a 22-mm stainless steel "sizer."[l]
- A "baseball" implant using a 20-mm hydroxyapatite sphere is usually the preferred size for an adult; however, the proper size of the implant must first be determined by using the stainless steel sizer set (available in 16, 18, 20, and 22 mm sizes).

- ○ Insert them sequentially until the supratarsal sulcus "fills out" and no tendency for spontaneous extrusion appears to occur.
- ○ Remember that a 20-mm hydroxyapatite sphere wrapped like a baseball is in actuality a 22-mm implant because of the wrap's thickness. Never obliterate the fornices, as ocularists must have some depth here to create a custom-made prosthetic eye that can later be "drilled out" for the integration peg.

> ## PITFALL
>
> Never cram a large implant into any orbit; otherwise, it is likely to extrude sooner or later.

- A "baseball" implant is created by wrapping the hydroxyapatite with a graft of autogenous posterior auricular muscle complex or autogenous fascia lata around the sphere.
- Impregnate the hydroxyapatite by placing the sphere in a 50-mL syringe filled with at least 20 mL of 0.75% Marcaine, and apply negative pressure by pulling on the plunger while occluding the syringe's tip, which causes the fluid to be sucked into the sphere's empty pores. This drug delivery system provides profound postoperative analgesia, anesthesia, and akinesia.
- Wrap the Marcaine-saturated ball with posterior auricular muscle complex graft or autogenous fascia lata, and suture the seams with 5-0 Vicryl sutures (P-3 needle). Just anterior to the equator of this complex wrap, cut four 2 × 5 mm windows 90 degrees apart to allow placement or suturing of the rectus muscles.

> **PEARL...** Autogenous material may provide a better wrap with less risk of transmission of infection. Alternative wrap materials include donor sclera, fascia lata, and dura (see Chapter 15).

- To encourage vascularization, drill shallow (1 to 2 mm) holes in the hydroxyapatite implant with an 18-gauge needle. These windows will allow vascular ingrowth to occur faster and also motility, thus enabling a peg to be inserted at a later date to complete the integration of prosthesis and implant.

---

[k] If the optic nerve is cut too short in the presence of an intraocular malignancy, such as malignant melanoma or retinoblastoma, and if the nerve is involved by the tumor, cells may spread beyond the cut section. This must obviously be avoided. Cutting the nerve under direct visualization ensures not only that an adequate section of the nerve is obtained but also that the posterior sclera is not inadvertently severed. If the latter happens, the remainder of the globe plus all extruded intraocular contents must be removed; an exenteration may be indicated if the eye harbors melanoma. In this hypothetical situation the patient's survival rate is uniformly poor. Conversely, cutting the nerve too long damages the posterior portion of Tenon's capsule, but this can be sutured without morbidity.

[l] Integrated Orbital Implants, Bio-Eye, San Diego, California.

- Insert the implant into Tenon's capsule and sequentially suture all four rectus muscles to the four corresponding windows located just anterior to its equator. Meticulously close Tenon's capsule with interrupted 4-0 Vicryl sutures (FS-2 needle); obtain generous bites of Tenon's capsule because this is the primary tissue barrier responsible for retaining the implant and preventing extrusion.
  - Never use nonabsorbable sutures (e.g., silk, nylon, Prolene, or Mersilene) as they will eventually extrude, leading to fistula formation and dehiscence of the Tenon's capsule and conjunctiva.
  - Avoid using traumatic suturing techniques such as pulling on the conjunctiva repeatedly with toothed forceps. Remember that Tenon's capsule is also traumatized and weakened by overzealous dissection of conjunctiva.
- The conjunctiva is closed with multiple 6-0 chromic gut and a conformer is inserted within the socket. Consider a 4-0 Frost suture of silk with rubber stints, "in and out through the gray line" of the eyelids for the first 7 to 10 postoperative days so that the conformer will not extrude.
  - If the conformer is too small or too large, ask an ocularist to customize one.
- At the end of the procedure, a 4-mL Duranest retrobulbar block for postoperative pain relief as well as regional blocks of the supraorbital, infratrochlear, and lacrimal nerves are necessary.
- Finally, pressure patch the orbit for 24 hours.

Auricular Muscle Complex Graft

Harvest the posterior auricular muscle complex graft on the same side as the enucleation so that the patient's head can move toward the opposite side during anesthesia.

- Instruct the patient to shampoo the scalp the night prior to surgery.
- Inject 1% lidocaine and epinephrine (1:100,000) subcutaneously 15 minutes prior to the onset of surgery in the retroauricular fold and into the helix.
- Place two 4-0 silk sutures at the upper and lower aspects of the helix and rotate the pinna anteriorly, fixating it in this position by attaching hemostats to them or suturing them to the preauricular skin.
- Perform a U-shaped skin incision with a No. 15 Bard-Parker blade at the posteromedial edge of the entire helix and extend it inferiorly toward the mastoid process. Use retractors and sharp dissection at the level of the "rete pegs" to reflect the posterior auricular skin. Dissect the skin in this plane past the entire pinna and extend it posteriorly over the mastoid process as needed according to size requirements.

  - Occasionally, a branch of the posterior auricular artery is cut and will need cautery. It lies near the hairline on the level of the external auditory canal.
- To elevate the posterior auricular muscle complex graft, start back at the helix and deepen the initial incision to the plane of the posterior auricular cartilage at the level of the perichondrium. Reflect this sheet of posterior auricular muscle complex graft with sharp dissection and harvest the appropriate size. It is permissible to include small superficial bites of auricular cartilage in the dissection if the graft's dissection becomes too thin.
  - Vary the graft in size, length, and width, depending on the size of the ear and diameter of the implant to be covered.
- Once harvested, arrange the posterior auricular muscle complex graft, placing thicker tissue that comes from the mastoid area and has greater tensile strength over the portion of the implant that will come to rest anteriorly in the orbit; this will reduce the chance of implant extrusion.
- Obtain meticulous hemostasis of this highly vascular donor bed with the bipolar or Bovie cautery, and follow by placing small bits of Gelfoam soaked in 0.25% Neo-Synephrine. These absorb in 4 to 7 days. Lightly cauterize or avoid cautery altogether on the dermal flap to prevent flap necrosis.
- Following hemostasis, close the auricular skin margin with interrupted sutures of 6-0 silk or nylon. Secure anterior and posterior Xeroform stints sandwiching the pinnae between them by double-armed sutures of 4-0 silk or Prolene passed full-thickness through the pinnae in two separate places to discourage cartilaginous hematoma. Tie these sutures with enough tension to prevent bleeding but not so tight as to cause cheese wiring compression necrosis.
- Caution the patient against aggressive manipulation of the scalp hair for 48 hours, which might stimulate bleeding or wound dehiscence.
- At the end of the procedure, apply a Glasscock mastoid splint[m] for 24 to 48 hours. A small Penrose drain placed between the helical sutures may be used if necessary. Use prophylactic antibiotics for 10 days.

> **PITFALL**
>
> Remember that in monocular persons wearing a prosthesis, the endophthalmitis rate is higher in case of open globe surgery; prophylaxis requires certain precautions (see Table 31-1).

[m]Oto-Med, Inc., Lake Havasu City, Arizona.

TABLE 31-1   PRECAUTIONS TO PREVENT ENDOPHTHALMITIS DEVELOPMENT IN THE PROSTHESIS-WEARING MONOCULAR PATIENT UNDERGOING OPEN GLOBE SURGERY[8]

Preoperatively
Examination of both the prosthetic and the operative sockets for any sign of infection or inflammation
Patient education with regard to personal hygiene and the rationale for the preoperative preparation
Preoperative cultures of both conjunctival fornices
Topical antibiotics: if the cultures are negative, broad-spectrum antibiotics for 48–72 hours; if the cultures are positive, appropriate antibiotic for as long as necessary to prove the operative field sterile by repeated cultures
Removal of the prosthesis as soon as antibiotic prophylaxis is instituted

Perioperatively
Preparation of the conjunctivae with povidone-iodine
Irrigation of the eye with saline solution
Microfiltration of all irrigation fluids
Preservation of an intact posterior capsule
Subconjunctival broad-spectrum antibiotics

Postoperatively
Antibiotic drops topically
Nonocclusive shield without patch
Appropriate instructions and careful follow-up with particular attention to complaints of pain or decreased visual acuity

Complications of enucleation include:

- dehiscence of the conjunctiva;
- extrusion of the orbital implant;
- ptosis;
- poor ocular motility;
- enophthalmos;
- orbital hemorrhage;
- orbital infection; and
- contracted socket syndrome.

PITFALL

Common factors leading to conjunctival dehiscence include poor surgical technique, improper suture material, and the use of an implant that is too large.

PEARL... If a dehiscence is small and noted within weeks of surgery, débridement and resuturing may salvage the procedure.

SUMMARY

Enucleation and evisceration are the most common options for treating patients who either present with severe eye injuries that cannot be anatomically reconstructed or have a permanently blind and painful eye following a serious ocular injury. The choice between these procedures is still controversial and has both anatomical and psychological implications. With the development of integratable orbital implants such as the hydroxyapatite and medpor, the cosmetic outcome of enucleation approaches that of evisceration, although the latter may be more physiological to the health of the orbit (see Chapter 36).

332 • SECTION III   MECHANICAL GLOBE INJURIES

REFERENCES

1. Ruedemann AD Jr. Sympathetic ophthalmic after evisceration. *Trans Am Ophthalmol Soc*. 1963;61:274–313.

2. Green WR, Maumenee AE, Sanders TE, et al. Sympathetic uveitis following evisceration. *Trans Am Acad Ophthalmol Otolaryngol*. 1972;76:625.

3. Albert DM, Diaz-Rohena R. A historical review of sympathetic ophthalmia and its epidemiology. *Surv Ophthalmol*. 1989:31:1.

4. Albert DM, Jakobiec FA. *Clinical Practice. Principles and Practice of Ophthalmology*. Philadelphia: WB Saunders; 1994.

5. Green WR. The uveal tract. In: Spencer WH, ed. *Ophthalmic Pathology: An Atlas and Textbook*. Philadelphia: WB Saunders; 1986:1915–1956.

6. Perry AC. Advances in enucleation. *Ophthalmol Clin North Am*. 1991;4:173–182.

7. Dutton JJ. Coralline hydroxyapatite as an ocular implant. *Ophthalmology*. 1991;98:370–377.

8. Morris R, Camesasca FI, Byrne J, John G. Postoperative endophthalmitis resulting from prosthesis contamination in a monocular patient. *Am J Ophthalmol*. 1993;116: 346–349.

ADDITIONAL READING

Callahan MA, Callahan A. *Ophthalmic Plastic and Orbital Surgery*. Birmingham, AL: Aesculapius Publishing Co; 1979.

Croxatto JO, Rao NA, McLean W, et al. Atypical histopathologic features in sympathetic ophthalmia: a study of 100 cases. *Int Ophthalmol Clin*. 1981;4:129.

Gass JDM. Sympathetic ophthalmia following vitrectomy. *Am J Ophthalmol*. 1982;93:552.

Jennings T, Tessier HH. Twenty cases of sympathetic ophthalmia. *Br J Ophthalmol*. 1989;73:140.

Lubin JR, Albert DM, Weinstein M. Sixty-five years of sympathetic ophthalmia: a clinicopathologic review of 105 cases (1913–1978). *Ophthalmology*. 1980;87:109–121.

Marak GE Jr. Recent advances in sympathetic ophthalmia. *Surv Ophthalmol*. 1979;24:141.

Michelson J. *Color Atlas of Uveitis*. 2nd ed. St. Louis: Mosby; 1992.

Nussenblatt RB, Whitcup SM, Palestine AG. *Uveitis. Fundamentals and Clinical Practice*. St. Louis: Mosby; 1996.

Remulla HD, Rubin PAD, Shore JW, et al. Complications of porous spherical orbital implants. *Ophthalmology*. 1995; 102:586–593.

Shields CL, Shields JA, De Potter P. Hydroxyapatite orbital implant after enucleation. Experience with initial 100 consecutive cases. *Arch Ophthalmol*. 1992;10:333–338.

Shields CL, Shields JA, De Potter P, et al. Lack of complications of the hydroxyapatite orbital implant in 250 consecutive cases. From the Oncology Service, Wills Eye Hospital, Thomas Jefferson University, Philadelphia.

Spencer WH. *Ophthalmic Pathology. An Atlas and Textbook*. Philadelphia: WB Saunders; 1986.

SECTION IV

NONMECHANICAL GLOBE INJURIES

Chapter 32

CHEMICAL INJURIES: CLINICAL COURSE AND MANAGEMENT

Michael D. Wagoner and Kenneth R. Kenyon

 The etiology and therapeutic strategies for acute management of chemical injuries of the eye were discussed in Chapter 11; here we focus on the pathophysiologic mechanisms that influence subsequent therapeutic strategies; the evolving clinical course; specific therapeutic recommendations during the acute, early repair, and late repair phases; and the visual rehabilitation of patients with severe chemical injuries.

PATHOPHYSIOLOGY

The management of chemical injuries after initial emergency intervention is based on an understanding of the complex interactions between:

- ocular surface regeneration;
- stromal matrix degradation and repair; and
- the inflammatory response.

Ocular Surface[a] Regeneration

Centripetal movement of cells from the peripheral cornea, limbus, or conjunctiva is responsible for the normal[2,3] or pathologic[4,5] replacement of the corneal epithelium. The limbal epithelial region serves as the generative tissue for corneal epithelial cells (Fig. 32–2).[6–8,b]

Following epithelial débridement of the entire corneal and limbal epithelium, the surrounding conjunctival epithelium not only resurfaces the cornea

---

[a] The term "ocular surface" emphasizes the interdependence of the stratified, nonkeratinizing epithelium of the cornea and conjunctiva (Fig. 32–1).[1]

[b] As proved by experimental studies, including specific immunolocalization.

but also evolves to resemble the normal corneal epithelium phenotypically.[9]

> **PEARL...** The process termed "transdifferentiation"[10] (i.e., the conjunctival epithelium evolving to become corneal epithelium) established the rationale for conjunctival autograft transplantation as a means of surgically restoring the ocular surface of chemically injured eyes.[11]

Transdifferentiation of the conjunctival epithelium is, however, rarely (if ever) complete, especially after *severe* chemical injury,[1,12,13] and is associated with:

- delayed reepithelialization[14];
- superficial and deep stromal neovascularization[12];
- persistence of goblet cells within the corneal epithelium[13]; and
- recurrent epithelial erosions due to abnormal epithelial basement membrane[14].

If the limbal stem cell loss is complete, severe superficial pannus invariably occurs, resulting in "conjunctivalization" of the resurfaced cornea.[15]

> **PEARL...** The limbal stem cells appear to be the most qualified cells to restore functional competence after extensive ocular surface as well as limbal stem cell injury.[16,17]

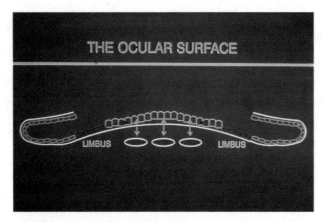

FIGURE 32–1 Schematic depiction of the ocular surface, demonstrating the continuity of the conjunctival (blue), limbal (red), and corneal (green) epithelium and the interactive relationship (arrows) between the corneal epithelium and stromal keratocytes. (From Wagoner MD. Chemical injuries of the eye: current concepts in pathophysiology and therapy. *Surv Ophthalmol.* 1997;41:275–313. Reprinted with permission from Elsevier Science.)

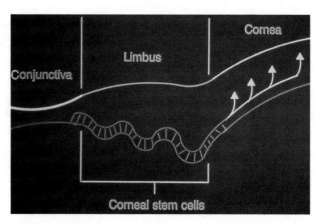

FIGURE 32–2 Schematic depiction of the corneal basal epithelial cells. Basal epithelial (stem) cells migrate centripetally along the basal epithelial layer and then anterior toward the surface. (From Wagoner MD, Kenyon KR, Shore JS. Ocular surface transplantation. In: Barrie J, Kirkness C, eds. *Recent Advances in Ophthalmology.* Vol 9. New York: Churchill Livingstone; 1995:59–90. Reprinted with permission from Churchill Livingstone.)

Corneal Stromal Degradation and Repair

> **PEARL...** The maintenance and regeneration of the corneal stroma are the primary function of the keratocyte.[18,19] Following chemical injury, keratocytes[c] are mobilized from adjacent regions to repopulate the area of injury.[24]

> **PITFALL**
>
> Keratocyte synthesis of collagen may be compromised by deficient levels of ascorbate in the aqueous following severe chemical injury[25] or by the injudicious use of topical corticosteroids.[26,27]

Type I collagen synthesis is maximum between days 7 and 56, with a peak at day 21.[24] It is essential to prevent stromal ulceration due to collagenolysis.

• MMPs (formerly known as collagenase) cause specific cleavage of the collagen molecule.[28,29] MMP-1

and MMP-8,[d] produced by keratocytes[21,22] and polymorphonuclear leukocytes,[30,31] respectively, can degrade type I, II, or III fibrillar collagen in the corneal stroma. These enzymes are not present in significant amounts until 14–21 days after chemical injury, corresponding to the period of maximal collagen synthesis and repair.[32]

Inflammatory Response

The association of inflammation with corneal ulceration and its cessation following exclusion of inflammatory cells are well recognized.[33–36]

Within 12–24 hours after chemical injury, infiltration of the peripheral cornea with inflammatory cells occurs.[37] If the injury is severe, a second wave of inflammatory cell infiltration:

• begins at 7 days; and
• peaks between 14 and 21 days when corneal repair and degradation are maximal.[37]

Persistent inflammation may delay reepithelialization[38] and perpetuate continued inflammatory cell recruitment, thereby initiating a vicious circle of progressive inflammatory cell-related destruction of the corneal stroma.

CLINICAL EVALUATION AND COURSE

Previous gradings of chemical injury severity[39,40] stressed the prognostic importance of vascular ischemia and necrosis in the limbal zone.

---

[c] These cells may perform multiple fibroblastic activities including phagocytosis of collagen fibrils,[20] synthesis of collagen,[20] collagenase,[21,22] and collagenase inhibitors.[22] These functions may be regulated by cytokines from epithelium[22] and inflammatory cells.[23]

[d] Formerly type I collagenase.

Table 32–1 shows the limbal stem cell based classification system[41] we propose to guide the intervention and predict the outcome.

The clinical course (see Table 32–2) after chemical injury progresses through three distinct phases:

- acute (0–7 days);
- early repair (7–21 days); and
- late repair (>21 days).[42]

The *healing pattern* occurring during these phases correlates with the original degree of limbal stem cell

TABLE 32–1   THE LIMBAL STEM CELL BASED CLASSIFICATION SYSTEM

Grade	Stem Cells	See Figure
Grade I	Little or no loss of stem cells	3A, C
Grade II	Subtotal stem cell loss	4A, C
Grade III	Complete stem cell loss	5A, C
Grade IV	Complete stem cell loss + loss of proximal conjunctival epithelium	6A, C

injury and provides support for subsequent therapeutic decisions.

THERAPEUTIC PRINCIPLES

Three-Step Approach
Our modified three-step approach to sterile corneal ulceration, (that is:

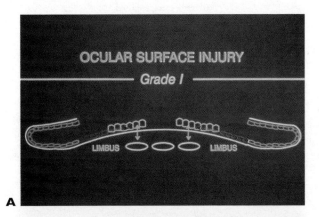
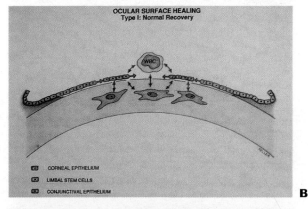
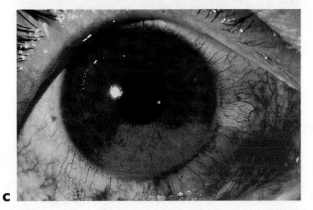
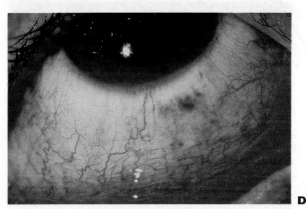

FIGURE 32–3 **(A)** Grade I chemical injury: schematic. The epithelial defect involves corneal epithelium but not limbal stem cells. **(B)** Type I healing pattern: schematic. During the brief period required for reepithelialization with normal phenotypic epithelium, all interactions between epithelium, inflammatory cells, and keratocytes are appropriate for repair. **(C)** Grade I chemical injury: clinical appearance. Epithelial defect involving one quadrant without significant limbal ischemia or evidence of limbal stem cell loss. **(D)** Type I healing pattern: clinical appearance. Prompt reepithelialization with normal corneal epithelial appearance without vascularization confirms that limbal stem cells adjacent to the corneal epithelial defect were unaffected by the chemical injury. (From Wagoner MD. Chemical injuries of the eye: current concepts in pathophysiology and therapy. *Surv Ophthalmol.* 1997;41:275–313. Reprinted with permission from Elsevier Science.)

Table 32–2   The Clinical Course after Chemical Injury

Phase (Days) and Type	Clinical Picture	See Figure
Acute (0–7)		
Type I	Reepithelialize without incident	3B, D
Type II	Delayed reepithelialization	4B
Type III	Little or no reepithelialization	5B
Type IV	Little or no reepithelialization	6B
Early repair (7–21)		
Type II	Delayed reepithelialization in deficient quadrant +/− vascularization	
Type III	Persistent epithelial defect	
Type IV	Persistent epithelial defect	
Late repair (21+)		
Type II	Persistent epitheliopathy with or without neovascularization in limbal stem cell–deficient quadrant	4D
Type III	Little or no reepithelialization, with progressive "conjunctivalization" of the corneal surface over a several month period	5D
Type IV	Continued absence of epithelium from both the proximal conjunctiva and cornea with development of sterile corneal ulceration	6D

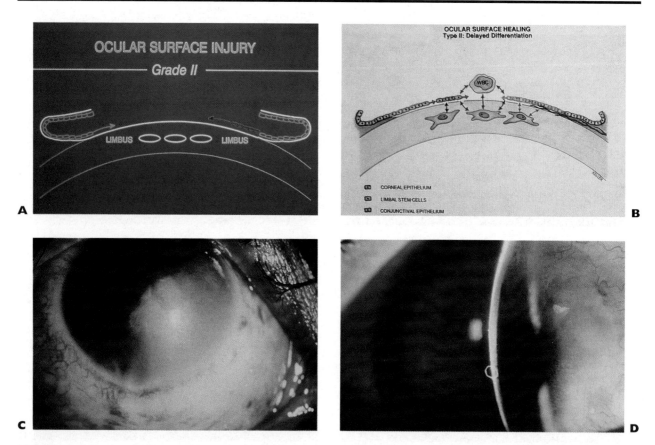

FIGURE 32–4   (A) Grade II chemical injury: schematic. Injury to the corneal epithelium and partial limbal stem cell loss. **(B)** Type II healing pattern: schematic. Reepithelialization from areas of normal limbal stem cells proceeds normally, while reepithelialization in areas of limbal stem cell loss is initially from conjunctival epithelium. Transient subepithelial vascularization may accompany the conjunctival epithelium. Interactions between epithelium, inflammatory cells, and keratocytes are usually appropriate for repair. **(C)** Grade II chemical injury: clinical appearance. In the quadrant with epithelial defect there is obvious limbal ischemia and probable loss of limbal stem cells (in contrast to the appearance in Fig. 32–5C). **(D)** Type II healing pattern: clinical appearance. Following reepithelialization, there are persistent epitheliopathy, subepithelial vascularization, and stromal haze. (From Wagoner MD. Chemical injuries of the eye: current concepts in pathophysiology and therapy. *Surv Ophthalmol*. 1997;41:275–313. Reprinted with permission from Elsevier Science.)

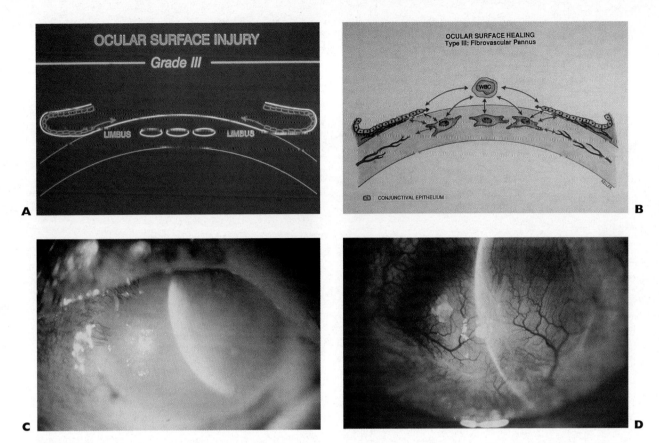

FIGURE 32–5   (A) Grade III chemical injury: schematic. There is loss of all corneal epithelium and limbal stem cells but preservation of the proximal conjunctiva. (B) Type III healing pattern: schematic. All reepithelialization must come from the conjunctival epithelium, which is usually considerably delayed. Interactions between the conjunctival epithelium, inflammatory cells, and keratocytes may or may not result in appropriate corneal repair. (C) Grade III chemical injury: clinical appearance. There is complete corneal and proximal conjunctival epithelial defect with loss of corneal stromal clarity. (D) Type III healing pattern: clinical appearance. There is complete coverage of the cornea with "conjunctivalized" epithelium and superficial and deep stromal vascularization. (A and B from Wagoner MD. Chemical injuries of the eye: current concepts in pathophysiology and therapy. *Surv Ophthalmol.* 1997;41:275–313. Reprinted with permission from Elsevier Science. C and D from Wagoner MD, Kenyon KR, Shore JS. Ocular surface transplantation. In: Barrie J, Kirkness C, eds. *Recent Advances in Ophthalmology.* Vol 9. New York: Churchill Livingstone; 1995:59–90. Reprinted with permission from Churchill Livingstone.)

1. promoting reepithelialization/transdifferentiation;
2. limbal stem cell transplantation; and
3. human amniotic membrane transplantation);

remains applicable to the entire clinical course following chemical injury.[34,35]

Step 1. Promoting Reepithelialization/ Transdifferentiation

The reestablishment of an intact and phenotypically normal corneal epithelium is the most important determinant of favorable outcome following chemical injury. In grade III or IV injuries,[e] surgical restora-

tion of a suitable stem cell population is mandatory to achieve this objective.

Step 2. Limbal Stem Cell Transplantation

Limbal autograft transplantation involves harvesting from the limbus of the patient's uninjured or less injured contralateral eye:

- two crescents of peripheral corneal limbal epithelium with
- a corresponding section of the conjunctiva (Fig. 32–7).[16]

This treatment is becoming standard even in the early clinical course of severe chemical injury, *prior to* the development of conjunctivalization of the cornea

---

[e] As confirmed by a type III or IV healing pattern.

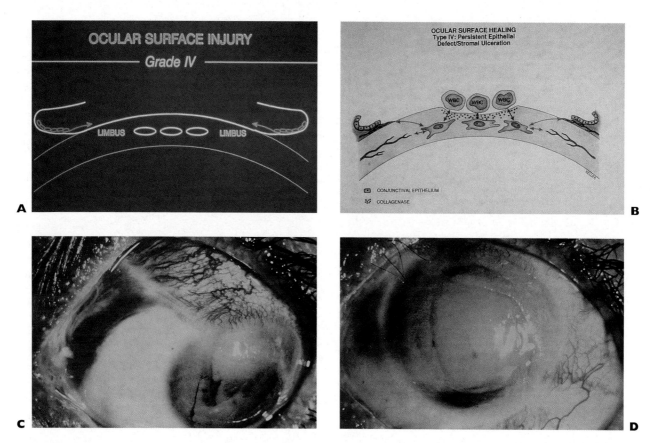

FIGURE 32-6   **(A)** Grade IV chemical injury: schematic. There is loss of all corneal epithelium and limbal stem cells and proximal conjunctiva. **(B)** Type IV healing pattern: schematic. Little or no reepithelialization is expected from the distal conjunctival epithelium. Interactions between inflammatory cells and keratocytes, in the absence of modulation by migrating epithelium, result in excessive collagenolysis instead of appropriate repair. **(C)** Grade IV chemical injury: clinical appearance. Complete corneal epithelial defect with limbal ischemia remains unchanged 4 months after the original injury. **(D)** Type IV healing pattern: clinical appearance. Sterile corneal ulceration with perforation and iris prolapse in the inferior cornea. A mature cataract is also present. (**A** and **B** from Wagoner MD. Chemical injuries of the eye: current concepts in pathophysiology and therapy. *Surv Ophthalmol*. 1997;41:275–313. Reprinted with permission from Elsevier Science. **D** from Mandel ER, Wagoner MD. *Atlas of Corneal Disease*. Philadelphia: WB Saunders; 1989:72. Reprinted with permission from WB Saunders.

surface in grade III injury (Fig. 32–8) or corneal stromal ulceration in grade IV injury (Fig. 32–9).

Limbal allograft transplantation with stem cells obtained from a living relative[43–45] or cadavers[46–49] is necessary in bilateral injuries.

- Limbal tissue may be harvested from the entire circumference of cadavers and transplanted to the entire limbal zone of the donor eye.[46,47]

- Limbal tissue harvested from living relatives is obtained in a manner identical to that described for limbal autografts, taking care not to excise more than 6 clock hours of limbal tissue.[43]

> **P**EARL... The remarkable proliferation and pluripotential differentiation characteristics of limbal stem cells provided the stimulus for investigation into the possibility that small numbers of harvested cells could be amplified in vitro and subsequently transplanted into a recipient eye.

- It has been demonstrated that human limbal stem cells can survive in animal models.[50,51]

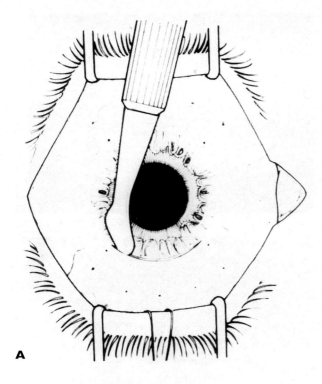

A

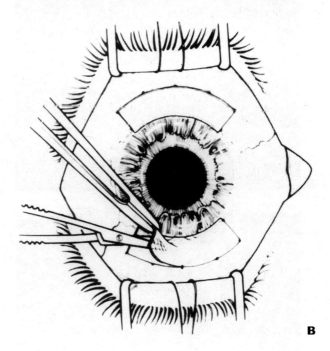

B

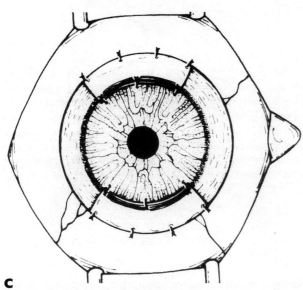

C

FIGURE 32–7 Technique of limbal stem cell transplantation. **(A)** Superior and inferior grafts limbal grafts are delineated with focal applications of cautery approximately 2 mm posterior to the limbus. The initial incision is made superficially within clear cornea and dissected posteriorly to the corneal limbus. **(B)** The bulbar conjunctival portion is undermined and thinly dissected anteriorly to its limbal attachment. The corneal portion of the dissection is then cut from the globe, with the limbal bulbar conjunctiva attached. **(C)** The limbal grafts are transferred to their corresponding sites in the recipient eye, where a corresponding dissection has been performed in the donor bed. The grafts are secured with 10-0 nylon sutures at the corneal edge and 7–0 Vicryl sutures at the conjunctival margin. (From Kenyon KR, Tseng SCG. Limbal autograft transplantation for ocular surface disorders. *Ophthalmology*. 1989;96:709–722. Reprinted with permission from Elsevier Science.)

- Autologously cultured corneal epithelium was able to restore the ocular surface in humans with unilateral alkali injury.[52]

- Transplantation of autologously and allogenically derived, cultured limbal stem cells on an amniotic membrane matrix was successful in humans.[53]

PEARL... This technology not only offers the prospect of providing larger numbers of limbal stem cells to severely injured eyes but also reduces the risk of potential complications related to limbal stem cell reduction in the donor eye.[52,53]

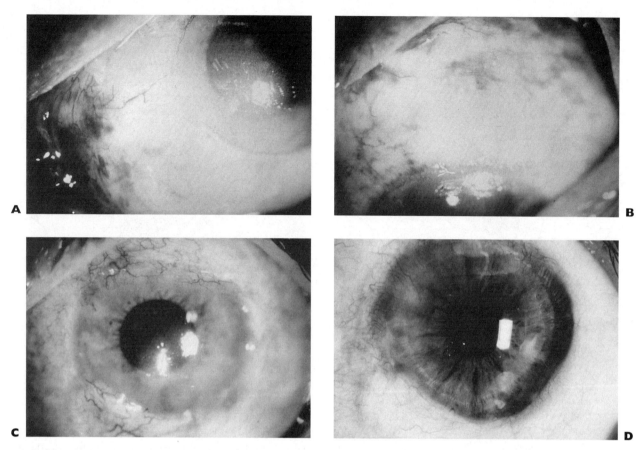

FIGURE 32–8   Limbal autograft, early intervention. (**A** and **B**) Preoperative appearance. Four weeks following an alkali injury, there is extensive limbal ischemia and no evidence of corneal epithelial recovery. (**C**) Postoperative appearance. Corneal epithelialization has been complete since 1 week. At 1 month, the corneal epithelium and stroma are clear and the visual acuity is 20/50, in contrast to the anticipated appearance of grade III injury, type III healing pattern without stem cell rehabilitation. (**D**) Postoperative appearance, 2 years. The corneal epithelial appearance remains normal, the stroma is clear and free of vascularization, and the visual acuity is 20/25. (From Wagoner MD, Kenyon KR, Shore JS. Ocular surface transplantation. In: Barrie J, Kirkness C, eds. *Recent Advances in Ophthalmology*. Vol 9. New York: Churchill Livingstone; 1995:59–90. Reprinted with permission from Churchill Livingstone.)

▼ PITFALL

The success of limbal allogenic stem cells, irrespective of source (cadaver vs. living relative) or transfer technique (direct vs. cell culture amplification), is compromised by immunologically mediated rejection of limbal allograft stem cells.[54,55]

The two factors contributing to the much higher rate of limbal stem cell rejection compared with PK are:

- a higher concentration of transplanted antigens in the peripheral cornea from which stem cells are harvested; and

- the transplantation of vascular tissue into a vascular bed.

PEARL... Topical and systemic immunosuppression results in a statistically significant increase in the rate of limbal allograft stem cell survival.[44,49]

One specific treatment recommendation is the use of:

- topical corticosteroids and cyclosporine indefinitely; and

- triple systemic immunosuppressive therapy (prednisone, cyclosporin A, and azathioprine) for at least 12–24 months.[55]

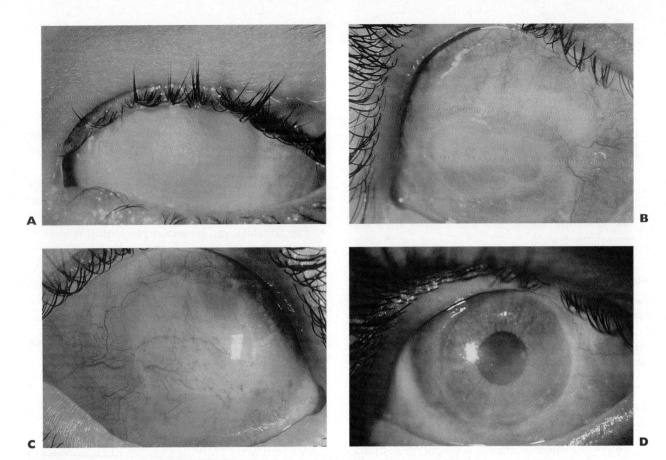

FIGURE 32-9 Limbal autograft (early intervention) with subsequent lamellar keratoplasty (late rehabilitation) in 5-year-old boy with alkali injury. **(A)** On injury day, the vision was light perception with marked corneal haze, 360 degrees of limbal ischemia, and loss of proximal conjunctiva, suggestive of grade IV injury. **(B)** When no corneal reepithelialization had occurred by 4 weeks, limbal autograft transplantation was performed to prevent sterile corneal ulceration, which characteristically occurs in the late repair phase with type IV healing patterns. **(C)** Nine months after limbal stem cell transplantation, the epithelium is intact, but the stroma remains opacified due to the original penetration of alkali with development of moderate stromal vascularization. **(D)** Fourteen months after limbal transplantation, a lamellar keratoplasty was performed. Nine years later the cornea has a healthy epithelial surface, the stroma is clear, and the visual acuity is 20/40. (From Wagoner MD, Kenyon KR, Shore JS. Ocular surface transplantation. In: Barrie J, Kirkness C, eds. *Recent Advances in Ophthalmology*. Vol 9. New York: Churchill Livingstone; 1995:59–90. Reprinted with permission from Churchill Livingstone.)

Step 3. Human Amniotic Membrane Transplantation

This membrane contains a thick basement membrane and serves as a strong and stable connective tissue substrate.[f]

> **PEARL...** Fresh or cryopreserved amniotic membrane transplantation has been successfully utilized to promote reepithelialization and prevent conjunctivalization of the ocular surface in experimental[57] and clinical[58] chemical injuries.

Advantages of the use of human amniotic membrane[g] include:

- lack of antigenicity; and
- ease of surgical manipulation.[58]

The amniotic membrane:

- provides an excellent matrix for epithelial migration;
- augments the function of existing stem cells; and

---

[f]Fresh membrane, obtained from the human placenta, was used as early as 1940 to repair conjunctival defects and symblepharon.[56]

[g]It can be prepared by separation from the chorion, flattening and placement on nitrocellulose paper, and storage at −80°C in Dulbecco's modified Eagle's medium and glycerol until used.[58] The amniotic membrane is peeled from the nitrocellulose paper at the time of surgery, placed on the recipient cornea to cover the deepithelialized surface, and sutured with 10-0 nylon sutures.[58]

- possibly enhances stem cell survival by reducing limbal inflammation,[61,62] although it does not replace limbal stem cell function.

The algorithm for use of amniotic membrane transplantation after chemical injury depends upon the concomitant status of the limbal stem cells.

- In case of incomplete stem cell loss with persistent epithelial defect (e.g., grade II injury), use amniotic membrane transplantation *alone*.
- In case of complete limbal stem cell loss with persistent epithelial defect (e.g., grade III or IV injury), use amniotic membrane *and* limbal stem cell transplantation.

Supportive Repair and Minimizing Ulceration

Successful restoration of a phenotypically normal, limbal stem cell–derived corneal epithelium has greatly reduced the need to resort to surgical intervention to address corneal ulceration with impending or actual perforation. Still, circumstances may arise where one of the following procedures may be required.

Tenoplasty

In grade IV injuries, the most immediate concerns are:

- the development of anterior segment necrosis due to loss of the limbal vascular blood supply; and
- the failure to reepithelialize with subsequent sterile corneal ulceration (Fig. 32–6).

> **P**EARL... **Advancement of Tenon's flaps may arrest or prevent sterile corneal ulceration in grade IV injuries.**

Tissue Adhesives

These are effective for the management of impending or actual perforation related to sterile ulceration of the corneal stroma following chemical injury.[33,36,60]

> **P**EARL... **In addition to providing immediate tectonic support, tissue adhesive arrests further ulceration by excluding inflammatory cells from the site and inducing fibrovascular scarring.[33,36]**

Tissue adhesives are best reserved for:

- impending perforations; or
- actual perforations of 1 mm or less.[60]

Details of application of tissue adhesives are listed below.

- Under the slit lamp/operating microscope, cyanoacrylate glue can easily be applied to the area of ulceration or perforation.
- A durable bandage soft contact lens is then usually used to provide comfort and reduce the chances of dislodgment of the glue.
- The adhesive can be left in place until it loosens spontaneously as a result of reepithelialization.
- It can be removed with jeweler's forceps after 6 to 8 weeks, when the inflammation has subsided and neovascularization of the area has eliminated the risk of recurrent ulceration.

> **PITFALL**
>
> Unfortunately, the fibrovascular scar results in poor visual acuity and worsens the prognosis of a PK. Still, repair with tissue adhesive remains vastly preferable to emergency tectonic keratoplasty.

Tectonic Keratoplasty

This may be required in the urgent setting of acute perforation not amenable to tissue adhesive.[61]

- A small tectonic keratoplasty can be used to "buy time" if the perforation is relatively small, until vascularization of the graft bed arrests further corneal ulceration.
- Until this occurs, it is often necessary to:
  - diligently replace sutures that loosen prematurely; and
  - treat recurrent ulceration in the graft or at the graft-host junction with cyanoacrylate glue.
- Rarely, multiple sequential tectonic keratoplasties are required to provide tectonic stability to the globe.

Large-Diameter Therapeutic PK

Encouraging results have been reported with the use of large-diameter (11–12 mm) PK in both the acute and chronic setting for the management of severe chemical injury.[62,63]

PEARL... Transferring not only corneal tissue for tectonic support but also limbal stem cells to restore and maintain a phenotypically normal corneal epithelium, large-diameter PK addresses the issues of both tectonic support and visual rehabilitation.

Topical and systemic immunosuppression is mandatory to help prevent immunologic rejection of the ocular surface epithelium.

Controlling Inflammation

Aggressive control of inflammation remains a high priority during the early and late repair phases.

PITFALL

It is important to recognize that continued use of topical corticosteroids may interfere with keratocyte migration and collagen synthesis during this period.[26,27] If corneal repair is insufficient to offset collagenolysis occurring in response to collagenolytic activity, progressive degradation ("melting") of the corneal stroma can occur.

PEARL... Progestational steroids do not significantly interfere with corneal repair[64] and can be substituted for corticosteroids at this time. Although not as potent anti-inflammatory agents as corticosteroids, progestational steroids have some anticollagenolytic properties[64] and may inhibit further ulceration after chemical injuries.[65,66]

SPECIFIC THERAPY

The most significant error made during the late repair phase is failure to proceed with surgical intervention to address the problems of persistent epithelial defects and stromal ulceration occurring as a consequence of limbal stem cell loss.

• Acute phase (days 0–7): see Chapter 11, Table 11–2.

• Early repair phase (days 7–21): see Table 32–3.

PITFALL

The most significant error during the late repair phase is failure to proceed with *surgical intervention* to address the problems of persistent epithelial defects related to either partial or complete limbal stem cell loss.

• Late repair phase (days >21):
  ○ Type II healing pattern: amniotic membrane transplantation +/− limbal stem cell transplantation.[h]
  ○ Type III or IV healing patterns: limbal stem cell transplantation +/− amniotic membrane transplantation.
  ○ Unilateral injury: autograft (contralateral eye).
  ○ Bilateral injury: allograft (living relative, cadaver, cultured stem cells).[i]
  ○ If the globe is tectonically unstable: large-diameter (11–12 mm) PK with systemic/topical immunosuppression.

Table 32–4 shows the elements of adjunctive medical treatment.

Late Rehabilitation (>3 Months)

Many times the severity of the initial injury and/or the failure to restore adequate limbal stem cell function results in:

• persistent epitheliopathy; or
• conjunctivalization of the ocular surface, with or without conjunctival cicatrization and distortion of normal globe–lid relationships.

PITFALL

The most frequent error in rehabilitative efforts is the failure to adequately restore limbal stem cell function and/or address conjunctival cicatricial abnormalities *before* proceeding with lamellar keratoplasty or PK.

---

[h] If persistent epithelial defect (especially if corneal thinning) develops.

[i] Adjunctive systemic/topical immunosuppression is required.

TABLE 32-3   EARLY PHASE TREATMENT OF THE CHEMICALLY INJURED EYE

Drugs in the Early Repair Phase (Days 7–21)	Dosage
Discontinue or taper (with careful observation) topical corticosteroids	
Substitute topical medroxyprogesterone 1%	Every hour while awake, every 2 hours at night
Topical sodium ascorbate 10%	Every 4 hours
Systemic sodium ascorbate 2 g	2 × daily p. os
Topical sodium citrate 10%	Every 4 hours
Topical tetracycline	4 × daily
Systemic doxycycline 100 mg	2 × daily p. os
Antiglaucoma	As needed

TABLE 32-4   ADJUNCTIVE MEDICAL TREATMENT DURING THE LATE REPAIR PHASE OF A CHEMICAL INJURY

Drug	Dosage
Topical medroxyprogesterone 1%*	Every 1 to 2 hours while awake
Topical sodium ascorbate 10%	4 × daily
Systemic sodium ascorbate 2 g	2 × daily p. os
Topical sodium citrate 10%	4 × daily
Topical tetracycline	4 × daily
Systemic doxycycline 100 mg	2 × daily p. os
Antiglaucoma	As needed

*May use topical corticosteroids if amniotic membrane transplantation has been used in conjunction with limbal stem cell transplantation.

PEARL... Mucosal tissue mechanically restores ocular surface anatomical relationships and reduces or eliminates the problems associated with mechanical disturbance of the fornical conjunctiva.

SPECIAL CONSIDERATION

Some authors[68] advocate the use of nasal mucosa with its goblet cell population, rather than buccal mucosa,[69] to restore some of the mucus secretion capabilities of the ocular surface. Not providing a source of phenotypically normal corneal epithelium, this technique is used in conjunction with limbal stem cell transplantation, prior to penetrating or lamellar keratoplasty.

Limbal Stem Cell Transplantation

It was originally described[16] for late rehabilitation following chemical injury of the scarred, vascularized cornea with complete limbal stem cell loss in one or more quadrants (Fig. 32–10). Following superficial keratectomy, transfer of donor limbal stem cells is performed.

- If the scarring and opacification are superficial, this procedure often provides dramatic improvement in visual acuity.
- If deeper corneal scarring and opacification are present, lamellar or penetrating keratoplasty may be performed.

Mucosal Membrane Grafts

Mucosal membrane grafts may be useful in fornix reconstruction associated with conjunctival cicatrization and restoration of normal globe–lid relationships.[67–69]

Lamellar/Penetrating Keratoplasty

The prognosis for successful PK is related to the original severity and sequelae of a chemical injury.[70] The prognosis is virtually hopeless if certain intraocular abnormalities have developed (e.g., glaucoma, hypotony, AC membrane formation). If intraocular abnormalities themselves do not preclude visual rehabilitation, the success rate of lamellar or penetrating keratoplasty can be improved if limbal stem cell function has been restored and conjunctival abnormalities have been corrected.[16]

Permanent Keratoprosthesis

It may be useful for bilateral, severe chemical injury where the prognosis is hopeless for PK because of:

- irreparable damage to the ocular surface; or
- repeated immunological rejection.[71–75]

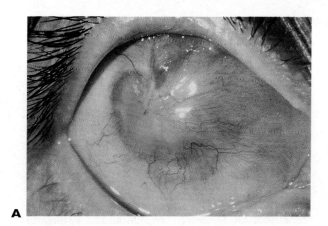

A

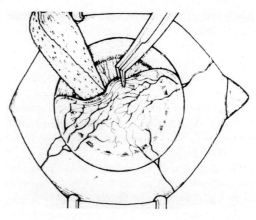

B

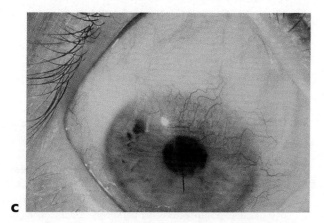

C

FIGURE 32–10   Limbal autograft, late intervention. **(A)** Preoperative appearance. One year after acid injury, there is extensive symblepharon of the superior fornix to the superior cornea, with associated corneal pannus and superficial stromal vasculature, poor cosmetic appearance, and counting fingers vision. **(B)** Technique of superficial keratectomy to remove symblepharon and corneal pannus in preparation for limbal autograft transfer from donor site. **(C)** Postoperative appearance, 1 year. There are dramatic improvements in cosmetic appearance, elimination of symblepharon and corneal pannus, and improved visual acuity to 20/50. Mild superficial vascular pannus persists. (**A** and **C** from Wagoner MD, Kenyon KR, Shore JS. Ocular surface transplantation. In: Barrie J, Kirkness C, eds. *Recent Advances in Ophthalmology*. Vol 9. New York: Churchill Livingstone; 1995:59–90. Reprinted with permission from Churchill Livingstone. **B** from Kenyon KR, Tseng SCG. Limbal autograft transplantation for ocular surface disorders. Ophthalmology. 1989;96:709–722. Reprinted with permission from Elsevier Science.)

Although the success rate has been variable in the past, improved keratoprosthesis design and postoperative management now offer a better prognosis.[74]

SUMMARY

For many years, the main focus of investigation and therapy for severe chemical injury was on control of inflammation and regulation of the delicate balance between collagen synthesis and collagenolytic activity with carefully selected *medical* intervention. In the past two decades, improved understanding of the importance of the ocular surface has added several *surgical* options. The development of ocular surface transplantation techniques, which restore depleted limbal stem cell populations and reestablish a normal corneal phenotype (limbal autograft and allograft transplantation) as well as enhance corneal epithelial migration, reduce limbal inflammation, and augment the function of surviving or transplanted limbal stem cells (amniotic membrane transplantation), has improved the early management and prognosis of the severely chemically injured eye.

REFERENCES

1. Friend J, Thoft RA. Functional competence of regenerating ocular surface epithelium. *Invest Ophthalmol Vis Sci*. 1978;17:134–139.

2. Thoft RA, Friend J. The X,Y,Z hypothesis of corneal epithelial maintenance. *Invest Ophthalmol Vis Sci*. 1983; 24:1442–1443.

3. Buck RC. Measurement of centripetal migration of normal corneal epithelial cells in the mouse. *Invest Ophthalmol Vis Sci*. 1985;26:1296–1299.

4. Friedenwald JS, Buschke W. Some factors concerned in the mitotic and wound-healing activities of the corneal epithelium. *Trans Am Ophthalmol Soc*. 1944;42:371–383.

5. Kinoshita S, Friend J, Thoft RA. Sex chromatin of donor corneal epithelium in rabbits. *Invest Ophthalmol Vis Sci.* 1981;21:434–441.

6. Davanger M, Evensen A. Role of the pericorneal papillary structure in renewal of corneal epithelium. *Nature.* 1971;229:560–561.

7. Schermer A, Galvin S, Sun TT. Differentiation-related expression of a major 64K corneal keratin in vivo and in culture suggests limbal location of corneal epithelial stem cells. *J Cell Biol.* 1986;103:49–62.

8. Zieske JD, Bukusoglu G, Yankauckas MA. Characterization of a potential marker of corneal epithelial stem cells. *Invest Ophthalmol Vis Sci.* 1992;33:143–152.

9. Shapiro MS, Friend J, Thoft RA. Corneal re-epithelialization from the conjunctiva. *Invest Ophthalmol Vis Sci.* 1981;21:135–142.

10. Thoft RA, Friend J. Biochemical transformation of regenerating ocular surface epithelium. *Invest Ophthalmol Vis Sci.* 1977;16:14–20.

11. Thoft RA. Conjunctival transplantation. *Arch Ophthalmol.* 1977;95:1425–1427.

12. Tseng SCG. Concept and application of limbal stem cells. *Eye.* 1989;3:141–157.

13. Tseng SCG, Hirst LW, Farazdaghi M, Green WR. Goblet cell density and vascularization during conjunctival transdifferentiation. *Invest Ophthalmol Vis Sci.* 1984;25:1168–1176.

14. Hirst LW, Fogle JA, Kenyon KR, Stark WJ. Corneal epithelial regeneration and adhesion following acid burns in the rhesus monkey. *Invest Ophthalmol Vis Sci.* 1982;23:764–773.

15. Geggel HS, Thoft RA, Friend J. Histology of human conjunctival transplantation. *Cornea.* 1984;3:11–15.

16. Kenyon KR, Tseng SCG. Limbal autograft transplantation for ocular surface disorders. *Ophthalmology.* 1989;96:709–722.

17. Tseng SCG, Tsai RJ. Limbal transplantation for ocular surface transplantation—a review. *Fortschr Ophthalmol.* 1991;88:236–242.

18. Cintron C, Hong BS, Covington HI, Kublin CL. Quantitative analysis of collagen from normal developing corneas and corneal scars. *Curr Eye Res.* 1981;1:1–8.

19. Sakai J, Hung J, Zhu G, et al. Collagen metabolism during healing of lacerated rabbit corneas. *Exp Eye Res.* 1991;52:237–244.

20. Ishizaki M, Zhu G, Haseba T, et al. Expression of collagen I, smooth muscle alpha-actin, and vimentin during the healing of alkali-burned and lacerated corneas. *Invest Ophthalmol Vis Sci.* 1993;34:3320–3328.

21. Johnson-Muller B, Gross J. Regulation of corneal collagenase production: epithelial–stromal cell interactions. *Proc Natl Acad Sci U S A.* 1978;75:4417–4421.

22. Johnson-Wint B. Regulation of stromal cell collagenase production in adult rabbit cornea: in vitro stimulation and inhibition by epithelial cell products. *Proc Natl Acad Sci U S A.* 1980;77:5531–5535.

23. Wagoner MD, Johnson-Wint B. Intact stromal explants in vitro behave like monolayers of primary stromal fibroblasts in their collagenase response to epithelial cytokines and interleukin-1. *Invest Ophthalmol Vis Sci.* 1987;28(suppl):222.

24. Fujisawa K, Katakami C, Yamamoto M. [Keratocyte activity during wound healing of alkali-burned cornea]. *Nippon Ganka Gakkai Zasshi.* 1991;95:59–66.

25. Pfister RR, Paterson CA. Additional clinical and morphological observations on the favorable effect of ascorbate in experimental ocular alkali burns. *Invest Ophthalmol Vis Sci.* 1977;16:478–487.

26. Beams R, Linabery L, Grayson M. Effect of topical corticosteroids on corneal wound strength. *Am J Ophthalmol.* 1968;66:1131–1133.

27. Gasset AR, Lorenzetti DW, Ellison EM, Kaufman HE. Quantitative corticosteroid effect on corneal wound healing. *Arch Ophthalmol.* 1969;81:589–591.

28. Gross J. An essay on biological degradation of collagen. In: Hay ED, ed. *Cell Biology of the Extracellular Matrix.* New York: Plenum; l982:217–258.

29. Harris ED Jr, Welgus HG, Krane SM. Regulation of mammalian collagenases. *Coll Relat Res.* 1984;4:493–512.

30. Lazarus GS, Brown RS, Daniels JR, et al. Human granulocyte collagenase. *Science.* 1968;159:1483–1485.

31. Macartney A, Tschesche H. Latent and active human polymorphonuclear leukocyte collagenases. *J Biochem.* 1983;130:71–78.

32. Gordon JM, Bauer EA, Eisen AZ. Collagenase in the human cornea: immunologic localization. *Arch Ophthalmol.* 1980;98:341–345.

33. Kenyon KR. Inflammatory mechanisms in corneal ulceration. *Trans Am Ophthalmol Soc.* 1985;83:610–663.

34. Kenyon KR. Decision making in the therapy of external eye disease: noninfected corneal ulcers. *Ophthalmology.* 1982;89:44–51.

35. Wagoner MD, Kenyon KR. Noninfected corneal ulceration. *Focal Points: Clinical Modules for Ophthalmologists.* Vol 3. San Francisco: American Academy of Ophthalmology; 1985:7.

36. Kenyon KR, Berman M, Rose J, Gage J. Prevention of stromal ulceration in the alkali-burned rabbit cornea by glued-on contact lens. Evidence for the role of polymorphonuclear leukocytes in collagen degradation. *Invest Ophthalmol Vis Sci.* 1979;18:570–587.

37. Paterson CA, Williams RN, Parker AW. Characteristics of polymorphonuclear leukocyte infiltration into the alkali-burned eye and influence of sodium citrate. *Exp Eye Res.* 1984;39:701–708.

38. Wagoner MD, Kenyon KR, Gipson IK, et al. Polymorphonuclear neutrophils delay corneal epithelial wound healing in vitro. *Invest Ophthalmol Vis Sci.* 1984;25:1217–1220.

39. Hughes WF. Alkali burns of the cornea. II. Clinical and pathologic course. *Arch Ophthalmol.* 1946;36:189–214.

40. Ballen PH. Mucous membrane grafts in chemical (lye) burns. *Am J Ophthalmol.* 1963;55:302–312.

41. Wagoner MD. Chemical injuries of the eye: current concepts in pathophysiology and therapy. *Surv Ophthalmol.* 1997;41:275–313.

42. McCulley JP. Chemical injuries. In: Smolin G, Thoft RA, eds. *The Cornea: Scientific Foundation and Clinical Practice.* 2nd ed. Boston: Little, Brown; 1987:527–542.

43. Kenyon KR, Rapoza PA. Limbal allograft transplantation for ocular surface disorders. *Ophthalmology.* 1995; 102(suppl):101–102.

44. Daya SM. Living-related conjunctivo-limbal allograft (lr-CLAL) for the treatment of stem cell deficiency: an analysis of long-term outcome [abstract]. *Ophthalmology.* 1995;106(suppl):102.

45. Rao SK, Rajagopal R, Sitalakshmi G, et al. Limbal allografting from related live donors for corneal surface reconstruction. *Ophthalmology.* 1999;106:822–828.

46. Tsai RJF, Tseng SCG. Human allograft limbal transplantation for corneal surface reconstruction. *Cornea.* 1994;13:389–400.

47. Tsubota K, Toda I, Saito H, et al. Reconstruction of the corneal epithelium by limbal allograft transplantation for severe ocular surface disorders. *Ophthalmology.* 1995;102:1486–1495.

48. Croasdale CR, Schwartz GS, Malling JV, et al. Keratolimbal allograft: recommendations for tissue procurement and preparation by eye banks, and standard surgical technique. *Cornea.* 1999;18:52–58.

49. Djalilian AR, Bagheri MM, Schwartz GS, et al. Keratolimbal allograft for the treatment of limbal stem cell deficiency. Presented at: The Scientific Program of the Castroviejo Society; October 23, 1999; Orlando, FL.

50. Lindberg K, Brown ME, Chaves HV, et al. In vitro propagation of human ocular surface epithelial cells for transplantation. *Invest Ophthalmol Vis Sci.* 1993;34: 2672–2679.

51. He Y-G, Alizadeh H, Kinoshita K, McCulley JP. Experimental transplantation of cultured human limbal and amniotic epithelial cells onto the corneal surface. *Cornea.* 1999;18:570–579.

52. Pellegrini G, Traverso CE, Franzi AT, et al. Long-term restoration of damaged corneal surfaces with autologous cultured corneal epithelium. *Lancet.* 1997;349: 990–993.

53. Schwab IR, Reyes M, Isseroff RR. Successful transplantation of bioengineered tissue replacements in patients with ocular surface disease. *Cornea.* 2000;19:421–426.

54. Williams KA, Brereton HM, Aggarwal R, et al. Use of DNA polymorphisms and polymerase chain reaction to examine the survival of human limbal stem cell allograft. *Am J Ophthalmol.* 1995;120:342–350.

55. Holland EJ, Schwartz GS. Changing concepts in the management of severe ocular surface disease over twenty-five years. *Cornea.* 2000;19:688–698.

56. De Roth A. Plastic repair of conjunctival defects with fetal membrane. *Arch Ophthalmol.* 1996;23:522–525.

57. Kim JC, Tseng SCG. Transplantation of preserved human amniotic membrane for surface reconstruction in severely damaged rabbit corneas. *Cornea.* 1995;14: 473–484.

58. Tseng SCG, Prabhasawat P, Barton K, et al. Amniotic membrane transplantation with or without limbal autografts for corneal surface reconstruction in patients with limbal stem cell deficiency. *Arch Ophthalmol.* 1998;116:431–441.

59. Reim M, Overkamping B, Kuckelkorn R. [2 years experience with tenon-plasty]. *Ophthalmologe.* 1992;89: 524–530.

60. Fogle JA, Kenyon KR, Foster CS. Tissue adhesive arrests stromal melting in the human cornea. *Am J Ophthalmol.* 1980;89:795–802.

61. Abel R Jr, Binder PS, Polack FM, Kaufman HE. The results of penetrating keratoplasty after chemical burns. *Trans Am Acad Ophthalmol Otolaryngol.* 1975;79: OP584–595.

62. Kuckelkorn R, Redbrake C, Schrage NF, Reim M. [Keratoplasty with 11–12 mm diameter for management of severely chemically-burned eyes]. *Ophthalmologe* 1993; 90:683–687.

63. Redbrake C, Buchal V, Reim M. [Keratoplasty with a scleral rim after most severe eye burns]. *Klin Monatsbl Augenheilkd.* 1996;208:145–151.

64. Phillips K, Arffa R, Cintron C, et al. Effects of prednisolone and medroxyprogesterone on corneal wound healing, ulceration, and neovascularization. *Arch Ophthalmol.* 1983;101:640–643.

65. Newsome DA, Gross JA. Prevention by medroxyprogesterone of perforation of the alkali-burned rabbit cornea: inhibition of collagenolytic activity. *Invest Ophthalmol Vis Sci.* 1977;16:21–31.

66. Lass JH, Campbell RC, Rose J, et al. Medroxyprogesterone on corneal ulceration: its effects after alkali burns on rabbits. *Arch Ophthalmol.* 1981;99:673–676.

67. Ballen PH. Mucous membrane grafts in chemical (lye) burns. *Am J Ophthalmol.* 1963;55:302–312.

68. Naumann GOH, Lang GK, Rummelt V, Wigand ME. Autologous nasal mucosa transplantation in severe bilateral conjunctival mucus deficiency syndrome. *Ophthalmology.* 1990;97:1011–1017.

69. Shore JW, Foster CS, Westfall CT, Rubin PAD. Results of buccal mucosal grafting for patients with medically controlled ocular cicatrical pemphigoid. *Ophthalmology.* 1990;99:383–395.

70. Alldredge OC, Krachmer JH. Clinical types of corneal transplant rejection; their manifestations, frequency, preoperative correlates, and treatment. *Arch Ophthalmol.* 1981;99:599–604.

71. Dohlman CH, Schneider HA, Doane MG. Prosthokeratoplasty. *Am J Ophthalmol.* 1974;77:694–700.

72. Cardona H, DeVoe AG. Prosthokeratoplasty. *Trans Am Acad Ophthalmol Otolaryngol.* 1977;83:271–280.

73. Rao GN, Blatt HL, Aquavella JV. Results of keratoprosthesis. *Am J Ophthalmol.* 1979;88:190–196.

74. Yaghouti F, Nouri M, Abad JC, et al. Keratoprosthesis: preoperative diagnostic categories. *Cornea.* 2001;20: 19–23.

75. Wagoner MD, Kenyon KR, Shore JS. Ocular surface transplantation. In: Barrie J, Kirkness P, eds. *Recent Advances in Ophthalmology.* Vol 9. New York: Churchill Livingstone; 1995:59–90.

Chapter 33

OCULAR MANIFESTATIONS OF NONOPHTHALMIC CONDITIONS

Wolfgang Schrader

 Nonmechanical globe injuries may be caused by:

- chemicals (see Chapters 11 and 32);
- temperature;
- radiation (see Chapter 34); or
- mechanical impact elsewhere in the body.

Traumatic events not directly related to the eye rarely lead to ocular lesions; if they do, these are via:

- changes in rheologic conditions;
- hypoxia; or
- a sudden increase of the intravascular pressure.

CONTROVERSY

Because of the great variability of retinal findings and a still incompletely understood response of the retina to distant trauma, the pathomechanism remains under debate.

Three mechanisms have been proposed to explain the resulting fundus findings:

- retinal vascular endothelial cell damage by increased intraluminal pressure;
- damage by emboli (e.g., air, blood products, fat); and
- mechanical forces acting at the vitreoretinal interface.

PURTSCHER'S RETINOPATHY

This is a retinopathy resulting from various etiologies and consisting of:

- marked macular and generalized retinal edema;
- multiple patches of peripapillary superficial retinal whitening;
- intraretinal hemorrhages around the optic disk; and
- disk edema (see Fig. 33–1).

The first case was described in 1868;[1] however, no epidemiological data are available.

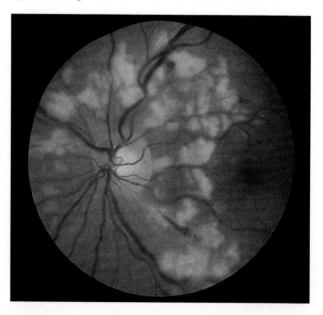

FIGURE 33–1 Purtscher's retinopathy (see the text for details).

Etiology

The most typical causes[2-6] follow:

- severe head trauma;
- fracture of (long) bones; or
- chest compression (typically in an MVC);

the condition has also been described, however, after:

- concussions of the liver;
- blow to the orbit;
- carotid surgery/angiography; and
- thoracic/renal surgery.

Pathophysiology

Various suggestions have been made with regard to the pathophysiology, such as:

- extravasation from retinal vessels during a sudden increase in the intracranial pressure[2];
- reflux venous shock waves produced from intra-thoracic chest compression[7];
- fat emboli in retinal arterioles[8,9]; and
- venous stasis.[9,10]

The underlying systemic condition generates various intravascular microparticles that occlude small peripapillary arterioles,[5,11-14] with the following mechanisms/materials contributing:

- fat embolization from long bone fractures or acute pancreatitis (due to enzymatic digestion of omental fat)[15];
- air emboli from compressive chest injuries[15];
- retinal venous wall trauma from venous reflux with endothelial cell swelling and capillary engorgement in the upper body[7];
- angiospastic response following a sudden increase in venous pressure[6,7];
- local retinal vascular coagulopathy or complement-induced granulocyte aggregation leading to multiple arteriolar occlusions[16]; and
- fibrin clots, aggregates of platelets and leukocytes.[15]

A Purtscher-like fundus picture may also occur in lupus erythematosus and at childbirth.[11,17]

Evaluation

The symptoms[a] are usually bilateral, although rarely symmetrical, and develop within 4 days.

- Unilateral cases have also been reported.[15,18]
- Patients complain of decreased vision, often from 20/200 to counting fingers.

- IBO (the peripheral retina is commonly spared):
  - numerous white retinal patches or confluent cotton-wool spots around the disk;
  - superficial retinal hemorrhages;
  - serous macular detachments, dilated and tortuous vasculature, and
  - disk edema.
- FA:
  - focal areas of arteriolar obstruction;
  - patchy capillary nonperfusion;
  - disk edema;
  - dye leakage from retinal arterioles, capillaries, and venules;[15]
  - the choroidal filling may be normal in the acute stages with some blockage of background choroidal fluorescence;
  - late perivenous staining and/or partial vein obstruction; and
  - optic disk edema.

Management

Management is by observation.

Complications

Lesions similar to those in Purtscher's retinopathy have been produced experimentally,[b] resulting in the clinical picture of Purtscher's retinopathy. It is thus obvious that the condition may be complicated by vascular occlusions in the retina and on the optic disk, leading to permanent functional impairment.

Prognosis and Outcome

The retinal lesions typically resolve in a few weeks to months. After resolution, the fundus may appear normal, but pigment migration and optic atrophy can occur.[4]

> **PEARL...** Both the visual acuity and the visual field[c] return to normal in most cases, although if optic atrophy occurs, the vision may be permanently reduced.[4]

Fundus features in Purtscher-type retinopathy are similar and may appear in many other conditions. History, associated systemic disease, and the interval

---

[a] It must be emphasized again that these appear in the absence of direct ocular trauma.

[b] Infusion into the carotid of 15- to 75-μm-diameter glass beads[19] and injection into the opthalmic artery of fibrin clots.

[c] Defects may originally vary from a central/paracentral/annular scotoma to large segmental defects.

between injury and onset of visual signs/symptoms may help in the differential diagnosis. Common etiologies include the following.

Fat embolism[20] is clinically recognized in up to 5% of patients with long bone fractures,[21,22] affects multiple organ systems,[23] and may be fatal in 20% of the severe cases.[24] Retinal lesions are present in 50–60% of patients, but they are more peripheral.[4,7]

Acute pancreatitis occurs when digestive enzymes released from the inflamed pancreas degrade omental fat, liberating into the general circulation free fat emboli that may eventually lodge in the retinal circulation.[15] A complement cascade may be activated by the release of pancreatic proteases, leading to leukoembolic retinal arteriolar occlusion.[16]

Compression cyanosis (or traumatic asphyxia) is accompanied by bluish discoloration of the chest, neck, face, and upper extremities.

Air embolization is a rare complication of chest/jugular vein surgery/injury. Distinguishing fundus features include a uniformly gray appearance of the fundus, a pale optic nerve, and intra-arterial air.[d]

Hydrostatic pressure syndrome occurs when a person is ejected from an aircraft traveling at very high speed. The high decelerating forces drive blood toward the head and create mental confusion, temporary loss of vision, periocular edema, ecchymosis of the lids, and subconjunctival and retinal hemorrhage.[7]

The nonophthalmologist should be aware of sight-threatening complications even in the absence of direct ocular involvement.

> **PEARL...** If the victim is unconscious or complains about visual loss during the first 4 days after severe trauma, an ophthalmologist should be called for consultation. The findings should be precisely documented and photographed because the patient may later seek compensation for the injury (see Chapter 7).

WHIPLASH SYNDROME

An energy transfer to the neck and head occurs via acceleration/deceleration; it is most common in rear-end collision MVCs[25] and may lead to a variety of clinical manifestations (whiplash-associated disorders). The predominant symptom is pain and discomfort, frequently in the absence of pathology on inspection or radiological investigation. There may be concussional injury to the brain.

Epidemiology and Prevention

In one study,[25] the driver-specific incidence rate was 96 per 100,000 licensed drivers per year. It varies with population density.[e]

Pathophysiology

A violent flexion is immediately followed by an extension of the neck, which may cause a mechanical injury to the sympathetic nerves.

> **PEARL...** The visual disturbance in whiplash syndrome may be caused by direct injury to the cervical/carotid artery or by an accompanying Purtscher type of injury; a true retinal excavation[26] may also exist, and the whiplash maculopathy may be related to vitreomacular traction.

Evaluation

The patients may have a wide range of complaints.

- The most common presenting symptoms are neck pain ($\leq 100\%$) and headache (54–66%).[25]
- Horner's syndrome[f] may be the most common ocular manifestation.[4]
- Visual complaints are reported in 8 to 26%.[25,27]
  - The reduction in visual acuity is rather acute but usually not worse than 20/30. The symptoms are bilateral and resolve over a period of a few days.
- On biomicroscopic examination, there is a gray swelling of the fovea. A crater-like depression less than 100 μm in diameter with slight RPE disturbance may remain unchanged even when the symptoms resolve.[26]
- FA may be normal or may show a tiny focal area of hyperfluorescence.[26]

Management

There is no known treatment.

Complications

An accompanying concussional injury to the brain may cause temporary palsy of the cranial nerves with diplopia.[4]

Prognosis and Outcome

The visual acuity usually, although not always, returns to normal. A similar clinical appearance and course may be seen after contusion and solar retinopathy (see Chapter 34).[11]

---

[d]This can be directly visualized as glistening white lines interrupting the blood column.[7]

[e]Higher in more populated regions.

[f]Miosis, ptosis, and pseudoenophthalmos.

The nonophthalmologist should be aware of sight-threatening complications even in the absence of direct ocular involvement. If the victim complains about visual loss after a whiplash injury, an ophthalmologist should be called for consultation. Accurate documentation is important.

SHAKEN BABY[g] SYNDROME

The 15% mortality rate underscores the importance of recognizing this form of child abuse.[29]

Epidemiology and Prevention

In central Europe, 3.5% of the parents confessed to having used so much violence on their children that it might have resulted in severe injury; 10% of traumatized children admitted to a hospital show evidence of physical violence.[30]

In a single year, 1120 instances of child abuse were registered by the police in western Germany[h]; the estimated number of cases was between 20,000 and 400,000.[30]

- Two thirds of the abused children are babies.
- The typical victim is a male infant, younger than 6 months of age, who is alone with the perpetrator at the time of the injury.[31]

SPECIAL CONSIDERATION

Certain anatomic features make the infant more likely to suffer from intracranial and intraocular bleeding as a result of shaking.[32] Relative to his body, the infant's head is disproportionately larger and heavier than that of an older child or adult and is less well stabilized by neck muscles. Furthermore, the smaller the child, the more acceleration-deceleration forces an adult can inflict.

- The incidence is unrelated to race, gender, socioeconomic status, or education.[31]
- The presenting sign is eye related in 4 to 6% of the cases.
- Whereas after accidental head injuries nearly all babies[i] have normal funduscopic examinations,

most babies with nonaccidental head injuries show varying degrees of retinal hemorrhages.

- ○ Retinal hemorrhages occur in 11 to 23% of all physically abused children and in 50 to 80% of shaken babies.[33–35]

Pathophysiology

The characteristic injuries include:

- subdural hemorrhages[j];
- retinal hemorrhages (Fig. 33–2); and
- fractures of the ribs or long bones.

PEARL...   The most severe brain injuries in shaken baby syndrome result from a forceful impact of the infant's or child's head against a firm surface.

The pathogenesis of the ocular hemorrhage is not as well understood.

- It may be related to an acute rise in the intracranial pressure after subdural hemorrhage (see later at Terson's syndrome).[32,36]
- The same acceleration and deceleration forces that cause intracranial hemorrhage also act on the vitreous.

---

[j] The vessels that bridge the cerebral cortices and venous sinuses may tear and bleed in response to repetitive acceleration and deceleration motion of the brain when the infant is shaken.

---

[g] Also called whiphash shaken infant syndrome,[28] battered child syndrome, or child abuse syndrome; see Chapters 10 and 30 for additional details.

[h] Population: 60 million.

[i] ≤ 3 years of age.

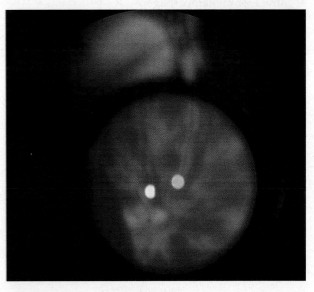

FIGURE 33–2   Retinal hemorrhages in shaken baby syndrome (see the text for details).

Some believe that these vitreous forces acting in a direction perpendicular to the plane of the retina might be strong enough to cause a separation of the ILM or a splitting of deeper retinal layers.[32,36,k]

- Retinal hemorrhage results from tearing of small retinal vessels and is therefore found in the ganglion cell or nerve fiber layer.[37]
- Increased venous pressure transmitted to the retina, akin to Valsalva retinopathy, may also occur.[l]

Evaluation

The most common *ocular* finding is intraocular hemorrhage (subretinal, intraretinal, preretinal [subhyaloid], and intravitreal).[38] Intra- and preretinal hemorrhages predominate, and, just as in Terson's syndrome, they are concentrated in the posterior pole and are usually bilateral.

Less common findings include:

- cotton-wool spots;
- white-centered hemorrhages;
- macular edema;
- papilledema; and
- "retinoschisis".[14,32,m]

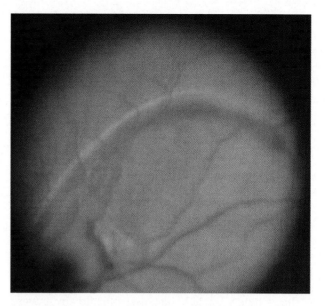

FIGURE 33–3   Perimacular ring caused by traumatic separation of the ILM. The ring is caused by elevation of the retina along the line where the ILM, hydrodissected by the submembranous (i.e., sub-ILM) hemorrhage, reinserts. (Courtesy F. Kuhn, MD.)

PEARL... The amount of intraocular blood correlates with the degree of acute neurologic damage.[39]

CT or MRI is required to diagnose the intracranial pathology. In selected cases, cerebrospinal fluid and subdural aspirations may be needed.

Intracranial findings include:

- subarachnoid hemorrhage;
- intracerebral hemorrhage;
- cerebral edema;
- cerebral atrophy;
- elevated intracranial pressure (often present); and
- a variety of consequential neurologic symptoms (e.g., irritability, lethargy, seizures, coma).

PEARL... The diagnosis of child abuse requires a high index of suspicion because it is rarely reported and there may be minimal external signs of trauma. Shaking, however, results in eye injuries in 35 to 46% of abused children[33,40,41] and may alone lead to trunk/limb bruises or fractures. Cervical cord hematomas are strongly suggestive,[42] as are retinal hemorrhages in a child with head injury.[43]

[k]However, it is even more likely that the ILM is elevated by intraretinal bleeding, causing the typical appearance of submembranous hemorrhagic macular cyst (see later and reference 53).

[l]Especially with a firm grip on the chest while shaking or even from direct choking of the victim.

[m]As mentioned before, this is probably ILM separation, not a true schisis (Fig. 33–3).

Although simple falls or normal playground activities in children 4 to 8 years old[38] do not cause retinal hemorrhages, a clinical picture similar to that seen in shaken baby syndrome can occur in infants from nontraumatic causes including:

- severe hypertension;
- vasculitis;

- meningitis;
- endocarditis;
- generalized sepsis;
- coagulopathy;
- hematologic disorders (e.g., leukemia); and
- blood dyscrasia.[38]

> **PEARL...** The indirect ocular signs may be accompanied by direct eye trauma (e.g., periorbital bruising, subconjunctival hemorrhage, neovascular glaucoma, cataract, retinal detachment). All children need high-resolution neuroradiological imaging.

Management

The suspicion of child abuse requires the initiation of a multidisciplinary approach, careful documentation, and reporting to authorities if required (see Chapters 7, 8, and 30).

> **PEARL...** The ophthalmologist must be familiar with the retinal manifestations of child abuse to act as an expert witness if necessary. The treatment of the retinal manifestations of shaken baby syndrome is mostly supportive as most hemorrhages and other acute changes resolve within several months.

Complications

Perimacular retinal folds, chorioretinal atrophy/scarring, optic atrophy, nonclearing vitreous hemorrhage, and retinal detachment may occur.[38,44] The last two conditions may require surgical treatment; enzyme-assisted vitrectomy (see Chapter 30 and the Appendix) can facilitate the creation of posterior vitreous detachment, which is otherwise very difficult in these infants.

Prognosis and Outcome

The clinical course ranges from complete resolution of the ocular symptoms to severe visual loss secondary to:

- optic nerve damage/atrophy[n];
- or macular scarring[45]; or
- or brain damage.

> ### PITFALL
>
> Cerebral cortical injury may leave the survivor blind or severely handicapped (e.g., with motor and cognitive disabilities): a 50% incidence of gazing disorders is reported.[29] Even without evidence of retinal damage, visual loss occurs in 35% of children.[47]

The Nonophthalmologist's Role

Because ≤46% of abused children have eye injuries,[33,40,41] an ophthalmologic consultation is required whenever child abuse is suspected. Furthermore, all children under 2 years of age who present with unexplained seizures, altered mental status, or hydrocephalus should also have an ophthalmic examination.[38]

TERSON'S SYNDROME

Terson's syndrome describes vitreous hemorrhage occurring in association with subarachnoid or subdural hemorrhage.

Epidemiology and Prevention

Intraocular hemorrhage is seen in about 20% of patients with acute intracranial hemorrhage[14,48]; vitreous hemorrhage is seen in ≤8% of patients with subarachnoidal bleeding. The intracranial hemorrhage can be subdural, subarachnoidal, theoretically even intracerebral. Whereas subarachnoidal bleeding originates from a cerebral aneurysm,[48,o] subdural hemorrhages are caused by trauma.

---

[n]Postmortem examination of the optic nerves in shaken babies often reveals perineural hemorrhage, which may contribute by nerve fiber compression to the development of optic atrophy in survivors.[37,46]

[o]Usually the anterior communicating artery.

Pathophysiology

The mechanism of how the intraocular hemorrhage occurs is controversial.[49,50,p]

> ## PEARL... The severity of the vitreous hemorrhage correlates directly with the rapidity and magnitude of intracranial pressure elevation and shows a correlation with the severity of the systemic condition.[51,52]

Evaluation

In the acute stage, vitreous hemorrhage often precludes visualization of the posterior pole, but after the blood begins to resorb, multiple preretinal, intraretinal, and subretinal hemorrhages can be seen. In the macula, a hemorrhagic cyst is seen in one third of the eyes; the blood is twice as likely to be under the ILM as in front of it.[52,53]

Management

The visual outcome is excellent after vitrectomy[52] if the blood does not spontaneously resorb.[54] The indication for, and timing of, vitrectomy for the vitreous hemorrhage in Terson's syndrome is controversial.

Early vitrectomy has been proposed to hasten visual recovery, and several reports have demonstrated good visual recovery after surgery.[52–54] This is also the experience of the author of this chapter.

Observation remains a viable option,[54] but visual recovery is much faster in eyes undergoing vitrectomy.

> ## PEARL... The surgically induced rapid visual recovery is very much appreciated by the patient, who commonly suffers from neurological handicaps as well; it also aids in the neurological rehabilitation of the patient.

Vitrectomy is not always as easy a procedure as it may appear, and the ILM rather commonly has to be peeled[53]; complications are not uncommon.[55]

Anesthesia is also a difficult question.

- General anesthesia may be risky.

- Conversely, some of these patients may be unable to understand the need for, and benefit of, surgery and might become excited during the procedure if operated under local anesthesia.[q]

> ## PEARL... Whether the patient should undergo vitrectomy or be observed requires the involvement in the decision making of the patient, the family, the neurologist, and the physical therapist. An individual, case-by-case evaluation of the risks and benefits is necessary.

Complications

Untreated, the intraocular hemorrhage may persist for many months—another argument for early surgery.[52,56] The development of PVR has been described with[55] and without[51] vitreoretinal surgery.

Prognosis and Outcome

Unless PVR or EMP formation occurs, the visual outcome is usually good.

The nonophthalmologist should request an ophthalmological consultation for *all* patients with subarachnoidal/subdural hemorrhage.[52]

VALSALVA RETINOPATHY

A hemorrhagic retinopathy may develop in response to a Valsalva maneuver,[r] which may occur during straining activities (e.g., heavy lifting, coughing, vomiting, blowing balloons[57]). The development of hemorrhages may be facilitated by underlying diseases/conditions of the retinal vessels (e.g., diabetic retinopathy,[58] retinal teleangiectasia,[59] arterial macroaneurysm,[60] pregnancy,[61] and sickle cell disease[62]).

There are no epidemiological data available.

Pathophysiology

The veins above the heart have no valves. A rapid rise in the abdominal pressure induces a rapid rise in the intravenous pressure, and various vessels inside or around the eye (e.g., subconjunctivally) may rupture. The Valsalva maneuver may be the cause of intraoperative ECH, see Chapter 22.

---

[p]Most likely a papillary/peripapillary/retinal capillary rupture, following a rapid rise of the intraocular venous pressure due to venous stasis via compression and stretching of the orbital veins.

[q]The author's personal observation.

[r]A rapid rise in abdominal pressure, especially against a closed glottis.

Evaluation

An accurate history is crucial. The amount of visual impairment depends on the location of the hemorrhage with regard to the fovea. The anterior segment is usually normal, although there may be conjunctival hemorrhage (hyposphagma). IBO most commonly reveals a red, dome-shaped hemorrhage underneath the ILM.[11]

Management

The hemorrhage usually clears spontaneously; if not, drainage using a pulsed Nd:YAG laser can be considered.[63,64] Surgery is another option and may require removal of the macular ILM (see Chapter 23).

HIGH-ALTITUDE RETINOPATHY

A condition similar to Valsalva retinopathy may occur at high altitudes (e.g., above 4000 m [12,000 feet]) in 20 to 60% of mountaineers.[65]

> **PEARL...** The hypoxia at high altitudes causes increased retinal blood flow and blood volume possibly via autoregulatory mechanisms. Furthermore, the retinal venous pressure can be increased by extreme physical exertion and Valsalva maneuvers during mountain climbing; the condition can then lead to intraretinal hemorrhages.

Retinal changes include:

- marked increase of the retinal vessel diameter with tortuosity of arterioles/venules; and
- hyperemia/edema of the disk.

The intra- and preretinal hemorrhages often spare the macular area. The person does not notice debilitating symptoms unless macular/vitreous hemorrhage occurs, which may be potentially hazardous when the patient is still high on the mountain. Clinically, all of these retinal changes are reversible within weeks.

> **PEARL...** To prevent high-altitude retinopathy, slow ascent and use of supplemental oxygen are recommended.

SPECIAL CONSIDERATION

Similar conditions (i.e., vasodilatation and intraocular hemorrhages) can occur when the cabin pressure suddenly decreases in airplanes. Vascular occlusions can develop in divers who develop caisson disease after a quick decompression: if the intracorporal air pressure decreases by more than 1 bar, air bubbles may develop in the vessels.[4]

SUMMARY

The conditions described in this chapter represent retinal consequences that are caused by trauma elsewhere in the body. These conditions are usually not severe, and most of them do not require treatment. Close cooperation (teamwork) between ophthalmologists and those working in other appropriate specialties is needed, as is counseling of the patient and family (see Chapter 5).

Table 33–1 provides an overview of the differential diagnostics of traumatic retinopathies.

TABLE 33–1 Differential Diagnosis of Traumatic Retinopathy

	Commotio Retinae (Berlin's Edema)	Purtscher's Retinopathy	Fat Embolism	Traumatic Asphyxia	Valsalva Retinopathy
Type of trauma	Direct globe contusion	Chest compression, head injury	Fracture of long bones, multiple injuries	Chest compression	Valsalva maneuver
Accompanying systemic picture	None	None	Pulmonary and cerebral signs, petechial hemorrhages	Blue-black discoloration of upper body	None
Onset of systemic picture	None	None	Symptom free interval of 1 or 2 days	Immediate	None
Initial vision	~20/200	Variable	Normal	Normal to NLP	Normal to finger counting
Duration of reduced vision	Several days	Several weeks	Several days	Several weeks	Several weeks
Final vision	Usually normal, sometimes impaired	Usually normal, sometimes impaired	Normal	Normal to NLP	Usually normal, sometimes impaired
Eyes externally	Contused	Normal	Normal to petechial conjunctival hemorrhages	Subconjunctival hemorrhages	Normal to conjunctival hemorrhages
Fundus picture	Retinal whitening	Exudates and hemorrhages	Exudates and hemorrhages, retinal edema	Normal or hemorrhages, rarely exudates	Hemorrhage under ILM; vitreous and retinal hemorrhages
Development of fundus picture	Within a few hours	Within 4 days	After 1 or 2 days	Immediate to 2 days	Immediate

Modified after Duke-Elder and MacFaul[4] and Marr and Marr.[7]

REFERENCES

1. Jacobi L. Ophthalmologischer Befund bei fractura basis cranii. *Graefes Arch Ophthalmol.* 1868;14:147–149.

2. Purtscher O. Angiopathia traumatica retinae. Lymphorrhagien des Augenhintergrundes. *Arch Ophthalmol.* 1912;82:347–371.

3. Purtscher O. Noch unbekannte Befunde nach Schädeltrauma. *Ber Versamml Dtsch Ophthalmol Ges.* 1910;36:294–301.

4. Duke-Elder S, MacFaul PA. Injuries, part I: mechanical injuries. In: Duke-Elder S. *System of Ophthalmology.* London: Henry Klimpton; 1972.

5. Roden D, Odonghue FGH, Phelan D. Purtscher's retinopathy and fat embolism. *Br J Ophthalmol.* 1989;73:677–679.

6. Pratt MV, DeVenecia G. Purtscher's retinopathy: a clinicopathological correlation. *Surv Ophthalmol.* 1970;14:417–423.

7. Marr WG, Marr EG. Some observations on Purtscher's disease: traumatic retinal angiography. *Am J Ophthalmol.* 1962;54:693–705.

8. Wagner W. *Zum Morbus Purtscher.* Stuttgart: Enke; 1968.

9. Archer DB. Traumatic retinal vasculopathy. *Trans Ophthalmol Soc UK.* 1986;105:361–389.

10. Schmidt JGH. Angiopathia retinae traumatica (Purtscher und Fettembolie). *Klin Monatsbl Augenheilkd.* 1968;152:672–679.

11. Gass JDM. *Stereoscopic Atlas of Macular Disease: Diagnosis and Treatment.* St. Louis: Mosby; 1987.

12. Power MH, Regillo CD, Custis PH. Thrombotic thrombocytopenic purpura associated with Purtscher retinopathy. *Arch Ophthalmol.* 1997;115:128–129.

13. Behrens-Baumann W, Scheurer G, Schroer H. Pathogenesis of Purtscher's retinopathy: an experimental study. *Graefes Arch Clin Exp Ophthalmol.* 1992;230:286–291.

14. Williams DF, Mieler WF, Williams GA. Posterior segment manifestations of ocular trauma. *Retina.* 1990;10:S35–S44.

15. Burton TC. Unilateral Purtscher's retinopathy. *Ophthalmology.* 1980;87:1096–1105.

16. Jacob HS, Craddock PR, Hammerschmidt DE, Moldow CF. Complement induced granulocyte aggregation: an unsuspected mechanism of disease. *N Engl J Med.* 1980;302:789-794.

17. Blodi B, Johnson M, Gass D, Fine SL, Joffe LM. Purtscher's-like retinopathy after childbirth. *Ophthalmology.* 1990;97:1654–1659.

18. Fischbein F, Safir A. Monocular Purtscher's retinopathy. *Arch Ophthalmol.* 1971;85:480–84.

19. Ashton N, Henkind P. Experimental occlusion of retinal arterioles (using glass ballotini). *Br J Ophthalmol.* 1965;49:225–234.

20. Zenker FA. Beiträge zur Anatomie und Physiologie der Lunge. Dresden: Braunsdorf; 1861.

21. Donnell JM. Observations of clinical fat embolism. *Can Med Assoc J.* 1962;86:1060–1066.

22. Ross. *Ann R Coll Surg.* 1970;46:159.

23. Gurd AR, Wilson RI. The fat embolism syndrome. *J Bone Joint Surg Br.* 1974;56:408–416.

24. Beck JP, Collins JA. Theoretical and clinical aspects of posttraumatic fat embolism syndrome. In: Calandruccio RA. American Academy of Orthopedic Surgeons Instruction Course Lectures. St. Louis: CV Mosby; 1973.

25. Spitzer WO, Skovron ML, Salmi LR, et al. Scientific monograph of the Quebec Task Force on Whiplash-Associated Disorders: redefining "whiplash" and its management. *Spine.* 1995;20:1s–73s.

26. Kelley J, Hoover R, George T. Whiplash maculopathy. *Arch Ophthalmol.* 1978;96:834–835.

27. Burke JP, Orton HP, West J, Strachan IM, Hockey MS, Ferguson DG. Whiplash and its effect on the visual system. *Graefes Arch Clin Exp Ophthalmol.* 1992;230:335–339.

28. Caffey J. The whiplash shaken infant syndrome: manual shaking by the extremities with whiplash induced intracranial and intraocular bleedings, linked with residual permanent brain damage and mental retardation. *Pediatrics.* 1974;54:396–403.

29. Ludwig S, Warman M. Shaken baby syndrome: a review of 20 cases. *Ann Emerg Med.* 1984;13:104–107.

30. Remschmidt H, Müller-Luckmann E, Hacker F, Schmidt MH, Strunk P. Ursachen und Prävention von Gewalt aus psychiatrischer Sicht. Gutachten der Unterkommission Psychiatrie der Gewaltkommision der Bundesregierung.

31. Lancon JA, Haines DE, Parent AD. Anatomy of the shaken baby syndrome. *Anat Rec.* 1998;253:13–18.

32. Greenwald MJ. The shaken baby syndrome. *Ophthalmology.* 1990;107:1472.

33. Jensen A, Smith R, Olson M. Ocular clues to child abuse. *J Pediatr Ophthalmol.* 1971;8:270–272.

34. Levin D, Bell D. Traumatic retinal hemorrhages with angioid streaks. *Arch Ophthalmol.* 1977;95:1072.

35. Riffenburgh R, Sathyavagiswaran L. Ocular findings at autopsy of child abuse victims. *Ophthalmology.* 1991;98:1519–1524.

36. Greenwald MJ, Weiss A, Oesterle CS, Friendly DS. Traumatic retinoschisis in battered babies. *Ophthalmology.* 1986;93:618–624.

37. Rao N, Smith RE, Choi JH, Xu XH, Kornblum RN. Autopsy findings in the eyes of fourteen fatally abused children. *Forensic Sci Int.* 1988;39:293–299.

38. Levin AV. Ocular manifestations of child abuse. *Ophthalmol Clin North Am.* 1990;3:249–264.

39. Wilkinson WS, Han DP, Rappley MD, Owings CL. Retinal hemorrhage predicts neurologic injury in the shaken baby syndrome. *Arch Ophthalmol.* 1989;107:1472–1474.

40. Harley RD. Ocular manifestations of child abuse. *J Pediatr Ophthalmol Strabismus.* 1980;17:5.

41. Friendly DS. Ocular manifestations of physical child abuse. *Trans Am Acad Ophthalmol Otolaryngol.* 1971;75: 318–332.

42. Hadley MN, Sonntag VKH, Rekate HL, Murphy A. The infant whiplash-shake injury syndrome: a clinical and pathologic study. *Neurosurgery.* 1989;24:536–540.

43. Buys YM, Levin AV, Enzenauer RW, et al. Retinal findings after head trauma in infants and young children. *Ophthalmology.* 1992;99:1718–1723.

44. Han DP, Wilkinson WS. Late ophthalmic manifestations of the shaken baby syndrome. *J Pediatr Ophthalmol Strabismus.* 1990;27:299–303.

45. Mushin AS. Ocular damage in the battered-baby syndrome. *Br Med J.* 1971;3:402.

46. Lambert SR, Johnson TE, Hoyt CS. Optic nerve sheath hemorrhages associated with the shaken baby syndrome. *Arch Ophthalmol.* 1986;104:1509–1512.

47. Hollenhurst RW, Stein HA. Ocular signs and prognosis in subdural and subarachnoidal bleeding in young children. *Arch Ophthalmol.* 1958;60:187–192.

48. Garfinkle AM, Danys LR, Nicolle DA, et al. Terson's syndrome: a reversible cause of blindness following subarachnoid hemorrhage. *J Neurosurg.* 1992;76: 766–771.

49. Doubler FH, Marlow SB. A case of hemorrhage into the optic nerve sheaths as a direct extension from a diffuse intra-meningeal hemorrhage caused by rupture of aneurysm of a cerebral artery. *Arch Ophthalmol.* 1917; 8:290–301.

50. Weingeist TA, Goldmann EJ, Folk JC, Packer AJ, Ossoinig KC. Terson's syndrome: clinicopathologic correlations. *Ophthalmology.* 1986;93:1435–1442.

51. Velikay M, Datlinger P, Stolba U, et al. Retinal detachment with severe proliferative vitreoretinopathy in Terson syndrome. *Ophthalmology.* 1994;101:35–37.

52. Kuhn F, Morris R, Witherspoon CD, Mester V. Terson syndrome: results of vitrectomy and the significance of vitreous hemorrhage in patients with subarachnoid hemorrhage. *Ophthalmology.* 1998;105:472–477.

53. Morris R, Kuhn F, Witherspoon CD, Mester V, Dooner J. Hemorrhagic macular cysts in Terson's syndrome and its implications for macular surgery. *Dev Ophthalmol.* 1997;29:44–54.

54. Schultz PN, Sobol WM, Weingeist TA. Long-term visual outcome in Terson syndrome. *Ophthalmology.* 1991;98:1814–1819.

55. Daus W, Kasmann B, Alexandridis E, Institution UAH. Terson-Syndrom. Komplizierte klinische Verläufe. *Ophthalmologe.* 1992;89:77–81.

56. Korner F, Meier GF. Vitrektomie bei Terson-Syndrom. Bericht über 18 Fälle. *Klin Monatsbl Augenheilkd.* 1992; 200:468–471.

57. Georgiou T, Pearce IA, Taylor RH. Valsalva retinopathy associated with blowing balloons [letter]. *Eye.* 1999; 13:686–687.

58. Kassoff A, Catalano RA, Mehu M. Vitreous hemorrhage and the Valsalva maneuver in proliferative diabetic retinopathy. *Retina.* 1988;8:174–176.

59. Raymond LA, Sacks JG, Choromokos E. Hemorrhagic Valsalva retinopathy in Leber's optic neuropathy. *Ann-Ophthalmol.* 1985;17:553–554.

60. Avins LR, Krummenacher TK. Valsalva maculopathy due to a retinal arterial macroaneurysm. *Ann-Ophthalmol.* 1983;15:421–423.

61. Deane JS, Ziakas N. Valsalva retinopathy in pregnancy [letter]. *Eye.* 1997;11:137–138.

62. Konotey Ahulu F. Valsalva vitreous haemorrhage and retinopathy in sickle cell haemoglobin C disease [letter]. *Lancet.* 1997;349:1774.

63. Ulbig MW, Mangouritsas G, Rothbacher HH, Hamilton AM, McHugh JD. Long-term results after drainage of premacular subhyaloid hemorrhage into the vitreous with a pulsed Nd:YAG laser. *Arch Ophthalmol.* 1998;116:1465–1469.

64. Raymond LA. Neodymium:YAG laser treatment for hemorrhages under the internal limiting membrane and posterior hyaloid face in the macula. *Ophthalmology.* 1995;102:406–411.

65. McFadden DM, Houston CS, Sutton JR, Powles ACP, Gray GW, Roberts RS. High altitude retinopathy. *JAMA.* 1981;67:214–218.

Chapter 34

PHOTIC AND ELECTRICAL TRAUMA

Yaniv Barkana and Michael Belkin

It has long been recognized that abnormally high amounts of light can damage the retina (gazing at the sun resulted in visual loss). In addition, today there are *artificial* light sources capable of causing photic retinal injury (e.g., ophthalmic instruments produce increasingly intense light to meet the demands of ophthalmologists for better diagnostic and therapeutic tools). The occupational use of laser systems is growing, and there is grave concern about the application of lasers as weapons specifically targeted at the human eye.

In this chapter we outline the basic concepts concerning the interaction of light with the eye and describe the clinical course of different types of light-induced eye injuries. We also provide guidelines for prevention, which—in the absence of any effective treatment for retinal phototoxicity—currently appears to be the only realistic approach at our disposal. Electrical ocular injury is also discussed.

PHOTIC TRAUMA

Pathophysiology

Light radiation in the visible and near IR part of the electromagnetic spectrum enters the eye and is focused by the refractive media to a retinal image about 5–30 μm in diameter. Focusing increases the retinal irradiance (see Table 34–1) by a factor of well over 10,000 above the irradiance incident at the cornea.

TABLE 34–1   BASIC TERMS DESCRIBING LIGHT SOURCES

Energy	The capacity for doing work, measured in J. Energy is commonly used to express the output of pulsed lasers such as Nd:YAG
Power	The rate of energy delivery, expressed in watts (W; joules per second). Power is used to express the output of continuous-wave lasers such argon lasers
Irradiance	Radiant power per unit area incident upon a given surface, such as the retina, measured in watts per unit area (e.g., W/cm^2)

> **PEARL...** The nature and severity of photic damage depend on several factors related to the light source and the eye.

Source-Related Factors

Wavelength of the Radiation   Optical radiation (wavelength: 380–1400 nm) is transmitted and focused on the retina by the eye's media.[1,2] Retinal exposure to such radiation at an above-threshold dose will cause damage. Photons of shorter (UV) or longer (far IR) wavelengths are rapidly absorbed in organic tissues and may cause corneal injury.

Duration and Intensity of Exposure   Three distinct mechanisms of light-induced tissue injury have been described, although more than one might be responsible for damage under certain circumstances.

- *Thermal damage* occurs when excessive energy (see Table 34–1) is absorbed by a suitable chromophore[a] at an exposure ranging from microseconds to seconds. Heat is produced faster than it can be dissipated, and the temperature of the tissue is increased.[3–5] An increase of at least $10°C$[5,6] causes denaturation and coagulation of proteins, with ensuing necrotic cell death and scarring.
  - An example of such thermal damage is the retinal lesion caused by argon laser photocoagulation.
- *Mechanical tissue damage* is caused when energy is absorbed rapidly, at a pulse duration in the picosecond (10^{-12} s) to nanosecond (10^{-9} s) range. The result is a very fast increase in temperature by thousands of degrees, with disintegration of a small volume of tissue into a collection of ions and electrons called plasma.[3,6] Together with water vapor, this generates a compressive pressure pulse (explosion), which travels out from the site of exposure and disrupts the surrounding tissues.
  - This process is employed clinically by the Nd:YAG laser photodisruptor for posterior capsulotomy, iridotomy, and so forth. Contrary to thermal damage, this type of damage is not significantly dependent on tissue pigmentation.
- *Photochemical damage* occurs at exposures typically lasting several seconds or longer, with a slow delivery of energy not causing significant buildup of heat.[7] Rather, single photons induce chemical reactions in the molecules that absorb them.
  - Typical examples include solar retinopathy and photodynamic therapy.

PEARL... The effect of excimer lasers is a special case. In the UV range, each photon has a high energy and can directly break molecular bonds in nucleic acids and structural proteins. This process is utilized in refractive surgery, where the objective is to reshape the cornea precisely, without causing appreciable thermal effects in tissues surrounding the incision.

---

[a]Chromophore is a pigment with a color that absorbs light of a particular wavelength. The most important pigment in the retina is *melanin*, which absorbs light throughout the visible and near-infrared spectrum and is densely concentrated in the retinal pigment epithelium cells and in the choroid. It is in these tissues that the thermal damage is greatest. *Xanthophyll* and *hemoglobin* are present in the retina in smaller quantities and absorb light at more specific wavelengths than melanin.

Eye-Related Factors

Location of the Injury   The most important factor in determining the degree and persistence of functional damage resulting from an exposure to light at an above-threshold dose is the retinal location of the injury, that is, its proximity to the fovea.

- A *foveal* lesion immediately causes a significant reduction in visual acuity, proportional to the number of photoreceptor cells destroyed.
- *Parafoveal* lesions might temporarily involve the fovea through edema and inflammation, which can extend over a diameter several times that of the injury spot. These, however, subside over a period of days or weeks.[8,9]
  - Conversely, a parafoveal lesion might spread to the fovea because of secondary cell damage via the release of various noxious agents (e.g., excitotoxic amino acid glutamate) by the directly affected neurons. The spread of these agents injures the neighboring, primarily unaffected cells, resulting in considerable functional loss.
- *Extramacular* lesions farther away from the fovea do not cause appreciable or permanent functional damage; a local scotoma may be produced, but this usually goes unnoticed and may be completely asymptomatic. A sufficiently high energy may injure the nerve fiber layer, spreading the morphological and functional damage to retinal areas not affected by the original lesion.[10]

Other Factors   Other factors include:

- the *state of refraction* at the time of injury (e.g., uncorrected ametropia, by increasing the diameter of the retinal spot, reduces the damage from any given irradiation); and
- the activation (or voluntary suppression) of the *blink and aversion reflexes* to bright light, typically limiting the exposure to intense visible radiation to 0.1 to 1.5 seconds.

Clinical Conditions

Acute Solar Retinopathy

Eye injury caused by the sun has been known for millennia. Plato recognized that observers should not look directly at the sun during an eclipse.[11] Galileo was reportedly injured by observing the sun through a telescope.[12] Most cases occur as a result of looking without suitable eye protection directly at the sun during a solar eclipse.[13–18] Less common circumstances include gazing at the sun during religious rituals,[19,20] while under the influence of hallucinogenic drugs[21] or in other states of altered consciousness,[22] or as a means of self-inflicted injury.[23]

Solar retinopathy is believed to result from photo-chemical damage.[12,24,b] Ultrastructurally, the damage is confined to the photoreceptors and the RPE.[24,25] Most patients present within a few days of injury, allowing easy identification of the source. Depending on the manner of looking at the sun, the damage may be bilateral or unilateral (usually the dominant eye).

Common initial symptoms include:

- variably decreased visual acuity (although <20/80 is exceptional);
- central scotoma (even if the visual acuity is 20/20); and
- a negative afterimage of the sun, which may last several hours.

The typical ophthalmoscopic lesion is a small, yel-low-gray spot at or near the fovea, surrounded by macular edema. The edema resolves in a few days to weeks, after which the macula may look normal or show minor pigmentary disturbance.

Foveolar depression or pseudohole may be observed; a true macular hole is rare. The FA is usually normal. Rarely, a macular window defect is observed.

Early improvement of the visual acuity is the rule, mostly occurring within a few weeks but sometimes lasting a few months. The final vision is typically ≥20/25, but a small central or paracentral scotoma may persist. The outcome is less favorable in atypically severe cases with low initial acuity. Late complications are rare.

PITFALL

Although excellent final visual acuity occurs in most eyes with solar retinopathy, subjective symptoms in vision can persist.

There is no known therapy for acute solar retinopa-thy. Corticosteroids are sometimes given, but their effect is unknown. Solar retinal injury is best pre-vented. Public campaigns and education through the media have reduced but not eliminated its incidence.

Certain prophylactic measures are not recom-mended because they are ineffective; retinal damage has been reported following direct observation, last-ing only a few seconds, of the sun through:

- sunglasses;
- smoked glass; and
- film.

PEARL... The safest way to observe the sun (e.g., during eclipse) is indirect; looking at the sun's image projected through a pinhole aperture in a piece of cardboard onto a piece of paper.

Welding Arc Maculopathy

In marked contrast to the commonly encountered photokeratitis caused by exposure to radiation emit-ted by welding arcs, injury to the retina from such exposure is rare, with only sporadic case reports in the literature.[26-28] The clinical presentation, course, and ophthalmoscopic findings are very similar to those in acute solar retinopathy.

Laser-Related Eye Injuries

A laser device produces a light beam that, unlike ordi-nary light, is coherent, monochromatic, unidirectional, and minimally divergent. The first laser was produced in 1960.[29] Lasers were promptly put to use in medicine, science, industry, and the military, and the first reports of accidental laser eye injuries soon followed.[30-32]

Experiments have demonstrated that retinal laser injury affects mainly the RPE cells and the outer seg-ments of the photoreceptors.[33,34] With "suprathresh-old" exposures, which are responsible for most of the lesions encountered clinically, all retinal layers are disrupted and choroidal blood enters the retina or the vitreous (Fig. 34–1).[35,36] These observations are con-sistent with an injury combining mechanical and ther-mal components. The medical literature currently

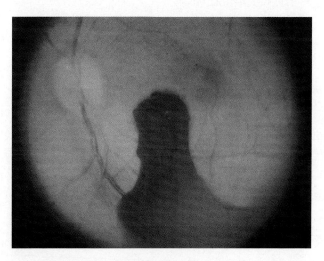

FIGURE 34–1 Vitreous hemorrhage induced by an Nd:YAG (1064 mm) Q-switched laser in a rhesus monkey eye. (Courtesy of the Medical Research Department, Walter Reed Army Institute of Research, San Antonio, Texas.)

---

[b] The retinal temperature increase is not high enough to cause thermal damage [photocoagulation].

contains nearly 200 such reports,[8,9,30–32,37–48] mostly from research laboratories and the industry. The reported injuries share several common elements.

- Almost all accidents could have been avoided by following standard laser safety practices; most victims did not wear eye protection because of lack of comfort.
- The injuries typically occurred during alignment of the laser beam or other adjustment procedures.
- Most of the reported injuries have been parafoveal, indicating that the victim was not looking directly into the laser source.
- Occasionally, the beam took an unexpected path, for example, unintentionally reflected by a mirror or nearby object such as photographic paper or a plastic membrane.
- Unexpected discharge of the laser device is rare.
- Almost all of the reported injuries were caused by short-pulse lasers, mostly Nd:YAG, operating in the visible and near-infrared spectrum and emitting a few mJ to tens of mJ per pulse of duration in the tens of nanoseconds range.

The clinical findings include the following.

- The victim experiences a sudden and severe disturbance of vision in one eye, often preceded by a visible flash of bright-colored light; occasionally, there is an audible "pop".
- Pain is unusual[37–39].
- The visual acuity is markedly decreased, commonly 20/200 or worse.
- Visual field defects are present.
- The anterior segment is typically unaffected.
- The IOP is normal.
- Ophthalmoscopy shows a single or multiple localized lesions of retinal edema, burns, or holes, typically in the macula, with hemorrhage (subretinal, subhyaloid, or vitreous).

The clinical course is usually the following.

- In the next few days/weeks after the injury, there is marked functional improvement, mainly due to the clearing of hemorrhage and subsidence of the inflammation at the site of injury.
- Vision may remain stable or deteriorate because of late complications such as chorioretinal scarring (Fig. 34–2), macular hole, or EMP. Long-term follow-up is thus warranted.

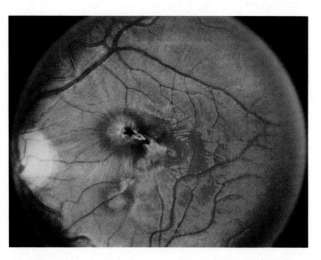

FIGURE 34–2   A case of four, accidental, 5-mJ exposures to an Nd:YAG laser, 1 year after the injury. Scarring and contraction around the scars are evident. (Courtesy of the Medical Research Department, Walter Reed Army Institute of Research, San Antonio, Texas.)

PITFALL

In laser workers, ophthalmoscopy may reveal peripheral retinal lesions consistent with old laser injuries, although the patient may have no recollection of such events (Fig. 34–3).[37,39–41] Presumably, laser injuries to the peripheral retina went unrecognized.

SPECIAL CONSIDERATION

It is recommended that individuals who are at high risk of laser exposure should undergo ophthalmoscopic examination before starting a potentially hazardous occupation and after its termination, mainly for medicolegal reasons (see Chapter 7). In view of the symptomatic nature of visually significant laser injuries and the unavailability of treatment for laser-induced retinal injuries, we do not think that periodic eye examinations are indicated, although the optimal sequence of examinations for laser workers remains controversial.

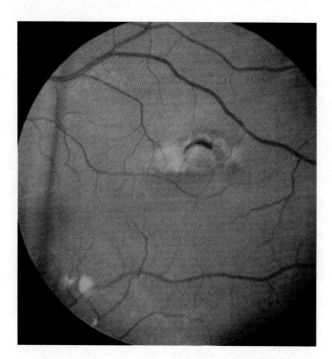

FIGURE 34–3 Probable laser scar in the retinal periphery discovered on routine examination. Patient stated that he "occasionally did not use eye protection" when working with various lasers. There were no symptoms during the probable exposure or later. The case illustrates the importance of ophthalmoscopic examination before starting to work at occupations that entail laser exposure hazards.

Hand-held laser pointers have become very popular, and their potential for eye damage has given cause for concern.

- They emit a continuous narrow beam of visible light (most commonly red; 670 nm for diode and 632.8 nm for helium-neon laser). The output power (see Table 34–1) is usually 1–5 mW.

- The likelihood that accidental exposure of the eye to such a device will result in permanent retinal injury is very small.[25,49–51]

- If shone directly at the eye, the retinal irradiance is similar to that caused by staring directly at the sun.[50] Under normal circumstances, however, where exposure is limited by the blink reflex and aversion response, this is incapable of causing retinal damage.

- Thermal damage may occur following prolonged (>10–20 s) staring into the beam.[52–54]

> **P**EARL... The ophthalmologist caring for patients complaining about laser pointer exposure should bear in mind that visible radiation is not absorbed by tissues at the front of the eye; consequently, symptoms such as pain or irritation are most probably caused by rubbing.

Laser range finders and target designators are commonly used in the military. Accidental exposures[39,41–43,47] generally follow a clinical course similar to that described previously.

Injuries have occurred mainly as a result of careless operation or in the course of military peacetime activities. There is only one report of an eye injury allegedly caused by an enemy laser during actual combat.[46]

Laser devices may be used deliberately to cause visual incapacitation and eye damage. Damage can potentially be inflicted from a long distance with relative ease. If these weapons, currently being developed by military industries,[55] are massively deployed in future battlefields, retinal injuries may be inflicted in large number. Although these laser weapons were named "blinding," they are better regarded as visually incapacitating, since true blindness is usually not expected to be inflicted. Eye protection against laser radiation is difficult on the battlefield because the wavelength of the enemy laser may not be known. In addition, more than one wavelength can be employed in a laser weapon system or tunable lasers may be used.

> **PITFALL**
>
> An optimal laser protection system is transparent under normal circumstances and switched on within a few nanoseconds, blocking light transmission when encountering coherent radiation. This type of protective device is not currently available and is unlikely to be developed in the near future.

Treatment Corticosteroids are often administered with the rationale of reducing the cellular inflammatory response to injury and thus limiting the extent of damage. However, this approach has not been properly evaluated in clinical studies. In animal models, corticosteroids have been reported as beneficial,[56–59] ineffective,[60,61] and even harmful.[62,63]

In recent years, neuroprotective compounds have been introduced, aimed at decreasing the secondary spread of damage in neuronal tissues, including the retina.[64–67] Compounds such as glutamate receptor blockers are currently being evaluated in clinical trials.

Complete protection against accidental laser injury is possible only if the characteristics of the instrument and its mode of employment are known. In the civilian environment this is relatively simple, and protection can be achieved by wearing goggles containing wavelength-specific filters. The main limitation of these protective devices is the reluctance of the operating personnel to wear them. There have been cases in which retinal injury has been inflicted when the persons were wearing a filter inappropriate for the laser being used.[34,48]

Photic Injury from Ophthalmic Light Sources

Macular damage from the operating microscope's light was first reported in 1983[68]; such injuries are rather commonly sustained in cataract or other anterior segment surgeries but in rare cases may be inflicted with the endoilluminator during vitrectomy.[69–81]

Injury from the Operating Microscope   In one study of 135 consecutive cataract operations, the incidence was 7.4%.[74] Prolonged operation time is a significant risk factor (in all but one patient the operation had lasted over 100 minutes, much longer than the typical duration of modern phacoemulsification surgery).[74] In a more recent series of 37 consecutive patients, no phototoxic injury was noted.[77]

The visual consequences depend on the lesion's proximity to the fovea, size, and severity of the lesion. Following anterior segment surgery, the visual acuity is usually not significantly decreased by the phototoxic lesion, and improvement with time has been documented even when the scotoma is paracentral.[75]

Injury from the Endoilluminator   The outcome of these lesions may be substantially worse.[76,78,79] These lesions are larger, more often involve the fovea, and may be responsible for significantly decreased visual acuity. Prevention is recommended, and various measures during vitrectomy have been described.[78]

The findings generally include the following.

- The ophthalmoscopic appearance of such injuries is a perifoveal, round to oval lesion of the RPE. The shape of the retinal lesion corresponds to the shape of the illuminating source used during surgery (e.g., a horizontal oval lesion could be caused by a horizontally oriented filament inside the microscope lamp). The lesion is usually inferior to the fovea and outside the avascular zone. Progressive pigmentation of the lesion may be observed over several months, distinguishing the acute maculopathy from an old scar.

- The FA shows a sharply demarcated, mottled hyperfluorescent lesion.

- Experiments on phakic eyes of living humans have confirmed the direct cause-and-effect relationship between light exposure and macular lesions as well as the observed clinical course.[82–84] The injury site 24 hours after exposure was described as a gray lesion at the level of the RPE, one to two disk areas in size. The visual acuity was minimally affected and a small paracentral scotoma could be demonstrated. Pigment migration within the lesion was noted after 1 week, and pigment clumping after 3 weeks. These findings are consistent with a photochemical injury mechanism. The use of UV and/or IR filters did not prevent the development of retinopathy.[83–84]

> **PEARL...** Visible lesions have been produced by exposure to the *IBO* in animal experiments[85–87] but are unlikely to occur in clinical practice. The threshold of histological retinal light injury, however, is lower than that of visible lesions.[88] It is prudent to use the lowest level of IBO illumination consistent with a satisfactory examination, especially if repeated examinations are required.

As in other types of photic trauma, prevention is the key. The risk of photic retinopathy can most probably be reduced by the following rational methods,[78] none of which has been properly substantiated:

- minimize the length of surgery;
- reduce the intensity of light used whenever possible;
- use noncoaxial light if feasible (oblique illumination places the intense image of the illuminating beam at the retinal periphery rather than in the foveal area);
- use appropriate filters to eliminate the unnecessary UV and IR wavelengths;
- place shields on the cornea to prevent retinal exposure when possible; and
- when using an endoilluminator for posterior segment procedures, minimize direct exposure to the fovea whenever possible by:

○ reducing the power;
○ increasing the distance between the probe and the retina; and
○ directing the light away from the fovea.

> **PEARL...** Visible light accounts for most of a person's sensory input, but at high intensities light may damage the very organ that makes the sensory use of such energy possible. Simple, common sense prevention practices can minimize such light-induced trauma.

ELECTRICAL TRAUMA

Eye injury from high-voltage electrocution is another uncommon type of nonmechanical trauma. It may be caused by passage of the current through ocular tissues or secondarily through heat. In one series, 3% of 159 consecutive patients with high-voltage burns had ophthalmic changes.[89]

- The most frequent occurrence is bilateral (anterior-subcapsular) cataract formation.[89–95] This has been observed as early as few hours after electrical injury but may take years to develop. The damage to other ocular tissues is not significant, and the prognosis following cataract extraction is good.
- Other ocular effects have been reported anecdotally and include retinal vascular changes[89] and macular hole.[89,96] In exceptionally severe cases, extensive thermal coagulative injury may necessitate enucleation.[93]

SUMMARY

Light is an uncommon but potentially serious cause of ocular injury. Sources of photic injury may include the sun, laser devices, and ophthalmic equipment. Although photic injury is an uncommon form of ocular trauma, it can have disastrous results, particularly when the macula is injured. Prevention is critical since treatment options are limited, and the natural history of such injuries is often poor.

REFERENCES

1. Boettner EA, Wolter JR. Transmission of the ocular media. *Invest Ophthalmol Vis Sci.* 1962;1:776–783.

2. Geeraets WJ, Berry ER. Ocular spectral characteristics as related to hazards from lasers and other light sources. *Am J Ophthalmol.* 1968;66:15–20.

3. Marshall J. Thermal and mechanical mechanisms in laser damage to the retina. *Invest Ophthalmol.* 1970;9:97–115.

4. Mellerio J. The thermal nature of retinal laser photocoagulation. *Exp Eye Res.* 1966;5:242–248.

5. Priebe LA, Cain CP, Welch AJ. Temperature rise required for the production of minimal lesions in the *Macaca mulatta* retina. *Am J Ophthalmol.* 1975;79:405–413.

6. Mainster MA, Sliney DH, Belcher CD, Buzney SM. Laser photodisruptors: damage mechanisms, instrument design and safety. *Ophthalmology.* 1983;90:973–991.

7. Ham WT, Ruffolo JJ, Mueller HA, Guerry S. The nature of retinal radiation damage: dependence on wavelength, power level and exposure time. *Vision Res.* 1980;20:1105–1111.

8. Hirsch DR, Booth DG, Schocket S, Sliney DH. Recovery from pulsed-dye laser retinal injury. *Arch Ophthalmol.* 1992;110:1688.

9. Toshihiro A. Accidental YAG laser burn. *Am J Ophthalmol.* 1984;98:116–117.

10. Zwick H, Gagliano D, Zuchlich JA, Stuck BE, Belkin M. Laser induced retinal nerve fiber layer (NFL) damage. In: Parel JM, ed. *Ophthalmic Techniques.* Bellingham, WA: SPIE; 1995:330–337.

11. L'esperance FA, ed. *Ophthalmic Lasers,* 2nd ed. St. Louis: CV Mosby; 1983:3.

12. Mainster MA, Khan JA. Photic retinal injury. In Ryan SJ, ed. *Retina,* 2nd ed. Philadelphia: Mosby–Year Book; 1994:1768.

13. Ridgway AEA. Solar retinopathy. *Br Med J.* 1967;3:212–214.

14. Penner R, McNair JN. Eclipse blindness. *Am J Ophthalmol.* 1966;61:1452–1457.

15. Rothkoff L, Kushelensky A, Blumenthal M. Solar retinopathy: visual prognosis in 20 cases. *Isr J Med Sci.* 1978;14:238–243.

16. Atmaca LS, Idil Aysun, Can Deniz. Early and late visual prognosis in solar retinopathy. *Graefes Arch Clin Exp Ophthalmol.* 1995;233:801–804.

17. Dhir SP, Gupta A, Jain IS. Eclipse retinopathy. *Br J Ophthalmol.* 1981;65:42–45.

18. Jacobs NA, Headon M, Rosen ES. Solar retinopathy in the Manchester area. *Trans Ophthalmol Soc UK.* 1985;104:625–628.

19. Cangelosi GC, Newsome DA. Solar retinopathy in persons on religious pilgrimage. *Am J Ophthalmol.* 1988;105:95–97.

20. Hope-Ross M, Travers S, Mooney D. Solar retinopathy following religious rituals. *Br J Ophthalmol.* 1988;72:931–934.

21. Schatz H, Mendelblatt F. Solar retinopathy from sun-gazing under the influence of LSD. *Br J Ophthalmol*. 1973;57:270–273.

22. Aiello LP, Arrigg PG, Shah ST, et al. Solar retinopathy associated with hypoglycemic insulin reaction. *Arch Ophthalmol*. 1994;112:982–983.

23. Ewald RA, Ritchey CL. Sun gazing as the cause of foveomacular retinitis. *Am J Ophthalmol*. 1970;70:491–497.

24. Hope-Ross MW, Gardiner MTA, Archer DB. Ultra-structural findings in solar retinopathy. *Eye*. 1993;7:29–33.

25. Mainster MA, Timberlake GT, Warren KA, Sliney DH. Pointers on laser pointers. *Ophthalmology*. 1997;104:1213–1214.

26. Naidoff MA, Sliney DH. Retinal injury from a welding arc. *Am J Ophthalmol*. 1974;77:663–668.

27. Uniat L, Olk RJ, Hanish SJ. Welding arc maculopathy. *Am J Ophthalmol*. 1986;102:394–395.

28. Romanchuk KG, Pollak V, Schneider RJ. Retinal burn from a welding arc. *Can J Ophthalmol*. 1978;13:120–122.

29. Maiman TH. Stimulated optical radiation in ruby. *Nature*. 1960;187:493.

30. Curtin TL, Boyden DG. Reflected laser beam causing accidental burn of the retina. *Am J Ophthalmol*. 1968;65:188–189.

31. Rathkey AS. Accidental laser burn of the macula. *Arch Ophthalmol*. 1965;74:346–348.

32. Jacobson JH. Accidental laser retinal burns. *Arch Ophthalmol*. 1965;74:882.

33. Goldman AI, Ham WT, Mueller HA. Mechanisms of retinal damage resulting from the exposure of rhesus monkeys to ultrashort laser pulses. *Exp Eye Res*. 1975;21:457–469.

34. Goldman AI, Ham WT, Mueller HA. Ocular damage thresholds and mechanisms for ultrashort pulses of both visible and infrared laser radiation in the rhesus monkey. *Exp Eye Res*. 1977;27:45–56.

35. Manning JR, Davidorf FH, Keates RH, Strange AE. Neodymium:YAG laser lesion in the human retina: accidental/experimental. *Contemp Ophthalmic Forum*. 1986;4(3):86–91.

36. Blankenstein MF, Zuchlich J, Allen RG, Davis H, Thomas SJ, Harrison RF. Retinal hemorrhage thresholds for Q-switched neodymium-YAG laser exposures. *Invest Ophthalmol Vis Sci*. 1986;27:1176–1179.

37. Boldrey EE, Little HL, Flocks M, Vassiliadis A. Retinal injury due to industrial laser burns. *Ophthalmology*. 1981;88:101–107.

38. Decker CD. Accident victim's view. *Laser Focus*. Aug 1977, p. 6.

39. Wolfe JA. Laser retinal injury. *Mil Med*. 1985;150:177.

40. Cai Y, Xu D, Mo X. Clinical, pathological and photo-chemical studies of laser injury of the retina. *Health Phys*. 1989;56:643–646.

41. Gabel VP, Birngruber R, Lorenz B, Lang GK. Clinical observations of six cases of laser injury to the eye. *Health Phys*. 1989;56:705–710.

42. Alhalel A, Glovinski Y, Treister G, et al. Long-term follow up of accidental parafoveal laser burns. *Retina*. 1993;13:152–154.

43. Gorsuch GM. Laser injury. *Navy Med*. 1996;March–April:23–26.

44. Kearney JJ, Cohen HB, Stuck BE, Rudd GP. Laser injury to multiple retinal foci. *Lasers Surg Med*. 1987;7:499–502.

45. Lang GK, Lang G, Naumann GOH. Accidental bilateral asymmetric maculopathy caused by a ruby laser. *Klin Monatsbl Augenheilkd*. 1985;186:366–370.

46. Mader TH, Aragones JV, Chandler AC, et al. Ocular and ocular adnexal injuries treated by United States military ophthalmologists during Operation Desert Shield and Desert Storm. *Ophthalmology*. 1993;100:1462–1467.

47. Modarres-Zadeh M, Parvaresh MM, Pourbabak S, Peyman GA. Accidental parafoveal laser burn from a standard military ruby range finder. *Retina*. 1995;15:356–358.

48. Lam TT, Tso MOM. Retinal injury by neodymium:YAG laser. *Retina*. 1996;16:42–46.

49. Mensah E, Vafidis G, Marshall J. Laser pointers: the facts, media hype, and hysteria. *Lancet*. 1998;351:1291.

50. Sliney DH, Dennis JE. Safety concerns about laser pointers. *J Laser Appl*. 1994;6:159–164.

51. Marshall J. The safety of laser pointers: myths and realities. *Br J Ophthalmol*. 1998;82:1335–1338.

52. Luttrull JK, Hallisey J. Laser pointer–induced macular injury. *Am J Ophthalmol*. 1999;127:95–96.

53. Zamir E, Kaiseman I, Chowers I. Laser pointer maculopathy. *Am J Ophthalmol*. 1999;127:728–729.

54. Sell CH, Bryan JS. Maculopathy from handheld diode laser pointer. *Arch Ophthalmol*. 1999;117:1557–1558.

55. Barkana Y, Belkin M. Laser eye injuries. *Surv Ophthalmol*. 2000;44:459–478.

56. Lam TT, Fu J, Takahashi K, Tso MOM. Methylprednisolone therapy in laser injury of the retina. *Graefes Arch Clin Exp Ophthalmol*. 1993;231:729–736.

57. Naveh N, Weissman C. Corticosteroid treatment of laser retinal damage affects prostaglandin E_2 response. *Invest Ophthalmol Vis Sci*. 1990;31:9–13.

58. Wilson CA, Berkowitz BA, Sato Y, et al. Treatment with intravitreal steroid reduces blood-retinal breakdown due to retinal photocoagulation. *Arch Ophthalmol*. 1992;110:1155–1159.

59. Ishibashi T, Miki K, Sorgente N, et al. Effects of intravitreal administration of steroids on experimental subretinal neovascularization in the subhuman primate. *Arch Ophthalmol*. 1985;103:708–711.

60. Rosner M, Solberg Y, Turetz J, Belkin M. Neuroprotective therapy for argon-laser induced retinal injury. *Exp Eye Res*. 1997;65:485–495.

61. Solberg Y, Dubinski G, Tchirkov M, Belkin M, Rosner M. Methylprednisolone therapy for retinal laser injury. *Surv Ophthalmol*. 1999;44(suppl 1):S85–S92.

62. Marshall J. Structural aspects of laser induced damage and their functional implications. *Health Phys*. 1989;56:617–624.

63. Schuschereba ST, Cross ME, Pizarro JAM, et al. High dose methylprednisolone treatment of laser-induced retinal injury exacerbates acute inflammation and long-term scarring [abstract]. *Int Symp Biomed Opt*. 1999:40.

64. Meldru B, Garthwaite J. Excitatory amino acid neurotoxicity and neurodegenerative disease. *Trends Pharmacol Sci*. 1990;11:379–387.

65. Faden AI, Salzman S. Pharmacological strategies in CNS trauma. *Trends Pharmacol Sci*. 1992;13:29–35.

66. Choi DW. The role of glutamate neurotoxicity in hypoxic-ischemic neuronal death: *Annu Rev Neurosci*. 1990;13:171–182.

67. Solberg Y, Rosner M, Belkin M. MK-801 has neuroprotection and antiproliferative effects in retinal laser injury. *Invest Ophthmol Vis Sci*. 1997;38:1380–1389.

68. McDonald HR, Irvine AR. Light-induced maculopathy from the operating microscope in extracapsular cataract extraction and intraocular lens implantation. *Ophthalmology*. 1983;90:945–951.

69. Ross WH. Light-induced maculopathy. *Am J Ophthalmol*. 1984;98:488–493.

70. Khwarg SG, Geoghegan M, Handcom TA. Light-induced maculopathy from the operating microscope. *Am J Ophthalmol*. 1984;98:628–630.

71. Boldrey EE, Ho BT, Griffith RD. Retinal burns occurring at cataract extraction. *Ophthalmology*. 1984;91:1297–1302.

72. Delaey JJ, DeWachter, Van Oye R, Verbraeken H. Retinal phototrauma during intraocular lens implantation. *Int Ophthalmol*. 1984;7:109.

73. Brod RD, Barron BA, Sueflow JA, Franklin RM, Packer AJ. Phototoxic retinal damage during refractive surgery. *Am J Ophthalmol*. 1986;102:121–123.

74. Khwarg SG, Linstone FA, Daniels SA, et al. Incidence, risk factors and morphology in operating microscope light retinopathy. *Am J Ophthalmol*. 1987;103:255–263.

75. Lindquist TD, Grutzmacher RD, Gofman JD. Light-induced maculopathy—potential for recovery. *Arch Ophthalmol*. 1986;104:1641–1647.

76. Postel EA, Pulido JS, Byrnes GA, et al. Long-term follow-up of iatrogenic phototoxicity. *Arch Ophthalmol*. 1998;116:753–757.

77. Byrnes GA, Chang B, Loose I, Miller SA, Benson WE. Prospective incidence of photic maculopathy after cataract surgery. *Am J Ophthalmol*. 1995;119:231–232.

78. Kuhn F, Morris R, Massey M. Photic retinal injury from endoillumination during vitrectomy. *Am J Ophthalmol*. 1991;111:42.

79. Michels M, Lewis H, Abrams GW. Macular phototoxicity caused by fiberoptic endoillumination during pars plana vitrectomy. *Am J Ophthalmol*. 1992;114:287.

80. Cech JM, Choromokos EA, Sanitato JA. Light-induced maculopathy following penetrating keratoplasty and lens implantation. *Arch Ophthalmol*. 1987;105:751.

81. Kingham JD. Photic maculopathy in young males with intraocular foreign body. *Mil Med*. 1991;156:44–47.

82. Green WR, Robertson DM. Pathologic findings of photic retinopathy in the human eye. *Am J Ophthalmol*. 1991;112:520–527.

83. Robertson DM, McLaren JW. Photic retinopathy from the operating room microscope. Study with filters. *Arch Ophthalmol*. 1989;107:373–375.

84. Robertson DM, Feldman RB. Photic retinopathy from the operating room microscope. *Am J Ophthalmol*. 1986;101:561–569.

85. Tso MOM, Fine BS, Zimmerman LE. Photic maculopathy produced by the indirect ophthalmoscope. I. Clinical and histopathologic study. *Am J Ophthalmol*. 1972;73:686–699.

86. Tso MOM. Photic maculopathy in rhesus monkey: a light and electron microscopic study. *Invest Ophthalmol*. 1973;12:17–34.

87. Tso MOM, Woodford BJ. Effect of photic injury on the retinal tissues. *Ophthalmology*. 1983;90:952–963.

88. Adams DO, Beatrice ES, Bedell RB. Retina: ultrastructural alterations produced by extremely low levels of coherent radiation. *Science*. 1972;177:58–60.

89. Boozalis GT, Purdue GF, Hunt JL, McCulley JP. Ocular changes from electrical burn injuries. A literature review and report of cases. *J Burn Care Rehabil*. 1991;12:458–462.

90. Oleszewski SC, Nyman JS. Electric cataract: a rare clinical entity. *Am J Optom Physiol Opt*. 1984;61:279–283.

91. Saffle J, Crandall A, Warden G. Cataracts: a long-term complication of electrical injury. *J Trauma*. 1985;25:17–21.

92. Van Johnson E, Kline LB, Skalka HW. Electrical cataracts: a case report and review of the literature. *Ophthalmic Surg*. 1987;18:283–285.

93. Al Rabiah SM, Archer DB, Millar R, Collins AD, Shepherd WF. Electrical injury of the eye. *Int Ophthalmol*. 1987;11:31–40.

94. Reddy SC. Electric cataract: a case report and review of the literature. *Eur J Ophthalmol*. 1999;9:134–138.

95. Fraunfelder F, Hanna C. Electrical cataracts. I. Sequential changes, visual and prognostic findings. *Arch Ophthalmol*. 1972;87:179–183.

96. Campo R, Lewis R. Lightning-induced macular hole. *Am J Ophthalmol*. 1984;97:792–794.

SECTION V

NONGLOBE INJURIES

Chapter 35

EYELID AND LACRIMAL TRAUMA

John A. Long and Thomas M. Tann

Eyelid trauma has been a part of human history since ancient times. Sharp sticks, flint knives, and animal bites have commonly led to substantial eyelid trauma. Phillip of Macedonia, the father of Alexander the Great, suffered extensive eyelid wounds yet lived long enough to launch his son. Archaeological evidence suggests, however, that eyelid wounds could signal fatal trauma. Harold of England suffered eyelid trauma during the Battle of Hastings. The Bayeux tapestry and legend claim that he was killed by an arrow, which entered his skull through his eyelid.

Repair of eyelid wounds is documented in ancient Egyptian and Greek writings. Bandages and sutures were available when words were first written to describe surgical techniques.

In modern times trauma is still common because of sharp objects, animal bites, fighting, and burns; in addition newer sources such as high-speed missiles, and MVCs have also emerged. This chapter reviews the current management concepts in treating patients with trauma to the eyelids and lacrimal system.

EPIDEMIOLOGY (USEIR DATA)

Rate of lid and lacrimal system involvement among all serious injuries: 5%; breakdown:

- lacrimal laceration: 81%;
- periocular laceration: 70%;
- lid erythema: 19%;
- lacrimal obstruction: <1%.;
- lid deformity: <1%.

Age (years):
- range: 0–90;
- average: 23;
- rate of 0- to 9-year-olds among the total: 23%;
- rate of 10- to 19-year-olds among the total: 18%;
- rate of ≥60-year-olds among the total: 6%.

Sex: 77% male.

Place of injury:
- home: 37%;
- street and highway: 21%;
- recreation and sport: 11%;
- industrial premises: 8%;
- public building: 5%;
- school: 3%.

Source of injury:
- various blunt objects: 28%;
- various sharp objects: 16%.
- MVC: 14%;
- fall: 8%
- gunshot: 6%;
- fireworks: 4%;
- BB/pellet gun: 3%;

Globe involvement among the total: 61%.

Rate of animal bites among the total: 9%.

Prevention

Through history and into modern times, clever devices have been developed to provide protection for the eyelids and eyeballs. From the hoplite helmet to shatterproof windshield glass, technology has continued to improve eye safety. In the 20th century, laws and regulations at the workplace have been very helpful; this tendency is not apparent in the home (see Chapter 4).

Eyelid Lacerations

Pathophysiology

Eyelid trauma can be quite dramatic, and the evaluation of eyelid trauma requires a thorough understanding of the anatomy of the eyelid and the adjacent structures. The eyelid's primary function is to provide protection to the eyeballs.

> **PEARL...** Because globe injury and eyelid trauma commonly occur concurrently, any investigation of eyelid trauma must include to a detailed examination of the eyeballs.

> **PEARL...** When orbital fat is present in the wound, an orbital injury has occurred.

The eyelid margin is in contact with both the tear film and the outside environment. The mucoepithelial junction is an important anatomic landmark.

The eyelid is also an important part of the *tear pump*. The action of the lid margin pushes tears toward the punctum for removal. Disruption of the eyelid margin may lead to an impaired tear pump. This can occur with notching of the eyelid margin or with traumatically induced laxity. The inability of the eyelids to properly move the tears may lead to:

- epiphora;
- dellen formation; or even
- corneal ulceration.

The canalicular system carries tears from the puncta to the lacrimal sac. Evidence suggests that the lower canalicular system is primarily responsible; however, in some people, the superior part of the system removes most of the tears.[1]

> **PEARL...** Patients with canalicular laceration always require repair. It is impossible to determine preoperatively whether the superior or lower canalicular system is dominant in the injured individual.

The canalicular system is very close to the conjunctival surface. An extremely medial cutaneous eyelid laceration may not involve the canalicular system if the wound is superficial.

> **PEARL...** A conjunctival laceration in the medial aspect of the eyelids probably involves the canalicular system.[2,3]

The levator muscle is the primary elevator of the upper eyelids. The levator aponeurosis is the tendon of the levator muscle. The levator muscle has numerous attachments in the eyelid, all of which may be involved with trauma. Insertions of the levator include:

- conjunctiva;
- superior tarsus;
- anterior tarsus;
- orbital septum; and
- skin.

The levator attaches to the conjunctiva at the superior fornix, the superior border of the tarsus through Müller's muscle, and the anterior face of the tarsus through the levator aponeurosis. Attachments to the orbital septum and skin are also consistently found. Eyelid trauma can lacerate or contuse the levator muscle or stretch and break the levator aponeurosis.

Eyelid trauma can compromise the levator function. Lacerations or contusive trauma may lead to traumatic ptosis. The ptosis may persist for a variable period of time and often resolves spontaneously only long after the other manifestations of trauma have healed.

Traumatic ptosis caused by contusion often improves spontaneously.[4] Characteristics of such a ptosis are:

- history of eyelid trauma;
- poor levator function; and
- slow but almost always full recovery.

The initial treatment for traumatic ptosis, which has been caused by contusion, is observation. It is not unusual to see complete recovery 6 months following the accident. If full recovery does not occur, exploration of the eyelid and repair of the ptosis are indicated.

Evaluation

The evaluation and diagnosis of eyelid trauma begin with a history and physical examination and observation. For the ophthalmologist, it is of paramount importance that a thorough eye examination be performed. Eyelid lacerations are often accompanied by severe globe injuries and retained orbital foreign bodies (see Chapters 24 and 36).[5–7]

> **PEARL...** Dramatic eyelid injuries may conceal dangerous ocular, orbital, and/or neurologic injuries (see Chapter 10).

- Even very small eyelid lacerations may involve the canalicular system. A high index of suspicion is important when evaluating the medial eyelids. Medial conjunctival lacerations often involve the canalicular system. Probing the canalicular system is easily accomplished in the ER.

> **PEARL...** For complex lacerations, irrigation of the lacrimal system with sterile saline can be performed. Saline exiting from the wound is a sure sign of canalicular laceration.

The levator muscle is evaluated by observing the excursions of the upper eyelids. Traumatic ptosis or mechanical ptosis may be documented. If possible, a lacerated levator aponeurosis should be repaired primarily. Mechanical ptosis, when seen without eyelid lacerations, may be due to:

- eyelid swelling;
- contusion to the levator aponeurosis;
- neurologic damage; and
- levator damage.

Without a laceration present, it is often wise simply to observe the ptosis for a period of time. Exploration of the levator muscle is not indicated unless an eyelid laceration and potential levator muscle or aponeurosis damage are observed.

Effective emergency evaluation of *children* is sometimes impossible in the ER (see Chapters 9 and 30). Probing and irrigation of a potentially lacerated canalicular system is contraindicated in the young or uncooperative patient. An examination under anesthesia is commonly needed to arrive at a definitive diagnosis.

> ▼ **PITFALL**
>
> Patient care should never be compromised for lack of an adequate examination.

Radiology has limited importance in the evaluation of eyelid trauma. An orbital CT scan should be ordered when the suspicion of a retained orbital foreign body is present (see Chapter 36).

Eyelid lacerations often occur due to animal bites.[8,9] The history of an animal bite should be reported to the authorities so that the animal can be observed for rabies.[7] Medical personnel may be required by local law to file the report of an animal bite injury (see in more detail later in this chapter).

Appropriate use of antibiotics, tetanus toxoid, and all prophylactic measures apply in case of eyelid trauma (see Chapters 8, 9, and 28 and the Appendix).[10]

Timing

Eyelid margin lacerations do not require immediate repair. Injuries of inebriated patients, presenting at night or on the weekend, can be repaired when experienced personnel become available during "regular business hours." After a thorough examination, antibiotic ointment and a patch will stabilize the patient until a definitive repair can be performed in 24 to 48 hours. It is usually not wise to delay the repair for over 48 hours.[4]

> **PEARL...** Eyelid lacerations do not have to be repaired immediately.

Management

Eyelid margin lacerations are commonly seen in ERs.

- Simple eyelid margin lacerations can usually be repaired in the ER under local anesthesia (see Chapter 8). To perform an adequate repair, proper equipment, lights, and support personnel must be present.
- Children and uncooperative patients and those with more complex injuries must be repaired in the operating room under general anesthesia.

The anatomy of the upper and lower eyelids guides the techniques for repair. Traditionally, the eyelid has been described as having two layers:

- an anterior lamella, consisting of the skin and the orbicularis muscle; and

- a posterior lamella consisting of the conjunctiva and the tarsus.

The approximation of these lamellae forms the basis for eyelid repair. By meticulous and precise closure, the overall goal is to restore the eyelid's:

- contour;
- function; and
- anatomy.

The eyelid has several anatomic structures that help to achieve the proper alignment:

- the eyelash line;
- the gray line; and
- the meibomian gland orifices.

The *eyelash line* is a consistent landmark, which will help with the proper suture placement and alignment of the eyelid. There are normally three linear rows of lashes on the upper eyelid and two linear rows of lashes on the lower eyelid.

PITFALL

Proper alignment of the eyelashes and proper orientation of the eyelashes are important. Suture imbrication of the eyelashes can lead to trichiasis once healing has occurred.

The *meibomian gland orifices* are another invariable eyelid margin landmark. The meibomian gland orifices arise in the tarsus and extend throughout the length of the tarsus. Placing eyelid margin sutures through the meibomian orifice line will provide a firm reapproximation.

The *gray line* is the surface projection of the muscle of Riolan. This invariable anatomic landmark is usually the location of the most posterior eyelid margin suture. The eyelid margin sutures, when properly placed, can be secured away from the conjunctiva with one additional skin suture.

The typical surgical process is the following:

- The first suture to place when repairing an eyelid margin laceration is at the eyelid margin. A 6-0 silk suture through the meibomian gland orifices will align the eyelid margin. The first well-placed suture will help with the placement of all subsequent sutures. By pulling on the lid margin suture, the tarsus will become aligned and aid in deep

suture placement. Silk sutures at the eyelid margin are preferred because they are soft, easy to work with, and have less memory than sutures composed of nylon or synthetic fibers.

PEARL... The eyelid margin sutures must not be in contact with the cornea.

- Once the eyelid margin is properly aligned, deeper sutures are introduced to secure the lacerated tarsus.[a]

PITFALL

When placing tarsal sutures, care must be taken that the suture does not penetrate through the full thickness of the tarsus, otherwise a suture-induced keratitis will develop.

- Similarly, the surgeon must protect the globe from inadvertent needle point injury. A corneal protector is usually available.[b]

- The upper eyelid tarsus can usually be reapproximated with two to three deep sutures. The lower eyelid tarsus requires one to two deep sutures. The deep suture knots should be tied in such a way that the knot is directed toward the skin surface. Fortunately, if the deep sutures extrude, they typically do so through the skin's surface instead of leading to suture keratitis.

- In many cases when an eyelid has been lacerated, the orbicularis muscle develops spasms, pulling the wound wide open.

PEARL... The contraction by the unopposed pull of the orbicularis muscle is one reason why lid margin lacerations look more severe than they usually are.

- It is very unusual for a lid margin to be missing in cases of simple lacerations. Careful reapproximation and firm support by the sutures allow adequate healing.

---

[a] A 5-0 Dexon suture with a D-1 needle is a good choice for eyelid margin lacerations. The needle is a spatulated, half-circle needle, and these characteristics allow precise lamellar placement through the lacerated tarsus.

[b] The corneal protector must not distort the eyelid's position.

- After the tarsal sutures have been placed, the orbicularis muscle is evaluated. If it appears to be gaped, the same 5-0 Dexon suture can be used to reapproximate the orbicularis muscle.
- The skin is usually in excellent approximation after the closure of the tarsus and orbicularis muscle.

Sutures of 6-0 silk can be used for eyelid margin and skin closure. For perpendicular lid margin lacerations, the skin sutures are typically placed deeper and wider than they are when closing lacerations that parallel the eyelid margin. Deeper and wider bites help stabilize the lid laceration and counteract the pull of the orbicularis muscle.

The silk eyelid margin sutures at the gray line and the meibomian gland line are reinforced by a 6-0 silk suture at the eyelash line. These sutures are carefully placed to prevent any imbrication of eyelashes. During the healing phase it is important that the lashes maintain a proper orientation because scarring and contraction may develop within the eyelid margin as it heals. After all the eyelid margin sutures have been placed, one additional skin suture can be placed on the anterior lamella, which pulls the eyelid margin sutures away from the cornea and secures them into an anterior position.

> **P**EARL... It is very unusual to have missing tissue from an eyelid laceration.[3]

Complications

The most common complication of eyelid margin lacerations is *lid notching*. This usually results from poor initial approximation or development of a wound gap, caused by postoperative eyelid swelling or orbicularis pull. Lid notching can disrupt the tear pump and tearing can occur. If the eyelid notching is a cosmetic detriment or symptomatic, a revision can be performed.

If eyelid margin revision is necessary due to either notching or *trichiasis*, a bloc of eyelid tissue may be taken, which includes the abnormal eyelid margin. The proper repair of an eyelid margin defect requires the full-thickness bloc excision of the corresponding tarsus. A full pentagonal bloc excision will allow proper eyelid reapproximation.

> **P**EARL... Pentagonal excisions of eyelid margins must include the full height of the tarsus.

Eyelid *alopecia* can develop when scarring and trauma destroy the eyelash follicles. In most patients,

focal eyelid margin alopecia is of little consequence. It may be camouflaged with makeup or permanently repaired with a bloc excision of the damaged eyelid margin.

Keloid formation after extensive eyelid lacerations is fortunately rare. The incidence of keloid formation increases in pigmented patients with severe trauma. As with so many problems in medicine, keloids tend to improve over time. The medical management of keloids involves judicious use of steroid injections, dermabrasions, and late wound revision.[11,12]

CANALICULAR LACERATIONS

Successful repair of canalicular lacerations (Fig. 35–1) requires the surgeon to be familiar with the canalicular system's anatomy and its relationship to the eyelid and the nasal structures. A lack of knowledge of these structures should prompt a referral to an oculoplastic surgeon who has experience in the area.

All lacerated canalicular systems should be repaired.

> **PITFALL**
>
> A persistent myth in medicine is that the upper canalicular systems do not need to be repaired. As mentioned previously, however, evidence shows that both the upper and lower canalicular systems are needed to carry away tears.[1]

> **P**EARL... *All* canalicular lacerations need to be repaired.

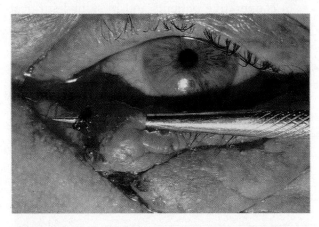

FIGURE 35-1   Left lower eyelid canalicular laceration.

The diagnosis of a lacerated canalicular system can be difficult. Very often, even relatively trivial eyelid lacerations involve the canalicular system. The nasolacrimal system can be gently probed and/or irrigated to establish the diagnosis. When examining children, an examination under anesthesia is often the only way to rule out the possibility of a canalicular laceration (see Chapter 9).

The canalicular system begins at the punctum at the upper and lower eyelid. A few facts that are helpful to remember are the following.

- The canalicular system has a short vertical component and then runs parallel to the medial eyelid margin on the conjunctival surface.
- The more medial the laceration of the canalicular system, the more posterior the cut edge of the canalicular system will be found.
- The canalicular system enters the lacrimal sac between the anterior and posterior halves of the medial canthal tendon.
- The nasolacrimal duct enters the lateral nose beneath the inferior turbinate. A stent passed through the nasolacrimal duct will enter the nose beneath the inferior turbinate. To retrieve this stent, its entry into the nose must be identified.

A variety of stents are available to facilitate canalicular system repair.[13–15] The authors prefer the *Crawford system*, which consists of silicone tubings attached to two malleable probes. The probes have a small bulb at the end, which facilitates their removal from the nose with a Crawford hook. Monocanalicular systems also exist for surgeons who are less familiar with the nasal anatomy. A bicanalicular intubation is preferred because it is less likely to become dislodged.

Surgical Technique

The repair of eyelid canalicular lacerations begins with adequate patient preparation.

- In cooperative patients and in skilled surgical hands, modified local anesthesia can be used.
- In all other instances general anesthesia should be used because some discomfort is involved, and epistaxis may lead to airway compromise in the nonintubated patient.[c]
- The identification of the proximal canaliculus is the most difficult aspect of canalicular laceration repair. With patients under general anesthesia, no local anesthesia should be used in the area of the canalicular laceration until the proximal cut edge

of the canalicular system has been found. A cotton applicator stick, patience, and gentle retracting exposure will often reward the surgeon with a cut canalicular edge. Gentle traction at the edge of the wound may help in the identification.

- If the canalicular system is difficult to identify, gentle irrigation of fluid into the uncut canalicular system may help in the identification of the laceration.[16] If the proximal canalicular system cannot be found, the eyelid should be closed without further manipulation.

PITFALL

The use of a pigtail probe is contraindicated because it has a high incidence of damage to the uninvolved canalicular system.[17]

- When the proximal and distal ends of the canalicular system laceration have been identified, stents can be passed through the canalicular system to bridge the laceration with tubing (Fig. 35–2). The injured canalicular system should be intubated prior to the uninjured canalicular system.[d]
- Once the silicone tubing is in place, the medial canthal tendon can be repaired. With the tendon reapproximated, there is no reason for a suture to be placed in the cut edge of the canalicular system. The stent will keep the canalicular system in good alignment and approximation.

---

[d]If it is impossible to intubate the injured canalicular system, at least the uninjured canalicular system can avoid iatrogenic damage.

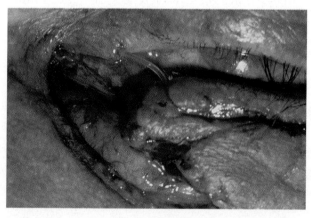

FIGURE 35–2 Bicanalicular silicone intubation of left lower eyelid canalicular laceration.

---

[c]LMA anesthesia is therefore not recommended; see Chapter 8.

- A properly placed bicanalicular stent does not need to be sutured into the nose. The nasal end of the tubing can be tied with five or six knots and allowed to retract back into the nose. The knots should be located at the tip of the inferior turbinate. The tubing should not exert any traction on the punctum or slitting of the punctum may occur.
- Once the stents are in good position and the medial canthal tendon has been closed, the eyelid laceration is repaired in a standard and layered manner.

Complications

The major complication of canalicular system repair is the failure to diagnose the problem and *failure to restore canalicular integrity*, which results in tearing. Inability to repair the canalicular system may lead to chronic tearing, which may require a reexploration of the eyelid or a conjunctivo-dacryocysto-rhinostomy with a Jones tube. Spontaneous early *dislocation of the stent* is a relatively frequent complication of bicanalicular silicone intubation.

PITFALL

Ideally, the stent should remain in place for 2 months. Earlier, inadvertent removal may lead to improper healing and long-term tearing.

PEARL... **Patients must be encouraged not to rub their eyes or to pull at the tube in the medial canthus.**

If the silicone tubing becomes dislodged and a loop is visible in the palpebral fissure, a decision must be made whether to replace or remove the tube. It is often possible simply to rethread the silicone tubing back through the canalicular system with a pair of forceps. Forcible nose blowing may at times help replace the tube within the nasolacrimal outflow tract. A 0-00 Bowman probe can be used to force the tube back through the system. If replacement of the tube is unsuccessful, early removal is the best option.

Two months is the usual time for stent removal. Patients may notice ocular irritation, mild tearing, and mucus formation at this time. The stent can be removed by cutting the loop of tubing in the palpebral fissure after the instillation of topical anesthetic. One edge of the cut tubing can be grasped with the forceps and the tubing can be pulled out through the previously undamaged canaliculus. Another option is to cut the tubing at the medial canthus and to have the patient forcibly blow the nose. The stent typically will fall out through the nasal vestibule, either immediately or over the next several days.

EYELID AVULSION

Severe eyelid avulsion injuries are frequently seen in MVCs and industrial injuries.

PITFALL

In most cases of severe avulsion injury, the eyelid remains on a vascular pedicle and can be replaced at the time of surgical repair. In no case should a potentially viable tissue be discarded.

During the initial evaluation of the patient with an avulsive injury, the tissues must be handled with care. Tension or pressure may compromise the tenuous vascular supply of the avulsed tissue and lead to tissue loss. When evaluation of the eyelid has been completed, the avulsed tissue may be protected under a patch.

The repair of eyelid avulsion injuries requires meticulous layered closure.

- In many cases, foreign body debris is present and needs to be thoroughly removed. Any organic foreign bodies need to be irrigated free, if possible; cultures may be obtained.
- The layered closure of an avulsion injury begins with deep closure of the medial or lateral canthal tendons.
- All canalicular lacerations must be addressed; see earlier in this Chapter.
- The levator muscle, if involved with the laceration, needs to be examined and, if possible, primarily repaired. In the area of the avulsion injury, not at the eyelid margin, 6-0 nylon sutures can be used to close the anterior lamella. This suture is a good choice because postoperative swelling and wound tension can be expected.

PITFALL

As a rule, absorbing sutures should not be used for this type of trauma repair. The tensile strength of an absorbing suture is simply not adequate for the postoperative swelling.

- As a rule, the conjunctiva and septum are *not* closed when repairing an eyelid avulsion. The conjunctiva will be in good approximation if the levator and tarsus are correctly reapproximated. Any conjunctival sutures will lead to corneal abrasion and pain (see Chapter 14).
- The orbital septum should *never* be closed because this may result in a restrictive ptosis or lagophthalmos. The septal attachments between the orbital rim and the levator should remain completely open as contraction of the septum during the healing phase is uncontrolled and may lead to restriction of the levator muscle. Leaving the septum open also allows easy egress of orbital hemorrhage and may prevent orbital injury due to postoperative swelling and bleeding.

PEARL...   Do *not* repair the orbital septum.

When avulsion injuries are accompanied by tissue loss, reconstructive surgery is more complicated. The initial goal is to stabilize the eyelid and protect the eyeball. Initial procedures, such as a tarsorrhaphy, may protect the eyeball until definitive reconstructive surgery can be performed. A variety of techniques for reconstructing missing eyelids is available. An oculoplastic surgeon who has experience in eyelid trauma or eyelid cancer surgery should be consulted in these complicated cases.

TRAUMATIC PTOSIS

Traumatic ptosis is not an uncommon consequence of eyelid trauma (Fig. 35–3). Ptosis may be seen both with lid lacerations and with contusion injuries.

The initial repair of a traumatic ptosis requires a careful and layered lid repair. If ptosis is present after meticulous lid closure, the treatment of choice is observation (Fig. 35–4).

PEARL...   Traumatic ptosis often improves spontaneously for up to 6 months after injury.[18–20]

Evaluation of the patient begins with careful history of the accident; special attention needs to be paid to the mechanism of injury. Scarring of the eyelid may produce a cicatricial ptosis with poor lid excursions. Evaluation of the eyelid may demonstrate a full-thickness scar. In these patients, an eyelid exploration with release of any scarring and special attention directed to the orbital septum, will often improve the situation. It is not uncommon for the levator function to remain poor after reconstructive surgery, due to neuromuscular damage.

In trauma patients in whom the levator function is normal, dehiscence of the levator aponeurosis is frequently found. Swelling caused by the accident can easily lead to a levator aponeurosis disinsertion. Repairing the levator aponeurosis should lead to a

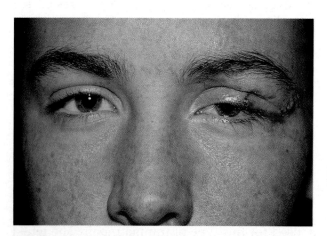

FIGURE 35–3   Traumatic left upper eyelid ptosis following eyelid trauma and laceration.

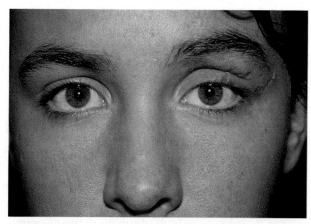

FIGURE 35–4   Spontaneous resolution of traumatic eyelid ptosis.

satisfactory lid height and contour. The levator function is the most accurate predictor of surgical success.

> **PEARL...** Patients with poor levator function often require more extensive ptosis surgery, including possible sling placement.

CICATRICIAL ECTROPION

A cicatricial ectropion of the eyelid may result from:

- tissue loss; or
- contraction of the septum.

Patients with cicatricial eyelid problems complain of:

- ocular pain and irritation due to incomplete lid closure or chronic exposure; and demonstrate
- scleral show and poor lid closure.

The evaluation of a patient with cicatricial changes involves determining which lamella of the eyelid is involved in the cicatrizing process.

- If ample skin is present, a posterior lamellar spacer (e.g., AlloDerm) or a hard palate graft will be needed to correct the defect.
- If inadequate skin is present, a full-thickness skin graft will be needed to correct the eyelid position.

Upper eyelid lagophthalmos is not an unusual finding following severe eyelid trauma. Treatment is directed at the involved lamella of the eyelid.

- In cases in which the orbital septum has been tethered to the eyelid, an eyelid exploration with a complete lysis of adhesions is necessary. Fat pads in the eyelid can be transposed or fat can be transplanted to the eyelid to provide a buffer between the septum and the underlying levator muscle.
- If the upper eyelid lagophthalmos is due to an anterior lamellar deficiency, a full-thickness skin graft may be necessary.

Skin grafts in the eyelid are often extremely well tolerated. The choice of a donor site for a full-thickness skin graft is unlimited.

- The most closely matched skin is from the opposite eyelid. In many patients, a blepharoplasty on the uninvolved eyelid will provide ample skin for reconstructive purposes.

- The retroauricular area is the second choice of skin donation. This skin is easily obtainable, and the donor site is readily hidden behind the ear. The retroauricular skin closely matches the eyelid skin in color and thickness.
- The third option for obtaining skin for eyelid reconstruction is from the supraclavicular area. This skin, however, is slightly thicker and the donor site is not as easily hidden.

BITE INJURIES

Bite injuries to the eyelid are not infrequent, especially in children. Eyelid evaluation of a dog bite victim often requires examination under anesthesia in this patient group. Special attention to the canalicular system must be paid because puncture wounds from the animal's teeth may produce deep damage to the canalicular system and lacrimal sacs.

> **PITFALL**
>
> When dealing with a dog bite injury, documentation of the dog's health and temperament is necessary. Reporting the injury to authorities may be required by law.

Meticulous repair of the injuries can often lead to complete functional and cosmetic recovery.[21,22] Although perfect results are possible in many cases, suboptimal results are often seen; they should be avoided by meticulous, layered closure of the eyelid and canalicular system in the operating room. Consider referral to a medical center where competent oculoplastic surgeons are available.

SUMMARY

Eyelid and canalicular injuries are frequent complications of severe trauma by blunt or sharp objects. Repairing these tissues is rarely emergent, and often can wait for careful intervention performed by someone intimately familiar with the anatomy and reconstruction of these structures. Improper initial repair can lead to significant and lasting visual as well as cosmetic side-effects.

REFERENCES

1. White WL, Glover AT, Buckner A, et al. Relative canalicular tear flow as assessed by dacryoscintigraphy. *Ophthalmology*. 1989;96:167–169.

2. Wulc AE, Arterberry JF. The pathogenesis of canalicular laceration. *Ophthalmology*. 1991;98:1243–1249.

3. Reifler DM: Management of canalicular laceration. *Surv Ophthalmol*. 1991;36:113–132.

4. Nelson C. Management of eyelid trauma. *Aust N Z J Ophthalmol*. 1991;19:357–363.

5. Goldberg MF, Tessler HH. Occult intraocular perforations from brow and lid lacerations. *Arch Ophthalmol*. 1971;86:145–149.

6. Siegel EB, Bastek JV, Mehringer CM, et al. Fatal intracranial extension of an orbital umbrella stab injury. *Ann Ophthalmol*. 1983;15:99–102.

7. Slonim CB. Dog bite–induced canalicular lacerations: a review of 17 cases. *Ophthalmic Plast Reconstr Surg*. 1996;12:218–222.

8. Tabbara KF, Al-Omar O. Eyelid laceration sustained in an attack by a rabid desert fox. *Am J Ophthalmol*. 1995; 119:651–652.

9. Kleimna DM, Dunne EF, Taravella MJ. Boa constrictor bite to the eye. *Arch Ophthalmol*. 1998;116:949–950.

10. American College of Surgeons Committee on Trauma. Prophylaxis against tetanus in wound management. *ACS Bull*. 1984;69(10):22–23.

11. Rockwell WB, Cohen IK, Ehrlich HP. Keloids and hypertrophic scars: a comprehensive review. *Plast Reconstr Surg*. 1989;84:827–837.

12. Ketchum LD, Cohen IK, Masters FW. Hypertrophic scars and keloids: a collective review. *Plast Reconstr Surg*. 1974;53:140–154.

13. Long JA. A method of monocanalicular silicone intubation. *Ophthalmic Surg*. 1988;19:204–205.

14. Crawford JS. Intubation of obstructions in the lacrimal system. *Can J Ophthalmol*. 1977;12:289–292.

15. Guibor P. Canaliculus intubation set. *Trans Am Acad Ophthalmol Otolaryngol*. 1975;79:419–420.

16. Seiff SR Ahn JC. Locating cut medial canaliculi by direct injection of sodium hyaluronate into the lacrimal sac. *Ophthalmic Surg*. 1989;20:176–178.

17. Kennedy RH, May J, Dailey J, et al. Canalicular laceration: an 11-year epidemiologic and clinical study. *Ophthalmic Plast Reconstr Surg*. 1990;6:46–53.

18. Silkiss RZ, Baylis HI. Management of traumatic ptosis. *Adv Ophthalmic Plast Reconstr Surg*. 1987;7:149–155.

19. Leone CR. Periorbital trauma. *Int Ophthalmol Clin*. 1995;35:1–24.

20. Serrano F, Starck T, Esquenazi S. Surgical treatment of human bites of the upper eyelid. *Ophthalmic Plast Reconstr Surg*. 1989;5:127–130.

21. Gonnering R. Ocular adnexal injury and complications in orbital dog bites. *Ophthalmic Plast Reconstr Surg*. 1987;3:231–235.

22. Herman DC, Bartley GB, Walker RC. The treatment of animal bite injuries of the eye and ocular adnexa. *Ophthalmic Plast Reconstr Surg*. 1987;3:237–241.

Chapter 36

ORBITAL TRAUMA

John A. Long and Thomas M. Tann

 The orbit is the cavity that houses, protects, and sustains the eyeball. It consists of seven bones (see Table 36–1), encompassing a pear-shaped area containing 30 mL^3 of volume. Some of the bones of the orbit are among the thickest in the skull, while others among the thinnest.

HISTORY

In prehistoric times there was ample evidence of orbital trauma and its sequelae. The remains of an Incan sacrifice has been found frozen in the Andes Mountains with orbital fractures that were probably associated with human sacrifice. Archaeological evidence from Europe demonstrates that Neanderthals could sustain extensive orbital trauma, yet survive and live for many years.

With modern life, new mechanisms of injury have developed, including high-speed missiles (bullets) and high-velocity impacts (e.g., in MVCs). These new mechanisms of injury require new methods of prevention and repair.

TABLE 36–1 THE SEVEN BONES OF THE ORBIT AND THEIR RESISTANCE

	Strong	Weak
Ethmoid		+
Frontal	+	
Lacrimal		+
Maxilla	+	
Palatine		+
Sphenoid	+	
Zygomatic	+	

EPIDEMIOLOGY (USEIR DATA)

Rate of orbital involvement among all serious injuries: 15%; breakdown:

- fracture: 78%;
- foreign body: 24%;
- hemorrhage: 1%.

Age (years):
- range: 0–103;
- average: 27;
- rate of 0- to 9-year-olds among the total: 8%;
- rate of 10- to 19-year-olds among the total: 22%;
- rate of ≥60-year-olds among the total: 7%.

Sex: 78% male.

Place of injury:
- street and highway: 29%;
- home: 28%;
- recreation and sport: 13%;
- industrial premises: 7%;
- public building: 5%.

Source of injury:
- various blunt objects: 36%;
- MVC: 23%;
- gunshot: 11%;
- BB/pellet gun: 11%;
- fall: 7%;
- various sharp objects: 4%.

Globe involvement among the total: 22%.

PREVENTION

Safety laws often specify ocular and orbital protection. The use of safety glasses (see Chapter 27), the development of shatterproof windshields[a] for cars, and motorcycle/bicycle helmets have all been beneficial for the reduction of orbital injuries. Federal, state, and local governments have enacted laws designed to protect workers. Increased awareness through education, advertising, and publicity has elevated the public's attention to accidents in general and orbital and ocular trauma in particular. Exercising common sense, however, remains the responsibility of the individual.

PATHOPHYSIOLOGY

The orbit's primary role is to protect the eyeball. The thick bones of the lateral and superior orbital rims provide firm protection; conversely, bones constituting the medial wall and the floor of the orbit are the thinnest and weakest in the human skull.

> **PEARL...** The combination of superior and lateral strength with medial and inferior wall weakness allows dissipation of energy when the orbit is struck.

The ability of the orbital floor to fracture selectively when the orbit is struck is an evolutionary masterpiece, a feature that is similar to a safety valve. When the energy from a blow to the orbit is dissipated through the fractured bone, it commonly saves the eyeball from rupturing.

> **PEARL...** It must always be remembered that through the orbital bones course the nerves and vessels needed to sustain the orbit and the eye, and on the other side of the orbital bones are other, vital, organs, such as the brain.

EVALUATION

The evaluation of a patient with suspected orbital trauma begins with a general examination to determine whether the nervous system is intact and what the patient's general medical condition is (see Chapter 10).

> ▼ **PITFALL**
>
> Injuries to the orbit are often associated with severe neurologic injuries, which are life threatening and take precedence over the orbital treatment.[1,2]

Presence or absence of enophthalmos or exophthalmos can be confirmed during *physical examination*. Evaluation of extraocular muscle movements may be performed and documented to check for restriction. Elements of an orbital examination include:

- Hertel exophthalmometry;
- extraocular muscle movement evaluation;
- visual acuity;
- sensory examination in the distribution of the supra- and infraorbital nerves;
- APD;
- palpation of the orbital rims; and
- auscultation for bruits.

A variety of imaging options (see Chapters 9 and 24) is available to assist with the evaluation of orbital trauma. They are always used in conjunction with an adequate physical examination. CT scan, MRI, and ultrasound all have advantages and disadvantages, and the initial physical examination will determine which tests to obtain and which are unnecessary (see Chapter 8).[3]

Orbital CT scans provide the best images of the relationship between the bone and soft tissue. This study is usually cheaper, faster, and more readily available than the MRI scan. The following are indications for ordering a CT scan:

- suspected orbital fractures;
- palpable bone step-offs;
- restricted extraocular muscle movements; and
- metallic orbital foreign bodies.

An *MRI scan* is best at differentiating soft tissue and may be the best diagnostic choice in cases of:

- associated neurologic damage; and
- wooden foreign bodies.[4]

---

[a] That is, laminated glass: when shattered, the two sheets of glass remain glued to a plastic sheet they sandwich, preventing the glass fragments from scattering (see Chapter 4).

PEARL... Specific contraindications for MRI scan include known or suspected ferrous intraorbital foreign bodies.[5]

An *ultrasound* examination is often not available in an ER setting, although it is helpful in identifying orbital abscess.

PEARL... The single most important test to perform when evaluating orbital trauma is visual acuity testing. With visual acuity loss, the orbital trauma becomes an orbital *emergency* (see Chapter 12).

The loss of vision implies pressure or impingement on the optic nerve or the eyeball. Emergency imaging and intervention should be anticipated. True orbital emergencies include:

- orbital abscess;
- optic nerve sheath hematoma;
- orbital foreign body in contact with the optic nerve; and
- open globe injury in conjunction with orbital injuries.

TYPES OF TRAUMA AND THEIR MANAGEMENT

Orbital Blowout Fracture

It is one of the most common orbital injuries encountered in an ER. Antecedent history often confirms a blow to the orbit with an object larger than the opening of the orbit itself, typically a fist or a softball. The classical clinical triad of a blowout fracture (Fig. 36–1) includes:

- diplopia caused by restrictive strabismus;
- infraorbital numbness caused by interruption of the inferior orbital nerve; and
- periocular ecchymosis.

Blowout fractures are caused by fractures of the bones in the inferior medial orbit.[b] There are two theories concerning the cause of blowout fractures.[6]

1. The *direct injury theory* describes a sudden compression of the globe with a fracture of the floor caused by increased orbital and ocular pressure.

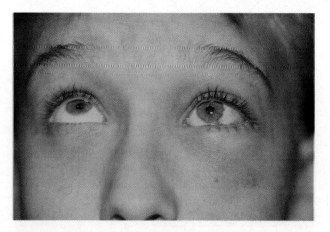

FIGURE 36–1 Left orbital blowout fracture; the patient presented with diplopia, infraorbital numbness, and periocular ecchymosis.

2. The *indirect injury theory* postulates that a blow to the inferior orbital rim causes a ripple effect in the orbital bones, which leads to fracture at their weakest point.

Both mechanisms of injury are probably involved in blowout fractures.

- The *ecchymosis* seen in conjunction with blowout fractures is caused by direct damage to the skin and orbicularis muscle.
- The *restricted extraocular muscle movements* typically seen with blowout fracture involve the bony entrapment of the *inferior rectus muscle* or *suspensory ligaments*. The entrapment leads to limited vertical eye muscle movements. Restrictive strabismus can be confirmed with a forced duction test.
  - *Forced duction testing* requires topical anesthesia and small forceps. Once the conjunctiva is anesthetized, the insertion of the inferior rectus muscle is purchased with forceps.[c]
  - A positive forced duction test indicates that there is palpable restriction to rotating the eyeball superiorly. A positive forced duction test is strong evidence that a blowout fracture is present with entrapment of the inferior rectus muscle.

PEARL... Entrapment is a clinical sign and cannot be diagnosed on CT examination.

---

[b] As mentioned earlier, these bones are among the thinnest in the body, designed to break as a pressure wave extends across the orbit; this potentially spares the globe from rupturing.

[c] Remember, this test is contraindicated if open globe injury is present or cannot be ruled out.

PEARL... Numbness along the distribution of the inferior orbital nerve is strong clinical evidence of an orbital blowout fracture. The most common location of blowout fracture is along the course of the inferior orbital nerve in the orbit. Typically, the nerve is not torn; it is simply stretched and/or contused at the time of injury. The numbness that results from this type of injury often resolves spontaneously in a matter of weeks to months.

For patients who present with an isolated blowout fracture, there are two options:

1. initially they can often be followed clinically[d]; or
2. if surgery is needed, it is usually (see the exceptions below) planned for 7 to 14 days after the trauma.[7]

Waiting allows time for:

• spontaneous improvement;
• resolution of the swelling associated with the initial trauma; and
• precise surgical planning.

PITFALL

Delaying surgery for over 14 days often results in increased scarring of the orbit.

Radiological evaluation of blowout fractures is necessary for adequate operative planning.[8] The location, severity, and adjacent anatomy can best be visualized with an orbital CT scan (Fig. 36–2). Both direct and coronal views should be obtained.

In some instances, *early repair* of blowout fractures is necessary. Indications include:

• associated craniofacial trauma;
• marked enophthalmos and hypoglobus; and
• complete disruption of the orbital floor.

Conversely, many patients with blowout fractures present months to years after the initial accident. There are several reasons for delayed presentation:

• the patient had life-threatening injuries at the time of the initial trauma, which took precedence over blowout fracture repair;

---
[d]Signs of extraocular muscle restriction, ecchymosis, and numbness often resolve spontaneously.

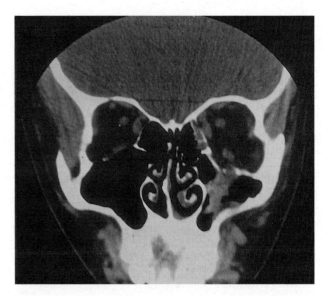

FIGURE 36–2 Orbital CT scan demonstrating discontinuity of the left orbital floor with prolapse of orbital contents into the left maxillary sinus.

• many craniofacial surgeons who repair fractures soon after the initial accident do not explore the orbit and do not repair blowout fractures; or
• during the acute phase of the injury the orbits may simply be too edematous to allow effective repair.

PEARL... It is not uncommon for enophthalmos and hypoglobus to develop and become a problem years after the initial accident.

The repair of old blowout fractures is often satisfactory. Late surgery requires the same guidelines for evaluation and treatment as fractures that occur acutely.

Surgical Technique

The usual approach to blowout fractures is the *transconjunctival approach,*[9] which:

• allows excellent exposure;
• conceals the incision; and
• prevents postoperative lid retraction.

The incision can be made with a scalpel, a cautery, or a laser. Access to the inferior orbital rim allows the periorbita to be opened and the orbital floor to be exposed.

Orbital floor implants come in a variety of shapes, sizes, and configurations.[10–13] Many choices are possible, and many materials have been successfully utilized. The best material for orbital implants is Supramid.

> **PEARL...** For simple blowout fractures, there is no need to place autogenous bone grafts, due to problems with variable resorption, scarring, and an increased incidence of strabismus.[14]

Autogenous bone grafts also increase the complication rate at the donor site. If simple materials are safe and effective, they should be the material of choice. A properly placed *Supramid orbital floor implant* has a minimal risk of extrusion.

> **PEARL...** The key to successful orbital blowout fracture repair is complete visualization of the entire length of the fracture.

Often the posterior aspect of the fracture lies near the orbital apex. The posterior aspect of the fracture may be responsible for the restrictive strabismus. Reducing the orbital contents under direct visualization along the entire length of the fracture will lead to the best results.

> **PITFALL**
>
> Orbital blowout fractures in children often present as a "greenstick fracture."[15,16] There may be ample evidence of a blowout fracture (e.g., restrictive strabismus and numbness along the distribution of the inferior orbital nerve), but the CT scan may not show a fracture at the orbital floor.

Orbital bones of children are much more aplastic than adult bones. These bones may fracture and simply snap back into place after the pressure wave has passed by. Radiological examinations may find the bones to be in perfect position. If a fracture has occurred, there may be entrapment of orbital tissue and restrictive strabismus. If clinical signs of a blowout fracture are present, exploratory surgery should be planned.

> **PEARL...** The recovery from blowout fracture surgery may take weeks to months. Often the last thing to recover from is the numbness along the distribution of the inferior orbital nerve. It is not unusual to see complete recovery as late as 6 months after the initial trauma.

Expanded Orbit Syndrome

Multiple fractures in and around the orbit may lead to the expanded orbit syndrome. If poor fracture approximation and bone disunion occur, the orbital volume can be dramatically expanded. An expanded orbit implies that one or more of the bony walls of the orbit have been broken and healed in an abnormal location (Fig. 36–3). This expansion can be seen in tripod and Le Fort III fractures.

Clinical signs and symptoms of an expanded orbit include:

- enophthalmos;
- deep superior sulcus;
- hypoglobus;
- eyelid asymmetry;
- diplopia; and
- associated cutaneous scarring.

The *radiological* findings of an expanded orbit syndrome typically include:

- evidence of broken bones healed in poor alignment;
- plating material along the orbital rims where repair attempts have been made; and, occasionally,
- material previously placed in the orbital floor.

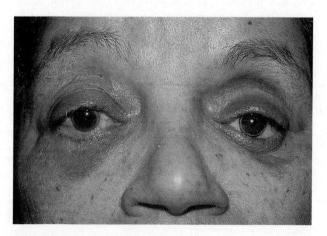

FIGURE 36–3 Expanded left orbit with enophthalmos, deep superior sulcus, hypoglobus, and eyelid asymmetry.

The repair of an expanded orbit may require either augmentation of the orbital volume or osteotomies and realignment of the orbital bones. Often orbital volume augmentation is the procedure of choice.

An expanded orbit presents for the surgeon a volumetric three-dimensional problem, which is complicated by gravity. The eyeball is displaced medially, inferiorly, and posteriorly. Orbital volume augmentation will ideally move the eyeball back into a symmetrical and appropriate position.

- The first choice of material for orbital volume augmentation is *autogenous orbital material*. In cases in which old blowout fractures are present,[e] the orbital tissue can be replaced into its normal position and the blowout fracture repaired in a routine manner.

- In cases with severe orbital expansion and severe globe dislocation, additional material may be added to the orbit to augment the volume. A variety of materials have been used in orbital volume augmentation.[17–22] Many of these materials are only of *historical* interest:
  ○ autogenous fat;
  ○ glass beads;
  ○ dermis fat; and
  ○ RTV silicone;

- The best material for orbital volume augmentation is *cranioplast*, a methyl methacrylate polymer widely used in orthopedic surgery and neurosurgery. When it is mixed, the material is moldable and modifiable; when the material hardens, it is no longer easily modifiable.

Surgical Technique

Orbital volume augmentation begins with exposure of the orbital floor, medial wall, and lateral wall. Wide exposure allows maximal use of the cranioplast to move the globe in three dimensions. The exposure should keep the periorbita intact if possible.

The mixing of cranioplast requires a well-ventilated room. After the cranioplast begins to harden, it can be placed into the potential space created by the orbital exploration. When the ideal amount of material is placed into the orbit, the cranioplast is allowed to harden there.

Once the cranioplast has hardened, it can be removed and revised with a bone bur. With modification, the cranioplast orbital floor implant can be

---

[e]Producing a volume problem.

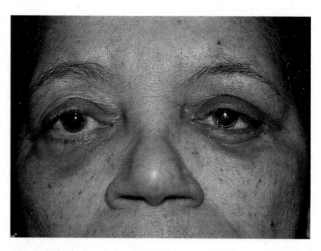

FIGURE 36–4   Same patient as on Fig. 36–3. Improved appearance following left orbital volume augmentation.

specifically modified to move the eyeball in three dimensions. Because the cranioplast has been allowed to harden in the orbit, the configuration of the orbital walls is mirrored by it, allowing the cranioplast to fit snugly into the orbit (Fig. 36–4). It is not necessary to suture or plate the material for fixation.

Complications of orbital volume augmentation are historically high. Many of the earlier techniques (e.g., glass beads and RTV silicone) have therefore been abandoned. Cranioplast orbital volume augmentation also can lead to complications such as:

- overcorrection;
- undercorrection;
- extrusion of cranioplast orbital implant; and
- diplopia.

> **PEARL...**   New orbital volume materials made of hydroxyapatite are now available. These materials have the advantage of biointegration, but they are not as easy to use or as easily modifiable as the cranioplast.

Orbital Foreign Bodies

The management of orbital foreign bodies is dependent upon the type of material in the orbit and its location. Some materials, such as wood, copper, and plant material, need to be removed if at all possible.[23] Materials such as BBs and shrapnel can be allowed to remain in the orbit, depending upon the location. Orbital foreign bodies that have penetrated adjacent structures, such as the cranial cavity or sinuses, need to be removed.

A careful patient *history* will often be suggestive of an orbital foreign body. A high-speed impact followed by pain and an entry wound on *inspection* are suggestive.

> **PEARL...** The examiner must be vigilant for associated neurologic, ocular, and sinus injuries.[24,25]

Initial evaluation for orbital foreign bodies should include a *CT scan* if a metallic foreign body is suspected. An *MRI* is the test of choice for glass or vegetative matter objects.

> **PEARL...** Remember that an intraorbital foreign body may have caused a perforating eye injury or a contusion, and additional ocular tissue lesions may also have been caused.

In summary, foreign bodies that need to be removed include:

- vegetative material;
- wood;
- copper;
- objects causing ocular or nerve damage; and
- foreign bodies that have penetrated adjacent structures.

The removal of foreign bodies is often through the entry wound. The wound track can be followed into the orbit by gentle retraction until the object is found. In cases of ferrous foreign bodies, a strong intraocular or electromagnet (see Chapter 24) can help with the localization and removal of the object (Fig. 36–5).

> **PEARL...** Most BBs are magnetic, composed of a steel sphere coated with bronze.

At the time of foreign body removal, a culture should be obtained and the wound should be irrigated with an appropriate antibiotic solution. With late removal, and

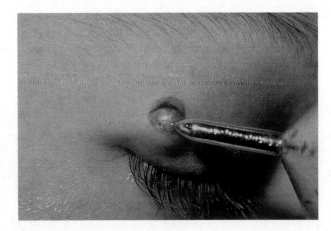

FIGURE 36–5 Magnetic BB being removed through the entry site with an EEM.

in foreign bodies associated with orbital abscess, the placement of a drain and/or packing material may be needed. Proper antibiotic treatment is also necessary.

> **PEARL...** In many cases, more than one foreign body is found.

Many foreign bodies do not need to be removed from the orbit. If vision is intact and the clinical situation is stable, surgery can be deferred or forgone.

> **PEARL...** As a general rule, if the risk of removing the object is higher than the risk of leaving the object in place, surgery should be avoided.

Orbital foreign bodies left in place are often remarkably stable. It is unlikely that they will be a nidus for infection or cause problems due to migration. In cases in which foreign body migration occurs, migration tends to be anteriorly, out of the orbit.

Anophthalmos

Orbital trauma and ocular trauma often lead to anophthalmos. The loss of an eye is a terrible and tragic event. This terrible loss can be mitigated by proper patient management and counseling (see Chapter 5). The restoration of the natural appearance of the orbit and its contents and amelioration of pain are the main goals of management.

The correct management of the anophthalmic patient begins before the eye is removed. The surgery to remove an eye must be performed in accordance with the type and timing of the injury; see Chapters 8 and 29 for decision making concerning whether or not to perform enucleation or evisceration and Chapter 31 on how to determine which of these two surgeries should be chosen as well as for the surgical techniques.

> **PITFALL**
>
> In many residency training programs, the evaluation and treatment (i.e., removal) of acutely traumatized, blind, painful eyes are often the responsibility of the junior resident. Enucleation of an eye, however, is not an operation for beginners. Technically, ocular extraction procedures are not difficult; but improper techniques will lead to lifelong problems for the patient because of the poor cosmetic outcome and the need for surgical revision(s). Close supervision of inexperienced residents is always advised, especially with enucleation.

An improperly performed surgery may lead to socket ptosis. Characteristic clinical findings of socket ptosis include:

- ectropion;
- deep superior sulcus;
- poor motility;
- contraction; and
- inability to retain an ocular prosthesis.

> **PEARL...** Enucleation should be considered as a complicated orbital surgery.

Problems with the anophthalmic socket can be difficult to remedy. With time, the problems of the anophthalmic socket become more severe. The anophthalmic socket conceptually can be thought of as aging more rapidly than the uninvolved side. Following ocular trauma and enucleation, the orbital suspensory ligaments may be disrupted and the orbital contents begin to descend because of gravity. Socket ptosis can be prevented by minimal disruption of the orbital suspensory ligaments at the time of the initial surgery.

> **PEARL...** The aesthetic long-term result of evisceration is superior to that of enucleation producing better long-term stability of the orbit.

SUMMARY

The main function of the bony structures surrounding the globe is to protect the eye against injury. It should be no surprise that these structures are frequently damaged following severe trauma, particularly by blunt objects. Injury to the orbital bones not only leads to disfigurement, but also may result in visually significant disability, particularly diplopia.

When both severe ocular and orbital injuries are present the eye must be stabilized prior to orbital surgery, which in most cases can be safely delayed for weeks following the injury. In the haste to diagnosis and repair the *globe* one must not forget about the periocular structures since the best management strategies must consider all injuries.

REFERENCES

1. Siegel EB, Bastek MD, Mehringer CM, et al. Fatal intracranial extension of an orbital umbrella stab injury. *Ann Ophthalmol.* 1983;15:99–101.

2. Mutlukan E, Fleck BW, Cullen JF, et al. Case of penetrating orbitocranial injury caused by wood. *Br J Ophthalmol.* 1991;75:374–376.

3. Lagalla R. Plain film, CT and MRI sensibility in the evaluation of intraorbital foreign bodies in an in vitro model of the orbit in pig eyes. *Eur Radiol.* 2000;10: 1338–1341.

4. Woolfson JM, Wesley RE. Magnetic resonance imaging and computed tomographic scanning of fresh (green) foreign bodies in dog orbits. *Ophthalmic Plast Reconstr Surg.* 1990;6:237–240.

5. Kulshrestha M, Mission G. Magnetic resonance imaging and the dangers of orbital foreign bodies. *Br J Ophthalmol.* 1995;79:1149.

6. Warwar RE, Bullock JD, Ballal DR, et al. Mechanisms of orbital floor fractures. A clinical, experimental and theoretical study. *Ophthalmic Plast Reconstr Surg.* 2000;1: 188–200.

7. Dortzbach RK. Orbital floor fractures. *Ophthalmic Plast Reconstr Surg.* 1985;1:149–151.

8. Harris GJ, Garcia GH, Logani SC, et al. Correlation of preoperative computed tomography and postoperative ocular motility in orbital blowout fractures. *Ophthalmic Plast Reconstr Surg.* 2000;16:179–187.

9. Lorenz HP, Longaker MT, Kawamoto HK. Primary and secondary orbit surgery: the transconjunctival approach. *Ophthalmic Plast Reconstr Surg.* 1999;103: 1124–1128.

10. Chew M, Lim TC, Lim J, et al. New synthetic orbital implant for orbital floor repair [letter]. *Plast Reconstr Surg* 1998;101;1734.

11. Jordan DR. Microplate fixation of prefabricated subperiosteal orbital floor implants. *Ophthalmic Surg.* 1995;26: 78–79.

12. Mauriello JA, Antonacci R, Mostafavi R. Hinged silicone covered implant for repair of large fractures of the internal orbital skeleton. *Ophthalmic Plast Reconstr Surg.* 1995;11:59–65.

13. Lemke BN, Kikkawa DO. Repair or orbital floor fractures with hydroxyapatite block scaffolding. *Ophthalmic Reconstr Surg.* 1999;15:161–165.

14. Marin PC, Love T, Carpenter R, et al. Complications of orbital reconstruction: misplacement of bone grafts within the intramuscular cone. *Plast Reconstr Surg.* 1998;101:1323–1327.

15. Bansagi ZC, Meyer DR. Internal orbital fractures in the pediatric age group: characterization and management. *Ophthalmology.* 2000;107:829–836.

16. Egbert JE, May K, Kersten RC, et al. Pediatric orbital floor fracture: direct extraocular muscle involvement. *Ophthalmology.* 2000;107:1875–1879.

17. Hill JC, Savar D. Silicone augmentation of the enophthalmic socket: a 14 year review *Can J Ophthalmol.* 1978, 13:294–298.

18. Borghoutss JMHM, Otto AJ. Silicone sheet and bead implants to correct the deformities of inadequately healed orbital fractures. *Br J Plast Surg.* 1978;31:254–258.

19. Sihota R, Sujatha Y, Betharia SM. The fat pad in dermis fat grafts. *Ophthalmology.* 1994;101:231–234.

20. Adenis JP, Bertin P, Lasudry JGH, et al. treatment of the postenucleation socket syndrome with a new hydroxyapatite tricalcium phosphate ceramic implant. *Ophthalmic Plast Reconstr Surg.* 1999;15:277–283.

21. Dresner SC, Codère F, Corriveau C. Orbital volume augmentation with adjustable prefabricated methylmethacrylate subperiosteal implants. *Ophthalmic Surg.* 1991;22:53–56.

22. Cahill KV, Burns JA. Volume augmentation of the anophthalmic orbit with cross-linked collagen (Zyplast). *Arch Ophthalmol.* 1989;107:1684–1686.

23. Nasr AM, Haik BG, Fleming JC, et al. Penetrating orbital injury with organic foreign bodies. *Ophthalmology.* 1999;106:523–532.

24. Simonton JT, Arthurs BP. Penetrating injuries to the orbit. *Adv Ophthalmic Plast Reconstr Surg* 1988;7:217–227.

25. Fezza J, Wesley R. The importance of CT scans in planning the removal of orbital-frontal lobe foreign bodies. *Ophthalmic Plast Reconstr Surg.* 1999;15:366–368.

Chapter 37

OPTIC NERVE AND VISUAL PATHWAY

Christopher A. Girkin and Lanning B. Kline

Although injury of the optic nerves and afferent visual pathways may be associated with little evidence of head injury, often there is associated serious brain, facial, and orbital trauma (see Chapter 10). These cases can be especially challenging for the clinician as alterations in the state of consciousness make assessment of visual function difficult. If vision is found to be impaired, management depends upon localization of the site and mechanism of injury.

Trauma may affect any segment of the visual pathways; and accurate localization requires a complete neuroophthalmologic assessment.

- The optic radiations are generally not involved in closed head injury as they are well supported by deep white matter structures. Rarely, the occipital lobe may be injured by a blunt impact to the occiput. These patients exhibit highly congruous hemianopic visual field defects with no pupillary abnormality.

- Traumatic chiasmal injury, although rare, produces bitemporal hemianopic field defects, and may be associated with endocrine disorders due to hypothalamic involvement.[1–3]

PEARL... The optic nerves are by far the most common site of visual pathway trauma.[4]

For the purposes of management, TON can be classified into three types of injuries[5]:

1. *optic nerve evulsion*, where the optic nerve is partially or completely separated from the globe (Fig. 37-1);

2. *direct injury* caused by impact on the optic nerve or nerve sheath from a penetrating foreign body, a displaced bone fragment, or a retroorbital hematoma; and

3. *indirect injury*, in which forces are transmitted to the optic nerve within the optic canal.

This chapter focuses on the various forms of TON (additional details can be found in Chapter 38).

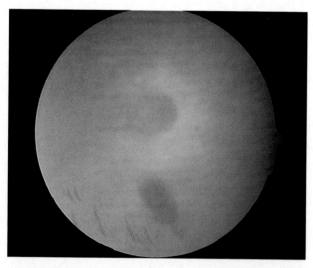

FIGURE 37-1 Typical appearance of an optic nerve evulsion with retinal hemorrhages and a nonrecognizable optic disk structure.

EPIDEMIOLOGY

Incidence. TON occurs in approximately 1.6% of cases of head trauma and 2.5% of cases of midface and maxillofacial trauma.

Age: 1–89 years (mean: 29).

Sex: the male-female ratio is 4:1.

Place: home is most common, followed by highway and workplace environments (USEIR data; see Table 37–1).

Cause: most often due to deceleration injury (see Table 37–2).

- MVCs and bicycle accidents are the most frequent cause (45% of the cases).
- Falls are the next most common cause (27%).
- Motorcycle crashes are a particularly high risk for TON (18% of the cases).
- In the USEIR, gunshot wounds are the most common source of injury (26%), followed by various blunt objects (see Table 37–3).

TABLE 37–I SITE OF OPTIC NERVE INJURY (USEIR DATA*)

Work/industrial	11%
Farm	2%
Home	33%
School	1%
Recreation/sport	12%
Street/highway	23%
Public building	3%
Unknown	12%
Other	3%

*Based on 427 cases.

Regardless of the type of TON, damage may occur via both primary and secondary mechanisms (see later in this chapter).[6] Undoubtedly, several of these mechanisms are interdependent and occur simultaneously or consecutively.

> **PEARL...** Indirect TON may occur after seemingly trivial injury to the head or superior orbital rim. Blunt impact to this region is transmitted along the orbital roof to the optic canal.

PATHOPHYSIOLOGY[a]

Primary Mechanisms

- *Shearing[a] injury*: the force generated by a blunt object's impact to the head, most commonly the forehead, can be transmitted to the optic nerve

[a] *Pathoanatomical considerations* (contributed by John A. Long, MD). The optic nerve extends 35 to 40 mm from the optic chiasm to the optic nerve head. It leads a slightly sinuous course and is well protected by orbital bones and fat. The primary biologic design flaw of the optic nerve is its vascular supply. The inner nerve receives blood supplied by the central retinal artery. The peripheral nerve receives its blood supply from the vasovasorum. When the inner or outer blood supply is disrupted, the optic nerve is damaged.

The optic nerve is firmly tethered within the optic canal. The canal is bony and swelling of the nerve in response to trauma is not possible beyond a certain extent: any trauma that leads to optic nerve edema may cause vascular compromise in the region of the optic canal. With rapid deceleration injuries or with coup/contrecoup injuries, the globe may move forward and stretch the optic nerve. With stretch injury, the vascular supply of the nerve can be damaged, and vision loss and an APD may develop.

TABLE 37–2 CAUSES OF TON (PUBLISHED STUDIES)

First Author, Year, Reference	Number of Cases	MVC	Bicycle	Fall	Assault	Other
Bodian, 1964[49]	6	—	1	3	—	2
Anderson, 1982[50]	7	3	1	3	—	—
Matsuzaki, 1982[51]	33	20	—	7	4	2
Nau, 1987[52]	18	7	2	5	1	3
Millesi, 1988[43]	29	18	—	6	5	—
Joseph, 1990[53]	14	2	3	4	3	2
Seiff, 1990[54]	36	15	—	13	4	4
Spoor, 1990[55]	21	9	—	3	4	5
Total	164	74 (45%)	7 (4%)	44 (27%)	21 (13%)	18 (11%)

TABLE 37-3   Causes of TON (USEIR Data*)

Hammer on metal	2%
Sharp object	5%
Nail	2%
Blunt object	24%
Fall	3%
Gunshot	26%
BB/pellet gun	10%
MVC	19%
Fireworks	2%
Explosion	2%
Lawn equipment	1%
Unknown	1%
Other	3%

*Based on 427 cases.

through the walls of the bony orbit and cause a shearing injury to the optic nerve (Fig. 37–2).[7] However, shearing of axons is no longer considered a common form of neurologic injury. Rather, trauma induces a focal disruption of axonal transport, which functionally separates the nerve leading to wallerian degeneration of the distal segment.[8]

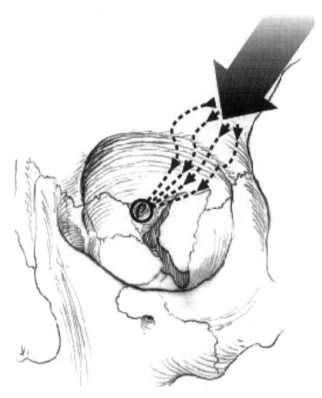

FIGURE 37-2   Transmission of lines of force from blunt frontal impact to the optic canal at the orbital apex.

- *Laceration*: either partial or complete laceration of the optic nerve or its sheath may occur due to a penetrating foreign body or a displaced bone fragment.
- *Compression*: penetrating foreign bodies or displaced bone fragments may compress the optic nerve as a primary mechanism of injury. Compression of the optic nerve may also occur as a secondary mechanism due to traumatic retroorbital or optic nerve sheath hematoma (see later in this Chapter).

Secondary Mechanisms

- *Ischemia*: interruption of the vascular supply may occur due to:
  - compression or laceration in direct TON; or
  - tearing of the microvasculature due to shearing forces in indirect TON.[6] This is perhaps the most important secondary injury following trauma.
- *Compression*: retroorbital and optic nerve sheath hematoma may occur after direct[9] or indirect TON[10] and may further damage the optic nerve. In addition, orbital emphysema following fractures of the paranasal sinuses is a rare cause of optic nerve compression.[12]

P I T F A L L

The detection of a compressive hematoma is critical because its evacuation may halt further visual decline and even improve vision.[11]

- *Reperfusion injury*: with resolution of the primary insult, subsequent reperfusion can generate oxygen-free radicals, which cause further injury by lipid peroxidation of axonal membranes and their supporting glial tissue.[13]
- *Edema*: bradykinin and related substances are activated following traumatic and ischemic brain injury.[6] Bradykinin initiates the release of arachidonic acid, producing a loss of vascular autoregulation and subsequent edema, which in the case of TON may produce a compartment syndrome within the optic canal that increases ischemic injury.[14] Bradykinin antagonists may in the future have a role in the management of TON.[15] Edema within the optic canal may elevate intracanalicular pressure and further exacerbate optic nerve injury.
- *Intracellular calcium* is increased after traumatic or ischemic damage to the nervous system and may lead to further cell death.[14]

• *Inflammation* is triggered by the release of inflammatory mediators due to the initial insult. First, polymorphonuclear cells arrive within 1–2 days of injury and release a broad array of toxic compounds.6 Within the first week, macrophages largely replace the polymorphonuclear cells and may promote reactive gliosis, which limits opportunities for axonal regeneration.[6]

Pathophysiology Specific to the Type of TON

Optic Nerve Evulsion

It is the rarest form of TON. Evulsion may occur secondary to both open and closed globe trauma. However, closed trauma (i.e., contusion) is more common, and evulsion is most commonly seen with severe blunt trauma to the orbit.

• *Total evulsion* of the optic nerve occurs when the vitreous and retina separate from the optic disk, and the lamina cribrosa is ripped from its attachments to the choroid and sclera. The retinal vessels may be partially or totally disrupted.[16]

• *Partial evulsion* involves a localized segment of the optic disk with incomplete disruption of laminar-scleral connections.

Three mechanisms have been postulated[17].

1. Traumatic compression of the globe rapidly raises the *IOP* to the point that the optic nerve is pneumatically disinserted.

2. Orbital trauma associated with a sudden rise in the *intraorbital pressure* stretches the optic nerve until it is evulsed from its scleral insertion.

3. Extreme *rotation* and *displacement* of the globe within the orbit disrupt the laminar region of the optic disk. This mechanism is seen with finger jab injuries into the orbit and is associated with optic nerve evulsion with minimal ocular damage.[b]

Direct TON

Direct optic nerve injury may be caused by penetrating impact from:

• blunt (e.g., a BB pellet), or sharp (e.g., a knife) foreign objects; or from a

• displaced fracture or spicule of bone in the region of the optic canal.[18]

Less commonly, compression of the optic nerve may occur following trauma due to a retroorbital or optic nerve sheath hematoma.[9] Orbital emphysema has rarely been associated with TON following orbital fractures and is due to air forced into the orbit through the fracture as a result of vomiting or nose blowing.[12]

Indirect TON

It is the most common form of TON.[6]

• The *intracanalicular* optic nerve is the most vulnerable to external blunt injury.[1] This 6- to 12-mm segment of the optic nerve passes through the optic canal, which lies between the two bases of the lesser wing of the sphenoid.[19]

SPECIAL CONSIDERATION

The optic canal contains the optic nerve, meninges, the ophthalmic arteries, and postganglionic sympathetic fibers. Within the canal, the optic nerve receives its blood supply from penetrating pial branches. It is immobilized by the dura in the canal, which is fixed to the surrounding periosteum and bone (see Fig. 37–3). About 4% of patients have no bone along the medial side of the optic canal; in such cases, the optic nerve is separated from the sphenoid sinus by only sinus mucosa and dura.[19]

• Indirect *intraorbital* optic nerve injury rarely occurs because of the laxity of the optic nerve in this area and the fact that it is well cushioned by surrounding orbital fat.

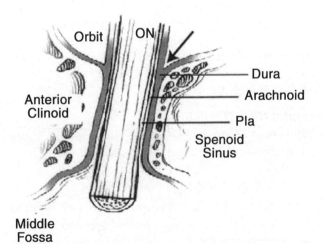

FIGURE 37–3 Anatomy of the optic nerve and canal illustrating the continuity of the orbital periosteum and dura surrounding the optic nerve (arrow).

---

[b] Both editors of this book have seen a case such as this: a young man's total optic nerve evulsion was caused by a fellow basketball player's finger accidentally poked into the orbit; shockingly, the external inspection revealed only minimal signs of injury.

- The *intracranial* optic nerve is also rarely damaged indirectly due to its mobility within the cranium and its cushioning by the surrounding cerebrospinal fluid.

Indirect injuries can be divided into anterior and posterior types.

- *Anterior indirect TON* denotes involvement of the optic disk and the segment of the retrobulbar optic nerve containing the central retinal artery.[20] In these cases, ophthalmoscopic abnormalities are present:
  - central retinal artery occlusion with an edematous retina, pale optic disk, threadlike arterioles, sludging of blood flow, and a cherry-red macular spot;
  - retinal vasospasm (may occur without total occlusion)[1];
  - diffuse swelling of the optic disk[21,c]; and
  - tears of the optic disk margin.

> **PEARL...** Optic disk margin tears are usually associated with hemorrhage of the optic disk of less than 120 degrees. Over a period of 1 to 4 weeks, these hemorrhages resolve, leaving a heavily pigmented scar at the disk margin and optic disk pallor. The visual field defects typically correlate well with the location of the optic disk injury.

- The diagnosis of *posterior indirect TON* requires:
  - signs of optic nerve dysfunction following trauma;
  - no ophthalmoscopic abnormalities; and
  - no evidence of chiasmal dysfunction.

Over 4 to 8 weeks, disk pallor develops. The site of injury in these cases may occur anywhere between the chiasm and the entry of the ophthalmic artery into the optic nerve. This is the most common type of indirect optic nerve injury.[18]

EVALUATION

Optic Nerve Evulsion

The visual acuity may be reduced to a variable degree in partial evulsion; in total evulsion, the eye's vision is NLP.
The fundus picture changes with time.

- Immediately after the injury, the disk is often obscured by overlying *vitreous hemorrhage*.
- Over time, as the view gradually improves, the disrupted disk contour becomes visible and in cases

of total evulsion, the scleral canal is seen devoid of the optic disk.

- This defect is gradually filled with *glial tissue*, which may extend into the vitreous.[17]
- The *differential diagnosis* of this fundus appearance includes staphyloma, optic pit, optic disk coloboma, and morning-glory syndrome.[d]
- In cases in which the disk is obscured by vitreous hemorrhage, orbital imaging with *ultrasound* or *CT scanning* may be useful in confirming the presence of optic nerve evulsion.[23]
- *Associated ocular findings* commonly include subconjunctival hemorrhage, limitation of extraocular movement, proptosis, and a dilated and amaurotic pupil.

Indirect TON

Examination of the visual system after head trauma may be difficult and measurement of the visual acuity may be impossible. However, every effort should be made to assess the visual function.

- In the alert verbal patient, a *visual acuity* measurement may be obtained at the bedside. Visual loss may range from a minimal decline to NLP. Absence of light perception should be carefully confirmed with the IBO by illuminating all four quadrants (see Chapter 9).

> **PEARL...** In the setting of indirect TON, the occurrence of NLP vision immediately following impact usually signals a permanent severe visual impairment.[e]

- *Pupillary responses* are of critical importance and provide an objective sign of optic nerve injury.[24] If possible, pupillary responses should be graded using neutral density filters.

> **PEARL...** Only one functional pupil is required to detect an APD with the swinging-flashlight test (see Chapter 9).

- *Color vision* provides another measure of optic nerve function. Asking the conscious patient to identify colored test objects is a useful bedside technique. Patients with an optic neuropathy describe colors as

---

[c]FA in these cases supports compromise of the posterior ciliary artery circulation.[22]

[d]Because of the history and the characteristic visual acuity change, differential diagnosis is rarely a problem.

[e]Clinically, the sequence of events is reversed; a patient presents with NLP vision and its cause must be identified.

"faded" or may be unable to identify the color. Color vision may also be evaluated using pseudoisochromatic plates.

- *IBO* should be performed to rule out other causes of visual loss (e.g., retinal detachment). In posterior TON, the fundus should appear normal.
- Confrontation techniques or perimetry should assess *visual fields* when possible. Optic nerve visual field defects fall into two general categories: central scotomas and nerve fiber bundle defects.

> **P**EARL... **Hemianopic defects, whether bitemporal or hemianopic, establish the site of injury as posterior to the optic nerve.**

- *Electrophysiology*, although limited in availability and often impractical in the setting of head trauma, can be useful in the evaluation of unresponsive patients. The VEP may be used to document conduction delays in comatose patients, and the initial VEP may correlate well with the final visual acuity.[25]
- High-resolution *CT* in both the coronal and axial planes should be performed to detect facial and optic canal fractures. There is a great variability in the reported incidence of canal fractures with indirect optic nerve injury, ranging from 1 to 92%.[26-28] The presence of canal fracture will help direct therapy.
  - Although inferior to CT in the detection of bone defects, *MRI* is occasionally a valuable adjunct to CT in imaging the intracanalicular and intracranial segments of the optic nerve for disruption or hematoma.
- Orbital *ultrasonography* should be performed in patients with anterior indirect optic neuropathy. Progressive visual loss associated with enlargement of the optic nerve sheath may respond to optic nerve sheath decompression.[20,29]

Direct Optic Nerve Injury

- *External inspection*: evaluation of the depth, direction, and extent of orbital and eyelid wounds from sharp objects is important no matter how minimal the external injury.
- *Imaging studies* should be obtained routinely to assess both orbital and intracranial injuries.
  - Within the orbit, *MRI* is generally superior for the detection of radiolucent material, which may have the same CT characteristics as orbital fat and air.[30]
  - However, *CT* should be used if there is a possibility of a ferromagnetic foreign body as the magnetic field of the MRI may cause the foreign body to shift, causing further visual loss[31] (see also Chapter 24).

> **▼ PITFALL ▼**
>
> Complete neurologic assessment is required as many of these patients have associated brain injuries.

MANAGEMENT STRATEGY

Optic Nerve Evulsion

The visual prognosis is generally poor. Medical therapy with intravenous megadose corticosteroids may be used, but to date there are no studies that document the efficacy of any form of treatment.

Indirect TON

Multiple factors are operative in the development of indirect optic nerve injury and visual recovery is unpredictable. This makes the interpretation of treatment modalities difficult, as many patients improve spontaneously without treatment.[32]

A literature review of case series of patients treated nonsurgically is summarized in Table 37–4; studies of patients treated surgically are presented in Table 37–5.

> **SPECIAL CONSIDERATION**
>
> **To date, there is no general consensus concerning the treatment of indirect optic nerve injury. It is up to the managing physicians to make a decision based on their own clinical experience.**

The following guidelines have been proposed in designing the treatment strategy.[6,33]

- If indirect optic neuropathy is diagnosed in the setting of closed head trauma and no medical contraindication exists, *intravenous megadose corticosteroids* should be given as soon as possible.
  - We define megadose steroids as greater than 250 mg per day in a single or divided dose. Various investigators have advocated doses ranging from 60 mg to 7 g per day.
- If the patient is taking steroids and continues to deteriorate, or improves and then deteriorates, *optic canal decompression* should be considered.
  - Decompression should not be performed as an elective procedure in an unconscious patient. Accurate visual assessment is impossible, and in this setting patients are unable to give informed consent.

TABLE 37-4 NONSURGICAL MANAGEMENT OF TON

First Author, Reference	Number of Cases	Improved	Not Improved	Treatment
Davidson[56]	37	11	26	—
Turner[57]	46	23	23	—
Hooper[58]	17	5	12	—
Anderson[50]	2	2	0	Megadose steroids
Tang[59]	13	5	8	No specific treatment
	5	1	4	Therapeutic dose of steroid
Millesi[43]	7	4	3	No specific treatment
	2	1	1	Intravenous steroids
Lessell[28]	25	5	20	No specific treatment
	4	1	3	Steroids (no dosage stated)
Wolin[60]	4	4	0	Megadose steroids × 3
Seiff[54]	15	5	10	Megadose steroids
	21	13	8	No specific treatment
Spoor[55]	22	19	3	Megadose steroids
Mauriello[61]	16	9	74	Megadose steroids

TABLE 37-5 SURGICAL MANAGEMENT OF TON

First Author, Reference	Number of Cases	Improved	Not Improved	Time between Injury and Surgery
Pringle[62]	3	0	3	2–4 weeks
Hooper[58]	4	1	3	18 hours–8 months
Niho[63]	7	5	2	5–263 days
Hughes[1]	5	0	5	20 hours–2 months
Edmund[24]	6	1	5	—
Imachi[64]	61	45	16	—
Niho[63]	25	20	5	—
Schmaltz[65]	13	1	12	—
Hammer[66]	4	4	0	<1 week
Fukado[26]	400	400	0	7–90 days
Goldware[67]	2	2	0	36 hours–10 weeks
Karnik[68]	10	2	8	1 week–1 month
Brihaye[69]	56	7	49	—
Anderson[50]	4	1	3	12–48 hours
Tang[59]	8	2	6	—
Fujitani[70]	28	7	21	—
Waga[71]	22	11	11	<21 days
Millesi[43]	3	0	3	12–24 hours
Lessell[28]	4	3	1	36–72 hours
Joseph[53]	14	11	3	1–5 days
Mauriello[61]	7	3	4	24–72 hours

○ Decompression may be performed on an unconscious patient with indirect optic nerve injury if the patient is undergoing other craniofacial or neurosurgical procedures.

- If an obvious compressive lesion is present on imaging studies (e.g., bone fragment, hematoma), decompression should be considered.

- If total loss of vision occurred at the moment of impact, it is most likely permanent and irreversible.[34] However, recovery from NLP can occur spontaneously, and because it is often difficult to determine whether the visual loss occurred at the moment of impact, patients with NLP should be treated the same way as patients with residual optic nerve function (see Chapter 8).

- In performing optic canal decompression, transethmoidal surgery is as effective as the transcranial approach and is associated with less morbidity.

PITFALL

The *International Optic Nerve Trauma Study* was a prospective, randomized clinical trial that attempted to evaluate whether treatment of TON with *intravenous steroids followed by optic nerve decompression* improves visual outcome over treatment with *steroids alone*.[37] Unfortunately, the study lacked the statistical power required to draw any firm conclusions that could be used to guide the management of individual patients.

Direct TON

Treatment of patients with direct optic nerve injury is generally supportive and should follow an approach similar to that for indirect TON.

PEARL... A decision to remove orbital or canalicular foreign bodies must be made on a case-by-case basis. Gunshot pellets that lodge deep in the orbit and have already damaged the optic nerve are best left alone (see also Chapters 12 and 36).

Empirical use of intravenous megadose corticosteroids is indicated and surgical decompression may be warranted in individual cases that fail to respond to, or worsen with, medical therapy, or in patients with optic nerve compression by bone fragments or hemorrhage.

PITFALL

The prospects for visual recovery in patients with direct TON are worse than that of indirect TON.

PITFALL

It is of critical importance to establish a baseline measurement of the visual function prior to performing any facial, orbital, or neurosurgical procedure in the setting of head trauma. Occasionally, the diagnosis of TON is delayed until the patient is alert following such procedures.

TIMING

PEARL... Both direct and indirect TON should be considered a true emergency.[6]

In patients with spinal cord trauma, immediate treatment with intravenous megadose corticosteroids has led to improvement if initiated within 8 hours of injury. A similar window of opportunity may exist with TON. Therefore, if a decision to treat is made, it should be implemented as soon as possible.

If there is no visual improvement within 48 hours or the patient's vision worsens despite steroids, optic nerve decompression should be considered.

MANAGEMENT

Optic Canal Decompression

Decompression of the optic nerve within the optic canal may be performed through various approaches (e.g., transcranial, transorbital, transethmoidal, transantral-transethmoidal, endonasal-transethmoidal). The goal of surgery is to reverse any component of compression (edema, hematoma, bone fragment) of the intracanalicular portion of the optic nerve.

Although the instrumentation involved in decompression of the optic nerve is beyond the scope of this text, it is important to understand that:

- techniques that do not involve craniotomy are associated with less morbidity and mortality; transethmoidal surgery is generally as effective as transcranial surgery[35]; however,
- only transcranial surgery permits decompression when the anterior clinoid is fractured and allows unroofing of the canal with removal of the falciform dural ligament.[18]

The criteria for adequate decompression of the optic canal include[36]:

- removal of 50% or more of the circumference of the optic canal;
- removal that encompasses the entire length of the canal; and
- total longitudinal incision of the optic nerve sheath, including the annulus of Zinn as advocated by some surgeons.

Optic Nerve Sheath Decompression

The goal of surgery is to decompress the orbital portion of the optic nerve. Orbital optic nerve sheath decompression may be performed from a medial or lateral approach. The surgical approach is determined by clinical and imaging findings.

The *medial approach* is generally preferred because it is technically easier to perform and avoids removal of the lateral orbital wall. In addition, a medial approach is more appropriate with a medial subperiosteal hematoma causing optic nerve compression. For a medial approach, a lateral canthotomy is performed followed by a medial peritomy. The medial rectus is disinserted from the globe after being secured with double-armed 6-0 Vicryl suture.

The *lateral approach* may be preferable in the setting of a depressed lateral wall fracture that compromises the nerve. In such cases, reduction of the fracture may be performed in combination with optic nerve sheath fenestration. For a lateral approach, a lateral orbitotomy is performed and the lateral rectus is disinserted from the globe in a similar fashion.

With either technique, it is helpful to place two 5-0 Dacron sutures transsclerally in the superior and inferior nasal quadrants to aid in rotating the globe and exposing the optic nerve. Malleable orbital retractors and cotton-tipped applicators are used to retract orbital fat.

The intrascleral course of the long posterior ciliary artery leads to the optic nerve. Once exposed, an

MVR blade[f] is used to incise the nerve sheath and drain the hematoma. A window in the dura is usually created by connecting parallel incisions made with the MVR blade. The rectus muscles and conjunctiva are reattached to their anatomic positions with absorbable sutures.

Additional Issues

- Multiple treatments have been proposed in the literature. Corticosteroids have been used at dosages ranging from 60 mg to 7 g per day.[32] Surgical decompression of the optic canal has been advocated by some authors, whereas observation alone has been endorsed by others.
- Unfortunately, there is no proven therapy for TON. Until such data are available, we recommend that the clinician clearly inform the patient about current treatment options (see Chapters 5, 7, and 8).
- One approach is to give all patients high-dose methylprednisolone according to the *National Acute Spinal Cord Injury Study* dosing schedule[37] (30 mg/kg as a loading dose and 5.4 mg/kg/h thereafter).
- If there is no improvement with steroid treatment, or if there is deterioration of vision, surgical decompression of the optic canal should be considered.

PITFALL

Optic canal or optic nerve sheath decompression should not be carried out in a patient who cannot give informed consent because of associated head injuries, unless other facial or neurosurgical procedures are also planned.

- If there is improvement with steroids, the patient may be given oral prednisone in a tapered dose. We generally maintain the patient with iv steroids for 3–5 days, followed by an oral steroid taper over 2–4 weeks. If vision declines when the patient is switched to oral steroids, the iv steroids should be reinstituted.
- If radiologic evidence exists of impingement of the optic nerve from a bone fragment or foreign body, especially if there is a continuing decline in vision, surgical intervention should be considered (see Chapter 12).
- The management of compressive TON from an orbital or optic nerve sheath hematoma is less

[f]Unitome 5560, Beaver Surgical, Waltham, MA.

controversial. Orbital hematomas in the presence of TON should be treated with a lateral canthotomy and cantholysis to permit expansion of the confined orbital contents. If there is little improvement in vision, orbital decompression may be attempted[38] or, if a subperiosteal collection of blood is found on imaging, it should be evacuated.

  ○ There is *no* role for AC paracentesis in this condition.

• In patients with TON who have an optic nerve sheath hematoma, fenestration should be considered. Orbital ultrasonography may reveal progressive enlargement of the optic nerve sheath in association with anterior TON and venous obstructive retinopathy. In these cases, sheath fenestration of the intraorbital optic nerve has been followed by visual improvement.[20]

Evacuation of an Orbital Hematoma
See Chapter 12.

ALTERNATIVE TO TREATMENT

Because there is no proven therapy for TON, an alternative is to follow the patient without treatment.

PITFALL

Because of the theoretical benefits of steroids, observation is not a commonly recommended therapy for TON. However, if steroids are contraindicated, observation does remain an option.

COMPLICATIONS

In most cases, high-dose steroids in the range recommended by the *National Acute Spinal Cord Injury Study* are well tolerated, without significant side effects.[37]

• Concomitant treatment with H_2 antagonists and antacids may be warranted to avoid gastrointestinal complications of steroids.

• Steroid-induced depression and psychosis, cardiac conduction abnormalities, and seizures can occur even with short-term steroids.

• The serum glucose should be monitored in all patients.

• Long-term side effects of steroid use such as aseptic necrosis, impaired wound healing, and immunosuppression are generally not an issue.[32]

SPECIAL ISSUE OF IMPORTANCE

The *International Optic Nerve Trauma Study* failed to demonstrate a clear benefit with either steroid treatment or optic nerve decompression in indirect TON. Although the number of patients studied was sufficient to determine differences in outcome between these two groups, clinically significant treatment effects for different subgroups of patients in this study could be missed.

The conclusion of this comparative nonrandomized intervention study was that treatment decisions should be made on a case-by-case basis.[32]

PROGNOSIS AND OUTCOME

Optic Nerve Evulsion

With complete evulsion, permanent blindness occurs. With partial evulsion, the final vision is dependent upon the extent and location of injury. In general, the visual outcome is poor.

Direct TON

If immediate blindness follows a direct injury, it is usually permanent.[8]

Dramatic visual improvement has been reported following transethmoidal optic canal decompression. This surgical approach was employed following a stab wound to the orbital apex in one case[41] and a canal fracture in another.[42] In general, the prognosis of direct TON is worse than that of indirect TON.

Indirect TON

Visual recovery following indirect TON is highly unpredictable whether or not therapy is administered. The reported rates of visual recovery range from 0 to 100%.[26,43] The results of studies of nonsurgical management are summarized in Table 37-4 and of surgical therapy in Table 37–5.

If complete loss of vision occurs at the moment of impact, the damage is usually permanent.[34]

CONTROVERSIES AND FUTURE TRENDS

As mentioned previously, the efficacy of any treatment for TON has not been demonstrated. Because therapeutic approaches to TON are empirical and based largely upon theoretical data from spinal cord injury, definitive recommendations must await the result of collaborative, prospective studies. However,

---

[8] In rare cases of direct optic nerve injury, recovery from NLP vision has been reported.[39,40] Visual recovery was spontaneous in both cases and the final acuity ranged from counting fingers to 20/100.

because of the infrequency of TON and difficulties in constructing a randomized trial, such helpful information is unlikely to be forthcoming.

Many alternative methods of treatment are currently being explored. Aminosteroids (lazaroids), apolipoprotein E, GM_1 gangliosides, and thromboxane receptor antagonist may induce neural regeneration in spinal cord injury and may prove useful in the management of TON.[44]

Bradykinin antagonists may provide an additional mechanism of treatment in the future by blocking other mechanisms of secondary injury.[15]

Several neuroprotective agents have demonstrated some promise in optic nerve crush models of glaucoma, which are similar in many respects to TON, and may prove useful in the future.[45-48]

SUMMARY

Until solid clinical data are available, the treatment of traumatic injuries to the optic nerve injuries will remain empirical. However, there is ample theoretical evidence to warrant aggressive treatment with iv megadose corticosteroids and surgical intervention for these injuries, which are potentially devastating for vision. The clinician must weigh the risks of intervention against these theoretical benefits in deciding when to institute therapy.

THE NONOPHTHALMOLOGIST'S ROLE

The management of TON involves a team approach with cooperation between the ophthalmologist, otolaryngologist, neurosurgeon, and neuroradiologist, as many of these patients have associated facial, cranial, and cerebral injuries.

PEARL... The results of serial ophthalmologic examinations should be used to guide the timing and course of medical treatment and to decide when surgical intervention is warranted.

REFERENCES

1. Hughes B. Indirect injury to the optic nerve and chiasma. *Bull Johns Hopkins Hosp.* 1962;111:98–126.

2. Heinz GW, Nunery WR, Grossman CB. Traumatic chiasmal syndrome associated with midline basilar skull fractures. *Am J Ophthalmol.* 1994;117:90–96.

3. Goh KY, Schatz NJ, Glaser JS. Traumatic chiasmal syndrome: a feature photograph. *Ann Acad Med Singapore.* 1996;25:614–615.

4. Lagreze WA. Neuro-ophthalmology of trauma. *Curr Opin Ophthalmol.* 1998;9:33–39.

5. Steinsapir KD. Traumatic optic neuropathy. *Curr Opin Ophthalmol.* 1999;10:340–342.

6. Steinsapir KD, Goldberg RA. Traumatic optic neuropathy. *Surv Ophthalmol.* 1994;38:487–518.

7. Strich S. Shearing of nerve fibers as a cause of brain damage due to head injury. *Lancet.* 1961;2:443–448.

8. Cheng CL, Povlishock JT. The effect of traumatic brain injury on the visual system: a morphologic characterization of reactive axonal change. *J Neurotrauma.* 1988;5:47–60.

9. Stonecipher KG, Conway MD, Karcioglu ZA, Haik BG. Hematoma of the optic nerve sheath after penetrating trauma. *South Med J.* 1990;83:1230–1231.

10. Wolter JR, Leenhouts JA, Coulthard SW. Clinical picture and management of subperiosteal hematoma of the orbit. *J Pediatr Ophthalmol.* 1976;13:136–138.

11. Kersten RC, Rice CD. Subperiosteal orbital hematoma: visual recovery following delayed drainage. *Ophthalmic Surg.* 1987;18:423–427.

12. Carter KD, Nerad JA. Fluctuating visual loss secondary to orbital emphysema. *Am J Ophthalmol.* 1987;104:664–665.

13. Flamm ES, Schiffer J, Viau AT, Naftchi NE. Alterations of cyclic AMP in cerebral ischemia. *Stroke.* 1978;9:400–402.

14. Flamm ES, Demopoulos HB, Seligman ML, Poser RG, Ransohoff J. Free radicals in cerebral ischemia. *Stroke.* 1978;9:445–447.

15. Braas KM, Manning DC, Perry DC, Snyder SH. Bradykinin analogues: differential agonist and antagonist activities suggesting multiple receptors. *Br J Pharmacol.* 1988;94:3–5.

16. Williams DF, Williams GA, Abrams GW, Jesmanowicz A, Hyde JS. Evulsion of the retina associated with optic nerve evulsion [published erratum appears in *Am J Ophthalmol* 1987;104:following 206]. Am J Ophthalmol. 1987;104:5–9.

17. Sanborn GE, Gonder JR, Goldberg RE, Benson WE, Kessler S. Evulsion of the optic nerve: a clinicopathological study. *Can J Ophthalmol.* 1984;19:10–16.

18. Steinsapir KD, Goldberg RA. *Traumatic Optic Neuropathy.* 5th ed. Baltimore: William & Wilkins; 1998:5.

19. Maniscalco JE, Habal MB. Microanatomy of the optic canal. *J Neurosurg.* 1978;48:402–406.

20. Hupp SL, Buckley EG, Byrne SF, Tenzel RR, Glaser JS, Schatz NS. Posttraumatic venous obstructive retinopathy associated with enlarged optic nerve sheath. *Arch Ophthalmol.* 1984;102:254–256.

21. Wyllie AM, McLeod D, Cullen JF. Traumatic ischaemic optic neuropathy. *Br J Ophthalmol.* 1972;56:851–853.

22. Hedges TRD, Gragoudas ES. Traumatic anterior ischemic optic neuropathy. *Ann Ophthalmol.* 1981;13: 625–628.

23. Kline LB, McCluskey MM, Skalka HW. Imaging techniques in optic nerve evulsion. *J Clin Neuroophthalmol.* 1988;8:281–282.

24. Edmund J, Godtfredsen E. Unilateral optic atrophy. *Acta Ophthalmol.* 1963;41:693–697.

25. Feinsod M, Auerbach E. Electrophysiological examinations of the visual system in the acute phase after head injury. *Eur Neurol.* 1973;9:56–64.

26. Fukado Y. Results in 400 cases of surgical decompression of the optic nerve. *Mod Probl Ophthalmol.* 1975;14: 474–481.

27. Kline LB, Morawetz RB, Swaid SN. Indirect injury of the optic nerve. *Neurosurgery.* 1984;14:756–764.

28. Lessell S. Indirect optic nerve trauma. *Arch Ophthalmol.* 1989;107:382–386.

29. Guy J, Sherwood M, Day AL. Surgical treatment of progressive visual loss in traumatic optic neuropathy. Report of two cases. *J Neurosurg.* 1989;70:799–801.

30. Specht CS, Varga JH, Jalali MM, Edelstein JP. Orbitocranial wooden foreign body diagnosed by magnetic resonance imaging. Dry wood can be isodense with air and orbital fat by computed tomography. *Surv Ophthalmol.* 1992;36:341–344.

31. Kelly WM, Paglen PG, Pearson JA, San Diego AG, Soloman MA. Ferromagnetism of intraocular foreign body causes unilateral blindness after MR study. *AJNR* 1986;7:243–245.

32. Levin LA, Beck RW, Joseph MP, Seiff S, Kraker R. The treatment of traumatic optic neuropathy: the International Optic Nerve Trauma Study. *Ophthalmology.* 1999: 106:1268–1277.

33. Volpe N, Lessel S, Kline L. Traumatic optic neuropathy: diagnosis and management. *Ophthalmol* Clin. 1991; 31:142–156.

34. Walsh F. Trauma Involving the Anterior Visual Pathways. New York: Appleton-Century-Crofts; 1979: 335–351.

35. Kline L. *Traumatic Optic Neuropathy.* San Francisco: American Academy of Ophthalmology; 1996:179–197.

36. Sofferman RA. Sphenoethmoid approach to the optic nerve. *Laryngoscope.* 1981;91:184–196.

37. Bracken MB, Shepard MJ, Collins WF, et al. A randomized, controlled trial of methylprednisolone or naloxone in the treatment of acute spinal-cord injury. Results of the Second National Acute Spinal Cord Injury Study. *N Engl J Med.* 1990;322:1405–1411.

38. Liu D. A simplified technique of orbital decompression for severe retrobulbar hemorrhage. *Am J Ophthalmol.* 1993;116:34–37.

39. Marouf L, Azar DT. Reversible visual loss following optic nerve injury. Ann Ophthalmol. 1985;17:582–584.

40. Feist RM, Kline LB, Morris RE, Witherspoon CD, Michelson MA. Recovery of vision after presumed direct optic nerve injury. *Ophthalmology.* 1987;94: 1567–1569

41. Spoor TC, Mathog RH. Restoration of vision after optic canal decompression [letter]. *Arch Ophthalmol.* 1986;104: 804, 806.

42. Kennerdell JS, Amsbaugh GA, Myers EN. Transantral-ethmoidal decompression of optic canal fracture. *Arch Ophthalmol.* 1976;94:1040–1043.

43. Millesi W, Hollmann K, Funder J. Traumatic lesion of the optic nerve. *Acta Neurochir (Wien).* 1988;93:50–54.

44. Schaffer M, Slamovits T, Burde R. *Traumatic Optic Neuropathy: Mechanisms and Treatment.* St Louis: Mosby; 1994:89–124.

45. Yoles E, Belkin M, Schwartz M. HU-211, a nonpsychotropic cannabinoid, produces short- and long-term neuroprotection after optic nerve axotomy. *J Neurotrauma.* 1996;13:49–57.

46. Schwartz M, Belkin M, Yoles E, Solomon A. Potential treatment modalities for glaucomatous neuropathy: neuroprotection and neuroregeneration. *J Glaucoma.* 1996;5:427–432.

47. Schwartz M, Yoles E. Optic nerve degeneration and potential neuroprotection: implications for glaucoma. *Eur J Ophthalmol.* 1999;9(suppl 1):S9–S11.

48. Wheeler LA, Lai R, Woldemussie E. From the lab to the clinic: activation of an alpha-2 agonist pathway is neuroprotective in models of retinal and optic nerve injury. *Eur J Ophthalmol.* 1999;9(suppl 1):S17–S21.

49. Bodian M. Transient loss of vision following head trauma. *N Y State J Med.* 1964;64:916–920.

50. Anderson RL, Panje WR, Gross CE. Optic nerve blindness following blunt forehead trauma. *Ophthalmology.* 1982;89:445–455.

51. Matsuzaki H, Kunita M, Kawai K. Optic nerve damage in head trauma: clinical and experimental studies. *Jpn J Ophthalmol.* 1982;26:447–461.

52. Nau H, Gerhard L, Foerster M. Optic nerve trauma: clinical, electrophysiological, and histological remarks. *Acta Neurochir (Wien).* 1987;89:16–27.

53. Joseph MP, Lessell S, Rizzo J, Momose KJ. Extracranial optic nerve decompression for traumatic optic neuropathy. *Arch Ophthalmol.* 1990;108:1091–1093.

54. Seiff SR. High dose corticosteroids for treatment of vision loss due to indirect injury to the optic nerve. *Ophthalmic Surg.* 1990;21:389–395.

55. Spoor TC, Hartel WC, Lensink DB, Wilkinson MJ. Treatment of traumatic optic neuropathy with corticosteroids [published erratum appears in Am J Ophthalmol 1991;111:526]. *Am J Ophthalmol.* 1990;110: 665–669.

56. Davidson M. The indirect traumatic optic atrophies. *Am J Ophthalmol.* 1938;21:7–21.

57. Turner J. Indirect injuries of the optic nerves. *Brain.* 1943;66:140–151.

58. Hooper R. Orbital complications of head injury. *Br J Surg*. 1951;39:126–138.

59. Tang R, Li H, Regner L. Traumatic optic neuropathy: analysis of 37 cases. *Invest Ophthalmol Vis Sci (Suppl)*. 1986;27:102.

60. Wolin MJ, Lavin PJ. Spontaneous visual recovery from traumatic optic neuropathy after blunt head injury. *Am J Ophthalmol*. 1990;109:430–435.

61. Mauriello JA, DeLuca J, Krieger A, Schulder M, Frohman L. Management of traumatic optic neuropathy—a study of 23 patients. *Br J Ophthalmol*. 1992;76:349–352.

62. Pringle J. Atrophy of the optic nerve following diffused violence to the skull. *Br Med J*. 1922;2:1156–1157.

63. Niho S, Niho M, Niho K. Decompression of the optic canal by the transethmoidal route and decompression of the superior orbital fissure. *Can J Ophthalmol*. 1970;5:22–40.

64. Imachi Y. [Clinical and patho-histological investigations on optic nerve lesions caused by head injuries]. *Nippon Ganka Gakkai Zasshi*. 1967;71:1874–1908.

65. Schmaltz B, Schurmann K. [Traumatic damages of the optic nerve. Problems of etiology and operative therapy]. *Klin Monatsbl Augenheilkd*. 1971;159:33–51.

66. Hammer G, Ambos E. [Traumatic hematoma of the optic nerve sheath and the possibilities of its surgical treatment]. *Klin Monatsbl Augenheilkd*. 1971;159:818–819.

67. Goldware S, Sylvester R, Baker L. Delayed post-traumatic optic neuropathy with recovery after unroofing the optic canal. *Neuroophthalmology*. 1980;1:77–78.

68. Karnik PP, Maskati BT, Kirtane MV, Tonsekar KS. Optic nerve decompression in head injuries. *J Laryngol Otol*. 1981;95:1135–1140.

69. Brihaye J. *Transcranial Decompression in Head Injuries*. New York: Springer-Verlag; 1981:116–124.

70. Fujitani T, Inoue K, Takahashi T, Ikushima K, Asai T. Indirect traumatic optic neuropathy—visual outcome of operative and nonoperative cases. *Jpn J Ophthalmol*. 1986;30:125–134.

71. Waga S, Kubo Y, Sakakura M. Transfrontal intradural microsurgical decompression for traumatic optic nerve injury. *Acta Neurochir (Wien)*. 1988;91:42–46.

Chapter 38

OCULAR MOTOR SYSTEM

John A. Long and Thomas M. Tann

 Ocular and orbital trauma frequently involves neurologic damage. In addition to containing the eye, the orbit is tightly packed with ocular support structures, including nerves, blood vessels, muscles, and fat. Concurrent trauma to the globe and orbit may easily become an "orbital multisystem trauma." The treatment of orbital and globe injuries requires a thorough knowledge of the ocular motor systems.

EPIDEMIOLOGY (USEIR DATA)

Rate of extraocular muscle involvement among all serious injuries: 3%.

Age (years):
- range: 2–81;
- average: 26;
- rate of 0- to 9-year-olds among the total: 10%;
- rate of 10- to 19-year-olds among the total: 20%;
- rate of ≥60-year-olds among the total: 6%.

Sex: 80% male.

Place of injury:
- home: 32%;
- street and highway: 22%;
- recreation and sport: 14%;
- industrial premises: 13%;
- public building: 5%.

Source of injury:
- various blunt objects: 32%;
- various sharp objects: 15%;
- MVC: 15%;
- gunshot: 14%;
- BB/pellet gun: 6%;
- fall: 5%.

Globe involvement among the total: 50%.

PATHOPHYSIOLOGY

The globe and orbit are innervated by 6 of the 12 cranial nerves. The anatomy of the nerve pathways and origins has been well described and may be significant for the evaluation of patients and their management. The involved nerves are:

- II (optic);
- III (oculomotor);
- IV (trochlear);
- V (trigemineal);
- VI (abducens); and
- VII (facial)

EVALUATION

Examination of patients in an ER setting always involves an assessment of the neurologic system.

- A detailed *history* will often guide subsequent steps of the examination. In patients with orbital injuries, extra care must be taken to evaluate for nerve damage.

- The *visual acuity* is crucial to take in the orbital trauma victim. Vision testing and the swinging-flashlight test (see Chapters 9 and 37) will establish whether the optic nerve is functioning, and whether symmetrically.

- An equally important neurologic test is the *pupillary examination* (see Chapter 3, 9, and 37). An APD indicates that the optic nerve is disrupted somewhere anterior to the chiasm; this should instigate further investigation, including an orbital *CT scan*.
- Evaluation of the *extraocular muscles' movement* can reveal information about cranial nerves III, IV, and VI.

> **PEARL…** A complete extraocular muscle examination, which takes seconds to perform, will establish the function of both the muscles and the nerves.

- If extraocular muscle movement abnormalities are seen in a traumatic setting, further radiologic investigation should be initiated. One exception to this is the simple blowout fracture, which may be diagnosed clinically (see Chapter 36). Radiologic examination of patients with obvious blowout fractures may be delayed for 1 week, pending the spontaneous resolution of symptoms. If the diplopia and restrictive strabismus seen in simple blowout fractures resolve, then an orbital CT scan is not necessary (see Chapter 36).
- In cases of orbital injury involving neurologic damage, a *CT scan* is the radiologic test of choice. The relationship between the bones and soft tissues of the orbits is best delineated with a CT scan. The CT scan is also the most useful radiologic test for preoperative surgical planning.

> **PEARL…** An *MRI scan* is the test of choice when orbital injury is accompanied by CNS trauma.

- Neurological injury to the orbit is almost always associated with trauma to the surrounding tissue(s). The neurological assessment of the globe and orbital injuries must be part of a *comprehensive* evaluation of the patient.

> **▼ PITFALL**
>
> The risk of CNS injuries must be meticulously evaluated.

CLINICAL CONDITIONS

TON

See Chapter 37.

Bell's Palsy

Pathophysiology

Because it has an extensive superficial plexus, the facial nerve is rather susceptible to trauma. The nerve exits the skull at the stylomastoid foramen and innervates the muscles of facial expression. The facial nerve innervates the orbicularis oculi muscle, and its dysfunction leads to Bell's palsy.

Diagnosis

The clinical appearance is one of facial paralysis. In traumatic cases, lacerations or evidence of contusion trauma are usually found. Ocular manifestations of Bell's palsy include:

- ectropion;
- lagophthalmos;
- brow ptosis; and
- ocular exposure symptoms.

Management

In the *early* phases, a search for the underlying cause is indicated. The initial treatment of the ocular manifestations of Bell's palsy is supportive (Fig. 38–1). The use of ocular lubricants and patching may significantly improve the patient's comfort. Spontaneous improvement and resolution of Bell's palsy are common. Supportive measures should be maintained for 6 months prior to contemplating surgical intervention. Surgical repair of a lacerated facial nerve may be attempted.[1] The use of steroids to modulate swelling and protect the nerve is controversial.

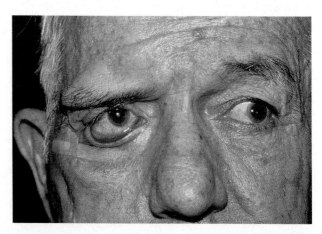

FIGURE 38–1 Right Bell's palsy manifest by brow ptosis, ectropion, and lagophthalmos.

For the first 6 months following the onset of Bell's palsy, the goal of treatment is the patient's comfort and safety.

- The use of artificial tears and ocular lubricants is often sufficient to provide improvement regarding the symptoms.
- Occasional patching of the eye at night may be necessary.

If simple remedies such as artificial tears and ocular lubricants are sufficient, then further treatment can be avoided or evaluated from an aesthetic perspective.

In *chronic* cases (patients who have had Bell's palsy for over 6 months), surgery is recommended. In reconstructive surgery[2], both functional and cosmetic considerations need to be addressed; the primary goal is to provide improved ocular function and comfort; the second goal is to improve the appearance.

▼ PITFALL

A stepwise approach to the surgical management of chronic Bell's palsy is usually followed to avoid overtreatment.

The surgical steps/goals are the following:

- optimize ocular lubrication;
- correct lower eyelid ectropion;
- repair brow ptosis;
- gold weight implant if symptomatic lagophthalmos is present; and
- tarsorrhaphy.

Additional noteworthy details are listed below.

- Lacking seventh-nerve innervation, the eyebrow and lower eyelid become ptotic.
- Any laxity already present will be exaggerated, and brow ptosis and ectropion will become manifest.
- The lower eyelid ectropion may lead to a worsening of exposure symptoms, ocular irritation, and tearing. If symptomatic ectropion is present, a horizontal eyelid-tightening procedure often improves patient comfort.

PEARL... *Brow ptosis* may not only produce dramatic facial asymmetry, which is aesthetically unappealing, but also affect the superior visual field, whose loss can easily be documented by visual field testing.

- The repair of brow ptosis is usually performed by removing an adjacent strip of skin superior to the eyebrow. An adjacent brow lift will restore the superior visual field and enhance facial symmetry (Fig. 38–2).
- A gold weight implant remained the "gold standard"[a] for the treatment of *paralytic lagophthalmos*.[3] A 6- to 16-g gold weight implant sewn to the superior tarsal border provides enough weight to augment gravity in the closure of the eyelid (Fig. 38–3).

---

[a] A variety of other devices have been described over the years, including springs, magnets, and slings.[4–9]

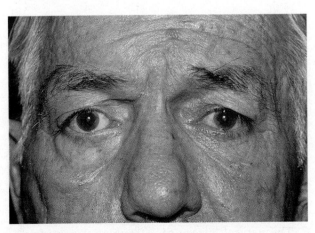

FIGURE 38–2 Right Bell's palsy following correction of brow ptosis and right lower eyelid ectropion.

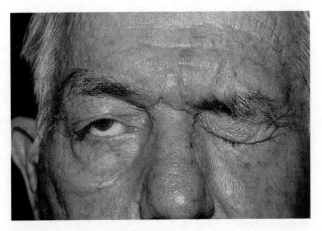

FIGURE 38–3 Right lagophthalmos caused by Bell's palsy.

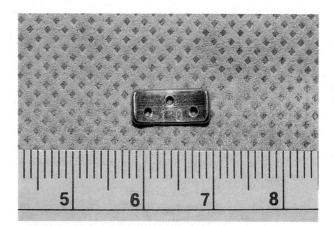

FIGURE 38–4 A 10-gram gold weight implant for treatment of paralytic lagophthalmos.

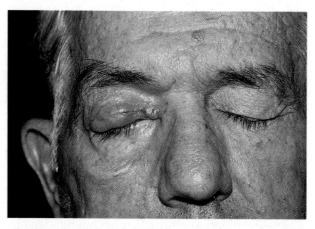

FIGURE 38–5 Improved eyelid closure following implantation of a gold weight implant in a Bell's palsy patient.

- If the patient is symptomatic in spite of the maximal use of the measures outlined previously (i.e., ocular lubricants, correction of lower eyelid laxity and brow ptosis, gold weight implants), tarsorrhaphy is effective at relieving pain associated with ocular exposure (Figs. 38–4 and 38–5).

PITFALL

The major disadvantage of tarsorrhaphy is that it causes a noticeable facial asymmetry, which can be rather distracting. If control of the pain is needed and/or the health of the cornea is compromised, a tarsorrhaphy should be performed as a last resort in the treatment of Bell's palsy.

Neurogenic Ptosis

The development of ptosis after eyelid or orbital trauma is quite common. In some cases the superior division of the third nerve is damaged, leading to neurogenic ptosis. This type of ptosis may be indistinguishable from other forms of ptosis (see Chapter 35) during the initial phase of recovery.

Traumatic ptosis often improves spontaneously weeks to months following the initial injury.[10] Associated swelling of the eyelid and orbit may lead to a dehiscence of the levator aponeurosis. The *diagnosis* of a neurogenic ptosis must encompass the following physical findings:

- poor levator function;
- history of eyelid or orbital trauma; and
- no lid function recovery after 6 months.

If the lid function does not recover by 6 months after injury, reconstructive surgery may be contemplated.

A *sling procedure* is usually necessary to elevate the eyelid margin. The Supramid sling ptosis repair is often the procedure of choice.[11] This sling is easy to place and also easy to remove.

The most frequent *complication* of sling procedures in older patients is the development of dry eyes, caused by iatrogenic lagophthalmos. In severe and refractory cases, the Supramid sling can be easily removed to allow the eyelid to return to its ptotic position and protect the cornea.

PEARL... If the Supramid sling is well tolerated over the years, it can be replaced with an autogenous fascia lata implant.

Traumatic Carotid Cavernous Fistula

A communication between the cavernous sinus and the carotid artery can develop following trauma. The fistula leads to the arterialization of the orbital vein.

Clinical signs of a traumatic carotid cavernous fistula are:
- pulsating proptosis;
- diplopia;
- elevated IOP; and
- dilated conjunctival vessels.

The *natural history* of a traumatic carotid cavernous fistula is often spontaneous embolization and resolution.

PITFALL

A persistent carotid cavernous fistula can lead to vision loss, primarily due to IOP.

Treatment of the traumatic carotid cavernous sinus fistula is indicated if prolonged elevation of the IOP is detected and visual field loss is developing. Two embolization options are available.

1. In most cases, embolization of the carotid cavernous sinus fistula is performed via a *femoral approach*.

PEARL... Prior to treatment, an arteriogram is required to pinpoint the location of the fistula.

2. In difficult cases in which the fistula is not accessible by the femoral approach, the best access can be achieved by cannulating the *superior ophthalmic vein*.[12–15] With the arterialization of the orbital veins caused by the carotid cavernous fistula, the superior ophthalmic vein is often quite large. The vein can be accessed by a superior medial anterior orbitotomy. A cannula for embolization is placed into the superior ophthalmic vein to provide access for the interventional radiologist. The cannula is removed following effective embolization.

SUMMARY

Orbital and ocular damage involving neurologic injury is relatively common. Unlike the approach to most problems in ophthalmology, one of the main "treatments" for neurologic injury is stabilization and observation because repair of trauma-related neurologic damage is often unavailable. We support the human body and allow nature to take its course. This ancient and traditional treatment may yield to more aggressive and invasive treatments in the years ahead.

REFERENCES

1. Hoffman WY. Reanimation of the paralyzed face. *Otolaryngol Clin North Am.* 1992;25:649–667.
2. Kinney SE, Seeley BM, Seeley MZ, Foster JA. Oculoplastic surgical techniques for protection of the eye in facial nerve paralysis. *Am J Otol.* 2000;21:275–283.
3. Kaplan C, Sela M, Peled I, Rousso M, Wexler MR. Gold implant to upper eyelid for correction of lagophthalmos. *Ann Ophthalmol.* 1980;12:1214–1215.
4. D'Hooge PJ, Hendrickx EM. Upper lid loading with dermis graft and levator weakening. Management of lagophthalmos due to facial palsy. *Ophthalmologica.* 1975;171:419–424.
5. Duetinger M, Freilinger G. Temporalis transfer for correction of lagophthalmos. *Eur Arch Otorhinolaryngol Suppl.* 1994:S142–S144.
6. Goumain AJ, Fevrier JC. Treatment of lagophthalmos in facial paralysis by Morel-Fatio's Aspring insertion operation. *J Med Bord.* 1965;142:797–801.
7. Lessa S, Carreirae S. Use of an encircling silicone rubber string for the correction of lagophthalmos. *Plast Reconstr Surg.* 1978;61:719–723.
8. McNeill JI, Oh YH. An improved palpebral spring for the management of paralytic lagophthalmos. *Ophthalmology.* 1991;98:715–719.
9. Sen DK. Temporalis transplantation for paralytic lagophthalmos. *Br J Ophthalmol.* 1970;54:680–682.
10. Silkiss RZ, Baylis HI. Management of traumatic ptosis. *Adv Ophthalmic Plast Reconstr Surg.* 1988;7:149–155.
11. Katowitz JA. Frontalis suspension in congenital ptosis using a polyfilament, cable-type suture. *Arch Ophthalmol.* 1979;97:1659–1663.
12. Derang J, Ying H, Long Y, et al. Treatment of carotid-cavernous sinus fistulas retrograde via the superior ophthalmic vein (SOV). *Surg Neurol.* 1999;52:286–292.
13. Gioulekas J, Mitchell P, Tress B, McNab AA. Embolization of carotid cavernous fistulas via the superior ophthalmic vein. *Aust N Z J Ophthalmol.* 1997;25:47–53.
14. Liang CC, Michon JJ, Cheng KM, Chan CM, Cheung YL. Ophthalmologic outcome of transvenous embolization of spontaneous carotid-cavernous fistulas: a preliminary report. *Int Ophthalmol.* 1999;23:43–47.
15. Monsein LH, Debrun GM, Miller NR, Nauta HJ, Chazaly JR. Treatment of dural carotid-cavernous fistulas via the superior ophthalmic vein. *AJNR.* 1991;12:435–439.

SECTION VI

APPENDICES

INSTRUMENTATION

Suzanne Nelson

TABLE A1–1 BASIC LIST OF INSTRUMENTATION*

Beaver blade handle
Blades, disposable
BSS for irrigation
Caliper
Corneal glue
Corneal shield—collagen shield
Cotton-tipped applicators
Culture media
Forceps, assorted (0.12, 0.3, 0.5, tying)
Foreign body forceps, assorted
Frazier suction tip
Healon
Iris spatula
Irrigating cannulas
Lacrimal intubation sets
Lid retractor
Mosquito clamps
Muscle hooks, fenestrated, Jameson
Needle holders, assorted (fine, locking, nonlocking;
    highly curved for posterior ruptures)
Ophthalgan
Permanent intraocular magnet (for IOFB extraction)
Retractor (Schepens)
Scissors, assorted (Barraquer, Stephens tenotomy, Vannas,
    sharp and dull Westcott)
Serafins
Speculums, assorted adult/pediatric
Sponges, 4 × 4
Suction tubing
Sutures and needles, assorted: curved and straight needles
    10-0 prolene
    10-0 nylon
    9-0 nylon
    6-0 Vicryl
    7-0 Vicryl
Weck spears
Wire cutters to cut items such as a fish hook imbedded
    into tissue

*Access to pharmacy is advised to have the intravitreal injections
properly prepared.

TABLE A1–2 EXPANDED LIST OF INSTRUMENTATION

Flute needles (straight, tapered)
Foreign body forceps, assorted
Gonio lens
Haptic cutters
Healon
Infusion cannulas, assorted (4 mm, 6 mm)
Infusion contact lens, assorted
Instruments to implant IOL
Instruments to remove IOL
Intraocular forceps, assorted
Intraocular gases and filters
Intraocular scissors, assorted
Iris retractors
PFCL
Plug forceps
Retinal tacks and forceps
Retractors, assorted
Scleral buckles, assorted
Scleral depressors
Scleral plugs
Silicone oil
Subretinal instruments
TKPs, assorted
Tonometer
Trephines to correspond to TKP size

TABLE A1–3 MACHINES

Cryo machine with assorted probes
Laser machine with IBO attachments and assorted probes
Ultrasonography machine (B scan)
Vitrectomy machine and disposable accessory packs

ENDOSCOPY

Claude Boscher

The endoscope, inserted through a small opening into a body cavity, provides a clear and up-close image. It serves diagnostic purposes but also aids in treatment. It might become an integral part of the ophthalmologist's armamentarium, and the indications for its use might grow in the future.

In addition to viewing ability behind the anterior segment of the eye, crucial areas in which the endoscope offers new hope are the prevention/treatment of ciliary body and vitreous base conditions leading to *phthisis* and *anterior PVR* (see Chapters 19 and 25).

This appendix reviews the potentials of endoscopy for the surgeon treating patients with eye injuries.

HISTORY[a]

By the 1980s, endoscopy had become a routine diagnostic and therapeutic tool in various fields of medicine (e.g., gastroenterology, otorhinolaryngology, gynecology, pneumotology, urology, arthroscopy).

Endoscopy in ophthalmology was actually first reported for trauma.[2] Subsequent studies[3–5] included evaluation and surgery of the globe and orbit for various conditions. Miniaturization of optic wave-guides and the development of electronic videoendoscopy made the technique available for ophthalmic microsurgery by the 1990s,[6] and a few series of patients have now been reported with various ophthalmic conditions.[b]

THE RATIONALE FOR ENDOSCOPE USE

Endoscopy allows undistorted intraoperative visualization of anatomical regions of the eye that are otherwise:

- inaccessible (e.g., behind the iris root); or
- difficult to visualize (e.g., lens zonules, ciliary processes, anterior part of the pars plana and of the vitreous base, subretinal space).

> **PEARL...** A major advantage of the endoscope is that it can be used even in eyes in which media opacity (e.g., hyphema, cataract) interferes with or prevents traditional transpupillary viewing.

Additional advantages of the endoscope include:

- high magnification; and a
- tangential approach.

---

[a]See reference 1 for additional details on the history of endoscopy in ophthalmology.

[b]For example, cyclophotocoagulation of the ciliary processes for primary open angle, congenital, and neovascular glaucomas,[7,8] PVR and peripheral retinal photocoagulation,[9] sulcus fixation of IOLs,[10–12] lens disclocation,[13] severe proliferative diabetic retinopathy,[14] laser-assisted endonasal and transcanalicular dacryocystorhinostomy.[15]

These allow a unique opportunity to evaluate:

- the ciliary body; and
- the depth of the anterior (zonular) part of the vitreous base.

INSTRUMENTATION

Two types of devices are available currently:

- fiberoptic bundles; and
- solid-state, GRIN rod lens.

In both systems, illumination of the field is provided by a bundle of glass pipes surrounding the endoscopic canal and connected to a light source. The objective is made of a GRIN lens; a coupling optic lens system enlarges and focuses the image on a CCD camera, which converts it into a video signal; this in turn is displayed on a video monitor and observed by the surgeon. Table A2-1 provides a practical overview of the two available transmission systems.

CLINICAL APPLICATIONS

Endoscopy in the Vitreous Cavity

Endoscopic viewing has the following *advantages*:

- *evaluation of the vitreous cavity* is:
  - *immediate,*
  - *complete*[c] (e.g., the posterior surface of the posterior lens capsule, Wieger's ligament, the back of

the iris, the anterior and posterior parts of the zonular system, the ciliary processes and epithelium, the vitreous base and its connections with the posterior lens capsule and zonules), and
  - *undistorted* (i.e., no scleral depression is necessary);
- *applicability for both the phakic and aphakic eyes;*
- *media opacity does not preclude its use;*
- *high magnification* (5× to 20×, compared with the microscope, depending on probe technology and the distance from the area observed).

PEARL... The axis of visualization of tissues observed in front of the endoscopy probe at the vitreous base is tangential/sagittal.

PEARL... More accurate evaluation of the "anatomical" depth and orientation of the vitreous fibers[d] or membranes is possible than that allowed by the frontal approach and even the highest magnification provided through the microscope.

---

[c]360 degrees.

[d]That is, circumferential; anteroposterior; parallel to the surface of the ciliary epithelium.

TABLE A2-1   COMPARATIVE CHARACTERISTICS OF BOTH TRANSMISSION SYSTEMS*

Variable	Fiberoptic Bundle	Quartz Rod
Image transmission	Fragmented in each micropipe ("honeycomb" effect)	Transmitted in entirety, without fragmentation
Magnification compared with microscope	~5×	~10×–20×
Resolution	Adequate for vitreoretinal procedures	Superior (intravascular cell flow can be observed; great future potential)
Field of view	110°	50° and 110° probes
Focus	Stationary	Adjustable with foot pedal
Distance from tissues observed	Image lost if the probe touches the tissue observed (however, an initial advantage at start: pseudostereopsis)	Image still transmitted even if the probe touches the tissue observed (advantage for subretinal work)
Presence of additional empty channel	None: probe includes laser pipe or not Sterilization	Yes
Weight of probe	Lighter	Heavier

*See reference 1 for more technical details.

Table A2-2 lists the specific advantages of endoscopy during *vitreoretinal surgery*.

Endoscopic viewing also has *disadvantages*:

- *requires training for video control;*
- *requires training for lack of stereoscopy[e]; and*
- *bimanual surgery is not possible.*

Endoscopy for Trauma

Exploratory (Diagnostic) Endoscopy

Visualization in the injured eye is often inadequate because of (or the combination of) several factors:

- media opacity (e.g., corneal laceration, edema, hyphema, hypopyon, cataract); and

- narrow pupil (e.g., posterior synechiae).

In such cases, if comprehensive reconstructive surgery cannot be performed (see Chapter 25), the endoscope offers diagnostic advantages[f]:

- differential diagnosis between a detached retina and a detached, thick posterior hyaloid (see Chapter 25)[g];
- assessment of the condition of the macula and its prognosis;
- rapid assessment of the feasibility and prognosis of a secondary procedure; and
- assessment of the condition of the ciliary body (i.e., phthisis development).

---

[e]In reality, as previously demonstrated by colleagues in other medical fields, the brain relatively rapidly acquires pseudostereoscopy and a perception of orientation and localization with respect to the lens and retina. In our experience, a few tens of cases are sufficient to achieve this. A new endoscope has been developed[10] (although commercially it is not available yet) that allows the surgeon to observe the images in the binoculars of the microscope.

---

[f]With potential medicolegal implications (see Chapters 5, 7, and 8).

[g]Even by trained personnel and using high-resolution B-scan ultrasonography, this may be difficult otherwise.

TABLE A2-2 The Advantages of Endoscopy during Vitreoretinal Surgery

Surgical Maneuver	*Advantage*
Entry of surgical tools	Avoiding incorrect instrument path (e.g., subciliary/subretinal infusion; perforation of anteriorly displaced retina)
Vitreous removal from sclerotomy sites	Prevention of secondary development of tear(s), re/detachment, anterior PVR
Removal of vitreous from behind the posterior capsule	Possible, even in the phakic eye; prophylaxis of hyaloidal fibrovascular proliferation
Anterior zonular vitreous base peeling	Possible, even in the phakic eye to:
	• identify/evaluate potential tractional forces (anteroposterior, circumferential);
	• remove vitreous behind the zonules, ciliary epithelium, and processes;
	• prevent vitreous base avulsion and retinal traction by close peeling of the vitreous cortex in between the anterior from the posterior attachments of the vitreous base;
	• forgo endolaser treatment in the area of the remaining vitreous cortex
Removal of dislocated/fragmented lens	Enhanced visual control during pars plana phacoemulsification/removal of lens particles trapped under PFCL
Sulcus-fixating of an IOL	Enhanced visual control
Fluid/air, PFCL/air, PFCL/silicone oil exchanges	• Enhanced visual control (the probe is kept in the fluid until reaching the optic disk)
	• Easy identification of residual PFCL bubbles in the vitreous cavity/subretinal space under air
Maneuvers under air	Enhanced visual control
Working under silicone oil	Better visualization of anterior reproliferations, of residual emulsified silicone bubbles
Visual control of unplanned incidents	

Exploratory endoscopy should *not* be performed unless the surgeon is also experienced both in the management of injured eyes and manipulation of the endoscope; the lack of stereopsis and the orientation difficulties in the vitreous cavity make such attempts dangerous.

Surgical (Therapeutic) Endoscopy

The goals of endoscope-assisted vitreoretinal surgery for the traumatized eye include (but are obviously not limited to) the *prevention of PVR development*, the leading cause of surgical failure after trauma, via retinal/ciliary detachment and ciliary body scarring. The tactical goals are:

- early removal of the vitreous blood and scaffold;
- removal of the anterior vitreous base; and
- prevention/treatment of tissue incarcerations in the wound(s).

In eyes in which early vitrectomy is not possible[h] without removal of the cornea, the endoscope offers an obvious solution.

PEARL... Endoscopy provides *timely* intervention via "bypassing" the media opacity, allowing the surgeon to perform, rather than to defer, maneuvers such as complete (anterior/posterior) vitrectomy and removal of scar tissue.

Practical advantages of endoscopy in the *early* management of the injured eye include the following.

- *Prevention of entry site complications during vitrectomy* (which can occur because of visualization problems, hypotony, ciliary body or retinal detachment, and anterior displacement of tissues—even when performing a sclerotomy at 2.5 mm from the limbus).
- *Rapid access to the posterior pole* through consecutive pockets of opaque, organized vitreous lacunae (see Chapter 25) containing blood/fibrin (e.g., to permit early evaluation of the macula; early PFCL injection to stabilize the retina [see Appendix A 4] and/or protect the macula from secondary injury).

- *Improved differential diagnosis* between detached retina and organized posterior hyaloid detachment.
- *Improved surgical control over* removal of a dislocated lens.
- *Close-up view of subretinal maneuvers* (e.g., removal of blood, membranes, IOFBs).
- *Improved visualization* under air or during air–fluid or air–PFC, exchanges.
- *Visual control* of any unplanned incident.

Endoscopy in trauma also has limitations; see Table A2-3.

ENDOSCOPY FOR THE BEGINNER

Until you gain more experience with the technology, use:

- *the panoramic probe;*
- *the endoscope as a regular illumination probe* and train yourself by alternating between endoscopic viewing on the video monitor and your standard visualization system;
- *the endoscope in easy cases* (e.g., vitreous hemorrhage in a pseudophakic eye and with an attached retina), avoiding complex, and especially trauma, cases.

Remember that:

- *orientation* is changed by rotating the probe between your fingers:
  ○ before entering the vitreous cavity, check the external view of the eye on the video to understand how you are oriented;
- *magnification* change is provided not by activating the microscope foot pedal but by pushing forward (i.e., approaching the target) or withdrawing the probe.

You have a risk of injuring the lens if you try to reach across the anterior vitreous (just as with any other mobile intraocular visualization system).

Helpful techniques to avoid lens touch include the following:

- if you have slit illumination on your microscope, utilize it to train your brain regarding the lens equator's position (invisible on the monitor but visible through the microscopic view);

---

[h] For example, inadequate visualization through the cornea in an eye that would otherwise not require PK; see Chapters 8, 23, 25, and 26),

Table A2–3   The Limitations of Endoscopy in Trauma

Variable	Difficulty
Fresh bleeding	The tip of the endoscope can be totally obscured by blood and fibrin; consequently, the image on the video monitor is red
Pars plana incision for the probe itself	The initial introduction of the endoscope itself may be dangerous if the ciliary body/retina are anteriorly displaced (introduction through the limbus and sacrificing a clear lens may be necessary)
Inherit characteristics of the current endoscope (orientation/probe manipulation difficulties; video control; lack of stereopsis; lack of bimanual manipulations)	Lack of experience/training makes endoscopy dangerous

- switch the sclerotomy sites around to gain access to all parts of the anterior vitreous.[i]

SUMMARY

Although the need for training and the initial expense may appear to be deterrents to endoscope use, this technology offers distinct advantages that other modalities cannot provide. The two major causes of surgical failure in trauma surgery today involve the development of anterior PVR and a nonfunctional or dysfunctional ciliary body; the endoscope allows the surgeon to visualize these areas. More thorough and earlier cleaning is thus possible, as well as the removal of vitreous, cells, scar tissue, and blood, increasing the chance of preventing late complications.

[i] A fourth sclerotomy may be necessary.

REFERENCES

1. Bocher C. Endoscopic vitreoretinal surgery of the injured eye. In: Alfaro DV III, Liggett PE. *Vitreoretinal Surgery of the Injured Eye.* Philadelphia: Lippincott-Raven; 1999:301–314.
2. Thorpe H. Ocular endoscope: instrument for removal of intravitreous nonmagnetic foreign bodies. *Trans Am Acad Ophthalmol Otolaryngol.* 1934;39:422–424.
3. Norris JL, Cleasby GW. An endoscope for ophthalmology. *Am J Ophthalmol.* 1978;85:420–422.
4. Norris JL, Cleasby GW. Endoscopic orbital surgery. *Am J Ophthalmol.* 1981;91:249–252.
5. Norris JL, Stewart WB. Bimanual endoscopic orbital biopsy. *Ophthalmology.* 1985;92:34–38.
6. Koch F, Spitznas M. Video endoscopic vitreous surgery. *Ophthalmol Chir.* 1990;2:71–78.
7. Uram M. Ophthalmic laser microendoscope endophotocoagulation. *Ophthalmology.* 1992;99:1829–1832.
8. Uram M. Ophthalmic laser microendoscope ciliary process ablation in the management of neovascular glaucoma. *Ophthalmology.* 1992;99:1823–1828.
9. Uram M. Laser endoscope in the management of proliferative vitreoretinopathy. *Ophthalmology.* 1993;101:1404–1408.
10. Leon C, Leon J, Rich WJ. From blind implantation to endoscopic control of posterior implantation : a new surgical concept. *Eur J Implant Refract Surg.* 1992;4:271–272.
11. Althaus C, Sundmacher R. Intraoperative intraocular endoscopy in transscleral suture fixation of posterior chamber lenses: consequences for suture technique, implantation procedure, and choice of PCL design. *Refract Corneal Surg.* 1993;9:333–339.
12. De Jesus G, Miyake Y, Miyake K. Endoscopic observation of fixation of posterior chamber lenses following pars plana vitrectomy. *Implants Ophthalmol.* 1987;1(3):98–100.
13. Boscher C, Lebuisson DA, Lean JS. Vitrectomy with endoscopy for management of retained lens fragments and/or posteriorly dislocated IOL. *Graefes Arch Clin Exp Ophthalmol.* 1998;236:115–121.
14. Boscher C, Cathelineau B, Cathelineau G. Endoscopy-assisted vitrectomy for severe proliferative diabetic retinopathy. *Ophtalmology Suppl.* 1999;106:165.
15. Hobson SR. Endoscopic surgery for lacrimal and orbital disease. *Curr Opin Ophthalmol.* 1994;5:32–38.

BASIC SURGICAL TECHNIQUES IN THE ANTERIOR SEGMENT

M. Bowes Hamill

Understanding some basic principles in the surgical management of tissue lesions helps the surgeon to comprehend not simply "how" but also "why" a procedure or a maneuver is (to be) done. This chapter satisfies this need by describing the principles and practice of handling a few of the most common injuries. Appendix 3 is intended for all ophthalmologists who treat patients with ocular trauma. Appendix 4 is intended for the specialist, explaining the basics of commonly performed procedures.

SURGICAL REPAIR OF CORNEAL WOUNDS

Introduction

The cornea is the major refractive service of the eye; hence, even small irregularities in curvature can result in significant visual disability. For this reason, repair of the injured cornea requires particular attention to detail in order to restore a smooth and optically effective refractive surface and thus maximize the patient's chances for good postoperative vision.

Whereas closure of most corneal wounds is fairly straightforward, stellate lacerations (e.g., wounds caused by high-velocity IOFBs) and certain ruptures can be difficult to piece together.

> **P**EARL... In general, it is best to do as much of the reconstruction as possible at the time of the primary closure.

Early repair:
- reduces the surgical problems caused by:
  - adhesion formation and
  - edema; and
- minimizes the chances of
  - ECH/SCH and
  - infection.

In most clinical settings, closure of corneal wounds is rather urgent; surgery should be performed as soon as possible, taking into consideration other factors (e.g., the time of patient's last meal and his medical status; see Chapter 8).

> **P**EARL... It should be appreciated that not all corneal lacerations require surgical repair for closure (see Chapter 14 and later in this Appendix).

Anatomic Reconstruction

Because of the critical nature of the corneal curvature to visual function, anatomic reconstruction of the cornea is key to achieving good postoperative vision.

- The first step in the restoration of the anatomy is the recognition and appreciation of anatomic landmarks and other features that will aid the physician in placing the apposing corneal edges in their correct relationship (Fig. A3–1). Such landmarks include:
  - limbus;
  - stellate edges; and
  - pigmentation lines in the epithelium.

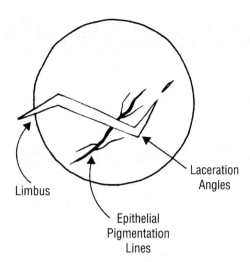

FIGURE A3–1 Corneal landmarks. Almost all corneal wounds contain some landmarks that facilitate anatomic realignment: the limbus, epithelial pigmentation lines (e.g., iron lines), and stellate would edges/angles of the wound itself.

> **PEARL...** By closing the landmarks as the initial step, the surgeon ensures that the apposition of the remainder of the corneal laceration will be anatomically correct.

- A careful examination of the *full* thickness of *each* of the wound edges must be undertaken to detect and reposition corneal fragments and/or flaps.

> **SPECIAL CONSIDERATION**
>
> Occasionally, it appears that there is also loss of corneal tissue. It is extremely rare, however; most frequently, pieces of cornea that appear to be missing are, in fact, folded under into the AC (see Chapter 14).

> **PEARL...** Loss of corneal tissue most commonly occurs as a result of trauma from high-speed IOFBs (e.g., gunshot wounds, explosions).

Basic Considerations and Steps

The surgeon needs to be aware of the effect the sutures have on the overlying corneal surface; this helps to avoid generating iatrogenic curvature abnormalities.

- Sutures close wounds by virtue of *tissue compression*; tightening of a suture results in tissue (and thus surface) distortion.[1]

> **PEARL...** Tissue compression caused by a corneal suture is mirrored on the overlying corneal surface.

- The compressive force generated by any individual suture is:
  ○ maximal in the plane of the suture but
  ○ extends some distance away from the suture (Fig. A3–2).

Different types of sutures result in different types of wound behavior.

Interrupted sutures have, as their most stable configuration when tightened, a planar circle (Fig. A3–3). To avoid tissue distortion by interrupted sutures, the suture should be placed and constructed in this configuration.

- Creation of an *interrupted*, round suture loop in a single plane is technically difficult. A compromise is the full-thickness "box" suture as illustrated in Figure A3–4.

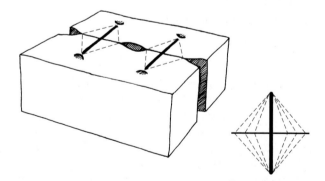

FIGURE A3–2 All sutures close the wound tissue by compression. The area of maximal compression is in the plane of the suture, but this compressive force also extends laterally to form a *zone* of compression. Tissue apposition occurs when the zone of compression is sufficient to close the tissue edges. Wound gape occurs at the areas where the compressive force is insufficient to appose the tissue edges. The size and extent of the zone of compression depend on suture length as well as on the tension of the suture material.

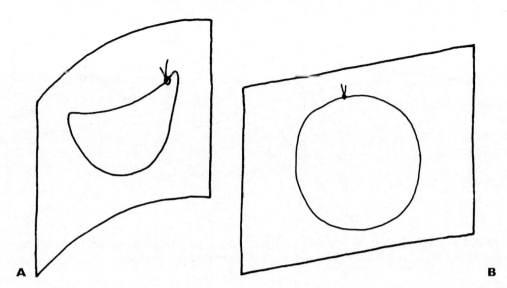

FIGURE A3–3   (**A** and **B**) The most stable configuration of an interrupted suture is a planar circle. With tightening, therefore, the suture, in an attempt to achieve this configuration, will distort the tissue contained within the loop and thus the corneal surface.

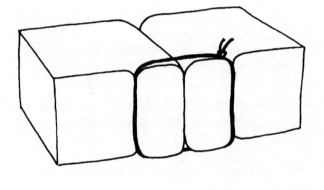

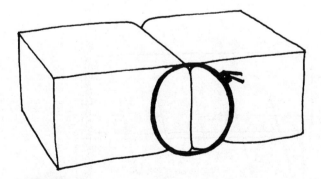

FIGURE A3–4   (Top and bottom) The "box" suture is a compromise structure for an interrupted suture. The suture is placed full thickness. With tightening, the tissue is compressed but the wound alignment is not altered. The surface effects of the suture are relieved with suture removal, whereas surface irregularities induced by *tissue misalignment* are permanent even after suture removal.

○ This configuration can be generated by pronation of the hand and passage of the needle directly posteriorly through the cornea, partial supination, and driving a needle exteriorly from the endothelial side of the opposite wound edge.

○ With tightening of the full-thickness box suture, the tissue is compressed but not inverted, everted, or shifted.

○ Use of *full-thickness* corneal sutures is recommended because these have minimal everting/inverting effects and facilitate closure of corneal wounds of different edge thicknesses.

PEARL...   Different edge thickness is frequently encountered in corneal wounds more than a few hours old: because of regional corneal edema, one wound edge may be significantly thicker than the opposing edge. By incorporating the full thickness of the cornea within the suture loop, these thickness differences are obviated, and closure with full-thickness suture bites will oppose identical layers across the defect (e.g., Descemet's with Descemet's; Bowman's with Bowman's).

○ Interrupted sutures should be placed at 90 degrees to the wound edge to avoid wound slippage (Fig. A3–5).

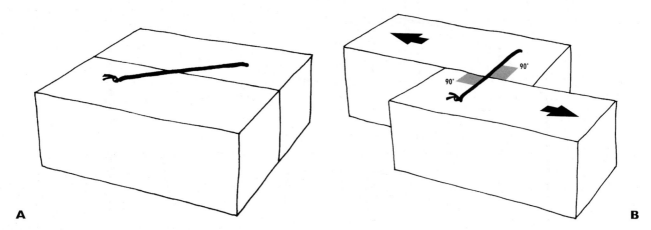

FIGURE A3–5   (**A** and **B**) Sutures should be placed at right angles to the wound at the point of the suture/wound intersection. Sutures at acute angles will cause wound slippage with tightening as illustrated.

• Once wound healing is complete and the suture has been removed, the compressive forces separated by the suture cease to exist.

PITFALL

If no anatomic distortion has occurred during wound healing and the flattening effect of the suture is relieved, the corneal curvature should return to normal. If, however, wound slippage or misalignment has occurred, this distortion is permanent (i.e., will *not* be alleviated by suture removal).

Running sutures have the benefit of a continuous zone of compression. This results in good wound apposition, but, unfortunately, they also have disadvantages:

• a large zone of compression (and thus flattening of the cornea);
• misalignment of wound edges due to suture-induced edge slippage[a] (Fig. A3–6.);
• straightening of curvilinear incisions; and
• rippling of the corneal surface if the sutures are not placed at the same depth or full thickness.

---

[a] Unless the sutures are placed in a bootlace or antitorque configuration.

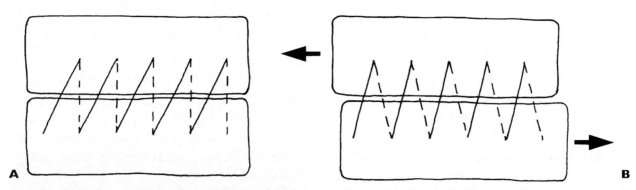

FIGURE A3–6   (**A** and **B**) Running sutures, unless placed in an antitorque configuration, will cause linear wound shift equal to approximately one half of the suture bite spacing.

Special Cases

Shelved Lacerations   As discussed earlier, surface abnormalities caused by wound slippage/misalignment are permanent, whereas surface flattening due to suture compression is relieved once the suture is removed.

> **PEARL...**   Shelved lacerations present a special situation: closure can cause wound slippage along the plane of the laceration.

- To prevent edge movement, the entire width of the laceration should be incorporated within the suture loop (Fig. A3–7A).
  - If this is not possible, the laceration can be closed in two layers (Fig. A3–7B), ensuring apposition of the wound edges while minimizing wound shift.[b]

Loose Fragments   As a principle, all loose fragments should be repositioned into their normal anatomic situation.

- If possible, the tissue edges should be *sutured* into place.

---

[b] It should be realized that the deeper suture is generally not removable.

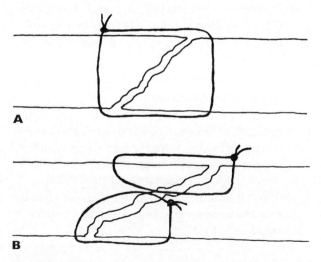

A

B

FIGURE A3–7   Shelved lacerations present a special problem. **(A)** If possible, the entire extent of the lacerations should be incorporated within the suture bite. **(B)** If the shelf is too long to allow closure with one suture, the cornea can be closed in two layers.

- If this is not feasible, the fragments can be secured either by:
  - oversewing; or
  - being splinted with a bandage soft contact lens.
- Occasionally, *corneal glue* can be of help in keeping the small corneal fragments in their normal position while healing progresses.

Restoration of Functional Architecture

After the normal anatomy has been restored, attention needs to be directed to recreating the functional anatomy.

> **PITFALL**
>
> A corneal wound and its repair act like a "double-edged sword": both the wound[c] and the treatment (i.e., suturing) cause corneal surface flattening.

Appropriately applied suture compression, however, can be used to restore the normal corneal contour: the Rowsey-Hays technique[2] utilizes compression of the *peripheral* sutures to effect change in the *central* corneal curvature.

- Peripheral compression is generated by the placement of:
  - multiple;
  - long; and
  - tight (i.e., with overlapping compression zones) sutures in the corneal periphery.
- The central cornea is therefore steepened and is *subsequently* closed with:
  - small;
  - more widely spaced; and
  - minimally compressive sutures.
- This suturing generates a spherical[d] corneal center with a relatively flat periphery (Fig. A3–8).

---

[c] As is clear from the purpose of, and experience with, refractive surgery.

[d] To ensure that the central cornea is indeed spherical, qualitative keratometry is recommended.

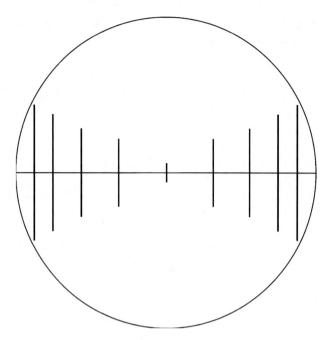

FIGURE A3–8   The Rowsey-Hays technique of corneal wound closure. The periphery of the wound is closed with long, tight, compressive suture bites. This results in flattening of the periphery and compensatory steepening of the corneal center. The center is then closed with short, spaced, minimally compressive suture bites to preserve the central steepening as much as possible. The result is a flattened periphery with a spherical center.

> **PEARL…   The refractive goal of corneal wound repair is not the restoration of a specific curvature but rather the reconstruction of a spherical corneal center.**

- A spherical central cornea:
  - maximizes the chances for rapid visual recovery postoperatively; and
  - facilitates contact lens fitting, if necessary.

Most *qualitative keratometric techniques* utilize a reflected image from the cornea to detect and estimate the axis of astigmatism.

- Several instruments are available; one of the simplest is the Flieringa ring.[e]

- The ring is held over the cornea and, utilizing coaxial illumination, its reflection from the epithelial surface is examined. The ideal reflection should be a round circle. The presence of corneal astigmatism causes the ring to appear oval.
- Sutures can then be either tightened or loosened so as to adjust the corneal curvature to the most spherical endpoint.
- Implied in this technique is the ability to adjust the suture tension while maintaining corneal closure. The sliding clove hitch or the sliding half-hitch[3,4] *slipknots* are extremely helpful in achieving this goal.

General Considerations

- The surgeon should minimize *handling* of the tissue:
  - repeated graspings result in maceration of the tissue edges and corneal edema, making anatomic reconstruction difficult;
  - suture placement should be first *planned* and *then* executed[f] rather than placing and replacing sutures on a trial-and-error basis.
- If watertight closure cannot be achieved with the use of sutures (see previously), several management options are available; the decision depends on the actual situation and the preference of the surgeon.
  - For *small* wounds, a bandage contact lens may be sufficient to seal the wound and allow healing.
  - For *larger* defects, tissue adhesive may be of benefit.
  - In *extreme* cases, a therapeutic corneal transplant (PK or lamellar keratoplasty) may be required.
- The *timing* of suture removal[g] is directed by the following:
  - the local wound healing response;
  - the corneal topography; and
  - the age of the patient. For instance, in young patients, sutures can be removed as early as 6–8 weeks following surgery (see Chapter 30); in older patients with large wounds, the sutures should be left in place for several months.
- *Healing* following corneal wounds is usually uneventful unless the patient develops an infection or other complications.

---

[e] The hinge spring of a safety pin can also be used.

[f] Mirroring the thought process described in Chapter 8.

[g] Remember that the cornea has no blood vessels; the healing process is slow.

- *Contact lens* fitting can be attempted 8–12 weeks following primary repair.
  - ◦ If the corneal center has been steepened and is fairly spherical, contact lens fitting is fairly straightforward.

PITFALL

A flat corneal apex with a steep periphery creates a difficult situation for contact lens fitting.

SUMMARY

With new developments in microsurgical technique and equipment, closure of corneal wounds with a good functional outcome is usually possible. The surgeon should pay attention to the restoration of both the anatomic relationships and the functional architecture of the tissue. Because of the importance of the corneal curvature for visual function, the effect of the suture closure on the overlying surface needs to be taken into consideration. Planning of all aspects of the intervention (see Chapter 8) helps to avoid many of the postoperative complications.

REFERENCES

1. Eisner G. *Eye Surgery*. New York: Springer-Verlag; 1980.

2. Rowsey JJ, Hays JC. Refractive reconstruction for acute eye injuries. *Ophthalmic Surg*. 1984;15:569–574.

3. Dangel ME, Kestes RH. The adjustable slide knot. An alternative technique. *Ophthalmic Surg*. 1980;12:843–846.

4. Terry C. The differentially adjustable slipknot. *Am IOL Implant Soc J*. 1977;3:197.

BASIC SURGICAL TECHNIQUES IN THE POSTERIOR SEGMENT

Wolfgang Schrader

Only a few decades ago, 75% of persons with serious ocular trauma became monocularly blind. Due to new surgical technology, this proportion has decreased significantly (see Chapter 8). Because the posterior segment is involved in 46% of open globe injuries (USEIR datum), we discuss here some of the basic principles and techniques used today to achieve retinal (re)attachment and a permanently transparent vitreous cavity.

CULTURING

Risk of Posttraumatic Endophthalmitis

After lacerating types of globe injuries, there is always a risk of endophthalmitis[1,2] (see Chapter 28). The risk depends heavily on the circumstances of the trauma: 30% incidence in rural trauma, compared with 11% in nonrural trauma in one study[3]; the presence of IOFBs also increases the risk[4]. We found[a] a 3.6% overall rate of posttraumatic endophthalmitis; it increased to 20% in an agricultural environment and to 38% if the injury was caused by fence wire contaminated with soil.

Principles

> **P**EARL... Although antibiotic treatment of endophthalmitis has to be initiated before microbiologic results are known, subsequent tailoring of the treatment requires identification of the organism.

Because the vitreous is an ideal place for most microbes to grow, this is the most rewarding site for culture taking.[b]

> **PITFALL**
>
> Never rely on a tap from the conjunctiva or the AC alone in case of a suspected endophthalmitis, even if the inflammation is limited to the anterior segment: the AC has a greater ability to resist an infecting agent than the posterior segment.[5,c]

- An AC culture fluid, even in aphakic eyes with a capsulotomy, may be negative in the presence of positive cultures from the vitreous, and only rarely is the AC sample positive in the presence of negative vitreous cultures.[6–9]

> **P**EARL... However, because organisms may occasionally be found in the aqueous in the presence of a negative vitreous culture, it is recommended that a sample of aqueous also be obtained.

---

[a] Retrospective review of 529 consecutive patients with open globe injuries seen at the University Eye Hospital in Freiburg, Germany, between 1981 and 1989.

[b] Even when the trauma or the focus of inflammation is apparently confined to the anterior segment or the lens appears to be intact.

[c] Even a large number of organisms injected into the aqueous of aphakic rabbits may not produce a progressive infection; a small number of organisms injected into the vitreous rapidly progresses to an endophthalmitis.

- Patients with an increased risk for developing post-traumatic endophthalmitis have to be monitored very closely[d] for signs and symptoms of intraocular inflammation

- Patients with suspected infectious endophthalmitis should be taken to the operating room to obtain diagnostic AC *and* vitreous samples for culture.

Diagnostic Techniques

- After a retrobulbar block, the AC aspirate is obtained via a paracentesis in the peripheral cornea using a 25- or 27-gauge needle attached to a tuberculin syringe to aspirate about 0.1 mL of aqueous.
  - The aqueous sample is immediately inoculated onto fresh, prelabeled culture media (see Chapter 28) to be incubated at 37°C (98.6°F) for bacterial isolation.[e]
  - Several drops of the specimen are placed onto slides for Gram and Giemsa staining for direct visualization of bacteria.
  - The AC usually reforms in 3 to 5 minutes.
- There are two ways to obtain the vitreous sample (the specimen is then treated as described previously).
  - If only a vitreous specimen is desired, one small sclerotomy incision 2.5 to 4 mm posterior to the limbus is performed.
  - If a pars plana vitrectomy is also planned, three standard incisions 3.5 to 4 mm posterior to the limbus are prepared. The infusion line is sutured to one of the incisions but not opened.[f]
  - A 22-gauge needle attached to a tuberculin syringe is then introduced through the sclerotomy incision into the midvitreous and 0.2 to 0.3 mL of liquid vitreous is aspirated.[g]

PEARL... If an adequate vitreous sample cannot be obtained with a needle, the pars plana incision is enlarged to introduce a vitreous cutter connected to a 2-mL Luer-Lok syringe instead of the machine consol. Under the operating microscope or the IBO, the vitrectomy probe is placed centrally in the anterior vitreous cavity and 0.25 to 0.5 mL of vitreous at a high cutting rate is aspirated into the syringe.

- If a therapeutic vitrectomy is necessary, it is performed in the standard fashion and the diluted vitreous specimen may be collected in a sterile container.

PITFALL

The fluid specimens collected with automated evacuation systems may be contaminated by bacteria[h] residing in the unsterile vacuum control manifold.[12]

  - The collected vitreous specimen has to be concentrated through a sterile membrane filter (≤ 0.45 μm pore size).[8] Filter transferred to a sterile Petri dish is cut into multiple sections with sterile instruments. Sections of filter paper are plated directly onto solid media and into liquid media for incubation. The surface of a portion of the filter paper can be scraped to prepare slides for staining. It is very important to prevent the vitrectomy specimen from coming in contact with any unsterile surface; for some vitrectomy instruments this requires suction with a sterile syringe rather than using the machine vacuum.
  - If trained personnel and a set of cultures are available in the operating room, direct inoculation of the cultures is preferred.[11,13]

---

[d] If necessary, hourly or every 2 hours in the first 24–48 hours, by a physician or trained nurse.

[e] Sabouraud agar and blood agar are inoculated and maintained at 25°C (room temperature) in cases of more indolent or delayed endophthalmitis in which a fungal cause is considered. Cultures for anaerobe bacteria are immediately sealed in a CO_2 atmosphere (Anaerocult ®P, Merck).[10,11]

[f] The intraocular infusion commonly contains antibiotics, which may interfere with the growth of organisms in the specimen obtained.

[g] Sometimes it is possible to get up to 1.0 mL of undiluted vitreous, but this should be tried only if an infusion line is sutured properly to restitute the IOP and prevent an ECH.

---

[h] *Pseudomonas*-related genera (*Stenotrophomonas maltophilia, Comamonas acidovorans, Chryseomonas* species), *Agrobacterium radiobacter, Flavobacterium* species, and *Micrococcus luteus* were found most frequently.

PEARL... The likelihood of successful culturing in cases of suspected endophthalmitis dramatically increases if the operating room has an "endophthalmitis set"[11]: *Columbia, hematine, modified fuchsine-disulfite-agar ENDO, yeast-cysteine-blood agar* (sealed in an anaerobe atmosphere, see earlier), and fungus media (*Sabouraud-bouillon*).[i] Intraocularly derived samples can thus be cultured in the operation room without delay.

PEARL... Polymerase chain reaction is highly successful in identifying suspected organisms.[14,15] The result is available within a few hours.[j] However, conventional cultures are still necessary for the antibiogram.

[i]The culture media should not be older than 1 week.

[j]A standardized test set for the most common organisms costs approximately US $80[15] (C. P. Lohmann, personal communication, 2000).

PARS PLANA INJECTIONS

Contrary to the anterior segment, the posterior segment cannot easily be reached by antibiotics without invasive measures. The best approach is injection via the pars plana.

- The volume of the injection generally should not exceed 0.1 mL.
  - Before the injection, the IOP may be lowered by a topical beta-blocker[k] and by oculopression.
- When several substances have to be injected, it is advisable to perform a paracentesis and drain some aqueous to further lower the IOP.
- The intraocular injection must be performed under antiseptic conditions.
- After topical anesthesia, the eye is rinsed with povidone-iodine.
- The antibiotic is administered using a tuberculin syringe and a 27-gauge needle.
- Usually a combination of intravitreal, subconjunctival, topical, and systemic antibiotics is given (see Chapter 28 and Appendix A 5; Table A4–1 summarizes the intravitreal dose, indications, and kinetics for different substances).[l]

[k]Administered 1 hour prior to injection.

[l]Note that in most cases, intravitreal application is not explicitly FDA approved.

TABLE A4–I INTRAVITREAL DOSAGES FOR VARIOUS CHEMOTHERAPEUTIC SUBSTANCES*

Generic Name	Intravitreal Dose	Vitreous Half-Time	Main Target
Penicillins			
Ampicillin	5 mg/0.1 mL	6 h	staphylococci, enterococci
Penicillin G	0.2–0.3 mg/0.1 mL	3 h	pneumococci, streptococci
Cephalosporins			
Cefazolin	0.5–2.0 mg/0.1 mL	7 h	streptococci Gr A–C. *Moraxella* sp.
Ceftazidime	2.25 mg/0.1 mL	16 h	*E. coli, Haemophilus influenzae, Moraxella* sp.
Ceftriaxone	2 mg/0.1 mL	12 h	*Haemophilus influenzae* (ampicillin-resistant), gonococci (penicillin-resistant)
Aminoglycosides			
Gentamicin	0.1 mg/0.1 mL	12–35 h	Enterobacteriaceae, *Pseudomonas aeruginosa*
Tobramycin	0.4 mg/0.1 mL	16 h	
Amikacin	0.4 mg/0.1 mL	24 h	
Miscellaneous			
Ciprofloxacin	0.1 mg/0.1 mL	NA	*Pseudomonas aeruginosa*
Clindamycin	1.0 mg/0.1 mL	7–8 h	staphylococci, pneumococci, anerobic sp.
Erythromycin	0.5 mg/0.1 mL	10	
Imipenem	0.5 mg/0.1 mL	NA	Anerobic sp., gonococci, pneumococci, Enterobacteriaceae, *Pseudomonas aeruginosa*
Vancomycin	1 mg/0.1 mL	30 h	Anerobic cocci, staphylococci, *Propionibacterium*
Amphotericin B	0.005–0.010 mg/0.1 mL	NA	*Aspergillus* sp., *Candida* sp.

*Adapted from references 16–18, and 20 (see also Chapter 28 and Appendix 5).

PEARL... The dosage has to be reevaluated in each individual case as retinal toxicity may vary. Initial intravitreal therapy usually consists of *vancomycin* 1.0 mg and *amikacin* 400 μg or *ceftazidime* 2.25 mg. Intravitreal *dexamethasone* 400 μg should also be considered.[17,19]

VITREOUS SUBSTITUTES AND THEIR REMOVAL[m]

Retinal Tamponade

Eyes with PVR require prolonged intraocular tamponade to permit adequate adhesion of the retina to the RPE. The two most commonly used modalities are intraocular gases (e.g., C_3F_8, SF_6) and silicone oil.

- A *gas tamponade has advantages* over silicone oil:
  ○ the duration of the tamponade can be varied depending on the eye's condition (Table A4–2);
  ○ it can be supplemented/removed as an office-based procedure; and
  ○ it dissipates spontaneously, thus obviating the need for additional surgery.

PEARL... Depending on the eye's aqueous production, a nonexpansile concentration (12[21] to 14%[22]) of C_3F_8 can last up to 8 weeks, and a nonexpansile concentration (18[22] to 20%[23]) of SF_6 usually lasts 2 to 3 weeks.

[m]See also Chapter 23.

- The major *disadvantages of gas tamponade* include:
  ○ the need for positioning;
  ○ a delay in visual rehabilitation;
  ○ the absence of a permanent tamponade; and
  ○ the patient's inability to travel by plane[24] until the gas bubble has resorbed.

Silicone oil is used when an internal tamponade longer than 4 weeks is desired, for example, in eyes with an attached retina but with PVR development. In all cases of traumatic retinal detachment or PVR, complete surgical relief of vitreoretinal traction has to be achieved: silicone oil is *not* a substitute for incomplete surgery.

PITFALL

Complete surgical relief of any vitreoretinal traction must first be achieved: silicone oil is not an alternative to, but an additional tool in, proper vitrectomy.

Intraocular Gases

History

Intraocular *air* has been used since 1911.[25] It has helped to increase dramatically the retinal reattachment rate when combined with drainage of the subretinal fluid and diathermy,[26] but it lost popularity when scleral buckling was introduced.[27] In 1969, SF_6 was described as achieving longer tamponades, particularly useful for giant tears.[28] Several *perfluorocarbon* gases were subsequently developed.[29-31]

TABLE A4–2 CLINICAL PROPERTIES OF INTRAOCULAR GASES[21,33]

Property	Air	Perfluoro-methane CF_4	SF_6	Perfluoro-n-ethane C_2F_6	Perfluoro-propane C_3F_8	Perfluoro-butane C_4F_{10}
Time to reach maximum bubble size	Immediate		2–4 days	2–4 days	4–5 days	
Half-life absorption phase			2.4–2.8 days		4.5–6 days	
Ratio of maximum volume to original volume of pure gas	1	2	2	3.25	4	5
Nonexpansile concentration	100%		18–20%	16%	10–16%	
Dwell time "therapeutic volume" of gas for pneumatic retinopexy	1 day	2 days	3–4 days	3	16 days	30 days

Physical Properties and Mode of Action of Intraocular Gases

The most important physical properties of gas use for retinal reattachment are:

- buoyancy[n]; and
- surface tension between the gas bubble and surrounding fluids.

> **PEARL...** The gas bubble is intended to occlude the retinal break[o] to prevent fluid flow from the vitreous through the hole, allowing reabsorption of the subretinal fluid and thus reattachment of the retina.

The solubility of a gas in the aqueous medium is the most important property determining the reabsorption rate of a gas bubble from the vitreous cavity.[32–34] If the gas bubble is less soluble than nitrogen, expansion of the bubble can occur.

> **PEARL...** Expansion can also occur with relatively soluble gases (e.g., air) when the patient under general anesthesia is breathing nitrous oxide, which is more soluble than air in water. To prevent IOP rise in the immediate postoperative period, nitrous oxide insufflation has to be discontinued when a fluid–gas exchange is performed.

The relationship between the bubble's volume and its arc of contact inside the eye is important to know for determining the size of gas bubble required to treat a retinal tear of a specific size and location.

- For a 90° arc of contact, [32,33]
  - 0.28 mL of gas for a 21-mm-diameter eye; and
  - 0.42 mL of gas for a 24-mm-diameter eye is required.
- For a 120° arc of contact,
  - 0.75 mL of gas for a 21-mm-diameter eye; and
  - 1.13 mL of gas for a 24-mm-diameter eye is required.

- For a 180° arc of contact,
  - 2.4 mL of gas for a 21-mm-diameter eye; and
  - 3.62 mL of gas for a 24-mm-diameter eye is required.[p]

Biocompatibility of Intraocular Gases

The gases are at least 99.8% pure; they are chemically nonreactive, colorless, odorless, and nontoxic. They do not cause significant flare or cell at the slit lamp[36] or vitreous inflammation (NEI data).

> **PEARL...** If the bubble is in apposition with the posterior lens capsule, a cataract develops unless the patient is positioned so that a layer of fluid is in between.[37,38] The cataract development is thought to result from drying or deprivation of nutrients rather than from a toxic effect of the gases.

When in contact with the corneal endothelium, gases cause persistent corneal edema and posterior corneal membrane formation.

Kinetics of Intraocular Gases

The kinetics of the less water-soluble gases (e.g., C_3F_8, SF_6) have been extensively studied.[23,29–31,39,40]

- Injection of 100% SF_6 or C_3F_8 leads to expansion of the bubble.
  - The volume continues to increase, reaching a maximum after 2 to 4 days for SF_6 and 4 to 5 days for C_3F_8.
  - Nitrogen is the main constituent responsible for the expansion. About 10% of the gas bubble concentration is carbon dioxide and oxygen, which remain at a fairly constant low concentration throughout the life of the gas bubble. The partial pressure of nitrogen in the bubble equilibrates roughly with the nitrogen's partial pressure in the capillary blood.
- The proportions of various gases in the bubble remain constant as the bubble volume gradually decreases, and all gases leave the eye at the same rate.
  - Because the long-acting gas is the slowest to leave the eye, it essentially controls the rate of clearance of the bubble volume until its final stage.
  - The half-life has been reported to be 2.4–2.8 days for SF_6 and 4.5–6 days for C_3F_8.

---

[n] Buoyancy is the result of the large difference in specific gravity between fluid and gas. A traction-free, superior tear tamponaded with a large air bubble will usually displace the fluid inferiorly/away from the tear, allowing the retina to flatten. Large bubbles and facedown positioning are required to tamponade inferior retinal breaks.

[o] At least most of the time.

[p] A later CT study found these gas volumes: 1.5 mL for an arc of 90° and 3 mL for 180°.

> **PEARL...** The gas is removed more rapidly when the eye is aphakic or pseudophakic. Conversely, the bubble lasts much longer in the presence of severe hypotony.[q] Clinically, these factors and the concentration/size of the injected gas bubble determine its clearance from the vitrectomized eye.[41]

- Excessive volumes of pure *expansile* gases can lead to a bubble size larger than the ocular volume; extremely high IOP resulting in central retinal artery occlusion and NLP vision follow.
  - The surgeon should keep the maximum size of the gas bubble slightly less than the vitreous volume to prevent cataract formation in phakic patients and corneal opacification in aphakic patients. The ratios of the maximum volume of the expanded gas bubble to the original volume of injected gas are shown in Table A4–2.
- Another option is to inject *nonexpansile* or slightly expansile concentrations of the gas, especially during a vitrectomy with a fluid–gas exchange.
  - Use of a nonexpansile 20% concentration of SF_6 (12% of C_3F_8) or, when attempting a total or near-total fluid–gas exchange at the conclusion of vitrectomy, is sufficient for a two-thirds tamponade for 1 week.[22] C_3F_8 concentrations of 10–16% are frequently used for large posterior segment tamponades.

Silicone Oil

History

Available since 1945, silicone oil was originally used for breast augmentation.

- It was first used, *without* vitrectomy, for retinal reattachment in 1962.[42,43]
- The permanent tamponade potential of silicone oil was utilized when applied as an *adjunct* to vitrectomy surgery.[44–46]
- The introduction of the 6 o'clock peripheral iridectomy[47] substantially reduced the incidence of silicone keratopathy and pupillary block glaucoma in aphakic patients.

---

[q] The *theoretical factors* determining how fast gas disappears are the molecular weight of the gas, the diffusion coefficient of the tissues, water solubility of the gas, IOP, the inflow rate of ciliary body secretion, phakic or aphakic status, hypotony, vitrectomy, stirring of vitreous fluid by ocular motion, outflow of aqueous through trabecular meshwork, posterior choroidal venous concentration of gases, and the vascular perfusion rate of the choroid.

- A multicenter, randomized study[48] in 1992 showed that silicone oil was superior to SF_6 and equal to C_3F_8 in repairing PVR detachments in conjunction with vitrectomy (see Chapter 23).

Physical and Chemical Properties, and Mode of Action of Silicone Oil

- Silicone oil is a polysiloxane polymer with a refractive index of 1.405 and a specific gravity of 0.96 to 0.98 g/cm^2: it is lighter than water and floats.
- Its buoyancy force and surface tension are less than those of gas.
- The viscosity of various silicone oils is dependent on their molecular weight, which is directly related to the length of the polymers constituting the oil.
- The commonly used oils today have viscosity coefficients between 1000 and 5000 centistokes.

The *advantages* of silicone oil tamponade include:

- a potentially permanent tamponade of constant size;
- a refractive index that permits optical correction, speeding visual rehabilitation;
- less stringent positioning requirements; and
- the ability of patients to travel by plane.

The *disadvantages* of oil are:

- the need for surgical removal; and
- a lower surface tension than gas.

Concepts for Surgical Use

It helps the surgeon to follow a certain protocol when introducing silicone oil.

- First flattening the retina with air, which has a much higher surface tension than silicone oil, makes it easier to recognize residual traction.

> **PEARL...** If the retina cannot be flattened by an air–fluid exchange because of residual traction, the surgeon cannot rely on silicone oil to achieve this because silicone oil's surface tension against the retina and choroid is less than that of air.

- At the defect, a small hemispheric bubble is formed on the subretinal side.[49] The maximum pressure difference that the surface of the bubble can sustain is reached when the radius of curvature of the bubble is equal to the radius of the break. Any further increase in pressure will force the silicone oil under the retina.

> **PEARL...** As a surgical rule, silicone oil will rarely become subretinal if the retina is closer to the choroid than the diameter of a 20-gauge cannula.[r]

Emulsification

The problem of silicone oil's decreasing surface tension over time is emulsification.[50]

> **PEARL...** Spontaneous emulsification, even without physical motion, occurs when the surface tension of the silicone oil approaches zero.

- Surfactants and ocular motion can lead to emulsification, especially as the surface tension decreases.
- Viscosity is also important: lower viscosity silicone oils emulsify more rapidly than higher viscosity silicone oils of the same purity.[51]
  - With a 20-centistoke viscosity, emulsification will occur within a few weeks/months.
  - If 1000-centistoke silicone oil is used, even if it is highly purified, tiny oil droplets (precursors of gross emulsification) are present in 100% of cases at 1 year.
  - With 12,500-centistoke silicone oil, no emulsification was found during a follow-up of 3 months to 2 years.

> **PEARL...** As soon as emulsification occurs, silicone oil should be either removed or replaced immediately; if the initial complications are not too severe, a slight delay is acceptable.

- Ocular fluid motion with instability at the interface leads to formation and separation of tiny droplets. Droplet formation decreases with increasing viscosity because increasing viscosity dampens unstable motion at the interface.
- Emulsification probably also depends on the relative purity of silicone oils.

Optics

The index of refraction of silicone oil varies between 1.400 and 1.405; this is slightly higher than that of aqueous or vitreous,[s] which causes refractive changes:

- in *phakic* eyes (Fig. A4–1A), a negative curvature between the posterior lens surface and silicone oil is formed, making
  - emmetropic eyes become hypermetropic by +6 to +7 diopters[45]; and
  - myopic eyes improve;
- in *aphakic* eyes (Fig. A4-1B),[t] the silicone oil meniscus has a positive curvature over the pupillary aperture and induces a hyperopia, which may make the eye nearly emmetropic. Because the silicone oil–aqueous interface is liquid, the curvature of this refractive surface is subject to change with posture[u];
- in *pseudophakic* eyes (Fig. A4-1C), the meniscus type of IOL is the preferred choice in the presence of silicone oil, as this minimizes the change in refractive power upon silicone oil removal.[54]

ERG

Silicone oil is a poor conductor of electrical current and has a high volume resistance.

> **PEARL...** Due to the increased resistance of silicone, ERG amplitudes are reduced in the presence of silicone oil but are normalized when the silicone oil is removed.

Ultrasound Image

The velocity of ultrasound in silicone oil at frequencies of 7 to 10 MHz is approximately 976 m/s.[55]

- It takes approximately 1.5 times longer for an ultrasound pulse to return through a vitreous cavity filled with silicone oil than in aqueous or vitreous: images thus appear farther away in silicone oil-filled eyes.

---

[r]Intraocular proteins and phospholipids act as surface-active agents and reduce the surface tension, enabling emulsification. The surface tension may become so low that the silicone oil can easily slip through a retinal break.

[s]1.33.

[t]Traumatized eyes requiring silicone oil often have lens damage as well[52]; 60% of the eyes are aphakic at the time of silicone oil filling and 100% become aphakic/pseudophakic eventually.[53]

[u]Patients who have good macular function often have significant improvement in visual acuity after silicone oil removal.

phakic eye + silicone oil: hyperopia

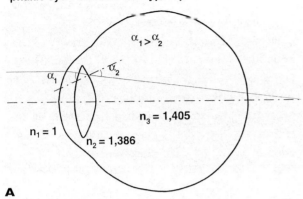

A

aphakic eye + silicone oil: hyperopia of variable extent

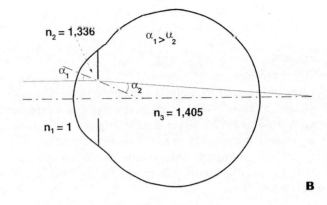

B

pseudophakic eye + silicone oil: emmetropia with meniscus type intraocular lens

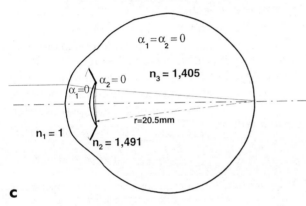

C

FIGURE A4–1 Refractive changes due to silicone oil in phakic, aphakic, and pseudophakic eyes (see the text for details).

- If the eye is partially filled with silicone oil, the silicone oil–water interface is highly reflective and is easily visualized on both the A and B scans.
- The lens transmits sounds faster in both aqueous fluids and silicone oil. However, the lens is more ultrasonically defocusing in silicone oil-filled eyes than in aqueous-filled eyes.
- The smoothness of the silicone oil–retina interface causes less scattering of the ultrasound pulse. Because the ultrasound pulse is reflected away from the transducer, loss of signal from the peripheral retina results.

PEARL... Silicone oil leads to an extremely distorted B-scan image, which requires caution in interpretation. Similarly, the A-scan time intervals in distance measurements require adjustment for adequate interpretation.

PFCLs

- PFCLs have specific gravities that are almost twice the density of water, permitting them to generate a tamponade force approaching that of gas.
- They have refractive indices close to saline, high interfacial tensions with water, and low viscosities (2 to 3 centistokes at 25°C).

PEARL... PFCLs are excellent for tamponading the retina in a supine position and forcing subretinal fluid/blood anteriorly through peripheral retinal breaks.

- Fluorochemicals are immiscible with silicone oil[v] and blood, enhancing visibility during exchanges.[56]

---

[v]Exception: perfluorohexyloctane C_6F_{13}-C_8H_{17} (F_6H_8).[64]

- Their potential for toxicity[57–59] is considered by most surgeons as prohibitive to their use as extended intraocular tamponades; they are generally removed at the end of the procedure.

History

Possible biologic applications of PFCL for oxygen-carrying ability and as a blood substitute were demonstrated in 1966.[60] They were first used as a vitreous substitute in 1982.[61] Beyond their original indication as a solely intraoperative tool,[56] more viscous liquids as short-term vitreous tamponade and lower specific weight liquids for longer tamponades have been developed.[62,63]

Physical and Chemical Properties, and Mode of Action of PFCL as a Vitreous Substitute

PFCLs have a surface tension against water comparable to that of silicone oil.

PEARL... The intraoperative uses of PFCLs depend on their higher specific gravity (see Table A4–3) because it enables the fluid to settle posteriorly, opening folds in the retina while expressing subretinal fluid anteriorly through preexisting retinal breaks.

PEARL... The tamponade pressure of PFCL on the inferior retina can be calculated by subtracting the specific gravity of the aqueous liquid from that of the PFCL and multiplying by the height of the overlying PFCL column. For equal-sized bubbles, the tamponade pressure in the downward direction of the PFCL is thus 12 to 14 times greater than that of silicone oil in the upward direction.

- The viscosity of the PFCL ranges from 0.8 to 8.0 mPas. The low viscosity allows the PFCL to be injected and removed easily from the eye with low-pressure gradients.
- The refractive index of PFCLs varies (1.42 for perfluorohexylhexane; 1.33 for perfluorophenanthrene; 1.27 for perfluoro-n-octane). The refractive index difference between perfluoro-n-octane/perfluorohexylhexane and aqueous is significant enough to allow easy visualization of a water-perfluorocarbon interface.[w]

---

[w] The refractive index for perfluorophenanthrene is the same as that of water: the interface is difficult to visualize.

TABLE A4–3   PROPERTIES OF SOME PFCLs

Property	Perfluoro-n-octane C_8F_{18}	Perfluoro-phenanthrene $C_{14}F_{24}$	Perfluoro-decaline $C_{10}F_{18}$	Perfluoro-hexyl-octane C_6F_{13}-C_8-H_{17} (F_6H_8)	Perfluoro-hexyl-hexane C_6F_{13}-C_6-H_{13} (F_6H_6)
Surface tension against air (mN/m)	14	16	19	21	20
Specific gravity	1.76	2.03	1.93	1.35	1.42
Vapor pressure (mm Hg at 37°C)	56	1	12.5		
Viscosity (mPas at 37°C)	0.8	8	2.9	3.2	1.85
Refractive index (refractive index of aqueous = 1.33)	1.27	1.33	1.31	1.34	1.42
Velocity of sound (m/s)	557				

- The velocity of sound for perfluoro-*n*-octane is 557 m/s, causing distortion and irregularities in the ultrasound image.
- Perfluorodecalin and perfluorophenanthrene have been shown to have high transparency to light in the visible spectrum. They present no obstacle to laser photocoagulation in the visible and infrared spectrum.

PEARL... The initial laser power settings should be kept low because the transmission of the PFCL is superior to that of Ringer's solution, which is a model for the aqueous- or vitreous-filled eye.[65]

Biocompatibility of PFCLs as Vitreous Substitutes

PFCLs are manufactured by fluorination of hydrocarbons. Hydrofluoric acid, perfluoroisobutylene, and similarly toxic hydrogen-containing compounds must be completely removed before the PFCL is used in the eye. PFCLs containing only fluorine and carbon atoms are the most biologically inert in the eye. Purified perfluoro-*n*-octane has essentially no contaminating hydrogen-containing perfluorocarbons.[66]

- The histologic effects of short-term use of intravitreal PFCL are relatively minor, but if left in the eye for a few weeks/months, relatively severe changes can occur:
  - cataract formation;
  - PFCL dispersion;
  - PFCL emulsification; and, if less purified products are retained for a longer time,
  - retinal detachment.

PITFALL

Within 2 months, macrophages ingest the smaller bubbles of both impure and pure grades of PFCLs. Dispersion is noted to some degree after 2 weeks of tamponade; after 3 to 4 months, the fundus is difficult to visualize. In addition, droplet division and fish-egging form around the surface of the main globule of the PFCL and in the AC within 6 weeks.[62]

CLINICAL USE OF VITREOUS SUBSTITUTES

Exchanges between Fluid, Gas, Silicone Oil, PFCL

- If PFCLs were used to reattach the retina and all retinal breaks have been treated with laser photocoagulation, the PFCL should be exchanged for BSS using a soft-tipped flute needle. PFCL should not be exchanged for air because visualization will be poor.
- Before a fluid–gas exchange, mark all retinal breaks with transvitreal diathermy to facilitate their visualization when the retina is flat.
- A fluid–gas exchange is performed using a soft silicone-tipped flute needle. Preexisting posterior breaks permit drainage of the subretinal fluid. If a retinal break is not already present or is very anterior and PFCL is unavailable, a posterior retinotomy is usually required.
  - The most advisable site for posterior retinotomy, if the specific conditions do not dictate otherwise, is the superonasal quadrant, not very far from the disk. Most surgeons use diathermy only, but the vitrectomy probe may also be used.
- If silicone oil is to be injected, the technique is the surgeon's preference. However, it is easier to perform a "double exchange," that is, first a fluid–gas exchange and then a gas–silicone oil exchange.[x]
- In aphakic patients or in pseudophakic patients with a defective iris/IOL diaphragm, an inferior peripheral iridectomy should be performed (see earlier).
- All exchanges are greatly facilitated when an automated air injector (GFLI; see Chapter 25) or a silicone oil pump is used.
- When the subretinal fluid is drained and air is injected, the surgeon needs to look for residual retinal traction[y] and monitor the IOP.
  - If there is persistent traction, it may result in enlargement of preexisting breaks, the creation of new breaks, and/or subretinal dislocation of silicone oil, PFCL, or even air.
  - If the traction cannot be resolved otherwise, a retinotomy/retinectomy must be performed.
- If retinopexy has not been performed earlier, this is the next step, using endolaser, indirect laser, transscleral laser, endocryopexy, or exocryopexy.

---

[x] The fluid-gas interface is easier to visualize than the fluid–silicone oil interface.

[y] This emphasizes the need for a wide-angle viewing system; see Chapter 8.

> **PEARL...** The most desirable method of retinopexy is laser; in addition to treatment around retinal breaks, a "new ora serrata" may be created with the indirect laser by performing treatment of 360 degrees, using moderately strong burns and applying less heavy treatment in the horizontal meridians.

Intraocular Gases

- Facedown positioning should be maintained for 8 to 11 days for firm adhesion between the neurosensory retina and the RPE to form after laser or cryopexy (see Chapter 24).
  - This is also important to prevent gas block glaucoma and to minimize the risk of peripheral anterior synechia formation. If patient compliance is good, cellular deposits can be seen on the lower corneal endothelium at the slit lamp "positional keratopathy."[z]
- Even if a nonexpansile or only slightly expansile gas concentration is used, it is important to monitor the IOP postoperatively.

> **PEARL...** Although applanation tonometry (e.g., Goldmann, electronic pen-like devices) is the most accurate method to detect IOP elevation, visual acuity monitoring for the loss of light perception by a nurse or the patient is also necessary as this may be the earliest sign of excessively high pressure. Large displacement tonometry (e.g., Schiøtz) gives falsely low values.

- Although intraocular gas bubbles result in better internal tamponade than silicone oil, the gas bubble is constantly decreasing in size. The gas bubble, however, can easily be supplemented in an outpatient fluid–gas exchange procedure if the bubble is too small or disappearing too rapidly.

> **PEARL...** If recurrent detachment from a new or previously undetected retinal break occurs in an eye that underwent vitrectomy (and scleral buckling), pars plana gas injection and indirect/slit-lamp laser photocoagulation[aa] can be performed. Laser is preferred because it is less prone to lead to PVR; in addition, cryopexy may be difficult because of an overlying buckle. If recurrent PVR is suspected, longer acting gases are preferred.

Complications of Intraocular Gases

Some of these are due to errors on the surgeon's part; others are caused by the patient's lack of or, paradoxically, excessive, positioning.

- Corneal decompensation, including positional keratopathy.
- Cataract formation resulting from the drying effect of the gas bubble.
- Glaucoma from overfilling of the eye with expansile gas; the consequent central retinal artery occlusion may lead to permanent blindness.[67]
- Peripheral anterior synechiae with total angle closure.
- Sharp IOP rise if the patient remains supine.[bb]
- Reduction in atmospheric pressure (e.g., air travel, driving rapidly up a steep mountain) can lead to painful IOP rise and loss of vision.
- IOLs may occasionally flatten against the cornea after fluid–gas exchange; this is less likely with rigid, angle-supported AC and PC IOLs.

> **PEARL...** Indirect and slit-lamp laser treatment can cause undesirable burns from reflections of internal fluid–air and air–fluid surfaces. To reduce this risk, the surgeon should avoid such treatment whenever possible.[68] When treatment through such an interface is unavoidable, it should be done as perpendicular to the interface as possible because the intensity of a reflected beam increases as the angle of incidence decreases. This can best be achieved using a wide-angle contact lens and a divergent beam. The location and intensity of internally reflected beams should be evaluated with the aiming beam *before* photocoagulating. Changes in beam intensity caused by reflectance and relative magnification encountered when switching from treating through a gas bubble to treating around it can lead to overintense burns and result in retinal and choroidal hemorrhages.

Gas for intraocular injection is aspirated through a 0.22-μm filter for sterilization. It is then injected through a second filter into the eye. Some surgeons use double filters to minimize the risk of contamination.

---

[z] A term coined by R. Morris, MD.

[aa] A modified pneumatic retinopexy procedure.

[bb] Aqueous continues to fill the posterior segment while the air bubble causes a pupillary block or prevents outflow through the trabecular meshwork.

Silicone Oil

Indications

- Severe PVR;
- vitreous and/or choroidal hemorrhage;
- traumatic retinal detachment failing previous vitreous surgery;
- large retinectomy;
- severe ciliary body destruction (see Chapters 8 and 19)[cc]; and
- severe injury to/disorganization of ocular tissues, especially if primary vitrectomy is performed.[70]

Removal

Silicone oil is essentially an IOFB (see Chapter 24); it is not reabsorbed by the eye, and the surgeon should, in general, intend to remove it.

> **PITFALL**
>
> Even in carefully selected cases, retinal redetachment occurs immediately or shortly after silicone oil removal in 3 to 33% of eyes.[71]

The silicone oil is removed to avoid the following complications associated with prolonged retention.

- Glaucoma due to emulsification
  - if the emulsified oil is removed in time, the glaucoma is manageable with medical therapy in only 70% of the eyes[72,73];
- band keratopathy due to silicone oil/cornea contact; and
- anisometropia, which often cannot be corrected by glasses/contact lens.

Silicone oil is temporarily or permanently *retained* in up to 40% of eyes because of the fear of redetachment.[74] Such cases include:

- peripheral tractional detachment or rhegmatogenous detachment if immediate redetachment upon silicone oil removal is feared[dd];
- having undergone several operations, the patient is reluctant to risk further surgery;
- phthisis is expected if the silicone oil is removed;
- patients who decline silicone oil removal until complications occur.

> **PEARL...** In cases of a hopelessly detached and atrophic retina with no further surgery warranted to restore vision, removal of the silicone oil may lead to immediate phthisis and severe cosmetic complications: retaining the oil may be the lesser of two evils (see Chapter 8).

> **PEARL...** When deciding whether to remove the silicone oil, the surgeon should carefully balance the period (under oil) with reduced visual acuity versus the threat of retinal redetachment. If the retina stays attached for approximately 2 months after silicone oil removal, it will probably remain attached.

Surgical Technique

- For less viscous (1000 centistokes) silicone oil:
  - insert through the pars plana an infusion cannula connected to BSS;
  - make an incision in the limbus in aphakic or through the pars plana[ee] in phakic eyes;
  - allow passive egress of the silicone oil while infusing BSS.
- For highly viscous (5000 centistokes) silicone oil:
  - introduce through a pars plana incision[ff] a 20-gauge needle, a rigid cannula, or a venous catheter, which is connected to a ≥ 10 mL syringe (Fig. A4-2) for aspiration;
  - introduce through a second pars plana incision a cannula connected to an infusion line.

> **PEARL...** Viscous silicone oil is preferably aspirated actively, using an automated suction unit. The syringe may be connected with a stopper for viscous fluid aspiration with tube connection to the vitrectomy suction unit.[gg] On the side of the syringe, a hole is prepared so that the syringe can be handled like a flute needle when active suction by the vitrectomy controlling system is applied.

[cc] An artificial iris diaphragm[69] may also become necessary (see Chapter 19).

[dd] The surgeon should offer these patients additional surgery or surgeries under silicone oil and silicone oil removal at a later date rather than leave an unstable anatomic situation.

[ee] This should be slightly larger than the standard incision would be; make sure that the choroid is adequately opened (e.g., using Vannas scissors).

[ff] Alternatively, active aspiration is used.

[gg] Geuder GmbH, Heidelberg, Germany.

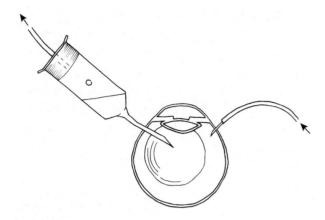

FIGURE A4-2   Silicone oil removal (see the text for details).

- As small silicone oil bubbles are always trapped in the peripheral retina or behind the iris, it is advisable to do an air–fluid exchange after completion of the silicone oil–fluid exchange. This pushes posteriorly the small anterior silicone oil bubbles, which can then be aspirated from the fluid surface or irrigated out of the eye. The exchanges should be repeated twice for a higher success rate.[hh]
- If the retina redetaches after silicone oil removal, repeat surgery is necessary.[75]

Complications

Complications, such as cataract, glaucoma, keratopathy, commonly occur. Retinopathy rarely develops even in long-standing cases.

CONTROVERSY

⬅➡

Although recurrent retinal detachment is the most frequent cause of failure in vitrectomy with silicone oil, it is still debated whether proliferation leading to redetachment is directly attributable to silicone oil.

Elevated IOP   Transient[ii] IOP increases (≥ 30 mm Hg) are common:

- in eyes with extensive surgical manipulations for severe PVR, especially in conjunction with lensectomy, scleral buckle, and judicious endolaser application;

- in aphakic eyes if the inferior iridectomy closes due to lens remnants or fibrosis because of inflammation;
  - Nd:YAG laser treatment opens the iridectomy usually only temporarily, requiring surgical intervention;
- as the result of inflammatory trabeculitis or external/internal obstruction of aqueous outflow by a scleral buckle or inflammatory debris (e.g., fibrin and cells, see Chapter 20);
- after extensive laser use, which may cause choroidal swelling, resulting in angle closure due to anterior rotation of the ciliary body[76];
- in the presence of even minimal emulsification,[jj] histopathologic examination has shown macrophages filled with silicone oil blocking the trabecular meshwork channels; and
- in aphakic patients who tend to sleep on their backs: the oil floats upward, pushing the peripheral iris against the trabecular meshwork and anterior synechiae form, slowly "zipping up" the entire angle.

> **PEARL...**   Emulsified silicone oil should be removed. If necessary, fresh high-purity silicone oil may be reinjected.

> **PEARL...**   If peripheral anterior synechiae cause the IOP elevation and the condition is detected early, facedown positioning may help. In severe cases, a filtering procedure with silicone oil removal or a (Molteno) valve procedure may be required.

Fibrin   Fibrin formation in the early postoperative period can act as a scaffold for future proliferations and may cause pupillary block glaucoma. The pupillary block can be managed by:

- laser "fibrinotomy" (argon or Nd:YAG);
- surgical removal; or
- TPA: intraocular injection of 6–25 μg results in clot dissolution within an hour.[78–80]

Severe posterior fibrin can also be managed with intraocular administration of TPA, but repeat injections may be required to prevent the reformation of fibrin.

Intraocular Hemorrhage   Intraocular hemorrhage in the immediate postoperative period is reported to occur most frequently in eyes that have had extensive

---

[hh] C. Eckardt, personal communication, 1998.

[ii] Persistent IOP elevation occurred in <1% of eyes in the Silicone Oil Study.[48,77]

[jj] Microdroplets in the AC or small creamy areas of emulsification seen in the superior equatorial retina.

relaxing retinotomies.[82,83] Occasionally, bleeding may occur during the closure of the sclerotomies. In gas-filled eyes, the blood frequently moves into the AC with patient positioning.

The blood, if not extensive, will be removed through the trabecular meshwork. If the hemorrhage fails to clear or hypotony is present,[kk] a fluid–gas exchange should be considered.

PITFALL

Hemorrhage occurring in an eye filled with silicone oil is an ominous sign. Frequently the bleeding originates at the edge of the retinotomy (mostly inferiorly[83]) and is confined there by the oil. Blood layered against the retina appears to stimulate reproliferation and is associated with recurrent retinal detachment.[83] If significant periretinal hemorrhage is noted, repeat surgery and removal of the blood should be considered.

Hypotony Hypotony occurred in 10 to 20% of eyes in the Silicone Oil Study,[48,77] due to:

- reduced aqueous production because of diminished blood supply to the ciliary processes secondary to
  - compression; or
  - destruction of the long ciliary vessels by a very large buckle or extensive retinopexy;
- traction on the ciliary body by anterior proliferation; or
- a large retinotomy.[82]

Unfortunately, no effective treatment has been identified, although early surgical removal of anterior proliferations has occasionally been successful (see Chapter 19).[84]

Cataract Because of a reduced supply of nutrients, cataract is an inevitable consequence of silicone oil being for an extended time in contact with the posterior lens capsule.[85]

PITFALL

Even if the silicone oil is removed early, the cataract will often continue to progress.

- If both the cataract and the silicone oil are removed, ECCE or phacoemulsification may be performed.[ll] See Chapter 21 for IOL implantation details.

PEARL... When cataract extraction is performed in an eye with (previous) silicone oil fill, it is advisable also to remove the central part of the posterior capsule in the same procedure, as the posterior capsule tends to form a dense and very strong opaque membrane, which is rather resistant to **YAG** laser capsulotomy.

- If the oil is retained, phacoemulsification, ECCE, or ICCE[mm] can be performed.[86]
- IOL is typically not implanted in an eye which has silicone oil.

Keratopathy Keratopathy (in the form of epithelial or stromal edema, band, or bullous keratopathy)[87] occurs in up to 45% of aphakic eyes filled with silicone oil after vitreous surgery for severe PVR; the frequency of keratopathy is related to the duration of internal tamponade[53] and is higher in eyes without retinal reattachment.[46,77]

- Bullous keratopathy[nn] is the manifestation of massive damage to, and loss of, corneal endothelial cells.

PEARL... Dehydration of the cornea by the waterproof silicone oil can maintain corneal clarity even in the absence of the corneal endothelium. However, when the silicone oil is removed, the cornea immediately opacifies as a result of stromal swelling (see **Chapter 8**).

- Band keratopathy is caused by long-term contact between silicone oil and the corneal endothelium,[53] probably as a consequence of inhibition of nutrient diffusion from the AC.
  - Early band keratopathy can be managed by removing the silicone oil; in advanced stages, the crystal deposits can be dissolved from Bowman´s layer with EDTA after epithelial abrasion.[53]

[kk] Indicating poor aqueous production and turnover.

[ll] We prefer ECCE because of the difficulties during phacoemulsification.

[mm] A 6 o'clock peripheral iridectomy should be performed if ICCE is the option chosen.

[nn] It can also occur after cataract surgery and after vitrectomy (2.8%[88]) without silicone oil use.

PITFALL

It must also be mentioned that emulsified or even intact silicone oil may appear in the AC in phakic eyes without visible damage to the zonules. Fortunately, this rarely leads to corneal complications, although the management is difficult: simple oil removal usually results in further oil prolapse; air is insufficient to hold the oil back; and viscoelastics may lead to IOP elevation postoperatively.

Recurrent Retinal Detachment Despite successful initial retinal reattachment in PVR, recurrent retinal detachment is common.[48,77]

PITFALL

The primary cause of retinal redetachment is a continuation of the proliferative process; with maturation and contraction of the new membranes, previously treated retinal breaks may reopen; new retinal breaks may occur; or the traction shortens/redetaches the retina. Unfortunately, the silicone oil bubble itself forces the proliferative factors to be concentrated near the retinal surface.

- If the macula remains reattached and the fibrous tissue stops contracting, no action is required.
- If removal of silicone oil is required or if the macula becomes detached, reoperation to remove the fibrous tissue is required.

Pharmacological inhibition of the proliferation is heavily investigated; in a randomized study, daunomycin has shown a significant reduction in the number of reoperations.[89,90]

PFCL

Technique

After complete peripheral vitrectomy and at least initial removal of posterior retinal membranes:

- the PFCL is slowly injected over the optic nerve head using a double-barrel cannula with a 24-gauge needle for injection and a 25-gauge needle for fluid drainage;

- the IOP must be monitored to avoid arterial pulsation/occlusion;
- keep the tip of the injection cannula within the initial PFCL bubble to prevent fish-egg formation.

PEARL... Do not inject PFCL if a large (posterior) retinal break is present and traction is not yet relieved: the PFCL will rapidly become subretinal.[91]

- Inject the PFCL up to the level of the most posterior break. If not all of the posterior subretinal fluid or blood is displaced anteriorly at this time, look for and remove all residual posterior membranes and traction.
- If no traction remains, more PFCL can be injected and the residual subretinal fluid be drained through the anterior break.

PEARL... Even complete PFCL fill (i.e., anteriorly to the most anterior break) can be performed if all retinal traction has been eliminated; this allows adequate peripheral laser coagulation. Evaporation of the PFCL is considerable; therefore the scleral incisions must be plugged if an IBO laser is used.

- Fluid–air exchange[92] can be performed by slowly aspirating the PFCL with a flute needle.
  - For the thin layer of PFCL remaining on the retina, inject 0.5 to 1 mL of BSS: the PFCL will develop small droplets and can be identified/removed easily.
- It is also possible to extract the PFCL with a flute needle first and perform a fluid-gas exchange subsequently, to ensure complete removal under better visualization.
- If silicone oil is used, the PFCL can be exchanged directly.

Indications

PFCL may be necessary in a large number of conditions:

- retinal detachment associated with giant tears;
- (traumatic) retinal detachment with complicated PVR; and to a lesser extent
- dislocated lens,[93] especially in the presence of retinal detachment;

- dislocated IOL;
- hemorrhagic detachment;
- retinal incarceration;
- extrusion of subretinal hemorrhage; and
- intraoperative hemorrhage.

Removal of Dislocated Lenses

Complete vitrectomy is performed (i.e., including removal of the peripheral vitreous). PFCL is then injected over the optic nerve head to float the dislocated lens off the retina and into the anterior vitreous cavity (see Chapter 21 for the use of viscoelastics). The lens can now be fragmented manually or with a phacofragmentor,[oo] or be extracted through a limbal incision (see Chapter 21).

Retinal Incarceration

As the PFCL fills the vitreous cavity,[95] the detached retina is flattened and stabilized, making the retinectomy and subsequent endophotocoagulation easier (see Chapter 16).

Expressing Subretinal Fluid

Submacular hemorrhage can be expressed through a posterior retinotomy:

- inject TPA through a small cannula into the subretinal space[96];
- wait 15 minutes;
- express the hemorrhage through a small posterior retinotomy using PFCL on the overlying retina.

Repeat the procedure as needed. Most surgeons do not perform laser retinopexy around the retinotomy site but use postoperative gas tamponade.

"Sandwich" Technique: PFCL and Silicone Oil

PFCL in combination with silicone oil in a sandwich technique has been used to control peripheral retinal bleeding.[97] The PFCL prevents blood from entering the subretinal space and restricts blood flow posteriorly; the silicone oil restricts blood flow anteriorly and provides a clear view for clot extraction and endodiathermy.

CONTROVERSY

The sandwich technique has also been proposed for prolonged internal tamponade to reduce the intraocular space available for PVR development.[98–100] Perfluorodecalin, because of its weight, may be less well tolerated than lighter PFCLs (see Table A4–3).

Complications

Because PFCL is used mostly as an intraoperative tool, the complications are fairly minor and related to:

- retained subretinal/intravitreal PFCL droplets;
- dispersion; or
- fish-egg formation.

PITFALL

In addition to interfering with visualization, there are reports on retinal degeneration, emulsification with foam cell formation, and macrophage ingestion of the PFCLs. Small droplets of retained subretinal perfluoro-*n*-octane and perfluorodecalin are slowly reabsorbed and leave a small localized retinal scotoma.

PEARL...   It appears that attempts to remove small droplets of subretinal PFCL (as long as they are not directly beneath the central macula) involve more risk than benefit.

PRIMARY VITRECTOMY IN SEVERELY TRAUMATIZED EYES

Consider primary[pp] vitrectomy[101–103] in the following cases:

- significant intraocular bleeding;
- large and posterior scleral wound if it can be closed first;
- perforating injury if the exit wound is small and self-sealing;
- major intraocular pathology;
- retinal incarceration;
- high risk for endophthalmitis, especially in the presence of certain types of IOFB (see Chapters 24 and 28); *and*
- a surgeon who is experienced in *all* techniques of vitreoretinal surgery.

Surgical Technique

- Close the traumatic wound(s).

[oo] The PFCL provides protection for the retina.[94]

[pp] Immediate or within 48 hours.

- Prepare the sclerotomies.[qq]

PITFALL

Do not open the infusion line before identifying the correct intravitreal position of the cannula (see Chapter 25).

- Perform a cautious anterior vitrectomy.
- The crystalline lens/IOL can rarely be saved (or may have been lost; see Chapter 21).
- If you try to preserve the lens, irrigate the AC as needed (see Chapter 17).
- Usually there is a posterior blood reserve, and a viscous tamponade is necessary to ensure visualization of the posterior segment.
- Carefully proceed with vitrectomy; use a combination of endo- and coaxial illumination as needed.

PEARL... Occasionally, oblique illumination from the fiberoptic through the peripheral cornea is superior to visualize structures in the anterior vitreous.

- If no retinal break with traction or retinal detachment is expected posteriorly and there is still bleeding, PFCL may be injected, even if a posterior vitreous detachment has not yet been achieved.[rr]
- Complete the vitrectomy, including detachment and removal of the posterior hyaloid face.
- Fill the eye with PFCL at least up to the equator and perform a laser cerclage.
- Many surgeons prefer an encircling band in addition.
- Finally, the PFCL is exchanged to silicone oil.

As an adjunct or, less preferably, as an alternative, the endoscope can also be used (see Appendix 2).

[qq] Unconventional regions of the anterior sclera may have to be selected.

[rr] The PFCL may even be helpful in detaching the posterior vitreous if a small area of posterior hyaloid separations exists and the PFCL can be injected through this hole.

RETINOPEXY

For creating chorioretinal adhesions, various options are available.

- Predominantly, laser (argon, diode) and cryopexy are used
- Laser and cryopexy can be delivered transvitreally or transsclerally; lasers may be used through the IBO.
- Lasers are preferred to cryopexy (see Chapters 8 and 24) because of cryopexy's risk of exacerbating PVR.[104–107]
- Diathermy and cyanoacrylate tissue adhesive are also available but are used only infrequently in vitreoretinal surgery for trauma.
- Retinopexy is typically used only after the retina has been reattached by gas, silicone oil, or PFCL.

PEARL... Occasionally, retinopexy can used in the presence of shallow retinal detachment; if within a few hours retinal reattachment is achieved, the chorioretinal scar will be just as effective.

SUMMARY

PVR remains the most common cause of failure in traumatized eyes with posterior segment involvement. PVR is the result of a complex series of events resulting in the abnormal proliferation of cells on available intraocular surfaces with membrane formation, cellular contraction, and retinal detachment.[108] Since the development of vitreous surgery almost 30 years ago, dramatic improvements have been made in surgical instrumentation and technique, permitting successful rehabilitation of previously unsalvageable eyes. Despite these advances, failure is still too common, the need for reoperation too high, and the visual results too frequently disappointing. The current focus of PVR management is primarily mechanical; future success depends on a clearer understanding of the underlying pathogenic mechanisms and perhaps on pharmacological prevention.[91,108]

REFERENCES

1. Barr CC. Prognostic factors in corneoscleral lacerations. *Arch Ophthalmol.* 1983;101:919–924.

2. Forster RK. Endophthalmitis. In: Duane TD, ed. *Clinical Ophthalmology.* Vol 4. Philadelphia: Harper & Row; 1985:24.

3. Boldt HC, Pulido JS, Blodi CF, Folk JC, Weingeist TA. Rural endophthalmitis. *Ophthalmology.* 1989;96:1722–1726.

4. Thompson JT, Parver LM, Enger CL, Mieler WF, Liggett PE. Infectious endophthalmitis after penetrating injuries with retained intraocular foreign bodies. *Ophthalmology.* 1993;100:1468–1474.

5. Maylath FR, Leopold JH. Study of experimental intraocular infection. *Am J Ophthalmol.* 1955;40:86–101.

6. Driebe WT, Mandelbaum S, Forster RK, Schwartz LK, Culbertson WW. Pseudophakic endophthalmitis. *Ophthalmology.* 1986;93:442–448.

7. Forster RK, Abbott RL, Gelender H. Management of infectious endophthalmitis. *Ophthalmology.* 1980;87:313–319.

8. Forster RK. Symposium: postoperative endophthalmitis: etiology and diagnosis of bacterial postoperative endophthalmitis. *Ophthalmology.* 1978;85:320–327.

9. Bohigian GM, Olk RJ. Factors associated with a poor visual result in endophthalmitis. *Am J Ophthalmol.* 1986;101:332–341.

10. Costin JD, Fischer W, Kappner M, Schmidt W, Schuchmann H. Kultivierung von anaeroben Mikroorganismen: Eine neue Methode zur Erzeugung eines anaeroben Milieus. *Forum Mikrobiol.* 5 1982;5:246–248.

11. Neß, Pelz K. Endophthalmitis, Verbesserung des Keimnachweises. *Ophthalmologe.* 2000;97:33–37.

12. Mino de Kaspar H, Grasbon T, Kampik A. Automated surgical equipment requires routine disinfection of vacuum control manifold to prevent postoperative endophthalmitis. *Ophthalmology.* 2000;107:685–690.

13. Minho de Kaspar H, Kollmann M, Klaus V. Endophthalmitis. Bedeutung mikrobiologischer Untersuchungen für die Therapie und Prognose. *Ophthalmologe.* 1993;90:726–736.

14. Lohmann CP, Linde HJ, Reischl U. Die Schnelldiagnostik einer infektiösen Endophthalmitis mittels Polymerase-Kettenreaktion (PCR): Eine Ergänzung zu den konventionellen mikrobiologischen Diagnostikverfahren. *Klin Monatsbl Augenheilkd.* 1997;211:22–27.

15. Lohmann CP, Linde HJ, Reischl U. Improved detection of microorganisms by polymerase chain reaction in delayed endophthalmitis after cataract surgery. *Ophthalmology.* 2000;107:1047–1051.

16. Gümbel H, Koch F. *Infektionen des Auges—Diagnostik und Therapie.* Bremen: UNI-med Verlag; 2000.

17. Heimann K. Vitrektomie bei Augenverletzungen. In: Mackensen G, Neubauer H. *Augenärztliche Operationen.* Heidelberg: Springer; 1989.

18. Lee VHI, Pince KJ, Frambach DA, Martemhed B. Drug delivery to the posterior segment. In: Ryan SJ. *Retina.* St. Louis: CV Mosby; 1994.

19. Alfaro V, Pastor JC, Meredith T. Posttraumatic endophthalmitis. In: Alfaro V, Ligett P. *Vitreoretinal Surgery of the Injured Eye.* Philadelphia: Lippincott; 1999.

20. Lesar TS, Fiscella RG. Antimicrobial drug delivery to the eye. *Drug Intell Clin Pharm.* 1985;19:642–654.

21. Peters MA, Abrams GW, Hamilton LH. The nonexpansile equilibrated concentration of perfluoropropane gas in the eye. *Am J Ophthalmol.* 1985;100:831–839.

22. Chang S. Intraocular gases. In: Ryan SJ. *Retina.* St. Louis: CV Mosby; 1989.

23. Abrams GW, Edelhauser HF, Aaberg TM, Hamilton LH. Dynamics of intravitreal sulfur hexafluoride gas. *Invest Ophthalmol Vis Sci.* 1974;13:863–868.

24. Dieckert JP, O'Connor PS, Schacklett DE, et al. Air travel and intraocular gas. *Ophthalmology.* 1986;93:642–645.

25. Ohm J. Über die Behandlung der Netzhautablösung durch operative Entleerung der subretinalen Flüssigkeit und Einspritzung von Luft in den Glaskörper. *Arch Ophthalmol.* 1911;79:442–450.

26. Rosengren B. Cases of retinal detachment treated with diathermy and injection of air into the vitreous body. *Acta Ophthalmol.* 1938;16:177.

27. Custodis E. Bedeutet die Plombenaufnähung auf die Sklera einen Fortschritt in der operativen Behandlung der Netzhautablösung? *Ber Dtsch Ophthalmol Ges.* 1953;58:102–105.

28. Norton EW, Aaberg T, Fung W, Curtin VT. Giant retinal tears: I. Clinical management with intravitreal air. *Am J Ophthalmol.* 1969;68:1011–1021.

29. Lincoff H, Moore D, Ramirez V, Deitch R, Long R. Long lasting gases as a substitute for intravitreal air in the treatment of retinal detachment. Read before the Cornell Alumni Meeting; New York; April 1967.

30. Lincoff H, Mardirossian J, Lincoff A, Liggett P, Iwamoto T, Jakobiec F. Intravitreal longevity of three perfluorocarbon gases. *Arch Ophthalmol.* 1980;98:1610–1611.

31. Lincoff H, Kreissig I, Brodie S, Wilcox L. Expanding gas bubbles for the repair of tears in the posterior pole. *Graefes Arch Clin Exp Ophthalmol.* 1982;219:193–197.

32. Parver LM, Lincoff H. Geometry of intraocular gas used in retinal surgery. *Mod Probl Ophthalmol.* 1977;18:338–343.

33. Parver LM, Lincoff H. Mechanism of intraocular gas. *Invest Ophthalmol Vis Sci.* 1978;17:77–79.

34. Thompson JT. Kinetics of intraocular gases: disappearance of air, sulfur hexafluoride, and perfluoropropane after pars plana vitrectomy. *Arch Ophthalmol.* 1989;107:687–691.

35. Hilton GF, Grizzard WS. Pneumatic Retinopexy: a two-step outpatient operation without conjunctival incision. *Ophthalmology.* 1986;93:626–641.

36. Tornambe PE. Pneumatic retinopexy. *Surv Ophthalmol.* 1988;32:270–281.

37. Fineberg E, Machemer R, Sullivan P. SF6 for retinal detachment surgery. *Mod Probl Ophthalmol.* 1974;12:173–176.

38. Miller B, Lean JS, Miller H, Ryan SJ. Intravitreal expanding gas bubble: a morphologic study in the rabbit eye. *Arch Ophthalmol.* 1984;102:1708–1711.

39. Lincoff H, Coleman J, Kreissig I, et al. The perfluorocarbon gases in the treatment of retinal detachment. *Ophthalmology.* 1983;90:546–551.

40. Lincoff H, Maisel JM, Lincoff A. Intravitreal disappearance rates of four perfluorocarbon gases. *Arch Ophthalmol.* 1984;102:928–929.

41. Meyers SM, Ambler JS, Fracs F, et al. Variation of perfluoropropane disappearance after vitrectomy. *Retina.* 1992;12:359–363.

42. Cibis PA, Becker B, Okun E, Canaan S. The use of liquid silicone in retinal detachment surgery. *Arch Ophthalmol.* 1962;68:590–599.

43. Armaly MF. Ocular tolerance to silicones. *Arch Ophthalmol.* 1962;68:390–395.

44. Haut J, Ullern M, VanEffenterre G, Chermet M. Utilisation du silicone intraoculaire a à propos de 200 cas. *Bull Soc Ophtalmol Fr.* 1979;79:797–799.

45. Haut J, Ullern M, Chermet M, VanEffenterre G. Complications of intraocular injections of silicone combined with vitrectomy. *Ophthalmologica.* 1980;180:29–35.

46. Zivojnovic R, Mertens AE, Barsma GS. Das flüssige Silikon in der Amotiochirurgie. Bericht über 90 Fälle. *Klin Monatsbl Augenheilkd.* 1981;179:17–22.

47. Ando F. Intraocular hypertension resulting from pupillary block by silicone oil. *Am J Ophthalmol.* 1985;99:87–88.

48. Silicone Study Group. Vitrectomy with silicone oil or sulfur hexafluoride gas in eyes with severe proliferative vitreoretinopathy: results of a randomized clinical trial—Silicone Study Report No. 1. *Arch Ophthalmol.* 1992;110:770–779.

49. Petersen J. The physical and surgical aspects of silicone oil in the vitreous cavity. *Graefes Arch Clin Exp Ophthalmol.* 1987;225:452–456.

50. Heidenkummer HP, Kampik A, Thierfelder S. Emulsification of silicone oils with specific physicochemical characteristics. *Graefes Arch Clin Exp Ophthalmol.* 1991;229:88–94.

51. Heidenkummer HP, Kampik A, Thierfelder S. Experimental evaluation of in vitro stability of purified polydimethylsiloxanes (silicone oil) in viscosity ranges from 1000 to 5000 centistokes. *Retina.* 1992;12:S28–S32.

52. Schrader W. Perforating injuries: causes and risks are changing. A retrospective study. *Ger J Ophthalmol.* 1993;2:76–82.

53. Lucke K, Laqua H. *Silicone Oil in the Treatment of Complicated Retinal Detachments.* New York: Springer; 1990.

54. McCartney DL, Miller KM, Stark WJ, Guyton DL, Michels RG. Intraocular lens style and refraction in eyes treated with silicone oil. *Arch Ophthalmol.* 1987;105:1385–1387.

55. Shugar JK, DeJuan E, McCuen BW, Tiedeman J, Landers MR 3d, Machemer R. Ultrasonic examination of the silicone filled eye: theoretical and practical considerations. *Graefes Arch Clin Exp Ophthalmol.* 1986;224:361–367.

56. Chang S. Low viscosity liquid fluorochemicals in vitreous surgery. *Am J Ophthalmol.* 1987;103:38–43.

57. Miyamoto K, Refojo MR, Tolentino FI. Perfluoroether liquid as a long-term vitreous substitute: an experimental study. *Retina.* 1984;4:264–268.

58. LoCasicio JA, Hammer M, Rinder D, et al. Effect of selected liquid perfluorochemicals compared to high and low viscosity silicone oil on corneal stroma and endothelium. *Invest Ophthalmol Vis Sci.* 1985;26:S145.

59. Chang S, Zimmerman NJ, Iwamoto T, Ortiz R, Faris D. Experimental vitreous replacement with perfluorotributylamine. *Am J Ophthalmol.* 1987;103:29–37.

60. Clark LCJ, Gollan F. Survival of mammals breathing organic liquids equilibrated with oxygen at atmospheric pressure. *Science.* 1966;152:1755–1756.

61. Haidt SJ, Clark LCJ, Ginsberg J. Liquid perfluorocarbon replacement of the eye. *Invest Ophthalmol Vis Sci.* 1982;22:S233.

62. Nabih M, Peyman GA, Clark LCJ, et al. Experimental evaluation of perfluorophenanthrene as a high specific gravity vitreous substitute: a preliminary report. *Ophthalmic Surg.* 1989;20:286–293.

63. Kirchhof B. Fluorkarbone in der Netzhaut-Glaskörperchirurgie. *Ophthalmo-Chir.* 1999;11:153–158.

64. Meinert H, Geisler U. Semifluorinated compounds in ophthalmology. *J Vitreoretina.* 1992;1:31–35.

65. Azzolini C, Docchio F, Brancato R, Trabucchi G. Interactions between light and vitreous fluid substitutes. *Arch Ophthalmol.* 1992;110:1468–1471.

66. Chang S, Sparrow JR, Iwamoto T, Gershbein A, Ross R, Ortiz R. Experimental studies of tolerance to intravitreal perfluoro-*n*-octane liquid. *Retina.* 1991;11:367–374.

67. Abrams GW, Swanson DE, Sabates WI, Goldman AI. The results of sulfur hexafluoride gas in vitreous surgery. *Am J Ophthalmol.* 1982;94:165–171.

68. Whitacre MM, Mainster MA. Hazards of laser beam reflections in eyes containing gas. *Am J Ophthalmol.* 1990;110:33–38.

69. Heimann K, Konen W. Artificial iris diaphragm and silicone oil surgery. *Retina.* 1992;12:S90–S94.

70. Lemmen KD, Heimann K. Früh-Vitrektomie mit primärer Silikonolinjektion bei schwerstverletzten Augen. *Klin Monatsbl Augenheilkd.* 1988;193:594–601.

71. Hammer ME. Vitreous substitutes. In: Tasman W, Jaeger EA. *Duane's Clinical Ophthalmology.* Philadelphia: Lippincott Williams & Wilkins; 2000.

72. Kampik A, Hoing C, Heidenkummer HP. Problems and timing in the removal of silicone oil. *Retina.* 1992;12(3 suppl):S11–S16.

73. Nguyen QH, Lloyd MA, Heuer DK, et al. Incidence and management of glaucoma after intravitreal silicone oil injection for complicated retinal detachments. *Ophthalmology.* 1992;99:1520.

74. Lucke KH, Foerster MH, Laqua H. Long-term results of vitrectomy and silicone oil in 500 cases of complicated retinal detachments. *Am J Ophthalmol.* 1987;104:624–633.

75. Leaver PK. Complications of intraocular silicone oil. In: Ryan SJ. *Retina.* St. Louis: CV Mosby; 1989.

76. McCuen BI, DeJuan EJ, Landers MBI, Machemer R. Silicone oil in vitreoretinal surgery: II. Results and complications. *Retina.* 1985;5:198–205.

77. Silicone Study Group. Vitrectomy with silicone oil or perfluoropropane gas in eyes with severe proliferative vitreoretinopathy: results of a randomized clinical trial—Silicone Study Report No. 2. *Arch Ophthalmol.* 1992;110:780–792.

78. Williams GA, Lambrou FH, Jaffe GJ, et al. Treatment of postvitrectomy fibrin formation with intraocular tissue plasminogen activator. *Arch Ophthalmol.* 1988;106:1055–1058.

79. Williams DF, Bennett SR, Abrams GW, et al. Low-dose intraocular tissue plasminogen activator for treatment of postvitrectomy fibrin formation. *Am J Ophthalmol.* 1990;109:606–607.

80. Snyder RW, Lambrou FH, Williams GA. Intraocular fibrinolysis with recombinant human tissue plasminogen activator. Experimental treatment in a rabbit model. *Arch Ophthalmol.* 1987;105:1277–1280.

81. Abrams GW. Retinotomies and retinectomies. In: Ryan SJ. *Retina.* St. Louis: CV Mosby; 1989.

82. Machemer R, McCuen BWI, DeJuan E Jr. Relaxing retinotomies and retinectomies. *Am J Ophthalmol.* 1986;102:7–12.

83. Morse LS, McCuen BWI, Machemer R. Relaxing retinotomies: analysis of anatomic and visual results. *Ophthalmology.* 1990;97:642–647.

84. Zarbin MA, Michels RG, Green RG. Dissection of epiciliary tissue to treat chronic hypotony after surgery for retinal detachment with proliferative vitreoretinopathy. *Retina.* 1991;11:208–213.

85. Leaver PK, Grey RHB, Garner A. Silicone oil injection in the treatment of massive preretinal retraction: II. Late complications in 93 eyes. *Br J Ophthalmol.* 1979;63:361–367.

86. Moisseiev J, Bartov E, Cahane M, et al. Cataract extraction in eyes filled with silicone oil. *Arch Ophthalmol.* 1992;110:1649–1651.

87. Lemmen KD, Dimopoulos S, Kirchhof B, Heimann K. Keratopathy following pars plana vitrectomy with silicone oil filling. *Dev Ophthalmol.* 1987;13:88–98.

88. Chung H, Tolentino F, Cajita VN, Acosta J, Refojo MF. Reevaluation of corneal complications after closed vitrectomy. *Arch Ophthalmol.* 1988;106:916–919.

89. Wiedemann P, Leinung C, Hilgers RD, Heimann K. Daunomycin and silicone oil for the treatment of proliferative vitreoretinopathy. *Graefes Arch Clin Exp Ophthalmol.* 1991;229:150–152.

90. Wiedemann P, Hilgers RD, Bauer P, Heimann K. Adjunctive daunorubicin in the treatment of proliferative vitreoretinopathy: results of a multicenter clinical trial. Daunomycin Study Group. *Am J Ophthalmol.* 1998;126:550–559.

91. Chang S, Reppucci V, Zimmerman NJ, Heinemann MH, Coleman DJ. Perfluorocarbon liquids in the management of traumatic retinal detachments. *Ophthalmology.* 1989;96:785–791.

92. Blinder KJ, Peyman GA, Paris CL, et al. Vitreon, a new perfluorocarbon. *Br J Ophthalmol.* 1991;75:240–244.

93. Lewis H, Blumenkranz MS, Chang S. Treatment of dislocated crystalline lens and retinal detachment with perfluorocarbon liquids. *Retina.* 1992;12:299–304.

94. Movshovich A, Berrocal MH, Chang S, et al. The protective properties of liquid perfluorocarbons in phacofragmentation. *Invest Ophthalmol Vis Sci.* 1992;33:1312.

95. Peyman GA, Alturki WA, Nelson NC. Surgical management of incarcerated retina in the sclerotomy. *Ophthalmic Surg.* 1992;23:628–629.

96. Vander JF. Tissue plasminogen activator irrigation to facilitate removal of subretinal hemorrhage during vitrectomy. *Ophthalmic Surg.* 1992;23:361–363.

97. Heimann K. Combined intraocular PFCL plus silicone oil tamponade for control of intraoperative hemorrhages (sandwich technique). *Vitreoretinal Surg Technol.* 1993;5:8.

98. Hegazy HM, Peyman GA, Liang C, Unal MH, Molinari LC, Kazi AA. Use of perfluorocarbon liquids, silicone oil, and 5-fluorouracil in the management of experimental PVR. *Int Ophthalmol.* 1998–99;22:239–246.

99. Sparrow JR, Jayakumar A, Berrocal M, Ozmert E, Chang S. Experimental studies of the combined use of vitreous substitutes of high and low specific gravity. *Retina.* 1992;12:134–140.

100. Meier P, Wiedemann P. Massive suprachoroidal hemorrhage: secondary treatment and outcome. *Graefes Arch Clin Exp Ophthalmol.* 2000;238:28–32.

101. Lemmen KD, Heimann K. Early vitrectomy with primary silicone oil filling in severely injured eyes. *Klin Monatsbl Augenheilkd.* 1988;193:594–601.

102. Cekic O, Batman C. Severe ocular trauma managed with primary pars plana vitrectomy and silicone oil [letter; comment]. *Retina.* 1998;18:287–288.

103. Spiegel D, Nasemann J, Nawrocki J, Gabel VP. Severe ocular trauma managed with primary pars plana vitrectomy and silicone oil. *Retina.* 1997;17:275–285.

104. Campochiaro PA, Bryan JAI, Conway BP, Jaccoma EH. Intravitreal chemotactic and mitogenic activity: implication of blood-retinal barrier breakdown. *Arch Ophthalmol.* 1986;104:1685–1687.

105. Campochiaro PA, Gaskins HC, Vinores SA. Retinal cryopexy stimulates traction retinal detachment formation in the presence of an ocular wound. *Arch Ophthalmol.* 1987;105:1567–1570.

106. Campochiaro PA, Kaden IH, Viduarri-Leal J, et al. Cryotherapy enhances intravitreal dispersion of viable retinal pigment epithelial cells. *Arch Ophthalmol.* 1985;103:434–436.

107. Singh AK, Glaser BM, Lemor M, Michels RG. Gravity-dependent distribution of retinal pigment epithelial cells dispersed into the vitreous cavity. *Retina.* 1986;6:77–80.

108. Wiedemann P. *Die medikamentöse Behandlung der proliferativen Vitreoretinopathie unter besonderer Berücksichtigung des Zytostatikums Daunomycin.* Stuttgart: Enke; 1988.

109. Marr WG, Marr EG. Some observations on Purtscher´s disease: traumatic retinal angiography. *Am J Ophthalmol.* 1962;54:693–705.

110. Duke-Elder S, MacFaul PA. Injuries, part I: mechanical injuries. In: Duke-Elder S. *System of Ophthalmology.* London: Henry Klimpton; 1972.

111. Morris R, Kuhn F, Witherspoon CD, Mester V, Dooner J. Hemorrhagic macular cysts in Terson's syndrome and its implications for macular surgery. *Dev Ophthalmol.* 1997;29:44–54.

PHARMACOLOGY

Martin L. Heredia-Elizondo,
Tamer A. Macky, D. Virgil Alfaro, and Joel H. Herring

Drug	Preparation	Dose
ANESTHETICS		
Lidocaine	0.5%, 1%, 1.5%, 2%, 4%, 10%, and 20% for injection	Extensive procedures: 10–20 mL of a 1% solution*
		Minor surgery: 2–10 mL of a 0.5% solution.
	0.5%, 1%, 1.5%, and 2% with epinephrine 1:200,000 for injection	Extensive time: up to 20 mL of a 1% solution with epinephrine
		Maximum dose:
		with epinephrine (7 mg/kg or 500 mg)
		without epinephrine (4.5 mg/kg or 300 mg)
Procaine	1%, 2%, and 10% for injection	Extensive procedures: <10 mL of the 2% solution
		Minor surgery: <20 mL of the 1% solution
ANTIBIOTICS		
Aminoglycosides		
Amikacin	50 and 250 mg/mL solution. (im and iv)	7.5 to 8.0 mg/kg every 12 h (iv)
		0.2 to 0.4 mg in 0.1 mL for intravitreal injection
Gentamicin	2 mg/mL solution (im, iv, and intrathecal)	1.5 to 2.0 mg/kg every 8 h
	10 and 40 mg/mL solution (im and iv)	0.1 mg in 0.1 mL for intravitreal injection
Neomycin	Neomycin sulfate 500 mg tablet	1 g every 4 h
	Neomycin-bacitracin-polymyxin ointment	One to four times daily
	Neomycin-dexamethasone 0.1% solution	Once or twice every h (topical)
Tobramycin	0.3% solution and ointment (topical)	Every 3–4 h (ointment)
	10 and 40 mg/mL solution (im and iv)	1–2 drops every 4 h , or 2 drops once or twice every h for severe infections (topical)
Cephalosporins		
Cefazolin	500 mg, 1 g, 10 g, and 20 g solution	133 mg/mL topical (one drop every 4–6 h)
		100 mg/mL subconjunctival
		2.25 mg intravitreal
		500 to 1000 mg every 6 h iv/im
Ceftazidime	500 mg, 1 g, and 2 g solution	50 mg/mL topical (one drop every 4–6 h)
		200 mg/mL subconjunctival
		2.2 mg intravitreal
		1–2 g every 12 h iv/im

---

*1% solution: 10 mg/mL.

continued

Drug	Preparation	Dose
Ceftriaxone	250 mg, 500 mg, 1 g, 2 g, and 10 g solution	3 mg intravitreal 1–2 g every 24 h iv/im
Penicillins		
Ampicillin	125 mg/5 mL and 250 mg/5 mL suspension (oral) 250 mg capsule (oral) 125 mg, 250 mg, 500 mg, 1 g, and 2 g solution (iv and im)	250–500 mg every 6 h (oral) 50 mg/mL topical (one drop every 4–6 h) 100 mg/mL subconjunctival 5000 μg intravitreal 1–3 g every 6 h (iv/im)
Methicillin	1 g, 4 g, and 6 g powder	1 g every 6 h (im, iv) Subconjunctival: 50–150 mg in 0.5 mL Intracameral: 1 mg in 0.2–0.5 mL
Oxacillin	250 mg and 500 mg capsule (oral) 250 mg/5 mL solution (oral) 500 mg, 1 g, and 2 g solution (iv)	50 mg/mL topical (one drop every 4–6 h) 75–100 mg subconjunctival 1 g every 6 h iv
Penicillin G	Benzathine: 600,000 U/mL suspension (im) Potassium: 20,000 U/mL suspension (iv, topical, subconjunctival) Procaine: 600,000 U/mL susp (im)	Topical: 100,000–333,000 U/mL Subconjunctival: 0.5–1.0 million U Intravitreal: 2000 U Oral: 400,000 U every 6 h iv: 2 to 6 million U every 4 h
Penicillin V	125 mg/5 mL and 250 mg/5 mL solution (oral) 250 mg and 500 mg tablet	250–500 mg every 6 h (oral)
Sulfonamides		
Sulfacetamide	10% suspension and ointment (topical) 10%, 15%, and 30% solution (topical) Same preparations and steroid: Prednisolone 0.2% and 0.5% Prednisone 0.25% Fluorometholone 0.1%	One or two drops every 2 to 3 h Ointment: one to four times daily
Trimethoprim/ sulfamethoxazole combination	80 mg trimethoprim, 400 mg sulfamethoxazole 160 mg trimethoprim, 800 mg sulfamethoxazole 40 mg trimethoprim, 200 mg sulfamethoxazole/5 mL oral suspension 80 mg trimethoprim, 400 mg sulfamethoxazole/5 mL infusion.	Tablet: 4 times daily Tablet: 2 times daily Suspension: 8 mg/kg daily trimethoprim and 4 mg/kg daily sulfamethoxazole in 2 divided doses iv: 20 mg/kg daily trimethoprim and 100 mg/kg daily sulfamethoxazole
Tetracyclines		
Tetracycline	1% solution and ointment (10 mg per mL and g) 125 mg/5 mL suspension and syrup 250 mg and 500 mg capsules 250 mg tablets 250 mg and 500 mg sterile powder (iv) 100 mg and 250 mg sterile powder (im)	3–4 times daily 1–2 g/daily adults and nonpregnant women, children aged more than 8 years should receive 25 to 50 mg/kg daily in two to four divided doses
Miscellaneous		
Bacitracin	500 U/g ophthalmic ointment 50,000 U vial (injection) 2500 U soluble tablet	2–6 times daily (topical) 10,000 U/0.5 mL subconjunctival 1000 U kg daily in 2–3 doses, not exceed 100,000 U daily
Chloramphenicol	0.5% solution (5 mg/mL) (topical) 1.0 % ointment (10 mg/mL) (topical) Capsules: 250 and 500 mg (oral) Palmitate: 150 mg/mL suspension (oral) Sodium succinate: 1 g (100 mg/mL) (injection)	One drop two to six times daily Every 3 h 1–3 g daily in systemic therapy (4g daily max)

continued

Drug	Preparation	Dose
Clindamycin	Hydrochloride: 75, 150, and 300 mg capsules	150 mg to 300 mg every 8 h (p.o.)
	Phosphate: 150 mg/mL solution (parenteral)	600 mg every 6 h (iv and im), not to exceed 8 g daily 1 mg for intravitreal injection
Erythromycin	0.5% ointment (5 mg/g) (topical)	One to six times daily
	250, 333, and 500 mg tablets	250 mg to 500 mg every 6 h
	Estolate: 125 and 250 mg capsules 125 and 250 mg/mL suspension 500 mg tablets	500 mg every 12 h
	Ethylsuccinate: 200 and 400 mg/5mL suspension or 400 mg tablets	600 mg every 8 h
	Stearate: 250 and 500 mg tablets	500 mg every 12 h
	Gluceptate: Powder 250 mg, 500 mg, and 1 g (iv)	1 to 4 g daily in iv
	Lactobionate: Powder 500 mg and 1 g (iv)	
Imipenem/Cilastatin	500–500 mg solution (injection)	500 mg/500 mg every 4 h, not to exceed 4 g daily
Polymyxin B	Ointment (in combination with other antibiotics and/or steroids)	Every half hour to hourly and then tapered (topical)
	Sterile powder U Vial: 500,000	25,000 to 40,000 U/kg daily for im 15,000 to 25,000 U/kg daily for iv
Vancomycin	500 mg, 1 g, and 10 g vials (iv) 1 g and 10 g (oral solution) 125 and 250 mg (powder)	1 g every 8 or 12 h 500 mg to 1 g every 6 h (oral) 25 mg/0.5 mL for subconjunctival injection 1.0 mg in 0.1 mL for intravitreal injection

ANTIFIBRINOLYTICS

Aminocaproic acid	Tablets: 500 mg Syrup and injection: 250 mg/mL	50 mg/kg every 4 h up to 30 g daily

ANTIFUNGALS

Amphotericin B	50 mg (lyophilized)	0.005 mg intravitreal 0.5–0.6 mg/kg daily iv (maximum of 1.5 mg/kg)
	3% ointment, cream, and lotion	3–4 times daily
Ketoconazole	1% and 3% solutions	1% solution subconjunctival
	200 mg tablets	200 mg daily
	2% cream and shampoo	
Miconazole	10 mg/mL sterile solution	300 mg daily (iv) 1% solution (topical) 0.25 mg intravitreal
	2% cream and lotion	

ANTIGLAUCOMA
Beta-blockers

Betaxolol	0.25% Suspension 0.5% Solution	One drop twice daily
Carteolol	1% Solution	One drop twice daily
Timolol	0.25% Solution 0.5% Solution	One drop twice daily One drop once daily (gel)

CAIs

Acetazolamide	Oral tablets: 125 mg and 250 mg Sustained-release capsules: 500 mg Lyophilized powder for iv injection: 500 mg	250 mg to 1000 mg daily, in four divided doses
Dichlorphenamide	Tablets: 50 mg	25 to 50 mg, one to four times daily
Dorzolamide	2% solution	One drop three times daily in the affected eye
Methazolamide	Tablets: 25 mg and 50 mg	25 to 50 mg, two or three times daily

Miotics

Carbachol	0.01%, 0.75%, 1.5%, and 3% solution	0.75% to 3.0% solution three times daily 0.01% solution intracamerally
Pilocarpine	0.5% to 10% solution, 4% usually maximal 4% gel	0.5% to 4.0% aqueous solution four times daily Once daily

continued

Drug	Preparation	Dose
	Ocusert: 20 µg/h and 40 µg/h sustained-release rate	Once every 7 days
Prostaglandins		
Latanoprost	0.005% solution	Once daily
Sympathomimetics		
Apraclonidine	0.5% and 1% solution	0.5% solution three times daily
Brimonidine	0.2% solution	One drop twice daily
Dipivefrin	0.1% solution	Once or twice daily
ANTI-INFLAMMATORY		
Nonsteroids		
Diclofenac	0.1% solution Tablets: 25, 50, and 75 mg	One drop four times daily postoperatively 25 to 50 mg three times daily
Flurbiprofen	0.03% solution Tablets: 50 and 100 mg	One drop every 30 minutes, for 2 h preoperatively
Indomethacin	0.5% and 1% suspension	One drop four times daily
Ketorolac	0.5% solution	One drop three times daily
Suprofen	1.0% solution	One drop 1, 2, and 3 h preoperatively or every 4 h while awake on the day of surgery
ANTI-IRON		
Deferoxamine	500 mg solution (injection)	1 g initial dose; followed by 0.5 g every 4 h, not exceed 6 g daily (systemic) 0.5 mL of a 10% solution twice a week (subconjunctival) 10% in 1% methylcellulose four daily (topical)
ANTIMETABOLITES		
5-Fluorouracil	500 mg/10 mL solution.	10 mg subconjunctival injection 1 mg intravitreal injection
Daunorubicin HCl	5 mg/mL solution (injection)	7.5 µg/mL solution infuse for 10 minutes
ANTITETANUS		
Antitoxin	10,000, 15,000, and 50,000 units (syringe or vial)	5000 to 10,000 U (prophylaxis) 40,000 to 100,000 U (iv treatment)
Immune globulin	250 units (syringe or vial)	250 U (prophylaxis) 5000 to 10,000 U (im treatment)
Tetanus toxoid	Adsorbed and ultrafined 5 Lf U solution	Three injections of 0.5 mL; second injection 5 weeks after the first one, the third 6–12 months later
CYCLOPLEGICS AND MYDRIATICS		
Atropine	0.5% and 1% sterile solution and ointment 0.1 mg/mL solution (indictable) 0.6 mg, 0.8 mg, and 1 mg tablets	Three times daily (solution), Once daily (ointment)
Cyclopentolate	0.5%, 1%, and 2% solution (topical)	One drop three or four times daily
Homatropine	2% and 5% sterile ophthalmic solution	Three times daily
Phenylephrine HCL	2.5% and 10% ophthalmic solution	One drop twice or three times daily
Tropicamide	0.5% and 1.0% ophthalmic solution	
CYTOTOXIC		
Azathioprine	50 mg tablets (oral) 100 mg lyophilized powder (iv)	2–3 mg/kg daily
Cyclosporin	100 mg/mL solution (oral) 25 mg and 100 mg soft gelatin capsules (oral) 50 mg and 1 mL vehicle (iv) 1% and 2% solution (topical)	2.5–5.0 mg/kg daily Topical solution 5 times daily

continued

Drug	Preparation	Dose
Cyclophosphamide	25 mg and 50 mg tablets 100 mg, 200 mg, 500 mg, 1 g, and 3 g powder (im, iv)	1–2 mg/kg daily
Chlorambucil	2 mg sugar-coated tablets (oral)	0.1 mg/kg daily
Methotrexate	2.5 mg tablets 2.5 and 25 mg/mL solution (im, iv, intrathecal) 20 mg, 50 mg, 100 mg, 250 mg, and 1 g powder (im, iv, intrathecal)	Weekly dose of 2.5 mg to 7.5 mg in a single or divided dose with a maximum dose of 15 mg/week

ENZYMES

Hyaluronidase	150 U/mL solution	5–7 U per mL of anesthetic solution
Urokinase	5000 U, 9000 U, and 250,000 U, solution	Intravitreal: 25,000 U in 0.3 mL iv: 4400 U/kg initially (90 mL/h every 10 min, then 15 mL/h every 12 h)

HYPEROSMOTICS

Glycerol	50% and 75% solution	1–1.5 g/kg every 6 h
Isosorbide	45% solution	1.5 g/kg every 6 h
Mannitol	10% and 20% solution	1–1.5 g/kg (3–5 mL per minute)
Topical osmotic:		
Glucose	40% and 50% solution	2–3 drops three times daily
Sodium chloride	2%, 5%, and 10% solution and ointment	Twice or three times daily

STERILIZING AND DISINFECTING

Providone-iodine	Swab stick with 10% solution	Apply to procedure site as needed

STEROIDS

Betamethasone	3 mg/mL suspension Tablet: 0.6 mg Syrup: 0.6 mg/5 mL	1 mg subconjunctival/Tenon, and transeptal Initial doses: 0.5 mg to 9 mg daily (systemic)
Dexamethasone	Alcohol: 0.1% suspension and 0.05% ointment	Individualized dose (topical)
	Sodium phosphate: 0.1% solution and 0.05% ointment	Individualized dose (topical)
	Sodium: 0.25 to 6 mg tablet 0.5 mg/5 mL oral suspension 0.5 mg/5 mL solution	0.75 mg to 9 mg p.o. daily
	Sodium phosphate: 4 to 24 mg/mL solution iv	0.75 mg to 9 mg iv or im daily
	Acetate: 8 mg/mL suspension im	4–8 mg subconjunctival/Tenon, and transeptal
	Acetate: 8 to 16 mg/mL suspension	0.4 mg intravitreal
	Sodium phosphate: 4, 10, 24 mg/mL solution	4 mg retrobulbar
Fluorometholone	0.25% and 0.1% suspension 0.1% ointment	Individualized dose (topical)
Hydrocortisone	5 to 20 mg tablet 10 mg/5 mL suspension 25 and 50 mg suspension im 50 mg/mL solution im/iv	20 to 240 mg systemic therapy
	Sodium succinate: 100 to 1000 mg powder	50–125 mg subconjunctival/Tenon
Methylprednisolone	2 to 32 mg tablet Sodium succinate: 40 to 1000 mg powder im/iv	20 to 80 mg systemic therapy
	Sodium succinate: 40 mg/mL, 125 mg/2 mL, 2g/30 mL solution	40–125 mg subconjunctival/Tenon
	Acetate: 20 to 80 mg/mL depot suspension	40–80 mg/0.5 mL transeptal, retrobulbar

continued

Drug	Preparation	Dose
Prednisolone	Phosphate: 0.5% solution and 0.25% ointment	Individualized dose (topical)
	Acetate: 0.12% and 1.0% suspension	5 mg to 50 mg (systemic therapy)
	Sodium phosphate: 0.12, 0.5, and 1% solution	
	1 to 5 mg tablet	
	15 mg/mL syrup	
	Acetate: 25 to 100 mg/mL suspension im	
	Sodium phosphate: 20 mg/mL solution im/iv	
Prednisone	1.0 to 50 mg tablet	1.0 to 1.5 mg/kg initial dose (systemic therapy)
	5 mg/mL oral solution	
Triamcinolone	Diacetate: 4 mg/mL syrup	4 mg to 48 mg daily (systemic)
	1 to 8 mg tablet	
	40 mg/mL suspension im	
	25 and 40 mg/mL suspension	40 mg subconjunctival/Tenon
	Acetonide: 10 and 40 mg/mL suspension	40 mg transeptal

VISCOELASTICS

Drug	Preparation	Dose
Chondroitin sulfate	4%	In surgery as needed
Hydroxypropyl methylcellulose	2%	In surgery as needed
Sodium hyaluronate	1%, 1.4%, and 1.6%	In surgery as needed

MYTHS AND TRUTHS ABOUT EYE INJURIES: ANSWERS TO COMMONLY ASKED QUESTIONS

Dante J. Pieramici and Ferenc Kuhn

In the management of ocular injuries, there are numerous examples of controversy. These controversies are gutturally argued at meetings and in the editorials of professional journals. The ophthalmologist's particular viewpoints are based, in large part, on the *opinions* of peers taught during residency training, rather than on solid *scientific* data. These viewpoints are stored in our brains and are inseparably under the influence of our feelings toward our mentors and teachers. In recalling such information, the clinical "fact" is intertwined with emotional memories, tainting it with righteousness. Separating *fact* from *myth* is particularly difficult given this emotional baggage. The study of ocular injuries has been particularly devoid of good scientific data to support many of our management decisions. This opens the door to speculation and the propagation of myth.

In the last decades, a number of investigators have attempted to answer many of the controversial points rationally. Although the data supporting some of these decisions may be fallible, they give the physician some guidance and are an improvement over the argument, "well that is how we have always done it." Throughout this book, the authors have attempted to support their clinical management decisions with scientific data rather than dogma. In the next few paragraphs we question a few of these controversial (if not dogmatic, axiom-like) points as the knowledge gained over the last several years has helped us understand that just because something has been in practice for a long time does not mean that it is correct or acceptable. We divided the list of myths into two categories, based on whether they are the primary concern of the ophthalmologist or of the patient.

THE OPHTHALMOLOGIST

MYTH: *NLP vision at the time of presentation following open globe injury is synonymous with permanent blindness.*
FACT: Useful vision can be recovered even when NLP vision is documented on proper preoperative testing with a bright light source (see Chapter 8).

MYTH: *If only minimal function can be restored to an eye after an injury and reconstruction may take several surgical sessions, it is better to leave the eye alone and not invest effort, time, and resources by offering intervention with so little to gain from it.*
FACT: The eye belongs to the patient, who must make the decision whether he or she wants the inconvenience of intervention(s) or the finality of blindness. Counseling therefore must be unbiased rather than one-sided; counseling must present what the options available for the patient are rather than what the ophthalmologist thinks the patient should do.[a]

MYTH: *All of the damage occurs at the time of impact during severe ocular injury, limiting the ophthalmologist's ability to affect the visual outcome.*
FACT: Following open globe trauma, the healing response may result in additional tissue injuries and the eye may deteriorate from excellent visual potential to becoming phthisical. Contusion injury probably results in a similar series of events, although this has not yet

---

[a] Remember that Murphy's law is all too commonly true: if another disease strikes in the future, it seems to prefer the fellow eye. Having even minimal vision in the injured eye might make all the difference for the patient (see Chapter 6).

been investigated in as much detail as the Ryan-Cleary model. Extrapolating from CNS models of contusion trauma would suggest that additional injury occurs as a result of the release of neurotransmitters.

MYTH: *Following injury by a blunt object, it is preferable if the eye opens (rupture) than if not (contusion) because the energy is released in the former case, as evidenced by the lower incidence of choroidal rupture in ruptured as opposed to contused eyes.*
FACT: While the incidence of certain tissue lesions may be lower in ruptured eyes than in those sustaining contusion, the overall anatomic damage is much more severe and the functional outcome much worse in ruptured eyes (see Chapter 27).

MYTH: *Traumatic corneal abrasions require patching to speed the healing process.*
FACT: In most cases, the corneal epithelium heals well without patching; in fact, patching may be counterproductive (see Chapter 14).

MYTH: *Following severe ocular injury, it is recommended that the patient be patched bilaterally to reduce ocular movement and further injury.*
FACT: There is no information to support this policy. In fact, patching both eyes in patients with a unilateral ocular injury will only increase their anxiety and fears about going blind. Only the injured eye should be shielded.

MYTH: *A breach in the lens capsule invariably necessitates the removal of the lens.*
FACT: Even if the injury results in violation of the peripheral lens capsule and an intralenticular foreign body is present, the developing cataract may remain localized and stationary so that the central lens is clear (see Chapter 21).

MYTH: *Dense vitreous hemorrhage following open globe injury can be followed with close observation.*
FACT: Vitreous hemorrhage is a key ingredient in the initiation and propagation of intraocular proliferation. Vitrectomy in the first few weeks following primary repair can interrupt this process and reduce the chance of retinal detachment and hypotony (see Chapter 23).

MYTH: *Retinal breaks associated with sclopetaria require treatment with laser or cryotherapy to prevent retinal detachment.*
FACT: Only rarely do retinal breaks associated with sclopetaria result in retinal detachment, and in most cases the eyes can be followed with close observation (see Chapter 23).

MYTH: *Applying blind cryopexy over a zone III (see Chapter 2) injury helps prevent retinal detachment.*
FACT: There is no evidence to support that blind cryopexy can prevent retinal detachment, but there is ample evidence that blind cryopexy can stimulate cellular proliferation and thus increase the risk of PVR (see Chapters 8, 23, and 24); it is therefore contraindicated to apply cryopexy unless performed under visual control.[b]

MYTH: *To be on the safe side, posterior retinal breaks are better treated with some type of "pexy."*
FACT: If the vitreous (i.e., traction) has been removed or severed around the area of the posterior retinal break, "pexy" is usually not necessary (see Chapter 24). Conversely, if the break is anterior, treatment is necessary to prevent the development of retinal detachment (see Chapter 23).

MYTH: *Orbital floor fractures invariably require surgical repair and this should be done as soon as possible.*
FACT: Many orbital floor fractures do not result in significant enophthalmos or diplopia and thus do not require surgical repair. Early repair of an orbital fracture when there is associated intraocular injury (i.e., posterior scleral wound) may result in additional iatrogenic trauma and should be deferred (see Chapter 36).

MYTH: *Orbital foreign bodies are best removed to avoid secondary complications.*
FACT: Removal of a deep orbital foreign body may cause more complication than retaining the object (see Chapters 30 and 36). An individual decision, carefully taking into consideration all risk factors, is necessary.

MYTH: *An eye that is blind (i.e., has NLP vision) following open globe injury runs a significant risk of inciting SO and thus enucleation should be recommended.*
FACT: With modern techniques of primary and secondary globe reconstruction, the incidence of SO is extremely low. For cosmetic and especially psychological considerations, most patients may be better served by retaining the eye. Extensive counseling and close follow-ups are necessary (see Chapters 8 and 31). Patients who do develop SO appear to respond favorably to steroid treatment in most cases.

MYTH: *Experienced ophthalmologists understand each other even if they do not use BETT.*
FACT: The language of ocular traumatology has nothing to do with experience. Without describing/typifying/categorizing an injury in a standardized fashion,[c] it is impossible to know whether a colleague

---

[b] Even in such cases, laser is preferred to cryopexy (see Chapters 8 and 23).

[c] The lack of standardization was the cause of one of the greatest ironies of our time: a spacecraft that successfully traveled hundreds of millions of miles only to crash at the last minute because some in the control room thought they were using the metric system while others used feet to measure the distance.

appreciates the description as intended. If "rupture" substitutes for all open globe injuries, how does one distinguish an injury that is truly a rupture? If an author uses the term "penetrating" in the article's title but indicates the term "perforating" as the key word, how should the reader determine what type of trauma is discussed?

THE PATIENT

MYTH: If vision in one eye (or the eye itself) is lost, the fellow eye gets "overused" and "strained."
FACT: The "workload" of one eye is independent of that of the fellow eye, just as the loss of one kidney does not exhaust the other kidney. Just because of becoming monocular, there is no need to change one's lifestyle in terms of the time spent on reading or watching television; but the person should consciously try to reduce the risk of injury to the remaining eye (i.e., wearing ocular protection as appropriate).

MYTH: Physical activities should be severely restricted if the patient suffered a serious eye injury.
FACT: There is no evidence to support this theory. The cause of post-traumatic retinal detachment is an unrecognized retinal break or the development of PVR, not jogging or lifting weights (see Chapter 27).

MYTH: Following open globe injury or severe closed globe injury, the patient should be counseled never to play sports again.
FACT: In reality, we do not have factual information to support this recommendation. Patients should be counseled in all cases about the importance of proper safety glass usage (see Chapter 27) and their legal implications (see Chapter 7). Likewise, little information exists to determine, with certainty, when it is safe to return to such activity following an injury.

MYTH: Deployment of an air bag during an MVC commonly results in severe ocular injury, supporting the argument that airbags should be deactivated.

FACT: Ocular injury during an MVC is 2.5 times more likely to occur if there is no air bag deployment. Air bags significantly reduce both the mortality and morbidity, even if occasionally they may be the cause of certain injuries.[d] Disengagement should be considered only in certain unique and specific circumstances (see Chapter 27).

MYTH: Unless the visual acuity drops to 20/50 in a patient with traumatic macular hole,[e] there is no indication to perform surgery.
FACT: There is no specific visual acuity that can be justified as a valid cutoff value. It is the patient's responsibility to determine whether the visual function allowed by the condition is sufficient. It is the ophthalmologist's responsibility to offer unbiased and reasonably accurate information regarding the risks and benefits of the procedure versus those of observation (see Chapters 5 and 8).

MYTH: Lacerations involving the upper canalicular systems do not need to be repaired since they do not play a role in the transport of tears.
FACT: In certain people the upper canalicular system plays a more important role in tear transport than the lower canalicular system. Because it is impossible to determine which of the two is more important in the injured person, the upper lid's laceration must also be properly repaired (see Chapter 35).

Future, well-designed studies of ocular injury will help us continue to debunk additional myths and offer better treatment recommendations to our patients. Ophthalmologists must keep an open mind and regularly analyze their own practice patterns to determine whether these hold up to the truth (e.g., evidence) or are just myths.

---

[d] In many cases, the reported link between air bag deployment and injury is assumed and has not been supported by evidence.

[e] The same can be said regarding other conditions (e.g., cataract, EMP).

THE NEED FOR STANDARDIZATION FOR PROTECTIVE EYEWEAR IN SPORTS

Paul F. Vinger

Ophthalmologists agree with the conclusion of the National Research Council that "Injury is probably the most under-recognized major health problem facing the Nation today." As the physicians who treat and see the consequences of trauma, U.S. ophthalmologists—working with the Safety Committee of the American Academy of Ophthalmology—are making a concerted effort to educate all eye care professionals and the general public as to which activities pose a risk for significant eye injury and how best to minimize the risk.

The following data were taken from the USEIR, and will be discussed in light of data gathered from a sampling of emergency rooms by the United States Consumer Products Safety Commission, through

NEISS. The NCAA injury rates (Table A7–1) apply only to sports played in participating colleges.

STUDY 1

The USEIR database contains 10,309 cases of serious eye injury from December 1988 to September 1999. Our analysis found the following.

- *Sex*: male 8284, female 1938, unknown 65, not stated 22.
- *Bilateral*: yes 757, no 9450, not stated 102.
- *Open globe*: yes 4798, no 5511, not stated 0.
- *Bystander*: yes 1626, no 5413, unknown 1185, not stated 2085.

TABLE A7–1   NCAA INJURY SURVEILLANCE SYSTEM. EYE INJURIES PER 1000 ATHLETE EXPOSURES THAT REQUIRE MEDICAL ATTENTION AND RESULT IN RESTRICTION OF THE STUDENT-ATHLETE'S PARTICIPATION FOR ONE OR MORE DAYS BEYOND THE DAY OF INJURY

	Football	Soccer		Volleyball	Field Hockey	Basketball		Baseball	Softball
	Men	*Men*	*Women*	*Women*	*Women*	*Men*	*Women*	*Men*	*Women*
1998–99	0.13	0.26	0.48	0.08	0.63	0.18	0.21	0.04	0.05
1997–98*	0.02	0.42	0.52	0	0.36	0	0.03	0.14	0.15
1995–96*	0.01	0.01	0.05	0.04	0.04	0.12	0.07	0.17	0.40
1994–95	0.02	0.06	0.06	0.03	0.10	0.14	0.07	0.20	0.36
1993–94	0.01	0.03	0.05	0.01	0.04	0.04	0.06	0.03	0.05
1992–93	0.01	0.07	0.02	0.01	0	0.10	0.03	0.01	0.03
1990–91	0	0.04	0.03		0.06			0.01	0.07
1989–90	0.02	0.07	0.06	0	0.06	0.10	0.04	0.01	0.03

*1996–97 missing.

455

- *Eyewear*: none 6359, regular 275, safety 144, sun 28, unknown 1321, other 24, not checked 2158.

- *Place of injury*: industrial 1278, farm 244, home 3888, school 255, *place for recreation and sport* 1261 (12%), street and highway 1299, public building 297, unknown 888, other 256, not stated 643.

- *Intent*: assault 1375, self-inflicted 90, unintentional 6385, unknown 509, not stated 1950.

- *Source*: hammer on metal 510, sharp object 1842, nail 565, blunt object 3148, gunshot 414, BB/pellet gun (includes paintball) 574, motor vehicle crash 954, fireworks 501, burn 236, explosion 296, lawn equipment 201, unknown 106, other 378, not stated 584.

- *Region*: Northeast 280, Southeast 5773, Midwest 2525, Southwest 809, West 846, Other 76.

STUDY 2

Because ASTM F8.57 is concerned with standards for sports, the USEIR injuries for sports and recreation were analyzed separately. Sufficient detailed data were present in 702 of the 1261 cases (56%). The well-documented 702 cases were studied in detail as a subset with the pertinent data imported for analysis into Data Desk. The results of the 702 cases are summarized in Table A7–2.

TABLE A7–2   USEIR SPORTS AND RECREATION INJURIES *n* = 702*

Sports Group	Total	Open Globe	Blind Eyes	Shattered Eyewear Lens	Sex (Percent Male)	Age (Median)	Protector Standard
Fishing	113	50	34	0/1	82.3%	27	None
Hunting/shooting	59	28	29	2/4	98.3%	32	None
Recreation	55	29	15	1/1	89.1%	17	None
Baseball	104	11	15	5/8	86.5%	14	ASTM F803
Softball	65	3	8	3/12	63.1%	29	None
Basketball	66	11	12	1/1	95.5%	24	ASTM F803
Racket sports	55	1	8	0/6	83.3%	25	ASTM F803
Hockey	13	2	0	0/0	100%	30	ASTM F513
Paintball	12	1	1	0/3	100%	17	ASTM F1776
Golf	29	12	12	4/6	72.4%	40	None
Soccer	24	0	1	0/1	66.7%	17	None
Ball sports, other	19	2	0	0/1	68.4%	12	None for most
Football	13	0	0	0/1	100%	15	NOCSAE
Water sports	15	3	5	0/0	66.7%	21	None
Sports, other	22	4	1	0/0	80.1%	22	None for most
Motor sports	11	5	5	0/0	81.9%	22	None for most
Fireworks	21	3	4	0/1	80.1%	20.5	None
Bungee cord	6	2	1	0/0	66.7%	21	ANSI Z87.1+
Total	702	167	151	16/46	83.3%	22.5 range 83	

*Blind eyes include final best corrected vision: NLP to <2/200.

Sex: In three cases the sex was not stated. Calculations based on 699 cases in which sex was specified.

Age: Injuries affected all age groups with a range of 2 to 85 years. The age median is given only to point to an age trend by sports group.

Motor sports include: 3 wheeler (1), 4 wheeler (2), auto racing (7), go-cart (1).

Hunting/shooting include: air rifle (4), BB gun (14), hunting (31), shooting (trap, skeet) (10).

Racket sports include: badminton (3), handball (2), racquetball (36), tennis (14).

Ball sports, other, include: play with ball (5), dodge ball (1), kickball (1), lacrosse (1), mud ball (1), stickball (1), volleyball (6), whiffle ball (3).

Water sports include: beach (1), boating (5), sailboat (1), surfing (3), swimming (1), water skiing (2).

Recreation includes: bicycle (1), camping (6), carnival (1), church function (1), darts (2), dirt bike (1), dog bite (1), fight (2), glass car window (1), hiking (5), home (1), motor vehicle crash (1), park (1), play (11), poker (1), recreation (11), sledding (1), sling shot (1), snowmobile (1), vacation house (1), water balloon (2), water hose (1), whirligig toy (1).

Golf includes: golf (28), putt-putt golf (1).

Sports, other, include: bow and arrow (1), boxing (4), frisbee (2), ice skating (1), karate (2), rodeo (3), roller skating (1), running (1), ice skating (1), skiing (3), wrestling (3).

Eyewear use: None 400, not stated 256, regular 35, safety 6, sun 5.

Eyewear failure (includes frame failure as well as shattered lens): Not applicable 656, no or uncertain 16, yes 30.

Of the 46 patients known to have been using eyewear at the time the injury occurred during sports and recreation, the eyewear shattered, often lacerating the globe, in 16 (35%). Eyewear use was none 400, unknown or not stated 256, regular 35, safety 6, and sun 5.

The Protector Standard column of Table A7–2 specifies the standard for eyewear that most likely would have prevented the injury. The + after ANSI Z87.1 in bungee cords refers to protectors that pass the high mass and high velocity sections of the standard. For such common sources of eye injury, as fishing, hunting, and golf, there are no standards. It is precisely for these sports with high risk of severe eye injury, and for which users would find protectors that meet the specifications of ASTM F803 too bulky, that the new ASTM moderate impact standard is intended. Note that 44% of fishing injuries, 47% of hunting injuries, and 41% of golf injuries are open globe. The high incidence of blinded eyes in fishing (30%), hunting (47%), and golf (41%) shows the need for appropriate eye protection and education in these sports. Table A7–3 shows the test energy specified in various standards.

STUDY 3

All cases in the entire database ($n = 10,309$) who were known to have been wearing eyewear ($n = 440^a$) at the time of injury were analyzed. In Table A7–4 "yes" means that definite shatter was specifically stated. "Probable" shatter was evident from the mechanism of injury and the actual injury. The shatter percentage ("yes" plus "probable"/total) was regular 20%, sun 18%, and safety 7%. Shattered eyewear accounted for over one sixth of the serious eye injuries to people wearing eyewear at the time of impact.

STUDY 4

Wound dehiscence is a major concern to ophthalmologists. 2.5 to 5.7% of patients who have had a PK can

---

^{a}This differs from $n = 471$ (regular 275, safety 144, sun 28, other 24) in study 1 because 31 of the cases in study 1 had inadequate information for inclusion.

TABLE A7–3   TEST OBJECTS, ENERGY OF EYEWEAR STANDARDS COMPARED WITH DROP HEIGHT OF A 19-oz (600 g WITH CAN WEIGHT ADDED) CAN OF BEANS

	Test Object	Mass (g)	Velocity (ft/s)	Joules	600-g Can of Beans Drop Height
ANSI Z80	5/8 inch steel ball	16	16.4	0.2	1.3 inches
ANSI Z87.1 basic	1 inch steel ball	68	16.4	0.9	6.0 inches
ANSI Z87.1 plus	1/4 inch steel ball	1.06	150	1.1	7.4 inches
	high mass	500	16.6	6.4	42.8 inches
ASTM moderate	same as ANSI Z87.1 plus				
ASTM F803	squash ball	24	132	19.4	10.8 feet
	racquetball	40	132	32.4	18.1 feet
	tennis ball	58	132	46.9	26.2 feet
	lacrosse	146	66	29.5	16.4 feet
	baseball <8 year	146	58.7	23.4	13.1 feet
	baseball 9–14 years	146	80.7	44.2	24.7 feet
	baseball over 15 years	146	102.7	71.5	39.8 feet
	baseball over 15 years	146	124.7	105.5	58.8 feet

TABLE A7–4   EYEWEAR SHATTER IN DATABASE (EYEWEAR $n = 440$, TOTAL USEIR DATABASE $n = 10,309$)

	No	Uncertain	Possibly	Probably	Yes	Total
Regular	133	80	1	5	49	268
Sun	8	15	0	2	3	28
Safety	110	15	0	1	8	134
Goggles	2	0	0	0	2	4
Face shield	3	0	0	0	1	4
Other	1	1	0	0	0	2
Total	257	111	1	8	63	440

expect traumatic dehiscence of the wound, on average 3.4 years after the PK but with no "safe" time (see Chapter 27). It is well recognized that the eyewall regains only approximately 50% of the original tensile strength when incisions have healed. An analysis of USEIR wound dehiscence data showed that, of the 126 cases of wound dehiscence in which eyewear use was known, 24 (19%) were wearing glasses (21 streetwear, 2 sunglasses, 1 safety glasses) and still developed globe rupture.

STUDY 5

The NEISS data that reflect approximately the same categories of sports and recreation injuries in the USEIR data are presented in Table A7–5.

TABLE A7–5   NEISS EYE INJURY DATA 1986 TO 1998

	1986	1987	1988	1989	1990	1991	1992	1993	1994	1995	1996	1997	1998
Eyewear*	6284	5342	5985	4711	8265	5629	8164	9375	8416	7212	7002	5314	8000
Fishing	586	1074	1146	478	1099	1017	856	1413	3223	1331	859	1173	925
Shooting	1883	2422	3189	2060	2370	2139	5515	2737	2330	2737	2446	2348	2720
Recreation	2123	2123	1963	2466	2590	2077	2916	2293	2721	2178	2308	2549	2566
Baseball	7644	6582	6280	5518	6379	6950	8083	6136	4227	3265	3837	2270	2635
Softball	0##	0	0	0	0	0	0	0	2480	1549	1192	1290	1394
Basketball	6049	7320	5492	5900	7705	6842	8304	8521	9117	8420	7852	7673	8723
Racket sports	4501	2994	2835	2674	3081	3890	4161	3183	2829	1692	2540	1562	2768
Hockey	722	728	330	151	514	1053	971	946	922	826	1034	756	1614
Golf	522	446	491	670	1263	927	1320	969	849	556	1076	636	827
Soccer	852	1009	892	1181	1492	1108	1469	1319	1330	1213	1407	864	1325
Ball sports other	2511	2660	1588	2119	1917	2547	2381	2492	2106	1472	1426	2761	1793
Football	2081	1964	2090	2310	1672	2930	2105	2197	2318	2412	1470	1776	1464
Water sports	2333	2817	2949	2376	2290	3310	3898	3187	3409	3938	2530	2513	3601
Sports other	1338	1028	1025	1099	1497	1549	2462	1706	1704	2915	2336	2486	1671
Motor sports	859	256	234	358	412	723	783	548	59100‡	281	680	411	639
Fireworks	1970	1673	1341	1332	1632	1542	2437	2933	2367	2406	1526	1526	1820
Stretch cords or straps	0†	0	0	0	0	0	0	0	554	323	894	788	458
Total	44244	42425	39818	37392	46168	46224	57817	51948	111996‡	46721	44411	40693	46941

1998 breakdown:

Eyewear includes: eyeglasses 2285, eye protection devices 4496, personal protection devices 1219.

Shooting includes: BBs or pellets 1012, gas, air or spring powered guns 1798, sheet shooting 0, gunpowder or ammunition, excl. BBs 0, other guns or firearms 0. NEISS does not have a separate eye injury category for paintball or hunting.

Recreation includes: camping equipment 134, tree houses or playhouses 66, bicycle 2135, sports recreation 231.

##Data were not collected for these years.

† *Softball and stretch cord:* data were not collected until 1994.

Racket sports include: handball 234, squash racquetball and paddleball 921, tennis 1613, badminton 0.

Hockey includes: ice hockey 319, field hockey 75, street hockey 233, hockey 987, roller hockey 0.

Motor sports includes all terrain vehicles. NEISS does not have an eye injury category for auto racing.

‡ 1994 figure includes a special study of all terrain vehicle injuries. Note the increase in the injury estimate when a study is targeted to one sport.

Ball sports, other, includes: lacrosse 76. volleyball 322, rugby 38. other ball sports 237, ball sports 1033, tetherball 87.

Water sports includes: swimming 1534, swimming pools 1853, swimming pool equipment 119, scuba diving 19, water skiing 0, water polo 0, powered personal watercraft 0.

Sports, other, includes: boxing 50, wrestling 50, skateboards 169, archery 38, horseback riding 537, sleds 303, snowmobile 75, snow skiing 154, trampolines 295.

Study 6

The SGMA estimates of sports participation are presented in Table A7–6.

Observations and Conclusions

1. When compared with the NEISS eye injury estimates, it is apparent that the USEIR captures approximately 0.3% of sports and recreation eye injuries (about 400,000 sports/recreation injuries over 10 years in NEISS, about 1300 sports/recreation injuries reported to USEIR). The databases supplement each other. NEISS gives national trends based on emergency room sampling, but the data are not detailed. USEIR is a slice of serious injuries treated by ophthalmologists for which detailed information is available. Because NEISS does not sample ophthalmologists' offices or eye hospitals, serious eye injuries, such as open globe injuries that go directly to the ophthalmology tertiary care center, this trauma is underrepresented in the NEISS database.

   The USEIR database has low representation from the Northeast and high representation from the Southeast, with one state (Alabama) having 4924 cases. The 47.8% representation of Alabama injuries may somewhat skew the injury data away from winter sports and more toward warm weather outdoor activities.

2. The NEISS data presented in Table A7–5 show that eye injuries are commonly related to eyewear. The eyewear numbers represent the entire NEISS database and are not limited to sports and recreational activities. A detailed analysis is not possible from the NEISS data at this time, but eyewear failure is a definite problem and requires more in-depth analysis.

3. USEIR data show that common sports-recreational activities, such as fishing, hunting, and golf, are associated with severe eye injury. There is no eyewear standard for these and other moderate impact sports such as frisbee and miscellaneous ball sports. Eyewear conforming to the moderate impact standard requirements can eliminate or decrease the severity of most moderate impact sports eye injuries. It must be realized that golf has such high impact energy concentration that moderate impact eyewear will permit contact of the protector to the eye. Hunting, mountain bicycling, and other sports also have the potential for extreme impacts, which will exceed the requirements of the proposed standard. The user will have more protection using high impact eyewear that conforms to ASTM F803, but complete protection from all possible hazards is not possible.

4. Shattered eyewear lenses and frame failure are relatively frequent causes of open globe injuries in moderate impact sports and recreational activities.

5. Postoperative wound dehiscence is common despite eyewear use at the time of injury. In order to protect eyes that are prone to rupture, it is necessary to have a lens that will not shatter held in a frame that has the ability to retain the lens and prevent contact with the eye.

6. The NEISS data are discouraging. We know that there has been a definite reduction in hockey injuries to players who wear protection. Hockey has an ASTM standard for protection, HECC, and the mandatory requirement for protector use in over 1 million players. There are now over 21 million player-years of HECC certified protector use without any significant eye injuries. Yet, as shown in Table A7–5, many hockey (ice, field, street) players still play without protection and suffer injuries.

7. Eye injuries can be reduced by a spectrum of standards combined with a strong education program. Standards range from fashion (Z80) to industrial (Z87) to moderate impact (ASTM proposed) to high impact (ASTM F803) with corresponding, clearly identifiable eyewear. The eyewear should be clearly labeled (Z87 markings for education and industry; PECC certification seal for ASTM standards) so that both the provider and the user are certain that the eyewear complies with the standard specifications.

8. Table A7–6 shows that many people participate in sports and recreational activities with moderate

TABLE A7–6 SGMA Sports Participation Trends: U.S. Population ≥ 6 Years, at Least Once in 1977 (millions)

Fishing	80.5
Hunting/shooting (target excluded)	21.6
Baseball	13.3
Softball	22.1
Basketball	45.1
Racket sports	33.3
Golf	26.3
Volleyball	34.1
Soccer	18.2
Football	30.3
Bicycling (fitness)	26.2
Mountain biking	8.4

impact eye hazard. A massive consumer and professional education program is essential. Sports with a high risk for eye injury, for which there is available certified protection, should have protection strongly recommended or mandated by sanctioning bodies; a good example is paintball.

9. The data support the need for a moderate impact standard for moderate impact sports. Eye care professionals may also specify eyewear that conforms to this standard as streetwear for patients who are functionally one-eyed or who have surgical or medical conditions that predispose to rupture of the eyewall.

10. ANSI Z80 and ANSI Z87 specifically state, in the scope of the standards, that they are not intended for sports. The can-of-beans test clearly displays that the test energies required to pass these standards are inadequate for most sports with the potential for moderate impact. The proposed ASTM moderate impact standard fills the gap between the ANSI standards and the high impact ASTM F803.

11. Eye care professionals and users are confused about eyewear appropriate for specific activities. A clear delineation of a spectrum of eyewear standards with an educational program should increase the awareness and use of protective eyewear and lead to a reduction in preventable injuries.

SUGGESTED READING

Jeffers J. An ongoing tragedy: pediatric sports-related eye injuries. *Semin Ophthalmol*. 1990;5:216–223.

Parver LM. Eye trauma: the neglected disorder. *Arch Ophthalmol*. 1986;104:1452–1453.

Schein OD, Hibberd PL, Shingleton BJ, et al. The spectrum and burden of ocular injury. *Ophthalmology*. 1988;95: 300–305.

Vinger PF. Eye safety testing and standards. *Ophthalmol Clin North Am*. 1999;12:345–358.

Vinger PF, Woods BA. Prescription safety eyewear: impact studies of lens and frame failure. *Optometry*. 2000;71: 91–103.

Vinger PF, Parver L, Alfaro DV, Woods T, Abrams BS. Shatter resistance of spectacle lenses. *JAMA*. 1997;277:142–144.

Index

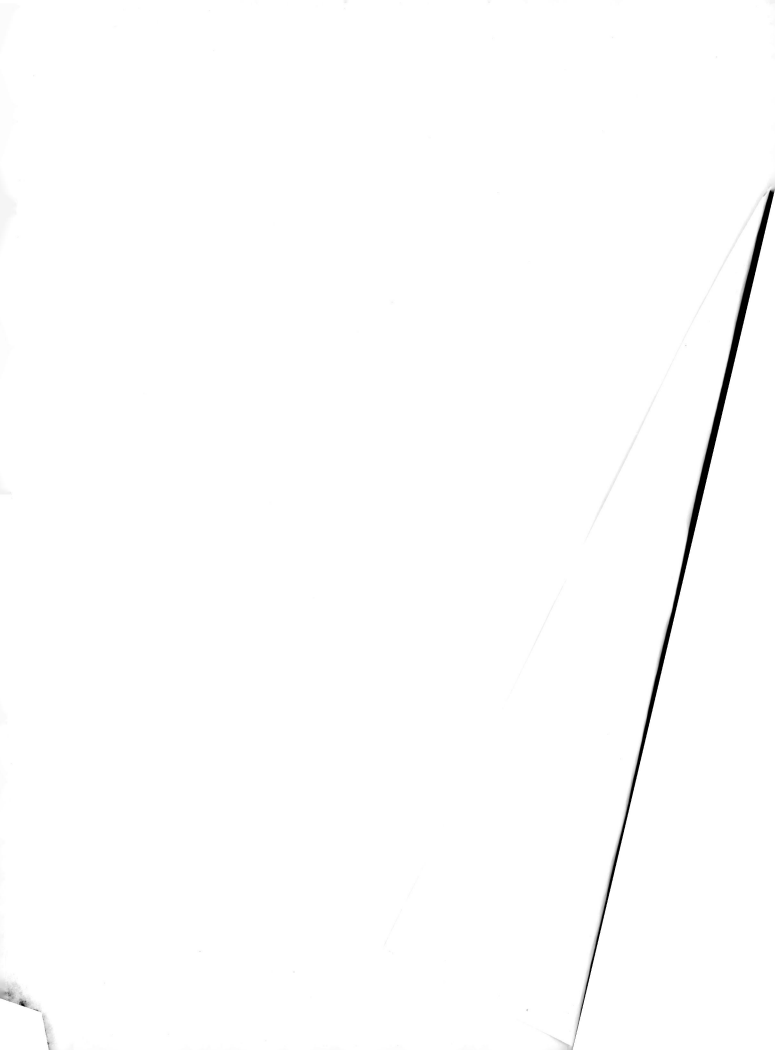